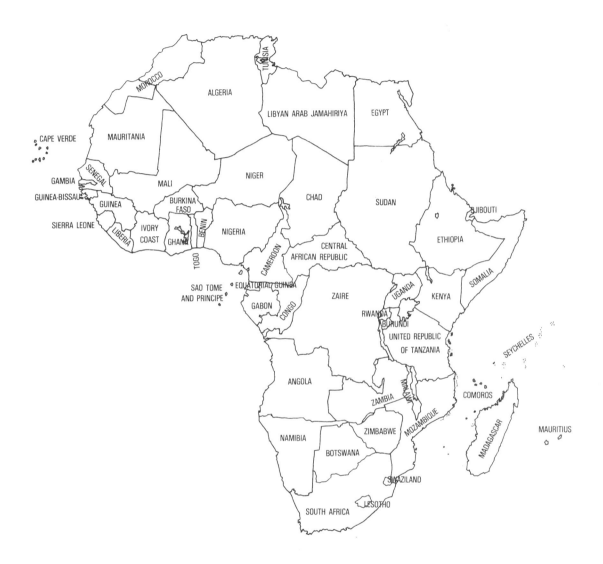

WORLD HEALTH ORGANIZATION
ORGANISATION MONDIALE DE LA SANTE

INTERNATIONAL AGENCY FOR RESEARCH ON CANCER
CENTRE INTERNATIONAL DE RECHERCHE SUR LE CANCER

ORGANIZATION OF AFRICAN UNITY
ORGANISATION DE L'UNITE AFRICAINE

SCIENTIFIC TECHNICAL & RESEARCH COMMISSION (STRC)
COMMISSION SCIENTIFIQUE TECHNIQUE ET DE LA RECHERCHE (CSTR)

VIRUS-ASSOCIATED CANCERS IN AFRICA

LES CANCERS ASSOCIES AUX VIRUS EN AFRIQUE

Proceedings of a Symposium organized by the Organization of African Unity/Scientific Technical Research Commission, World Health Organization Regional Office for Africa, the International Agency for Research on Cancer, the United Nations Environment Programme and the International Association for Study of Liver Disease and co-sponsored with Institut Pasteur Production, the International Union Against Cancer and the International Association for the Study and Prevention of Virus-associated Cancer

EDITORS/REDACTEURS

A. OLUFEMI WILLIAMS, GREGORY T. O'CONOR, GUY B. DE-THE & COUAVI A. JOHNSON

IARC SCIENTIFIC PUBLICATIONS NO. 63
OAU/STRC SCIENTIFIC PUBLICATIONS No. 1

INTERNATIONAL AGENCY FOR RESEARCH ON CANCER
LYON
FRANCE

The International Agency for Research on Cancer (IARC) was established in 1965 by the World Health Assembly as an independently financed organization within the framework of the World Health Organization. The headquarters of the Agency are at Lyon, France.

The Agency conducts a programme of research concentrating particularly on the epidemiology of cancer and the study of potential carcinogens in the human environment. Its field studies are supplemented by biological and chemical research carried out in the Agency's laboratories in Lyon and, through collaborative research agreements, in national research institutions in many countries. The Agency also conducts a programme for the education and training of personnel for cancer research.

The publications of the Agency are intended to contribute to the dissemination of authoritative information on different aspects of cancer research.

Oxford University Press, Walton Street, Oxford OX2 6DP

London New York Toronto
Delhi Bombay Calcutta Madras Karachi
Kuala Lumpur Singapore Hong Kong Tokyo
Nairobi Dar es Salaam Cape Town
Melbourne Auckland

and associated companies in
Beirut Berlin Ibadan Mexico City Nicosia

Oxford is a trade mark of Oxford University Press

Published in the United States
by Oxford University Press, New York

ISBN 0 19 723063 6
ISBN 92 832 0163 9 (Publisher)
ISBN 978 2453 00 5 (OAU/STRC)

Le Centre international de Recherche sur le Cancer (CIRC) a été créé en 1965 par l'Assemblée mondiale de la Santé et il est financé de manière indépendante dans le cadre de l'Organisation mondiale de la Santé. Son Siège est à Lyon, France.

Le CIRC exécute un programme de recherche qui porte particulièrement sur l'épidémiologie du cancer et l'étude des cancérogènes potentiels dans l'environnement humain. Ses études sur le terrain sont complétées par des recherches biologiques et chimiques effectuées dans les laboratoires du Centre, à Lyon, et, par le truchement d'accords de recherches collectives, dans des instituts nationaux de nombreux pays. Le Centre exécute également un programme d'enseignement et de formation de personnel à la recherche sur le cancer.

Les publications du Centre ont pour objet de contribuer à la diffusion d'informations faisant autorité sur divers aspects de la recherche cancérologique.

Oxford University Press, Walton Street, Oxford OX2 6DP

London New York Toronto
Delhi Bombay Calcutta Madras Karachi
Kuala Lumpur Singapore Hong Kong Tokyo
Nairobi Dar es Salaam Cape Town
Melbourne Auckland
and associated companies in
Beirut Berlin Ibadan Mexico City Nicosia

Oxford is a trade mark of Oxford University Press

Published in the United States
by Oxford University Press, New York

ISBN 0 19 723063 6
ISBN 92 832 0163 9 (Publisher)
ISBN 978 2453 00 5 (OAU/STRC)

CONTENTS

HEPATOCELLULAR CARCINOMA: ETIOLOGY

GENITAL CANCERS

KAPOSI'S SARCOMA

LYMPHOMAS, LEUKAEMIAS AND IMMUNODEFICIENCIES

FOREWORD

Since IARC was established in 1965, many countries of the African continent have participated actively in its collaborative research programmes. It may be said, in fact, that these programmes in Africa have contributed significantly to the success and scientific recognition that the Agency enjoys today.

Two of the initial research programmes of the Agency were concerned with cancers of great importance and high incidence in Africa: Burkitt's lymphoma and carcinoma of the liver. In addition, the Agency's first regional research center was developed in East Africa; and the first publication in the IARC Scientific Publications series dealt with liver cancer, including, in large part, related studies in Africa.

The programmes on Burkitt's lymphoma and liver cancer have proven to be highly productive in terms of scientific achievement, and both continue as major projects of the Agency. It is therefore with a renewed sense of anticipation that IARC welcomes yet another aspect of our collaboration with African colleagues.

The initiative for this Symposium comes from the Organization of African Unity, which has succeeded in bringing together for the first time scientists and physicians from many parts of Africa to consider specific approaches to the prevention and control of virus-associated cancers. The symposium addresses those tumours that occur in high incidence in Africa, and particular attention is given to ways in which multidisciplinary, multinational and multiregional cooperation may lead to a more rapid solution of problems and the attainment of ultimate goals.

The Agency is proud to be a partner in this new venture with OAU and the other co-sponsoring groups. We do believe that cancer research in Africa will continue as it has in the past to yield unique information, which will be of benefit not only to Africans but to all of the world.

L. Tomatis
Director
International Agency
for Research on Cancer

PREFACE

Depuis la création du CIRC en 1965, de nombreux pays du continent africain ont participé activement aux programmes de recherche que le Centre conduit avec d'autres partenaires. On peut dire en fait que ces programmes en Afrique ont contribué de façon majeure au succès et à la reconnaissance scientifique dont le Centre jouit actuellement.

Deux des programmes de recherche initiaux du Centre concernaient des cancers d'une grande importance et d'une incidence élevée en Afrique: le lymphome de Burkitt et l'épithélioma du foie. De plus, le premier centre de recherche régional du CIRC a été installé en Afrique de l'Est; et la première publication dans la collection des Publications Scientifiques du CIRC concernait le cancer du foie et comprenait, pour une grande part, les études afférentes menées en Afrique.

Les programmes sur le lymphome de Burkitt et le cancer du foie se sont avérés hautement productifs en succès scientifiques et la poursuite de ces deux programmes sont des projets majeurs du Centre. C'est donc avec un sens de l'anticipation renouvelé que le CIRC accueille maintenant une nouvelle étape de notre collaboration avec nos collègues africains.

L'initiative de ce Symposium revient à l'Organisation de l'Unité Africaine, qui a réussi à réunir pour la première fois scientifiques et médecins de nombreuses parties de l'Afrique pour réfléchir aux approches spécifiques en matière de prévention et de contrôle des cancers viro-associés. Le Symposium approche ces tumeurs, dont l'incidence est élevée en Afrique, et une attention particulière est accordée aux moyens par lesquels une coopération multidisciplinaire, multinationale et multirégionale peut conduire à résoudre plus rapidement les problèmes et à atteindre les objectifs fondamentaux.

PREFACE

Le Centre est fier d'être associé, dans cette nouvelle entreprise, à l'OUA et aux autres groupes qui la parrainent. Nous avons la conviction que la recherche sur le cancer en Afrique continuera, comme elle l'a fait dans le passé, à produire des informations exceptionnelles qui bénéficieront non seulement aux Africains, mais au monde entier.

L. Tomatis
Directeur
Centre International de Recherche
sur le Cancer

INTRODUCTION

It is now widely accepted that environmental factors play an essential role in the pathogenesis of many, if not most, human cancers. Viruses as a group must be considered as one of the most important of the environmental factors that influence the incidence and patterns of cancer in Africa.

Hepatocellular carcinoma, carcinoma of the cervix, carcinoma of the penis, Kaposi's sarcoma, nasopharyngeal cancer and certain types of lymphoma and leukaemia are known or believed to be associated with specific transforming viruses and are among the commonest tumours seen in African patients.

The major objectives of this Symposium were to review and exchange current information relating to the etiology and pathogenesis of these cancers in the different countries of Africa and to consider measures for their control and prevention.

The Symposium, which was organized jointly by the Scientific and Technical Research Commission of the Organization of African Unity, the International Agency for Research on Cancer, the World Health Organization African Regional Office, the United Nations Environmental Programme and Institut Pasteur Production, attracted participants from 25 African countries, eight European countries, the USA and China. The scientific contributions addressed the objectives from the point of view of many disciplines, ranging from descriptive epidemiology to molecular biology and potential clinical applications.

Some emphasis was given to chronic liver disease and liver cancer, and the ultimate control of these serious sequelae of hepatitis B infection was highlighted by several reports on effective control of the virus by vaccination. A report was drafted by an ad-hoc group convened at the meeting, to consider and encourage the development and widespread use of an affordable vaccine in Africa, for consideration by international agencies and action by the various national governments in Africa.

INTRODUCTION

The manuscripts included in this publication provide an informative record of the Symposium and are arranged under the general subject headings of: liver cancer, genital cancers (cervix and penis), cancer of the nasopharynx, Kaposi's sarcoma, lymphomas and leukaemias. The presentations covered many aspects of these virus-associated cancers, including recent research methods that may be expected to have an early application in diagnosis, treatment and prevention.

The opportunities in Africa for applied research and for making scientific contributions to the study of virus-associated cancers are limitless. Clinical material is abundant, and scientific competence, which exists in many of the African countries, must be encouraged and strengthened. Africa has in the past played a leading role in the geographic pathology of cancer, as well as in numerous other areas of biomedical research, and there is great potential for the existing scientific institutions to make further contributions to cancer research in general.

This international Symposium was unique in many ways and succeeded in bringing together active clinicians and scientists from all parts of Africa, as well as from other continents, to exchange information on virus-associated neoplasms which are of particular interest and importance in Africa. This type of scientific activity should be encouraged and supported in the future.

A. Olufemi Williams
Gregory T. O'Conor

INTRODUCTION

Il est maintenant largement admis que les facteurs de l'environnement jouent un rôle essentiel dans la pathogenèse de beaucoup, sinon de la plupart, des cancers humains. Les virus en tant que groupe doivent être considérés comme un des plus importants de ces facteurs de l'environnement qui influencent l'incidence et les modalités du cancer en Afrique.

On sait, ou l'on pense, que le cancer primitif du foie, l'épithélioma du col utérin, l'épithélioma du pénis, le sarcome de Kaposi, le cancer du nasopharynx, et certains types de lymphomes et de leucémies sont associés à des virus transformants spécifiques; ces cancers font partie des tumeurs les plus communes chez les patients Africains.

Les principaux objectifs de ce Symposium ont été de considérer et d'échanger les informations concernant l'étiologie et la pathogenèse de ces cancers dans les différents pays d'Afrique et d'envisager les mesures à prendre pour leur contrôle et leur prévention.

Le Symposium, qui a été organisé conjointement par la Commission Scientifique et Technique et de la Recherche de l'Organisation de l'Unité Africaine, le Centre International de Recherche sur le Cancer, le Bureau Régional pour l'Afrique de l'Organisation Mondiale de la Santé, le Programme des Nations Unies pour l'Environnement, et l'Institut Pasteur Production, a réuni des participants de 25 pays Africains, de huit pays Européens, des Etats-Unis et de la Chine. Les contributions scientifiques ont abordé les différents sujets sous l'angle de nombreuses disciplines, allant de l'épidémiologie descriptive à la biologie moléculaire et à ses applications cliniques potentielles.

Une certaine emphase a été apportée aux maladies chroniques du foie et au cancer du foie, et la prévention ultime des séquelles graves de l'hépatite B a été mise en lumière par plusieurs rapports sur le contrôle effectif du virus HB par la vaccination. Le rapport d'un groupe ad hoc réuni durant le meeting dans le but de considérer et d'encourager le développement d'un vaccin accessible pour l'Afrique, et son utilisation

INTRODUCTION

étendue, a été rédigé pour être soumis à la considération des centres internationaux et des différents gouvernements nationaux Africains.

Les manuscrits figurant dans cette publication fournissent un compte-rendu informatif du Symposium et sont groupés par thèmes: cancer du foie, cancers génitaux (col utérin et pénis), cancer du nasopharynx, sarcome de Kaposi, lymphomes et leucémies. Les présentations ont couvert de nombreux aspects de ces cancers viro-associés, y compris les méthodes récentes de recherche, dont on peut attendre pour bientôt des applications dans le diagnostic, le traitement et la prévention.

En Afrique, les occasions d'étude des cancers viro-associés sont sans limites. Le matériel clinique est abondant; la compétence scientifique existe dans beaucoup des pays Africains et mérite d'être encouragée et renforcée. Dans le passé, l'Afrique a joué un rôle moteur dans la pathologie géographique du cancer, aussi bien que dans de nombreux autres domaines de la recherche biomédicale. Ses institutions scientifiques constituent toujours un potentiel important dans la recherche sur le cancer.

Ce Symposium, unique par bien des aspects, a réussi à réunir cliniciens et scientifiques provenant de toutes les parties d'Afrique et des autres continents, et leur a permis d'échanger des informations sur les néoplasmes viro-associés qui présentent un intérêt et une importance particuliers en Afrique. Ce type d'activité scientifique devrait à l'avenir être encouragé et soutenu.

A. Olufemi Williams
Gregory T. O'Conor

LIST OF PARTICIPANTS

Y.A. ANGATE B.P. V156
Abidjan 01, Ivory Coast

P.P. ANTHONY Postgraduate Medical School
Barrack Road
Exeter EX2 5DY, UK

A. AYOOLA P.O. Box 7629
Ibadan, Nigeria

T. BENNIKE Strandboulevard G6 t.v.
2100 Copenhagen Ø, Denmark

J. BIRCHER Renelweg 20
3045 Meikirch, Switzerland

B.L.C. BLANCHET 2 Place A. Fournier
75010 Paris, France

B.S. BLUMBERG Balliol College, Eastman House
St Cross Road
Oxford OX13 BJ, UK

T.R. BOWRY P.O. Box 30588
Nairobi, Kenya

B. BROTMAN P.O. Box 31
Robertsfield, Liberia

G.R. BRUBAKER Shirati Hospital
Musoma, United Republic of
Tanzania

M.E. CHUWA WHO Regional Office for Africa
B.P. 6
Brazzaville, Congo

J.D. CHIPHANGWI P.O. Box 95
Blantyre, Malawi

P. COURSAGET 2bis Boulevard Tonnelli
37000 Tours, France

G. de THE	Laboratoire d'Epidémiologie et Immunovirologie des Tumeurs Université Claude Bernard Faculté de Médecine Alexis Carrel Lyon, France
N. EL GOULLI	147 Boulevard Heurteloup 37000 Tours, France
A. EL HAFED	B.P. 6213 RI Agbal Rabat, Morocco
H.E. AMBASSADOR FAKIH	P.O. Box 30551 Nairobi, Kenya
T.I. FRANCIS	Federal University of Technology Akure, Nigeria
L. GEBRESELASSIE	P.O. Box 1242 Addis Ababa, Ethiopia
P.L. GIGASE	Nationalestraat 155 2000 Anvers, Belgium
G. GIRALDO	Cassella dei Cangiani 80131 Naples, Italy
L. GISMANN	Im Neuenheimer Feld 6900 Heidelberg, Federal Republic of Germany
C.M. GOMBE	B.P. 32 Brazzaville, Congo
H.N.B. GOPALAN	P.O. Box 30197 Nairobi, Kenya
C. GREENFIELD	P.O. Box 41663 Nairobi, Kenya
H. GROSSMANN	K.C.M.C. Hospital Private Bag Moshi, United Republic of Tanzania

K. HAILE GIORGIS

Ministry of Health
P.O. Box 1234
Addis Ababa, Ethiopia

E. HESELTINE

International Agency for Research
on Cancer
150 cours Albert Thomas
69372 Lyon Cédex 08, France

J.C. HANSFORD

P.O. Box 30546
Nairobi, Kenya

A.O.K. JOHNSON

University of Ibadan
Ibadan, Nigeria

B. JOHNSTON

P.O. Box 20752
Nairobi, Kenya

E.G. KASILI

P.O. Box 30588
Nairobi, Kenya

M.M.R. KALENGAYI

P.O. Box 864
Kinshasa XI, Zaire

C. LEEVY

100 Bergen Street
Newark, N.J., USA

A. LINSELL

P.O. Box 20351
Nairobi, Kenya

C.G.H. LOUCQ

17 rue Bourgelat
69002 Lyon, France

Hon. P. LEAKEY

Ministry of Foreign Affairs
Nairobi, Kenya

M. LUTZNER

National Cancer Institute
Bethesda, MD 20205, USA

L.R. MBAE

P.O. Box 33551
Nairobi, Kenya

F.D. MARTINSON

University of Ibadan
Ibadan, Nigeria

J. MSIRIKALE	P.O. Box 3592 Dar-Es-Salaam, United Republic of Tanzania
S. MASINDET	P.O. Box 68133 Nairobi, Kenya
M.A.M. MPAT	B.P. 1508 Kinshasa I, Zaire
K. MUHOMBE	P.O. Box 20723 Nairobi, Kenya
L.V. MENESES	Maputo, Mozambique
A. MOSSI	B.P. 27 Niamey, Niger
J.K.G. MATI	P.O. Box 30588 Nairobi, Kenya
I. MANN	P.O. Box 20360 Nairobi, Kenya
P.M. NYARANG'O	P.O. Box 98 Kitale, Kenya
H. NSANZE	P.O. Box 30588 Nairobi, Kenya
F.K. NKRUMAH	P.O. Box A-178 Harare, Zimbabwe
F. NGOWI	K.C.M.S. Private Bag Moshi, United Republic of Tanzania
N. NKANZA	P.O. Box 50001 Lusaka, Zambia
J.N. ONYANGO	P.O. Box 20824 Nairobi, Kenya

G. O'CONOR

International Agency for Research
on Cancer
150 cours Albert-Thomas
69372 Lyon, Cédex 08, France

C. OLWENY

P.O. Box A178 Avondale
Harare, Zimbabwe

F. PLUMMER

P.O. Box 30588
Nairobi, Kenya

A.M. PRINCE

310 East 67th Street
New York, NY 10021, USA

H. RAVELOSON

B.P. 88
Tananarive, Madagascar

D. SERWADDA

P.O. Box 3935
Kampala, Uganda

T.F. SOLANKE

U.C.H.
Ibadan, Nigeria

R. SCHMAUZ

Institüt für Pathologie
Ratzeburger Alle 160
2400 Lübeck 1, Federal Republic of
Germany

O. SOBESLAVSKY

World Health Organization
Avenue Appia
1200 Geneva, Switzerland

M.F. SEBTI

2 Ain Takaout Monte des Zaers
Rabat, Morocco

G.H.W. SEILER

K.C.M.S.
Private Bag
Moshi, United Republic of Tanzania

P. TOURE

B.P. 5126
Dakar, Sénégal

P.M. TUKEI

P.O. Box 20752
Nairobi, Kenya

P.J. TIOLLAIS

28 rue du Dr Roux
75015 Paris, France

A. UWAIFO

University of Ibadan
Ibadan, Nigeria

H.J. WOLF

Max von Pettenkofer
Institut, Just. Pettenkofer
Strasse 9a, 800 Munich 2, Federal
Republic of Germany

C.K.O. WILLIAMS

Department of Haematology
U.C.H.
Ibadan, Nigeria

Y. ZENG

100 Ying Xing Jie
Beijing, China

Secretariat

A. O. WILLIAMS

Executive Secretary
OAU/STRC, PMB 2359,
Lagos, Nigeria

C.A. JOHNSON

Assistant Executive Secretary
OAU/STRC
Lagos, Nigeria

A.G. TALL

Director a.i.
IBAR Office
P.O. Box 30786
Nairobi, Kenya

A. AFEWORK

Chief Accountant
OAU/STRC
Lagos, Nigeria

B. OBILANA

Administrative Assistant
OAU/STRC
Lagos, Nigeria

M.A.S. OUGO   Document Officer
IBAR Office
P.O. Box 30786
Nairobi, Kenya

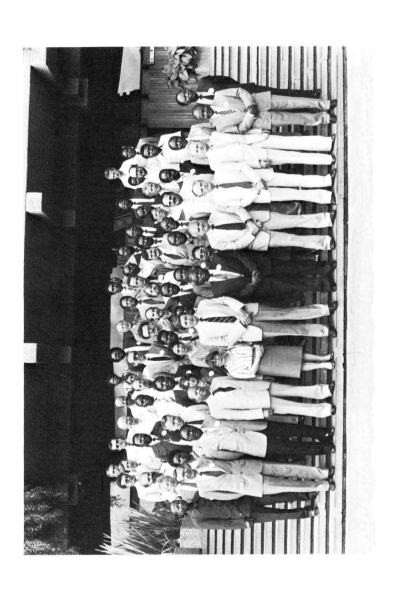

ADDRESS OF WELCOME

Professor A. Olufemi Williams

Executive Secretary, Organization of African Unity,
Scientific Technical and Research Commission
Lagos, Nigeria

Your Excellencies, Representative of the Government of Kenya, delegates, distinguished participants, colleagues, ladies and gentlemen, I have great pleasure in welcoming you to this Symposium which is being held in this beautiful capital city of Kenya, Nairobi. The interim Secretary-General of the Organization of African Unity, Dr Peter Onu, who is unable to be here with us today owing to other commitments, sends his best wishes to all here present and wishes the meeting every success. I should like to take this opportunity of expressing our gratitude to the Government of Kenya for their full cooperation in making available all the facilities for this meeting.

The Scientific Technical and Research Commission of the OAU has the responsibility and mandate for implementing activities in Africa related to science, technology and research. The importance of research in Africa, particularly in medical sciences, cannot be overemphasized in the development of any nation and its economic well-being. It is therefore appropriate that a Symposium of this nature should be held at this point in time, particularly as it relates to the possibility of preventing the development of liver cancer or other cancers by vaccination. In the overall field of health, it is possible to identify three phases in the evolution of a developing nation.

The first phase is the inflammatory or infective phase. The second phase is the degenerative phase and the third phase is the neoplastic phase or the phase of tumour growth. The second and third phase need not necessarily be consecutive.

The majority of diseases in Africa today belong to the first phase, where infections and communicable diseases are overwhelming and extremely common and are responsible for high frequencies of morbidity and mortality. The current Symposium is dealing with the sequelae and complications of infection with viruses in the African region. The most important sequel of this type of infection is chronicity followed by the development of cancer.

This historic Symposium will attempt for the next four days to present and discuss basic data from different parts of Africa in respect of cancers affecting the liver, the female and male genital organs (cervix and penis) lymph-nodes and skin. Considerable progress has been made in these areas of cancer research both in Africa and outside Africa. We are very fortunate in having experts in all these fields with us today both from Africa and from outside Africa. The response to the invitation has been most encouraging as we have representatives from 25 African countries and 10 non-African countries. This forum will provide a unique opportunity to obtain first-hand information from several parts of Africa which is not readily available in standard texts. Such invaluable information will help African policy-makers in the field of health administration to make decisions based on reliable data.

It is perhaps pertinent to stress at this point that there is a severe shortage of trained manpower in the fields of virology and oncology (cancer research) in Africa. It is therefore not surprising that there are very few virologists and oncologists at this meeting. If I were to hazard a guess, I would say that for the whole continent of Africa, which has a population of over 400 million, there is perhaps a ratio of one oncologist to 10 million people and one virologist to 1 million people. These figures may not even be realistic but they reflect the current situation in Africa. In addition to these shortages, there are extremely few institutes of virology or institutes or facilities for cancer research or training in Africa. To quote figures, there are less than 10 of these institutes throughout the 50 countries of Africa. It is therefore hoped that, when recommendations and future perspectives are considered, these factors will be taken into account.

We are grateful to our friends from friendly countries who have continued to help Africa in elucidating its problems in the area of virology and cancer. Four friendly countries deserve special mention, namely the USA, France, Belgium and the UK. They are not only represented here today but their products, in terms of African experts, are here to impart the benefits of their training in collaboration with others. I take this opportunity to express our gratitude to all the friendly countries and would like to encourage all, without exception, to continue with their efforts in transferring appropriate knowledge and technology to the Africans, who in turn, will use it to the benefit of their fellow men and mankind.

I wish to thank all the co-sponsoring organizations, namely the WHO Regional Office for Africa (Brazzaville), the International Agency for Research on Cancer (Lyon), UNEP, the Ministry of Cooperation of the Government of France and Institut Pasteur Production (France) for their generous support and cooperation in the successful organization of this meeting. As President of the International Association for the Study of Liver Disease, I wish to convey the best wishes of the Council to all of you and wish you a very successful meeting. I should also like to take this opportunity to thank all those who have either supported or co-operated in the organization of the meeting and particularly Dr Quenum, the WHO Regional Director for Africa, Dr Tolba, the Executive Director of UNEP, Dr Tomatis, the Director of IARC, Dr Weber, the Director of Institut Pasteur Production, and last but not least, the two consultants who are here with us, Dr Greg O'Conor and Dr Guy de-Thé.

It gives me great pleasure to welcome all participants, delegates, friends, distinguished ladies and gentlemen to this symposium. I hope that you will enjoy your stay in Kenya, even though the programme appears a rather full one.

Long live the OAU.

Long live international cooperation.

ALLOCUTION DE BIENVENUE

Professeur A. Olufemi Williams

Secrétaire Exécutif de l'Organisation de l'Unité Africaine, Commission Scientifique Technique et de la Recherche, Lagos, Nigéria

Excellences, qui représentez le Gouvernement du Kenya, Mesdames et Messieurs les Délégués, Mesdames et Messieurs les Congressistes, chers Collègues et Confrères, j'ai le très grand plaisir de vous accueillir à ce Symposium ici, à Nairobi, la magnifique capitale du Kenya. Le Secrétaire Général par interim de l'Organisation de l'Unité Africaine, le Dr Peter Onu, que d'autres obligations ont empêché d'être des nôtres aujourd'hui, vous adresse à tous ses meilleurs voeux pour le succès de cette rencontre. J'aimerais profiter de cette occasion pour exprimer notre gratitude au Gouvernement du Kenya dont la coopération sans faille a permis d'organiser cette réunion.

La Commission Scientifique Technique et de la Recherche de l'OUA a la responsabilité et le mandat de créer en Afrique des activités relatives à la science, à la technologie et à la recherche. On ne saurait trop insister sur l'importance de la recherche en Afrique, tout spécialement dans le domaine des sciences médicales, pour le développement d'une nation et le progrès de son bien-être économique. Il est donc légitime qu'un Symposium de cette nature se tienne en ce moment, précisément parce qu'il porte sur les possibilités de prévention vaccinale du cancer du foie et d'autres cancers. Dans le domaine général de la santé, on peut distinguer trois phases dans l'évolution d'une nation en voie de développement.

La première est la phase inflammatoire ou infectieuse. La second est la phase dégénérative et la troisième est la phase de la croissance tumorale. La seconde et la troisième ne sont pas forcément successives.

ALLOCUTION DE BIENVENUE

Aujourd'hui, la majorité des maladies qui surviennent en Afrique appartiennent à la première phase. Les infections et les maladies transmissibles, extrêmement répandues, sont accablantes et responsables d'une morbidité et d'une mortalité importantes. Dans ce Symposium, on traitera des séquelles et des complications de certaines infections virales dans la Région Afrique. La séquelle la plus importante de ce type d'infection tient à son caractère chronique qui entraîne le développement du cancer.

Ce Symposium historique s'efforcera pendant les quatre prochains jours de présenter et de discuter les données essentielles des différentes parties d'Afrique au sujet des cancers du foie, des organes génitaux féminins et masculins (col de l'utérus et pénis), des ganglions lymphatiques et de la peau. Dans la recherche sur ces cancers, des progrès considérables ont été réalisés, aussi bien en Afrique qu'hors d'Afrique. Nous bénéficions ici de la présence d'experts dans tous ces domaines, qui viennent aussi bien d'Afrique que de l'étranger. Il est tout-à-fait encourageant de constater qu'ont répondu à l'invitation des représentants de 25 nations africaines et de 10 nations non-africaines. Ce forum représente une occasion unique d'obtenir de différentes parties d'Afrique des informations de première main, qui ne sont pas encore disponibles dans les textes standard. Des informations aussi inestimables permettront aux législateurs africains de prendre en matière de santé publique des décisions qui reposent sur des données sûres.

Il faut peut-être souligner ici que les ressources humaines qualifiées dans les domaines de la virologie et de l'oncologie (recherche sur le cancer) sont sévèrement insuffisantes en Afrique. Il n'est donc pas surprenant qu'il y ait peu de virologistes et d'oncologistes à cette réunion. Si je devais avancer un chiffre, je dirais que pour le continent africain, qui a une population de plus de 400 millions d'habitants, il y a peut-être un oncologiste pour 10 millions de personnes et un virologiste pour 1 million. Ces chiffres sont peut-être même supérieurs à la réalité, mais ils reflètent cependant la situation courante en Afrique. De plus, il existe très peu d'instituts de virologie ou d'instituts ou d'équipements pour la recherche ou la formation dans le domaine du cancer. Pour citer des chiffres, il y a moins de 10 instituts de ce genre dans les 50 pays d'Afrique. On peut néanmoins souhaiter que ces facteurs seront pris en compte quant on considèrera les recommandations et les perspectives futures.

-XXX-

ALLOCUTION DE BIENVENUE

Nous sommes reconnaissants envers nos amis des pays amis qui ont continué d'aider l'Afrique à résoudre ses problèmes dans le domaine de la virologie et du cancer. Quatre d'entre eux méritent une mention spéciale, à savoir les Etats-Unis d'Amérique, la France, la Belgique et le Royaume-Uni. Ils sont non seulement représentés aujourd'hui, mais leurs produits, en terme d'experts africains, sont ici pour partager le bénéfice de leur formation en collaborant avec d'autres. Je saisis cette occasion pour exprimer notre gratitude à toutes les nations amies, et j'aimerais les encourager toutes, sans exception, à continuer leurs efforts pour le transfert des connaissances spécifiques et de la technologie vers les Africains qui, à leur tour, vont les utiliser au bénéfice de leurs concitoyens et de l'humanité.

Je désire remercier toutes les organisations qui ont parrainé ce Symposium, notamment le Bureau Régional pour l'Afrique de l'OMS (Brazzaville), le Centre International de Recherche sur le Cancer (Lyon), le PNUE, le Ministère de la Coopération du Gouvernement Français, et l'Institut Pasteur Production (France) pour leur soutien généreux et leur coopération dans la réussite de cette rencontre. En tant que Président de l'Association Internationale pour l'Etude des Maladies Hépatiques, je désire présenter les meilleurs voeux du Conseil à vous tous, et je vous souhaite une rencontre très fructueuse. Je désire également profiter de l'occasion pour remercier tous ceux qui ont apporté leur soutien ou leur coopération à l'organisation de cette rencontre, et en particulier le Dr Quenum, Directeur Régional de l'OMS pour l'Afrique, le Dr Tolba, Directeur Exécutif du PNUE, le Dr Tomatis, Directeur du CIRC, le Dr Weber, Directeur de l'Institut Pasteur Production, et enfin, mais ce ne sont pas les moindres, les deux Consultants qui sont ici avec nous - le Dr Greg O'Conor et le Dr Guy de-Thé.

Mesdames et Messieurs qui allez participer à ce Symposium, Mesdames et Messieurs les Délégués, mes Amis, j'ai le grand plaisir de vous accueillir. Je vous souhaite un excellent séjour au Kenya, bien que le programme du meeting paraisse plutôt rempli.

Vive l'OUA,

Vive la coopération internationale.

HEPATOCELLULAR CARCINOMA: ETIOLOGY

HEPATOCELLULAR CARCINOMA: AN OVERVIEW

P.P. Anthony

Postgraduate Medical School
University of Exeter
Exeter, United Kingdom

Liver tumours continue to attract an interest that may seem out of proportion when we consider their place amongst all cancers, not to mention infection, malnutrition and the many other scourges of mankind, but there are good reasons for this:

1. Hepatocellular carcinoma, which is the main type of neoplasm in the liver, is one of the commonest internal malignancies in sub-Saharan Africa, China and South-East Asia and it is the commonest in certain areas, e.g., Mozambique, Taiwan and parts of the Chinese People's Republic. Mortality is practically 100% and an estimated 250 000 people die annually, most of them young males. Moreover, the death toll is still rising even in low-incidence areas.

2. Carcinogenesis in the liver has been the most intensively studied experimental model for many years and the lessons learnt are applicable to cancers at most sites.
3. New developments continue to take place that are of universal interest: the probable etiological role of hepatitis B virus (HBV) and aflatoxins, the establishment of alpha-fetoprotein as a uniquely reliable tumour marker, the emergence of commonly used oral contraceptive steroids as an ominous risk factor of as yet unassessed significance are but a few of these.

The study of this cancer in Africa has not only opened up entirely new vistas in oncogenesis but may also lead to the first successful example of eradication of a tumour and stand, in years to come, as a monument to international cooperation.

EPIDEMIOLOGY

Our knowledge of the world-wide distribution of tumours is based on data provided by cancer registries in many parts of the world, published by the International Agency for Research on Cancer in successive volumes of the series Cancer Incidence in Five Continents. The most up to date of these appeared in 1982 and contains information from registries in 37 countries (Waterhouse et al., 1982). Liver tumours appear under the broad heading 'malignant neoplasms of the liver, primary site; (code number 155.0 of the International Classification of Diseases). This fails to distinguish between the various histological types, but detailed studies in many locations have established that the geographical variability is due largely to liver-cell or hepato-cellular carcinoma. The next commonest type, bile-duct carcinoma or cholangiocarcinoma, occurs with much the same low frequency everywhere, except in parts of South-east Asia where it is associated with infestation with liver flukes. As this is not relevant to Africa, it will not be discussed any further. All other liver tumours are extremely rare.

World-wide incidence

If all the available sources are used, a tabulation of the world-wide incidence of hepatocellular carcinoma is possible, and is likely to be accurate within broad limits (Table 1). The highest rates of all obtain in Mozambique, Southern China and Taiwan. Pockets of high incidence occur elsewhere, e.g., on the west coast of the United States, where it is confined to Oriental immigrants. Variations also occur in homogeneous populations within the same country, for example in Greece and Kenya. These relate to HBV carriage rates and/or differences in exposure to aflatoxin. In Europe and North America some differences are seen which may be explained by alcohol and occupational or industrial exposure to chemicals.

Studies in migrants

When individuals migrate from high- to low-incidence areas, e.g., Chinese to the United States, they tend to maintain their high frequency rates at least for the first and second generations. Blacks, who were forcibly carried across the Atlantic in slave ships from the 17th to the 19th centuries, now show a low frequency as compared with Blacks in Africa. Whites tend to

Table 1. World-wide incidence of liver tumours[a]

High (20 - 150)	Intermediate (5 -20)	Low (up to 5)
East, West, Central and Southern Africa Southern China South-east Asia	Mediterranean countries Japan	Europe North America India

[a] The figures indicate incidence per 100 000 population per year

maintain their low rates even after many years in a high-incidence area like South Africa. It has been suggested, and is most probably true, that they are protected from their new environment by rigidly maintaining the life-style and habits of their home countries in Europe.

Time trends

Data from successive volumes of Cancer Incidence in Five Continents have been analysed and generally show an upward trend (Saracci & Repetto, 1980). Some of the increase may be attributed to improvements in diagnosis and registration but prolonged survival of patients with cirrhosis is likely to be the most important factor.

ETIOLOGY

Any discussion of the etiology of hepatocellular carcinoma tends to concentrate increasingly on the role of HBV, but this is not meant to imply that this virus is directly oncogenic or that other factors, notably aflatoxin, may be dismissed from consideration. The interrelationships between tumour, virus, chemicals, hormones, alcohol, nutrition, presence or absence of cirrhosis and so on are complex and each or a number of them may play a part in the outcome. These have been discussed in great detail recently in many reviews (Cameron et al., 1976; Okuda & Peters, 1976; Cancer Research, 1976; Remmer et al., 1978; Lapis & Johannessen, 1979; Munoz & Linsell, 1982; Okuda & MacKay, 1982).

Age

The incidence of hepatocellular carcinoma increases with age in all populations but with a tendency to fall off in old age. In high-incidence areas, however, the peak is seen in the third and fourth decades whilst in low-incidence areas it is shifted to the sixth and seventh decades. In Mozambique, 50% of patients are less than 30 years old. The early onset of the disease in high-incidence areas has been explained by exposure to environmental carcinogens at or soon after birth. In experiments also, young animals are more susceptible.

Sex

The disease occurs predominantly in males in all parts of the world, particularly in those with a high incidence, and the same is true for experimental animals. We have no adequate explanation for this. HBV infection in South Africa is said to be equally prevalent in both sexes (Kew et al., 1983).

Racial differences

Chinese seem to have a high incidence of the tumour wherever they go, whilst this is true of Blacks only in Africa and not in the United States; Whites retain a low frequency everywhere. Indians, who have a low incidence in India, show a rise after they have been settled in Singapore, Hong Kong and South Africa. These racial differences are explained by variations in HBV carriage rates.

Genetics, congenital anomalies and metabolic disorders

Table 2 lists many seemingly disparate factors and conditions that have been alleged to carry an increased risk of hepatocellular carcinoma. Many are anecdotal and only a few need be considered. The subject has recently been reviewed by Weinberg and Finegold (1983).

Table 2. Putative and potential etiological factors that are or may be genetically determined

---

Genetic:

> Familial
> HLA types
> Blood groups

Congenital:

> Neonatal hepatitis/atresia
> Congenital hepatic fibrosis
> Situs inversus
> Polyposis coli
> Neurofibromatosis
> Soto's syndrome

Metabolic errors:

> Byler's disease
> Glycogen storage disease
> Tyrosinaemia
> Porphyria
> Alpha-1-antitrypsin deficiency
> Haemochromatosis

Other:

> Obstruction of inferior vena cava

No particular HLA type or blood group has been found to be associated with hepatocellular carcinoma. Family clusters of the tumour have invariably been associated with spread of HBV infection due to close contact (Tong et al., 1979). Hepatic tumours develop in up to 50% of cases of type 1 glycogen storage disease: most are adenomas and may regress on treatment. Hereditary tyrosinaemia seems to be the metabolic defect most commonly associated with malignancy, which occurs despite dietary control. Levels of alpha-fetoprotein are high in patients with tyrosinaemia, even in the absence of a tumour. This has also been documented in ataxia teleangiectasia, in which hepatic tumours also occur.

Deficiency of alpha-1-antitrypsin is a genetically determined condition associated with neonatal jaundice and cirrhosis in early childhood and with pulmonary emphysema and cirrhosis in adults (Sharp, 1982). The pattern of inheritance is complex and is under the control of Pi (protease inhibitor) genes of which PiZ is the most important in relation to disease, particularly when the individual is a homozygous, i.e., PiZZ, carrier. During the 1970s a number of reports appeared suggesting an increased incidence of hepatocellular carcinoma in PiZ carriers with low levels of alpha-1-antitrypsin (Eriksson & Hägerstrand, 1974). Moreover, Palmer and Wolfe (1976) showed that PAS-positive intracytoplasmic globules, representing alpha-1-antitrypsin and similar to those found in the liver cells of enzyme-deficient individuals, were also present in a proportion of hepatocellular carcinomas of patients who did not have the PiZ gene and were not deficient in the enzyme. It was suggested that the inability to discharge alpha-1-antitrypsin into the circulation, either by liver cells of Pi7 carriers or by liver-cancer cells in others, had a promoting effect on tumour growth by allowing a wide variety of proteases to destroy contact-inhibition amongst transformed liver cells. Some more recent studies have supported, while others have failed to confirm the association of hepatocellular carcinoma with alpha-1-antitrypsin deficiency, and the matter is far from settled (Cohen et al., 1982).

Idiopathic haemochromatosis predominantly affects men and has an autosomal recessive type of inheritance; hepatocellular carcinoma develops in up to 22% of cases (Purtilo & Gottlieb, 1973). The longer the patients live, the higher the risk. Malignancy is not seen in the precirrhotic phase of the disease, and removal of excess tissue iron does not prevent it. The relationship seems, quite clearly, to be between the male sex, cirrhosis and cancer and not between iron and cancer (MacSween, 1974). The high incidence of hepatocellular carcinoma in the South African Bantu is no longer thought to be related to haemosiderosis but to HBV and aflatoxin.

Recent reports indicate that obstruction of the inferior vena cava is present in a high proportion (up to 20%) of cases of hepatocellular carcinoma in South Africa and that this precedes the development of the tumour; the risk of malignant disease following hepatic venous outflow obstruction has been put as high

as 47.5% (Simson, 1982). Similar findings have been reported
from Japan, India and, occasionally, from other parts of the
world (Okuda, 1982). Two anatomical types of occlusion have been
described: a high membranous one where the vein joins the right
atrium, and a fibrous occlusion of variable length below this
level. It is disputed whether this lesion is congenital or
acquired but it is certainly long-standing. Chronic outflow
obstruction may act as a stimulant for the promotion process
without which cells initiated by a variety of agents would not
progress to neoplasia.

Alcohol and nutrition

     A history of chronic alcohol abuse is frequently found in
patients with hepatocellular carcinoma, particularly in low-
incidence areas where HBV infection is uncommon. In the
majority, cirrhosis is present and the risk of malignant change
is proportional to its duration, varying from 5 to 30%; this is
not reduced by giving up the habit (Lee, 1966).

     Postulated pathogenetic possibilities include: a mutagenic
effect of alcohol and its metabolites notably acetaldehyde, liver
enzyme induction resulting in altered biotransformation of potentially carcinogenic chemicals, and promotion through cirrhosis.
In addition, both alcohol and the often concomitant malnutrition
cause alterations in immune defence mechanisms (Leevy et al.,
1976) that may render the individual more susceptible to chronic
HBV infection. Several reports indicate an increased incidence
of HBV markers in alcoholics, and integrated HBV DNA was recently
found in the genome of tumour cells of all of a group of 20
patients with alcoholic cirrhosis and hepatocellular carcinoma
even though only 9 of 16 tested showed serological evidence of
infection (Bréchot et al., 1982).

     Malnutrition is common in most areas with a high incidence
of hepatocellular carcinoma and a low intake of protein with
associated immunodeficiency, diets low in lipotropic agents,
deficiencies of vitamins A, C and E and of the trace element
selenium may all play a part in the genesis of liver cancer (Kew
et al., 1982).

Parasites

It has been suggested that the immunosuppressive effect of chronic malaria infection may predispose to HBV infection and liver cancer but there is little factual evidence for this. In Vietnam, Welsh et al. (1976) found no difference in serological evidence of malaria between those with hepatocellular carcinoma and controls. Hepatic fibrosis is the result of heavy infestation with Schistosoma mansoni and S. japonicum, but this does not lead to carcinoma in the absence of HBV infection.

Chemicals and naturally occurring carcinogens

Table 3 lists those agents that have been most frequently considered in the etiology of hepatocellular carcinoma but few of these are seriously considered to be a risk for man (Okuda & MacKay, 1982).

N-Nitroso compounds are powerful carcinogens in fish, rodents and mammals (International Agency for Research on Cancer, 1978). Exposure of man may occur in two ways: through ingestion of preformed compounds (present in minute amounts in foodstuffs) or as a result of in vivo formation from secondary amines and nitrite. Solvents represent a minor hazard in certain occupations, e.g., in laundries and dry cleaners, as well as in the petrochemical industry. Azo dyes are largely of historical importance in that butter yellow was the first agent to produce liver tumours experimentally. Organochlorine pesticides are cancer promoters and are both widely used and extremely stable compounds; they tend to accumulate in body fat stores of animals and man. In China, an association was noted between hepatocellular carcinoma and the consumption of drinking-water from ditches and stagnant ponds but not from deep wells or free-flowing streams (Delong, 1979). This was attributed to contamination with pesticides but not proven. An analogous situation exists with polychlorinated biphenyls, also widely used and potentially hazardous, but no firm evidence has yet been produced of their harmful effect in man.

Pyrrolizidine alkaloids are proven hepatotoxins and the four listed in Table 3 are credited with the ability to induce tumours in the liver. Acute poisoning from drinking herbal teas and remedies results in liver failure whilst chronic ingestion leads to veno-occlusive disease, seen in Jamaica, India and Afghanistan. Cycasins are found in palm-like plants, the seeds

Table 3.   Chemicals and naturally occurring carcinogens in the etiology of liver-cell carcinoma

---

N-<u>Nitroso compounds</u>:

   <u>N</u>-Nitrosodiethylamine
   <u>N</u>-Nitrosodimethylamine
   <u>N</u>-Nitrosomethylurea

<u>Solvents</u>:

   Carbon tetrachloride
   Trichlorethylene
   Polycyclic hydrocarbons

<u>Organochlorine pesticides</u>:

   DDT
   Dieldrine
   Chlordane

<u>Pyrrolizidine alkaloids</u>:

   Isatidine
   Lasiocarpine
   Monocrotaline
   Retrorsin

<u>Mycotoxins</u>:

   Aflatoxin
   Sterigmatocystin
   Luteoskyrine
   Cyclochorotine

<u>Others</u>:

   Azo dyes
   Cycasin
   Polychlorinated biphenyls
   Safrole
   Tannic acid

---

and roots of which are used as food in times of drought and famine. The active principle is methylazoxymethanol, which is similar to N-nitrosodimethylamine. Fortunately, it is water-soluble and is normally removed during preparation for consumption. The use of safrole is no longer permitted and tannic acid has long been replaced as a topical agent in the treatment of burns.

Mycotoxins, of which aflatoxin is by far the most important, are second only to HBV in the list of environmental agents that are heavily implicated in the etiology of hepatocellular carcinoma in man. Aflatoxin is the metabolic product of the mould Aspergillus flavus, a common food-spoilage fungus in hot, humid climatic conditions and after prolonged storage. It exists in several forms of which B_1 is the most potent. The chemistry, toxicity and epidemiological evidence have been extensively reviewed (Wogan, 1976; US Department of Health, Education, and Welfare, 1978; Munoz & Linsell, 1982). The risk of dietary exposure to aflatoxin B_1 and a known high incidence of hepatocellular carcinoma coincide in many parts of Africa and Southeast Asia and a series of field studies have indicated a close relationship. Aflatoxin B_1 has also been found in the livers of a high proportion of patients with hepatocellular carcinoma and not in controls from the same locality (Onyemelukwe et al., 1980). A possible synergistic relationship between aflatoxin B_1 and HBV is strongly suggested. Other fungal metabolites listed in Table 3 are of doubtful significance.

Drugs

Many drugs (oxytetracycline, aminopyrine, tolazamide) contain amino groups that can, at least theoretically, undergo nitrosation in the body but there is no evidence to link them with liver tumours in man. Similarly, the experimental carcinogenic potential of phenobarbitone and hydantoin derivatives is yet to be seen, if it exists. Thorotrast and arsenic induce angiosarcoma of the liver and, rarely, cholangiocarcinoma and hepatocellular carcinoma. The most important drugs are 17-alkylated synthetic gonadal steroids, both androgenic/anabolic and oral contraceptive agents, the effects of which on the liver include the induction of tumours (Table 4). The evidence is fully discussed by Klatskin (1977), Huggins and Giuntoli (1979), Rooks et al. (1979), Mettlin and Natarajan (1981) and Ludwig (1983). Most tumours induced by both androgenic and oestrogenic compounds are hepatocellular adenomas, and carcinomas have been rare (Neuberger et al., 1980); some are known to have regressed after discontinuation of the drug. Peliosis has been seen only with androgenic/anabolic steroids. The number of cases is still small: 3.4 per 100 000 per year is expected in the United States. A co-carcinogenic effect in association with HBV infection or aflatoxin is a source of real concern for the future in Africa and South-east Asia.

Table 4. Hepatic side-effects of gonadal sex steroids

Steroid	Jaundice	Peliosis	Liver tumours
Androgenic/anabolic steroids:			
Methyltestosterone	+	+	+
Oxymethalone	+	+	+
Norethandrolone	+	+	+
Fluoxymesterone	+		
Oestrogens:			
Ethynil oestradiol	+	−	+
Mestranol	+	−	+
Progestogens:			
Norethisterone	±	−	?
Norethynodrel	±	−	?

Hepatitis B virus

The role of HBV in the genesis of hepatocellular carcinoma is one of the main subjects of this Symposium and only a brief outline of the evidence is called for here (see Table 5). The evidence for a causative role of the virus is growing steadily stronger but it is still incomplete, and the relationship may be more complex than one of simple cause and effect (Szmuness, 1978;

Kew, 1981; Maupas & Melnick, 1981; Beasley et al., 1982; Okuda & MacKay, 1982; Munoz & Linsell, 1982; Bassendine, 1983; Arthur et al., 1984).

It should be noted in passing that hepatitis A virus is not in any way linked to hepatocellular carcinoma in either high-incidence (Drucker et al., 1979) or low-incidence (Tabor et al., 1980) areas for the tumour. The explanation may lie in the fact that the liver cell is non-permissive to this virus and dies when infected: dead cells do not give rise to cancer. As we have no diagnostic markers for non-A, non-B hepatitis, we do not know what, if any, role it has to play. The recently discovered delta agent has not yet been adequately investigated for any contribution it may make to chronic liver disease and tumour genesis.

HBV carriage rate and tumour incidence match almost exactly throughout the world (Szmuness, 1978; Maupas & Melnick, 1981; Munoz & Linsell, 1982). Transmission in high-incidence areas is mainly vertical, namely mother-to-infant at or near birth, whilst in low-incidence areas it is horizontal, adult-to-adult. This partly explains the much earlier age peak of the tumour (20-40 years) in high-incidence than in low-incidence areas (40-60 years).

Case-control studies, first reported from Uganda (Vogel et al., 1970) and Taiwan (Tong et al., 1971) and subsequently from all parts of the world (Szmuness, 1978; Maupas & Melnick, 1981; Bassendine, 1983), have shown a strong and unequivocal relationship between presence of HBV infection and hepatocellular carcinoma. This is equally true in high- as well as in low-incidence areas. The markers most frequently associated with the tumour are the surface antigen are (HBsAg) and the antibody to the core antigen (anti-HBc).

Prospective studies, recently published, provide perhaps the strongest evidence yet of an association between HBV and hepatocellular carcinoma; they have also defined the magnitude of the risk, which is terrifying. A total of 22 707 male Chinese government employees in Taiwan were followed up for a mean of 4.7 years per man. They were chosen because of their known high HBV carrier rate and frequency of hepatocellular carcinoma and because, all being insured, an accurate record of causes of illness and death was guaranteed. Of 89 cases of hepatocellular carcinoma, 86 occurred in HBsAg carriers, the remaining 3 were positive for anti-HBc and 2 of these were also positive for

Table 5. Evidence for an etiological role of HBV in hepato-cellular carcinoma

---

HBV carriage rate matches tumour incidence

Strength of relationship in case-control studies

Prospective studies

Greater risk of malignancy in cirrhosis due to HBV

Liver-cell dysplasia and HBV

Presence of HBV antigens in tumour patients

Presence of integrated HBV DNA in tumour cells

Production of HBsAg by tumour cells in culture

HBV-like viruses in animals and tumours

---

anti-HBs. No case of carcinoma occurred amongst those without any virus markers. The relative risk for liver-cell carcinoma amongst carriers was 223, which is the highest for any risk factor for cancer ever recorded and far exceeds the relative risk of 20 for lung carcinoma in heavy smokers, for example. Carriers also showed a relative risk of 15 for cirrhosis. The life-time risk of death from hepatocellular carcinoma and/or cirrhosis in those infected with HBV was put at between 40% and 50% (Beasley et al., 1981, 1982). Other studies conducted in Japan and Hawaii produced similar results.

Cirrhosis associated with HBV infection has been repeatedly shown to carry a greater risk of malignant change than cirrhosis without HBV (Obata et al., 1980).

Liver-cell dysplasia, alleged to be a premalignant change (Anthony et al., 1973), is associated with cirrhosis and carriage of HBsAg. The original findings of this study were confirmed in Thailand, Japan and Hong Kong but disputed or refuted by others in Japan and South Africa.

HBV antigens have consistently been found in the non-tumorous liver of patients with hepatocellular carcinoma (Okuda & MacKay, 1982) but with difficulty or not at all in the tumour itself.   It seems that viral replication becomes increasingly defective during neoplastic transformation with loss of hepatitis B e antigen, HBeAg, HBsAg and HBcAg in this order in most cases.

HBV DNA is found integrated into the genome of neoplastic liver cells in nearly all cases studied to date, even in the absence of any serological marker and in patients apparently suffering from alcoholic cirrhosis (Shafritz & Kew, 1981; Shafritz et al., 1981; Bréchot et al., 1982).   These findings have been confirmed in Africa, China and Greece.   Details vary and no HBV oncogene has yet been demonstrated but integration precedes the development of the tumour.   A co-carcinogenic effect with aflatoxin has also been suggested.

Hepatocellular carcinoma cells in tissue culture have been shown to produce HBsAg but no other antigens much less the whole virus (Alexander et al., 1982); this, however, fits the observation of increasingly defective replication of HBV in hepato-cellular carcinoma tissue in vivo.

HBV-like viruses have been found in ducks, ground squirrels and woodchucks;   only the last named develop hepatocellular carcinoma and the tumour differs somewhat from that seen in man (Popper et al., 1981).

In brief, almost all the postulated criteria for an etiolo-gical role of any virus in oncogenesis have now been met, except for two: HBV has not yet produced hepatocellular carcinoma in subhuman primates, such as chimpanzees, to which it is trans-missible, and the effect of preventive vaccination on tumour incidence is yet to be seen.

PATHOGENESIS OF HEPATOCELLULAR CARCINOMA

Chemical carcinogenesis

The carcinogenic effects of hundreds of chemical compounds have been studied, mainly in rats, and much detailed information is now available on the probable steps involved in neoplastic transformation; these are shown in Table 6. Further details and references to the vast literature on the subject are found in many review articles and books (Cancer Research, 1976; Remmer et al., 1978; Lapis & Johannessen, 1979; Farber, 1981; Okuda & MacKay, 1981; Pitot, 1982).

Table 6. Probable steps in neoplastic transformation due to chemical agents

Step	Associated effects
Initiation	Metabolic conversion of proximate to ultimate carcinogen Damage to DNA, organelles and membranes Fixation of abnormality by cell proliferation
Promotion	Inhibition - selection Enzyme changes Hyperplastic nodules Autonomous neoplastic nodules
Overt malignant behaviour	Metastases and death

Most chemical carcinogens are inert in themselves and require metabolic conversion by the mixed-function oxygenase system, located in the endoplasmic reticulum, to produce highly reactive epoxides which damage DNA, organelles and membranes. The abnormality is 'fixed' by a round of cell proliferation and the cell is 'initiated'. Such cells have no autonomy and mostly revert to normal unless they are further 'promoted' by the same or other agents. As most carcinogenic compounds are cytotoxic, normal cells are inhibited and abnormal ones are selected in increasing numbers. Enzyme changes observed are mainly a loss of normal adult enzymes (ATPase, G6Pase, beta-glucuronidase) and an increase of foetal markers (gamma-glutamyl transpeptidase, alpha-fetoprotein, beta-chorionic gonadotrophin). Hyperplastic nodules appear which are often strikingly basophilic. These later become autonomous and eventually overt malignancy results with metastases and death of the animal. An increased cell turn-over state, e.g., partial hepatectomy or presence of cirrhosis, accelerates the course of events.

A peculiar phenomenon is the proliferation of 'oval cells' or stem cells, not seen in man, and experimental tumours are often different from those occurring spontaneously in humans; mixed hepatocellular and bile-duct carcinoma are often induced.

Viral oncogenesis

Experimental tumour viruses are either DNA or RNA viruses. The latter are also known as retroviruses because their RNA must be transcribed backwards, so to speak, into a DNA copy by the enzyme reverse transcriptase before replication can take place (Fig. 1). Most virus-induced tumours in animals are lymphomas, leukaemias and soft-tissue sarcomas; carcinomas are rare. Persistence of the viral genome in the host cell is essential for neoplastic transformation (Wyke, 1981; Essex & Gutensohn, 1981; Enrietto & Wyke, 1983).

Oncogenes

The discovery of specific DNA sequences associated with malignancy has created enormous interest in recent years (Hamlyn & Sikora, 1983; Robertson, 1983). Originally described in viruses (v-onc) they were subsequently found in experimental animal and, in some cases, spontaneously occurring human, tumours (C-onc). Many have been purified, sequenced and cloned and can readily be studied in transfection assays using tissue cultures

FIG. 1.   TRANSCRIPTION OF VIRAL NUCLEIC ACIDS
INTO HOST-CELL GENOME

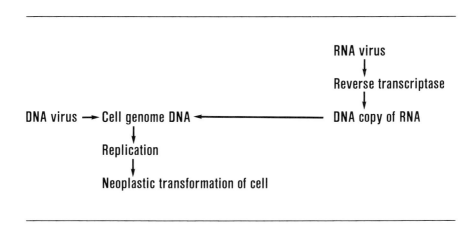

of suitable cell lines, such as the one derived from the NIH 3T3 mouse fibroblast.   Oncogenes are widespread in all vertebrate species and viruses pick them up as they pass through cells. Normally, they are present in small amounts and their physiological role is probably growth control.   They encode for phosphoproteins with protein kinase activity and produce growth-factor-like molecules or receptors for them.   If they are displaced, altered or overexpressed, uncontrolled cell proliferation may result.   Oncogenes are just beginning to be studied in liver regeneration and carcinogenesis (Fausto & Shank, 1983).   HBV is not known at present to possess an oncogene but the virus, or part of it, is known to be integrated into liver cells during infection and carcinogenesis and it could act by 'turning on' a cellular oncogene, a phenomenon usually referred to as 'promotional insertion'.   A virus, or several viruses and/or chemical carcinogens could act together through oncogenes.   This is now being studied and we may soon see a unified, coherent explanation of the seemingly disparate theories of carcinogenesis that have been based on epidemiological, chemical experimental and virological observations.

Precancerous changes in the human liver

Cirrhosis itself is a precancerous condition: it is usually
long-standing, macronodular and associated with HBV carriage.
Hyperplastic or autonomous nodules are rarely seen (Tezuka &
Sawai, 1983) but enzyme changes, similar to those seen during
experimental chemical carcinogenesis, have rarely been documented
(Uchida et al., 1981). It has been suggested that liver-cell
dysplasia (Anthony et al., 1973) is a precancerous change and
this has been both confirmed and denied since.

PATHOLOGY OF HEPATOCELLULAR CARCINOMA

The gross appearances, mode of spread and natural history
are well known. Table 7 summarizes the information on laboratory
diagnosis, paraneoplastic syndromes and tumour markers. The
histological appearances were reviewed by an international group
set up by the World Health Organization in 1978: this resulted
in a much needed, clear definition of the different types of
tumour that may arise in the liver, essential for epidemiological, clinical and basic scientific research (World Health
Organization, 1978). The WHO classificiation remains valid, but
a few modifications have become necessary and these concern mainly the gradual recognition of the so-called good-prognosis types.

The main contribution of the WHO group was the clear separation of hepatocellular carcinoma from cholangiocarcinoma and
the recommendation that all histological subtypes of hepatocellular carcinoma (trabecular, pseudoglandular, compact,
scirrhous, pleomorphic, clear-cell) be regarded as mere morphological variants of a single disease. We now have to recognize
that there are, in fact, exceptions to this rule.

Clear-cell carcinoma has been widely claimed to have a
better prognosis than is average for all other subtypes (Lai et
al., 1979).

Fibrolamellar carcinoma is now the accepted name of the
variant that has previously been described as compact or
scirrhous. This is a tumour that is seen in adolescents and
young adults of either sex, is commonly associated with hypercalcaemia and/or high levels of vitamin B12 binding protein and
carries a good prognosis (Berman et al., 1980; Craig et al.,
1980). The slow rate of growth allows surgical resection of a

Table 7. Laboratory diagnosis, paraneoplastic manifestations and tumour markers of hepatocellular carcinoma

---

Laboratory diagnosis:

Alkaline phosphatase↑
Gamma-glutamyl transpeptidase↑
Alpha-fetoprotein > 1000 ng/ml

Paraneoplastic syndromes and tumour markers:

Hypoglycaemia
Hypercalcaemia
Erythrocytosis
Dysfibrinogenaemia
Vitamin B12 binding protein
Hypercholesterolaemia
Human chorionic gonadotrophin
Proline hydroxylase
Porphyria cutanea tarda
Hypertrophic pulmonary osteoarthropathy

---

usually solitary mass. It is uncertain at present whether this tumour is truly of liver-cell origin and it may be derived from an endocrine cell in the liver.

Encapsulated or minute hepatocellular carcinoma was originally described in Japan (Okuda et al., 1977) but also occurs in parts of South-east Asia. It is often small, generally less than 5.0 cm, and is surrounded by a fibrous capsule which appears to contain it. It may be detected by a variety of imaging methods and by estimation of alpha-fetoprotein in the blood. A high rate of cure has been achieved by surgical resection.

Other morphological observations which were unexplained in 1978 have now been studied further. The occurrence of Mallory bodies in tumour cells of non-alcoholic patients is confirmed: it probably results from a disturbance of intermediate filament metabolism. The heterogeneity of the so-called globular hyaline bodies has been demonstrated by immunohistology: they may represent albumen, alpha-1-antitrypsin, alpha-fetoprotein, CEA, HCG, isoferritin and so on.

Finally, spontaneous regression of hepatocellular carcinoma has been reported in a small number of well documented cases (Gottfried et al., 1982) for no reason that could be detected.

CONCLUSIONS

It is difficult, in a few pages, even to summarize the enormous body of knowledge that has emerged in the last 10 years on the subject of hepatocellular carcinoma. Many questions remain unanswered but the prospects are bright. This merciless and lethal scourge of developing countries may be eliminated or its incidence at least reduced in our life-time. If so, it will be a success almost without parallel and one to which scientists in Africa will have made a unique and outstanding contribution.

REFERENCES

Alexander, J.J., Van der Merwe, C.F., Saunders, R.M., McElligott, S.E. & Desmyter, J. (1982) A comparison between in vitro experiments with a hepatoma cell line and in vivo studies. Hepatology, 2, 92-96

Anthony, P.P., Vogel, C.L. & Barker, L.F. (1973) Liver cell dysplasia: a premalignant condition. J. clin. Pathol., 26, 217-223

Arthur, M.J.P., Hall, A.J. & Wright, R. (1984) Hepatitis B, hepatocellular carcinoma and strategies for prevention. Lancet, 1, 607-610

Bassendine, M.F. (1983) Hepatitis B virus and liver cell carcinoma. Recent Adv. Histopathol., 12, 137-146

Beasley, R.P., Hwang, L.Y., Lin, C.C. & Chien, C.S. (1981) Hepatocellular carcinoma and hepatitis B virus. A prospective study of 22707 men in Taiwan. Lancet, 2, 1129-1133

Beasley, R.P., Blumberg, B., Popper, H. & Wain-Hobson, S. (1982) Hepatitis B virus and hepatocellular carcinoma. In: Okuda, K. & MacKay, I., eds, Hepatocellular carcinoma (UICC Technical Report Series, Vol. 74, No. 17), Geneva, UICC, pp. 60-93

Berman, M.M., Libbey, N.P. & Foster, J.H. (1980) Hepatocellular carcinoma polygonal cell type with fibrous stroma - an atypical variant with a favorable prognosis. Cancer, 46, 1448-1455

Bréchot, C., Nalpas, B., Courouce, A.-M., Duhamel, G., Gallard, P., Carnot, F., Tiollais, P. & Berthelot, P. (1982) Evidence that hepatitis B virus has a role in liver-cell carcinoma in alcoholic liver disease. New Engl. J. Med., 306, 1384-1387

Cameron, H.M., Linsell, D.A. & Warwick, G.P., eds (1976) Liver Cell Cancer, Amsterdam, Elsevier

Cancer Research (1976) Symposium: early lesions and the development of epithelial cancer. Cancer Res., 36, 2475-2706

Cohen, C., Berson, S.D. & Budgeon, R.B. (1982) Alpha-1-antitrypsin deficiency in Southern African hepatocellular carcinoma patients, an immunoperoxidase and histochemical study. Cancer, 49, 2537-2540

Craig, J.R., Peters, R.L., Edmondson, H.A. & Omata, M. (1980) Fibrolamellar carcinoma of the liver: a tumour of adolescents and young adults with distinctive clinicopathologic features. Cancer, 46, 372-379

Delong, S. (1979) Drinking water and liver cell cancer. Chin. med. J., 92, 748-756

Drucker, J.A., Coursaget, P., Maupas, P., Goudeau, A., Gerety, R.J., Chiron, J.P., Denis, F. & Diop-Mar I. (1979) Hepatitis A infection and primary hepatocellular carcinoma. Biomedicine, 31, 23-25

Enrietto, P.J. & Wyke, J.A. (1983) The pathogenesis of oncogenic avian retroviruses. Adv. Cancer Res., 39, 269-284

Eriksson, S. & Hägerstrand, I. (1974)   Cirrhosis and malignant hepatoma in alpha-1-antitrypsin deficiency.   Acta Med. Scand., 195, 451-458

Essex, M. & Gutenssohn, N. (1981)   A comparison of the pathobiology and epidemiology of cancers associated with viruses in humans and animals. Prog. med. Virol., 27, 114-126

Farber, E. (1981)   Chemical carcinogenesis.   New Engl. J. Med., 305, 1379-1389

Fausto, N. & Shank, P.R. (1983)   Oncogene expression in liver regeneration and hepatocarcinogenesis.   Hepatology, 3, 1016-1023

Gottfried, E.B., Steller, R., Paronetto, F. & Lieber, C.S. (1982) Spontaneous regression of hepatocellular carcinoma. Gastroenterology, 82, 770-774

Hamlyn, P. & Sikora, K. (1983) Oncogenes. Lancet, ii, 326-330

Huggins, G.R. & Giuntoli, R.L. (1979) Oral contraceptives and neoplasia. Fertil. Steril., 32, 1-23

International Agency for Research on Cancer (1978)   IARC Monographs on the Evaluation of the Carcinogenic Risk of Chemicals to Humans, Vol. 17, Some N-Nitroso Compounds, Lyon

Kew, M.C. (1981)   Clinical, pathologic and etiologic heterogeneity in hepatocellular carcinoma: evidence from Southern Africa. Hepatology, 1, 366-369

Kew, M.C., Newberne, P.M. & Popper, H. (1982) Other aetiological processes in hepatocellular carcinoma.   In: Okuda, K. & MacKay, I., eds, Hepatocellular Carcinoma (UICC Technical Report Series, Vol. 74, Report No. 17), Geneva, UICC, pp. 110-116

Kew, M.C., Rossouw, E., Paterson, A., Hodkinson, J., Whitcutt, M. & Dusheiko, G. (1983)   Hepatitis B virus status of black women with hepatocellular carcinoma. Gastroenterology, 84, 693-696

Klatskin, G. (1977) Hepatic tumours: possible relationship to use of oral contraceptives. Gastroenterology, 73, 386-394

Lai, C.L., Wu, P.C., Lam, K.C. & Todd, D. (1979) Histologic prognostic indicators in hepatocellular carcinoma. Cancer, 44, 1677-1683

Lapis, K. & Johannessen, J.V., eds (1979) Liver Carcinogenesis, Washington, DC, Hemisphere Publishing Co.

Lee, F.I. (1966) Cirrhosis and hepatoma in alcoholics. Gut, 7, 77-85

Leevy, C.M., Chen, T., Luisada-Opper, A., Kanagasundarum, V. & Zetterman, R. (1976) Liver disease of the alcoholic: role of immunologic abnormalities in pathogenesis, recognition and treatment. Prog. Liver Dis., 5, 516-530

Ludwig, J. (1983) Drug effects on the liver. A tabular compilation of drugs and drug-related hepatic diseases. Dig. Dis. Sci., 24, 785-796

MacSween, R.N.M. (1974) A clinico-pathological review of 100 cases of primary malignant tumours of the liver. J. clin. Pathol., 27, 669-682

Maupas, P. & Melnick, J.L. (1981) Hepatitis B infection and primary liver cancer. Prog. med. Virol., 27, 1-5

Mettlin, C. & Natarajan, N. (1981) Studies on the role of oral contraceptive use in the etiology of benign and malignant liver tumours. J. surg. Oncol., 18, 73-85

Munoz, N. & Linsell, A. (1982) Epidemiology of primary liver cancer. In: Correa, P. & Haenszel, W., eds, Epidemiology of Cancer of the Digestive Tract, The Hague, Nijhoff, pp. 161-195

Neuberger, J., Portmann, B., Nunnerley, H.B., Laws, J.W., Davis, M. & Williams, R. (1980) Oral contraceptive associated liver tumours: occurrence of malignancy and difficulties in diagnosis. Lancet, 1, 273-276

Obata, H., Hayashi, N., Motoike, Y., Hisamitsu, T., Okuda, H., Kobayashi, S. & Nishioka, K. (1980) A prospective study on the development of hepatocellular carcinoma from liver cirrhosis with persistent hepatitis B virus infection. Int. J. Cancer, 25, 741-747

Okuda, K. (1982) Membraneous obstruction of the inferior vena cava: etiology and relation to hepatocellular carcinoma. Gastroenterology, 82, 376-379

Okuda, K. & Peters, R.L., eds (1976) Hepatocellular carcinoma, New York, Wiley

Okuda, K. & MacKay, I. (1982) Hepatocellular Carcinoma (UICC Technical Report Series, Vol. 74, Report No. 17), Geneva, UICC

Okuda, K., Musha, H., Nakajima, Y., Kubo, Y., Shimokawa, Y., Nagasaki, Y., Sawe, Y., Jinnouchi, S., Kaneko, T., Obata, H., Hisamitsu, T., Motoike, Y., Okasaki, N., Kajiro, M., Sakamoto, K. & Nakashima, T. (1977) Clinicopathologic features of encapsulated hepatocellular carcinoma. A study of 26 cases. Cancer, 40, 1240-1245

Onyemelukwe, C.G., Nirodi, C. & West, C.E. (1980) Aflatoxin B[1] in hepatocellular carcinoma. Trop. geog. Med., 32, 237-242

Palmer, P.E. & Wolfe, H.J. (1976) Alpha-1-antitrypsin deposition in primary hepatic carcinomas. Arch. Pathol. lab. Med., 100, 232-236

Pitot, H.C. (1982) The natural history of neoplastic development: the relation of experimental models to human cancer. Cancer, 49, 1296-1304

Popper, H., Shih, J.W.K., Gerin, J.L., Wong, D.C., Hoyer, B.H., London, W.T., Sly, D.L. & Purcell, R.H. (1981) Woodchuck hepatitis and hepatocellular carcinoma: correlation of histologic with virologic observations. Hepatology, 2, 91-98

Purtilo, D.T. & Gottlieb, L.S. (1973) Cirrhosis and hepatoma occurring at Boston City Hospital (1917-1968) Cancer, 32, 458-462

Remmer, H., Bolt, H.M., Bannasch, P. & Popper, H., eds (1978) Primary Liver Tumours, Lancaster, MTP Press

Robertson, M. (1983) Oncogenes and multistep carcinogenesis. Br. med. J., 287, 1084-1086

Rooks, J.B., Ory, H.W., Ishak, K.G., Strauss, L.T., Greenspan, J.R., Hill, A.P. & Tyler, C.W. Jr (1979) Epidemiology of hepatocellular adenoma. The role of oral contraceptive use. J. Am. med. Assoc., 242, 644-648

Saracci, R. & Repetto, F. (1980) Time trends of primary liver cancer: indication of increased incidence in selected cancer registry populations. J. natl Cancer Inst., 65, 241-247

Shafritz, D.A. & Kew, M.C. (1981) Identification of integrated hepatitis B virus sequences in human hepatocellular carcinoma. Hepatology, 1, 1-8

Shafritz, D.A., Shouval, D., Sherman, H.I., Hadziyannis, S.J. & Kew, M.C. (1981) Integration of hepatitis B virus DNA into the genome of liver cells in chronic liver disease and hepatocellular carcinoma: Studies in percutaneous liver biopsies and post-mortem tissue specimens. New Engl. J. Med., 305, 1067-1073

Sharp, H.L. (1982) Alpha-1-antitrypsin: an ignored protein in understanding liver disease. Sem. Liver Dis., 2, 314-328

Simson, I.W. (1982) Membraneous obstruction of the inferior vena cava and hepatocellular carcinoma in South Africa. Gastroenterology, 82, 171-178

Szmuness, W. (1978) Hepatocellular carcinoma and the hepatitis B virus: evidence for a causal association. Prog. med. Virol., 24, 40-69

Tabor, E., Trichopoulos, D., Manousos, D., Zavitsanos, X., Drucker, J.A. & Gerety, R.J. (1980) Absence of an association between past infection with hepatitis A virus and hepatocellular carcinoma. Int. J. Epidemiol.. 9, 221-223

Tezuka, F. & Sawai, T. (1983) Hyperplasia of small hepatic cells in the precancerous condition of cirrhotic livers. _Tokohu J. exp. Med._, 139, 171–177

Tong, M.J., Sun, S.-C., Schaeffer, B.T., Chang, N.-K., Lo, K.-J. & Peters, R.L. (1971) Hepatitis-associated antigen and hepatocellular carcinoma in Taiwan. _Ann. intern. Med._, 75, 687–691

Tong, M.J., Weiner, J.M., Ashcavai, M.W. & Vyas, G.N. (1979) Evidence for clustering of hepatitis B virus infection in families of patients with primary hepatocellular carcinoma. _Cancer_, 44, 2338–2342

Uchida, T., Miyata, H. & Shikata, T. (1981) Human hepatocellular carcinoma and putative precancerous disorders. _Arch. Pathol. lab. Med._, 105, 180–186

US Department of Health, Education, and Welfare (1978) _Oncology Overview. Selected Abstracts on Aflatoxin and Other Mycotoxin Carcinogenesis_, Springfield, National Technical Information Service, International Cancer Research Data Bank

Vogel, C.L., Anthony, P.P., Mody, N. & Barker, L.F. (1970) Hepatitis-associated antigen in Ugandan patients with hepatocellular carcinoma. _Lancet_, 2, 621–624

Waterhouse, J., Muir, C., Shanmugaratnam, K. & Powell, J. (1982) _Cancer Incidence in Five Continents_, Vol. IV, Lyon, International Agency for Research on Cancer

Weinberg, A.G. & Finegold, M.J. (1983) Primary hepatic tumours of childhood. _Hum. Pathology_, 14, 512–537

Welsh, J.D., Brown, J.D., Arnold, K., Matthews, H.M. & Prince, A.M. (1976) Hepatitis B surface antigen, malaria titres and primary liver cancer in South Vietnam. _Gastroenterology_, 70, 392–396

Wogan, G.N. (1976) _Aflatoxins and their relationship to hepatocellular carcinoma_. In: Okuda, K. & Peters, R.L., eds, _Hepatocellular Carcinoma_, New York, Wiley, pp. 25–41

World Health Organization (1978) Histological Typing of Tumours of the Liver, Biliary Tract and Pancreas (International Histological Classification of Tumours No. 20), Geneva

Wyke, J.A. (1981) Oncogenic viruses. J. Pathol., 135, 39-85

CANCER PRIMITIF DU FOIE: VUE D'ENSEMBLE

P.P. Anthony

University of Exeter
Exeter, United Kingdom

Les tumeurs du foie suscitent toujours un intérêt qui peut paraître hors de proportion quanD on considère leur place parmi tous les cancers, pour ne pas parler des infections, de la malnutrition et des nombreux autres fléaux de l'humanité; mais il y a de bonnes raisons pour cela:

1. Le cancer primitif du foie, qui représente le principal type de cancer du foie, est un des cancers internes les plus communs en Afrique sub-Saharienne, en Chine, et en Asie du Sud-Est, et c'est le plus courant dans certaines régions telles que le Mozambique, Taïwan et certaines parties de la République Populaire de Chine. La mortalité est pratiquement de 100% et, selon les estimations, 250 000 personnes, pour la plupart des hommes jeunes, en meurent chaque année. De plus, cette mortalité est toujours en augmentation, même dans les régions de faible incidence.

2. La cancérogenèse du foie est depuis de nombreuses années le modèle expérimental le plus étudié, et les leçons qu'on en a apprises peuvent s'appliquer aux cancers survenant dans la plupart des localisations.

3. Cette étude connaît toujours de nouveaux développements, d'un intérêt universel: le rôle étiologique probable du virus de l'hépatite B (HBV) et des aflatoxines, la mise en évidence d'un marqueur tumoral unique et caractéristique, l'alpha-foetoprotéine, l'émergence des contraceptifs oraux stéroïdiens comme facteur de risque inquiétant mais dont l'importance n'est pas encore établie, n'en représentent que quelques uns.

L'étude de ce cancer en Afrique n'a pas seulement ouvert des perspectives tout-à-fait nouvelles dans l'oncogenèse, mais il est possible qu'elle aboutisse au premier succès dans l'éradication d'une tumeur, et qu'elle s'élève, dans les années à venir, comme un monument à la coopération internationale.

EPIDEMIOLOGIE

Notre connaissance de la distribution mondiale des tumeurs est basée sur les données des registres du cancer établis dans différentes parties du monde, et publiées par le Centre International de Recherche sur le Cancer dans les volumes consécutifs de la collection "Cancer Incidence in Five Continents". Le plus récent a été publié en 1982 et contient les informations provenant des registres de 37 pays (Waterhouse et coll., 1982). Les tumeurs du foie y figurent sous la dénomination large de "néoplasmes malins du foie, site primitif" (numéro de code: 155.0 de la Classification Internationale des Maladies). Cette dénomination ne permet pas de distinguer les différents types histologiques, mais des études détaillées réalisées dans plusieurs régions ont établi que la variabilité géographique est due en grande partie à l'épithélioma hépatocellulaire ou cancer primitif du foie. Le type de cancer du foie le plus commun après le cancer primitif du foie, l'épithélioma du canal cholédoque, ou épithélioma cholangiocellulaire, se retrouve partout avec à peu près la même fréquence, sauf dans certaines régions d'Asie du Sud-Est, où il est associé à l'infection par des douves du foie. Comme ceci ne s'applique pas à l'Afrique, nous n'en discuterons pas davantage. Toutes les autres tumeurs du foie sont extrêmement rares.

Incidence mondiale

Si l'on utilise toutes les sources disponibles, il est possible de dresser un tableau de l'incidence mondiale du cancer primitif du foie, et il est probable qu'il soit exact, à l'intérieur de larges limites (Tableau 1). Les taux les plus élevés de tous sont obtenus au Mozambique, en Chine du Sud et à Taiwan. Des enclaves de haute incidence se rencontrent dans d'autres régions, par exemple sur la côte ouest des Etats-Unis, où elle est limitée aux immigrants orientaux. Des variations se produisent également au sein de populations homogènes à l'intérieur d'un même pays, par exemple en Grèce et au Kenya. Elles sont liées aux taux de portage du virus de l'hépatite B (HBV) et/ou à des différences d'exposition à l'aflatoxine. En Europe et en Amérique du Nord, on observe des différences qui peuvent s'expliquer par la consommation d'alcool et l'exposition professionnelle ou industrielle à des produits chimiques.

Tableau 1. Incidence mondiale des tumeurs du foie[a]

Elevée (20-150)	Intermédiaire (5-20)	Basse (jusqu'à 5)
Afrique orientale, occidentale, centrale et méridionale	Pays Méditerranéens Japon	Europe Amérique du Nord Inde
Chine méridionale		
Asie du Sud-Est		

[a] Les chiffres indiquent l'incidence pour 100 000 personnes et par an.

Etude des migrants

Les individus qui migrent d'une région d'incidence élevée à une région de faible incidence, comme les Chinois aux Etats-Unis, tendent à conserver leurs taux d'incidence élevés, tout au moins pendant la première et la deuxième génération. Les Noirs, qui du 17ème au 19ème siècles ont été amenés de force de l'autre côté de l'Atlantique sur les bateaux négriers présentent maintenant une fréquence faible, comparée à celle des Noirs Africains. Les Blancs tendent à conserver leurs taux d'incidence faibles, même après de nombreuses années dans les zones d'incidence élevée telles que l'Afrique du Sud. On a suggéré, et c'est probablement exact, qu'ils sont protégés de leur nouvel environnement du fait qu'ils maintiennent de façon rigide le style de vie et les habitudes des pays européens dont ils sont originaires.

Variations dans le temps

L'analyse des données publiées dans les éditions successives de "Cancer Incidence in Five Continents" montrent en général une tendance à l'augmentation (Saracci & Repetto, 1980). Une partie de l'augmentation peut être attribuée aux améliorations dans le diagnostic et l'enregistrement, mais la survie prolongée des patients atteints de cirrhose est vraisemblablement le facteur le plus important.

ETIOLOGIE

Toute discussion sur l'étiologie du cancer primitif du foie tend à se concentrer de plus en plus sur le rôle du virus HB, mais cela ne signifie pas que ce virus soit directement oncogène, ou que d'autres facteurs, notamment l'aflatoxine, puissent être écartés. Les inter-relations entre tumeur, virus, produits chimiques, hormones, alcool, nutrition, présence ou absence de cirrhose, etc., sont complexes, et chacun ou un certain nombre de ces facteurs peuvent jouer un rôle dans le résultat final. Cela a été discuté récemment en détail dans plusieurs revues (Cameron et coll., 1976; Okuda & Peters, 1976; Cancer Research, 1976; Remmer et coll., 1978; Lapis & Johannessen, 1979; Munoz & Linsell, 1982; Okuda & MacKay, 1982).

Age

L'incidence du cancer primitif du foie augmente avec l'âge dans toutes les populations, mais elle tend à chuter aux âges plus avancés. Cependant, dans les zones d'incidence élevée, le pic se situe dans la 3ème et la 4ème décades, tandis que dans les zones de faible incidence, ce pic est décalé vers la 6ème et la 7ème décades. Au Mozambique, 50% des patients ont moins de 30 ans. On a expliqué l'apparition précoce de la maladie dans les zones d'incidence élevée par l'exposition à des cancérogènes de l'environnement dès la naissance ou peu après. Les études expérimentales ont également démontré que les jeunes animaux sont plus sensibles.

Sexe

Dans toutes les parties du monde, et en particulier dans celles où l'incidence du cancer primitif du foie est élevée, ce sont les sujets de sexe masculin qui sont les plus touchés. La même chose est vraie pour les animaux de laboratoire. Nous n'avons pas d'explication rationnelle pour ce fait. En Afrique du Sud, la prévalence de l'infection HBV est, d'après ce que l'on dit, la même dans les deux sexes (Kew et coll., 1983).

Différences raciales

Les Chinois semblent présenter une incidence élevée de cancer primitif du foie, où qu'ils aillent, alors que pour les Noirs cela est vrai seulement lorsqu'ils vivent en Afrique, et pas aux Etats-Unis. Les Blancs conservent partout une fréquence faible. Les Indiens, qui ont une incidence faible en Inde, présentent une augmentation après qu'ils se soient établis à Singapour, à Hong Kong, et en Afrique du Sud. Ces différences raciales peuvent s'expliquer par des variations dans les taux de portage du virus HB.

Génétique, anomalies congénitales et désordres métaboliques

Le Tableau 2 énumère des facteurs et des états apparemment assez disparates dont on a prétendu qu'ils entraînaient un risque accru de cancer primitif du foie. Beaucoup d'entre eux sont purement anecdotiques et seulement quelques uns méritent d'être considérés. Le sujet a récemment été passé en revue par Weinberg et Finegold (1983).

On n'a pas trouvé d'association entre un type HLA particulier, ou un groupe sanguin et le cancer primitif du foie. Des concentrations familiales de tumeur ont invariablement été associées à la diffusion de l'infection HBV due à des contacts étroits (Tong et coll., 1979). Des tumeurs hépatiques se développent jusque dans 50% des cas de glycogénose de type 1: la plupart de ces tumeurs sont des adénomes et peuvent régresser sous traitement. La tyrosinémie congénitale semble le déficit métabolique le plus communément associé à une tumeur maligne, qui se développe même si on contrôle la maladie par un régime. Les taux d'alpha-foetoprotéine sont élevés chez les sujets atteints de tyrosinémie, même en l'absence de tumeur. La même chose a été constatée dans l'ataxie-telangiectasie, dans laquelle des tumeurs hépatiques surviennent également.

Le déficit en alpha-1-antitrypsine est une maladie d'origine génétique caractérisée par une jaunisse néonatale et une cirrhose dans la petite enfance, et chez l'adulte par un emphysème pulmonaire et une cirrhose (Sharp, 1982). Le mode de transmission de

Tableau 2. Facteurs étiologiques potentiels et putatifs, étant
ou pouvant être d'origine génétique

Facteurs Génétiques

    Familiaux
    Types HLA
    Groupes sanguins

Facteurs Congénitaux

    Hépatite néonatale/atrésie
    Fibrose hépatique congénitale
    Situs inversus
    Polypose rectocolique
    Neurofibromatose
    Syndrome de Sotos

Erreurs du métabolisme

    Maladie de Byler
    Glycogénose de type 1
    Tyrosinémie
    Porphyrie
    Déficit en alpha-1-antitrypsine
    Hémochromatose

Autres facteurs

    Obstruction de la veine cave inférieure

---

la maladie est complexe, et sous le contrôle des gènes Pi (inhibiteurs des protéases); parmi ces gènes Pi le gène PiZ est le plus important par rapport à la maladie, en particulier quand l'individu est porteur homozygote du gène, c'est-à-dire porteur de PiZZ. Durant les années 1970, un certain nombre de rapports ont suggéré une incidence accrue de cancers primitifs du foie chez les sujets porteurs du gène PiZ et présentant des taux faibles d'alpha-1-antitrypsine (Eriksson & Hägerstrand, 1974). De plus, Palmer et Wolfe (1976) ont montré la présence de globules intracytoplasmiques positifs au PAS, constitués d'alpha-1-antitrypsine et semblables à ceux retrouvés dans les cellules hépatiques des individus atteints du déficit enzymatique dans un certain nombre de cancers primitifs du foie chez des patients qui ne possèdaient pas le gène PiZ et n'étaient pas déficitaires pour l'enzyme. On a suggéré que l'incapacité des cellules hépatiques des porteurs du gène PiZ, ou des cellules hépatiques cancéreuses des autres patients, à libérer l'alpha-1-antitrypsine dans la circulation avait un effet promoteur sur la croissance tumorale, en permettant la destruction, par toute variété de protéases, de l'inhibition de contact entre les cellules hépatiques transformées. Des études plus récentes ont tantôt confirmé et tantôt infirmé l'association du cancer primitif du foie avec le déficit en alpha-1-antitrypsine, et le problème est loin d'être résolu (Cohen et al., 1982).

L'hémochromatose primitive affecte surtout les sujets de sexe masculin, et est transmise de façon autosomique récessive; un cancer primitif du foie se développe dans jusqu'à 22% des cas (Purtilo & Gottlieb, 1973). Plus les patients vivent vieux, plus le risque est élevé. Le cancer ne se voit pas durant la phase pré-cirrhotique de la maladie et l'élimination du fer tissulaire excédentaire ne le prévient pas. Le cancer semble nettement lié au sexe masculin et à la cirrhose et non pas à l'accumulation de fer (MacSween, 1974). On ne pense plus à l'heure actuelle que l'incidence élevée du cancer primitif du foie chez les Bantous d'Afrique du Sud soit liée à l'hémosidérose, mais au virus HB et à l'aflatoxine.

Des rapports récents indiquent qu'une obstruction de la veine cave inférieure est présente dans une proportion importante (jusqu'à 20%) des cas de cancer primitif du foie en Afrique du Sud et que cette obstruction précède le développement de la tumeur; on a estimé à 47,5% le risque de tumeur maligne consécutif à l'obstruction du flux veineux hépatique (Simson, 1982). Des résultats similaires ont été rapportés au Japon, en Inde, et occasionnellement, dans d'autres parties du monde (Okuda, 1982). Deux types anatomiques d'occlusion ont été décrits: un type hautement membraneux, où la veine joint l'atrium droit, et une occlusion fibreuse, de longueur variable, se situant en dessous de ce niveau. Cette lésion est-elle congénitale ou acquise? La question est encore sujet à débat. Mais il est certain que la lésion est ancienne. L'obstruction chronique du flux veineux peut stimuler le processus de promotion, sans lequel les cellules initiées par différents agents ne peuvent pas progresser vers la malignité.

Alcool et nutrition

On retrouve fréquemment des antécédents d'alcoolisme chronique chez les sujets atteints de cancer primitif du foie, particulièrement dans les régions de faible incidence où l'infection HBV n'est pas fréquente. Dans la majorité des cas, il existe une cirrhose et le risque de transformation maligne est proportionnel à sa durée, et varie de 5 à 30%; le risque n'est pas réduit par le renoncement à cette habitude (Lee, 1966).

Plusieurs possibilités pathogéniques ont été avancées parmi lesquelles un effet mutagène de l'alcool et de ses métabolites, notamment de l'acétaldéhyde, une induction des enzymes hépatiques entraînant une altération de la biotransformation des produits chimiques potentiellement cancérogènes, et une promotion par la cirrhose. De plus, l'alcool et la malnutrition qui l'accompagne causent souvent tous les deux des altérations dans les mécanismes de défense immunitaire (Leevy et coll., 1976) qui peuvent rendre les individus plus sensibles à l'infection HBV chronique. Plusieurs rapports indiquent une incidence accrue des marqueurs du virus HB chez les alcooliques et, récemment, on a retrouvé l'ADN du virus HB intégré dans le génome de cellules tumorales de tous les 20 patients atteints de cirrhose alcoolique et de cancer primitif étudiés, bien que seulement 9 des 16 sujets testés aient présenté les marqueurs sériques de l'infection (Bréchot et coll., 1982).

La malnutrition est commune dans la plupart des régions où l'incidence de cancers primitifs du foie est élevée, et le faible apport protéique avec le déficit immunitaire qui lui est associé, les régimes pauvres en agents lipotropes, les carences en vitamines A, C et E et en sélénium peuvent tous jouer un rôle dans la genèse du cancer du foie (Kew et coll., 1982).

Parasites

On a suggéré que l'effet immunosuppresseur du paludisme chronique pourrait prédisposer à l'infection HBV et au cancer du foie, mais il y a peu de preuves concrètes pour confirmer cette hypothèse. Au Vietnam, Welsh et coll. (1976) n'ont pas trouvé de différence entre les sujets atteints de cancer primitif du foie et les témoins, au niveau des marqueurs sériques. L'infestation massive par Schistosoma mansoni et S. japonicum conduit à une fibrose hépatique mais cela n'entraîne pas le développement d'épithélioma en l'absence d'infection HBV.

Cancérogènes chimiques et d'origine naturelle

Le Tableau 3 montre les agents qui ont été le plus fréquemment examinés dans l'étiologie du cancer primitif du foie, mais on considère que peu d'entre eux représentent un risque sérieux pour l'homme (Okuda & MacKay, 1982). Les composés N-nitrosés sont des cancérogènes puissants chez les poissons, les rongeurs et les mammifères (Centre International de Recherche sur le Cancer, 1978). L'homme peut y être exposé de deux façons: par l'ingestion de composés pré-formés (présents en quantités minimes dans les aliments) ou à la suite de leur formation in vivo à partir d'amines secondaires et de nitrite. Les solvants représentent un risque mineur dans certaines professions, par exemple dans les blanchisseries et les pressings, aussi bien que dans l'industrie pétrochimique. Les colorants azoïques présentent surtout une importance historique, du fait que le "butter yellow" a été le premier agent a produire des tumeurs expérimentales du foie. Les pesticides organochlorés sont des promoteurs du cancer. Ce sont des composés largement utilisés et extrêmement stables; ils tendent à s'accumuler dans les réserves graisseuses des animaux et des humains. En Chine, on a observé que le cancer primitif du foie était associé à la consommation d'eau stagnante provenant de fossés et d'étangs, mais pas à la consommation d'eau provenant de puits profonds ou de cours d'eau courante (Delonq, 1979). Cela a été attribué à la contamination de l'eau par des pesticides, mais cela n'a pas été prouvé. Une situation analogue existe avec les polychlorobiphényls qui sont également largement utilisés et représentent un danger potentiel, mais aucune preuve de leur effet nocif chez l'homme n'a encore été produite.

Il a été prouvé que les alcaloïdes de la pyrrolizidine sont des hépatotoxines, et les quatre qui figurent au Tableau 3 ont la réputation de pouvoir induire des tumeurs du foie. L'empoisonnement aigu par des tisanes et des remèdes entraîne une insuffisance hépatique, tandis que leur ingestion chronique conduit à une maladie veino-occlusive qu'on voit à la Jamaique, en Inde et en Afghanistan. Les cycasines se trouvent dans des plantes apparentées aux palmiers, dont les graines et les racines sont consommées lors des sécheresses et des famines. Leur principe actif est le méthylazoxyméthanol, qui est semblable à la N-nitrosodiméthylamine. Heureusement, il est soluble dans l'eau, et il est normalement éliminé durant la préparation pour sa consommation. L'utilisation du safrole n'est plus autorisée et l'acide tannique a été remplacé depuis longtemps comme topique dans le traitement des brûlures.

Les mycotoxines, dont l'aflatoxine est de loin la plus importante, se situent seulement en seconde place derrière le virus HB dans la liste des facteurs de l'environnement qui sont fortement impliqués dans l'étiologie du cancer primitif du foie chez l'homme. L'aflatoxine est le métabolite de la moisissure Aspergillus flavus, qui se développe couramment dans la nourriture stockée de façon prolongée à la chaleur et à l'humidité. Elle existe sous plusieurs formes, dont la plus active est la forme B_1. La chimie, la toxicité et les preuves épidémiologiques ont été passées en revue de façon extensive (Wogan, 1976; US Department of Health, Education & Welfare, 1978; Munoz & Linsell, 1982). L'exposition alimentaire à l'aflatoxine B_1 coïncide avec l'incidence élevée de cancer primitif du foie dans de nombreuses régions d'Afrique et d'Asie du Sud-Est, et une série d'études sur le terrain a montré une relation étroite. L'aflatoxine B_1 a également été retrouvée dans le foie d'une proportion élevée de patients ayant un cancer primitif du foie mais pas chez les sujets témoins de la même région (Onyemelukwe et coll., 1980). Il a été suggéré que l'aflatoxine B et le virus HB pourraient agir de façon synergique. D'autres métabolites d'origine fongique, qui figurent au Tableau 3, ont une importance douteuse.

Médicaments

De nombreux médicaments (oxytétracycline, aminopyrine, tolazamide) contiennent des groupements aminés qui peuvent, du moins en théorie, subir une nitrosation dans l'organisme; mais on ne possède aucune preuve permettant de les rattacher aux tumeurs du foie chez l'homme. De même, s'il existe, l'éventuel pouvoir cancérogène expérimental du phénobarbital et des dérivés de l'hydantoïne n'a pas encore été démontré. Le thorotrast et l'arsenic induisent des angiosarcomes du foie et, rarement, des cholangioépithéliomas et des cancers primitifs du foie. Les médicaments les plus importants sont les stéroïdes gonadiques de synthèse alkylés en position 17, qui sont à la fois des androgènes/anabolisants et des contraceptifs oraux, dont les effets sur le foie comprennent l'induction de tumeurs (Tableau 4). Les preuves en ont été discutées de façon extensive par Klatskin (1977), Huggins et Giuntoli (1979), Rooks et coll. (1979), Mettlin et Natarajan (1981) et Ludwig (1983). La plupart des

Tableau 3. Cancérogènes chimiques et d'origine naturelle dans l'étiologie du cancer primitif du foie

---

Composés N-nitrosés

N-nitrosodiéthylamine
N-nitrosodiméthylamine
N-nitrosométhylurée

Solvants

Tétrachlorure de carbone
Trichloréthylène
Hydrocarbbures polycycliques

Pesticides organochlorés

DDT
Dieldrine
Chlordane

Alcaloïdes de la pyrrolizidine

Isatidine
Lasiocarpine
Monocrotaline
Rétrorsine

Mycotoxines

Aflatoxines
Stérigmatocystine
Lutéoskyrine
Cyclochorotine

Divers

Colorants azöques
Polychlorobiphényls
Safrole
Acide tannique

---

tumeurs induites par les composés à la fois androgènes et oestro-
gènes sont des adénomes du foie, et les épithéliomas sont rares
(Neuberger et coll., 1980); on sait que certains ont régressé
après l'arrêt du médicament. Une péliose a été observée seulement avec les stéroides androgènes/anabolisants. Le nombre de
cas est encore faible: on peut s'attendre à 3,4 cas pour 100 000
et par an aux Etats-Unis. La possibilité d'effet co-cancérogène
en association avec l'infection HBV ou avec l'aflatoxine est
source de réelles préoccupations pour l'avenir en Afrique et en
Asie du Sud-Est.

Le virus de l'hépatite B

Le rôle du virus HB dans la genèse du cancer primitif du
foie est un des principaux sujets de ce Symposium, et il convient
d'en donner ici seulement un bref aperçu (Tableau 5). Les
preuves du rôle étiologique du virus s'accumulent régulièrement,
mais elles sont encore incomplètes et il est possible que la
relation soit plus complexe qu'une simple relation de cause à
effet (Szmuness, 1978; Kew, 1981; Maupas & Melnick, 1981; Beasley
et coll., 1982; Okuda & MacKay, 1982; Munoz & Linsell, 1982;
Bassendine, 1983; Arthur et coll., 1984).

Il est à noter au passage que le virus de l'hépatite A n'est
en aucune façon lié au cancer primitif du foie, ni dans les zones
de haute incidence (Drucker et coll., 1979) ni dans celles de
faible incidence (Tabor et coll., 1980). Cela peut s'expliquer
par le fait que la cellule hépatique n'est pas permissive pour ce
virus, et meurt lorsqu'elle est infectée: des cellules mortes ne
peuvent pas donner naissance à un cancer. Comme on ne dispose
d'aucun marqueur diagnostic de l'hépatite non-A,non-B, on ne sait
pas si elle joue un rôle et lequel. On n'a pas encore étudié
convenablement la contribution que l'agent delta, découvert
récemment, pourrait apporter au développement de la maladie hépatique chronique et à la genèse de la tumeur.

Le taux de portage du virus HB et l'incidence des tumeurs se
superposent presque exactement partout dans le monde (Szmuness,
1978; Maupas & Melnick, 1981; Munoz & Linsell, 1982). Dans les
régions d'incidence élevée, la transmission est principalement
verticale, c'est-à-dire de la mère à l'enfant, à la naissance ou
peu après, tandis que dans les régions de faible incidence, elle
est horizontale, d'adulte à adulte. Cela explique en partie

Tableau 4. Effets secondaires au niveau du foie des stéroides
sexuels gonadiques

Stéroïde	Jaunisse	Péliose	Tumeurs du foie
Stéroïdes androgénes/anabolisants			
Méthyltestostérone	+	+	+
Oxyméthalone	+	+	+
Noréthandrolone	+	+	+
Fluoxymestérone	+		
Oestrogènes			
Ethynil oestradiol	+	−	+
Mestranol	+	−	+
Progestatifs			
Noréthistérone	±	−	?
Noréthynodrel	±	−	?

Tableau 5. Preuves du rôle étiologique du virus HB dans le
cancer primitif du foie

Taux de portage du virus HB correspondant à l'incidence de la
   tumeur
Solidité de la relation dans les études cas-témoins
Etudes prospectives
Risque de maladie maligne plus grand dans les cirrhoses causées
   par le virus HB
Dysplasie hépatique et HBV
Présence des antigènes du virus HB chez les patients cancéreux
Présence de l'ADN du virus HB intégré dans les cellules tumorales
Production de l'AgHBs par les cellules tumorales en culture
Virus semblable au virus HB chez les animaux et dans les tumeurs

pourquoi le pic d'âge se situe beaucoup plus tôt (20-40 ans) dans
les zones de haute incidence que dans les zones de faible incidence (40-60 ans).

Les études cas-contrôles, dont les premiers compte-rendus
venaient d'Ouganda (Vogel et coll., 1970) et de Taiwan (Tong et
coll., 1971) puis par la suite de toutes les parties du monde
(Szmuness, 1978; Maupas & Melnick, 1981; Bassendine, 1983) ont
montré une relation forte et sans équivoque entre la présence
d'une infection HBV et le cancer primitif du foie. C'est vrai
aussi bien dans les régions d'incidence élevée que dans les
régions de faible incidence. Les marqueurs les plus fréquemment
associés à la tumeur sont l'antigène de surface (AgHBs) et les
anticorps dirigés contre l'antigène central (anti-HBc).

Les études prospectives, publiées récemment, apportent
peut-être l'évidence la plus forte d'une association entre le
virus HB et le cancer primitif du foie; elles ont aussi permis
de définir la grandeur du risque, qui est terrifiante. Un total
de 22 707 Chinois de sexe masculin employés du Gouvernement à
Taiwan ont été suivis pendant une moyenne de 4,7 années par
individu. Ils avaient été choisis parce que l'on savait qu'il y
avait chez eux une proportion élevée de porteurs du virus HB et
que l'on connaissait leur fréquence de cancer primitif du foie,
et parce que, comme ils étaient tous assurés, on était sûr que
les causes de maladie et de décès seraient rapportées de façon
exacte. Des 89 cas de cancer primitif du foie, 86 sont survenus
chez des porteurs de l'AgHBs, et les 3 autres chez des sujets
possédant des anticorps anti-HBc, dont deux possédaient également
des anticorps anti-HBs. Aucun cas de cancer n'est survenu parmi
ceux qui n'avaient aucun des marqueurs du virus. Le risque
relatif de cancer primitif du foie chez les porteurs était de
223, ce qui est le plus élevé des facteurs de risque jamais enregistrés pour un cancer, et il dépasse de loin le risque relatif
de 20 pour le cancer du poumon chez les gros fumeurs, par exemple. Les porteurs présentaient également un risque relatif de 15
pour la cirrhose. Calculé sur la vie entière, ce risque de
mourir d'un cancer primitif du foie et/ou de cirrhose chez les
sujets infectés par le virus HB se situe entre 40 et 50% (Beasley
et coll., 1981, 1982). D'autres études menées au Japon et à
Hawai ont produit des résultats similaires.

On a montré à plusieurs reprises que <u>la cirrhose associée à l'infection HBV</u> comportait un plus grand risque de transformation maligne que la cirrhose sans HBV (Obata <u>et coll.</u>, 1980).

La dysplasie hépatocellulaire, dont on prétend qu'elle constitue un état précancéreux (Anthony <u>et coll.</u>, 1973), est associée à la cirrhose et au portage de l'AgHBs. Les résultats originaux de cette étude ont été confirmés en Thailande, au Japon, et à Hong-Kong, mais ont été discutés ou réfutés par d'autres au Japon et en Afrique du Sud.

Les <u>antigènes du virus HB</u> ont été retrouvés avec consistance dans les parties non-tumorales du foie de patients atteints de cancer primitif du foie (Okuda & MacKay, 1982), mais avec difficulté ou pas du tout dans la tumeur elle-même. Il semble que la réplication virale devienne de plus en plus défective durant la transformation néoplasique, avec dans la plupart des cas, la perte dans l'ordre chronologique de l'antigène e du virus HB (AgHBe) puis de l'AgHBs et enfin de l'AgHBc.

On a retrouvé l'<u>ADN du virus HB</u> intégré dans le génome des cellules hépatiques tumorales dans presque tous les cas étudiés jusqu'ici, même en l'absence de marqueurs sériques, et chez des patients souffrant apparemment d'une cirrhose alcoolique (Shafritz & Kew, 1981; Shafritz <u>et coll.</u>, 1981; Bréchot <u>et coll.</u>, 1982). Ces résultats ont été confirmés en Afrique, en Chine et en Grèce. On observe des variations portant sur des détails et aucun oncogène HBV n'a encore été mis en évidence, mais l'intégration précède le développement de la tumeur. On a également suggéré un effet co-cancérogène avec l'aflatoxine.

On a montré que <u>les cellules de cancer primitif du foie en culture</u> produisent l'AgHBs, mais aucun autre antigène, et beaucoup moins le virus entier (Alexander <u>et coll.</u>, 1982); ceci correspond à l'observation <u>in vivo</u> d'une réplication de plus en plus défective dans le tissu de cancer primitif du foie.

<u>Des virus semblables au virus HB</u> ont été retrouvés chez des canards, des écureuils et des marmottes; seules ces dernières développent des cancers primitifs du foie, et la tumeur diffère quelque peu de celle que l'on voit chez l'homme (Popper <u>et coll.</u>, 1981).

En résumé, presque tous les critères à remplir pour établir un rôle étiologique d'un virus dans l'oncogenèse ont maintenant été retrouvés, sauf deux: le virus HB n'a pas encore produit de cancer primitif du foie chez les primates, tels que les chimpanzés, à qui il est transmissible, et il reste à constater l'effet de la vaccination préventive sur l'incidence des tumeurs.

PATHOGENESE DU CANCER PRIMITIF DU FOIE

Cancérogenèse chimique

Les effets cancérogènes de centaines de composés chimiques ont été étudiés, principalement chez le rat, et des informations très détaillées sur les étapes probablement impliquées dans la transformation néoplasique sont maintenant disponibles. Elles sont exposées dans le Tableau 6. Des détails et des références complémentaires ayant trait à la littérature abondante sur le sujet peuvent être trouvés dans de nombreux articles de synthèse et livres (Cancer Research, 1976; Remmer et coll., 1978; Lapis & Johannessen, 1979; Farber, 1981; Okuda & MacKay, 1982; Pitot, 1982).

La plupart des produits chimiques sont inertes en eux-mêmes et doivent subir une conversion métabolique par le système d'oxygénase à fonction mixte, situé dans le réticulum endoplasmique, pour produire des époxydes hautement réactifs qui endommagent l'ADN, les organelles et les membranes. L'anomalie est "fixée" par un cycle de réplication cellulaire et la cellule est alors "initiée". De telles cellules n'ont pas d'autonomie et reviennent la plupart du temps à la normale, à moins qu'elles ne soient en plus "promues" par le même agent ou par d'autres. Comme la plupart des composés cancérogènes sont cytotoxiques, les cellules normales sont inhibées et les cellules anormales sont sélectionnées en nombres croissants. Les modifications enzymatiques observées consistent principalement en une perte des enzymes de la cellule adulte normale (ATPase, G6Pase, beta-glycuronidase) et en une augmentation des marqueurs foetaux (gamma-glutamyl transpeptidase, alpha-foetoprotéine, gonadotrophine beta-chorionique). Des nodules hyperplasiques apparaissent, qui sont souvent étonnamment basophiles. Ces derniers deviennent autonomes et il en résulte éventuellement une tumeur maligne patente avec des métastases et entraînant la mort de l'animal. Une situation de régénération cellulaire augmentée, par exemple une hépatectomie partielle ou la présence d'une cirrhose, accélère le cours des évènements.

Tableau 6. Etapes probables de la transformation néoplasique par des agents chimiques

Etape	Effets associés
Initiation	Conversion métabolique du carcinogène proximal en carcinogène ultime Altération de l'ADN, des organelles et des membranes Fixation de l'anomalie par la prolifération cellulaire
Promotion	Inhibition - sélection Modifications enzymatiques Nodules hyperplasiques Nodules néoplasiques autonomes
Comportement malin (patent)	Métastases et mort

Un phénomène particulier est la prolifération de "cellules ovales" ou cellules souches, que l'on n' observe pas chez l'homme; les tumeurs expérimentales sont souvent différentes de celles qui surviennent spontanément chez les humains; souvent on induit des épithéliomas du foie à cellules mixtes et des épithéliomas du canal cholédoque.

Oncogenèse virale

Les virus produisant des tumeurs expérimentales sont soit des virus à ADN, soit des virus à ARN. Ces derniers sont également connus sous le nom de rétrovirus, parce que leur ARN doit être transcrit pour ainsi dire en marche arrière, en une copie ADN par l'enzyme transcriptase réverse avant que la replication puisse avoir lieu (Fig. 1). La plupart des tumeurs induites par des virus chez les animaux sont des lymphomes, des leucémies et des sarcomes des tissus mous; les épithéliomas sont rares. La

persistance du génome viral dans la cellule-hôte est essentielle
pour la transformation néoplasique (Wyke, 1981; Essex &
Gutensohn, 1981; Enrietto & Wyke, 1983).

FIG. 1. TRANSCRIPTION DES ACIES NUCLEIQUES VIRAUX
DANS LE GENOME DE LA CELLULE-HOTE

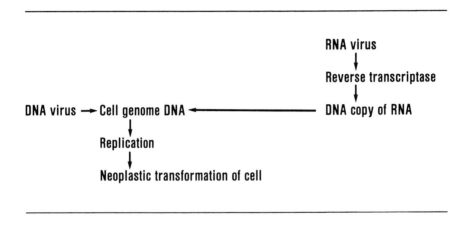

Oncogènes

La découverte de séquences d'ADN spécifiques associées au
cancer a suscité un intérêt considérable ces dernières années
(Hamlyn & Sikora, 1983; Robertson, 1983). Décrits à l'origine
dans les virus (v-onc), les oncogènes ont été par la suite
retrouvés dans les tumeurs expérimentales de l'animal et, dans
certains cas, dans les tumeurs spontanées de l'homme (c-onc).
Beaucoup ont été purifiés, séquencés et clonés et peuvent être
étudiés facilement par des essais de transfection utilisant des
cultures de lignées cellulaires appropriées, telles que celle qui
est dérivée des fibroblastes de souris NIH 3T3. Les oncogènes
sont répandus chez tous les vertébrés, et les virus les emportent
lors de leur passage dans les cellules. Normalement, ils sont
présents en petites quantités, et ils jouent probablement un rôle
physiologique dans le contrôle de la croissance. Ils codent pour
des phosphoprotéines à activité protéine kinase, et produisent
des molécules semblables aux facteurs de croissance ou à leurs
récepteurs. S'ils sont déplacés, altérés ou surexprimés, il peut

en résulter une prolifération cellulaire incontrôlée. On commence juste à étudier le rôle des oncogènes dans la régénération et la cancérogenèse du foie (Fausto & Shank, 1983). Pour l'instant, on n'a pas identifié d'oncogène dans le virus HB, mais on sait que le virus, ou une partie du virus, est intégré dans les cellules hépatiques durant l'infection et la cancérogenèse, et il pourrait agir en "activant" un oncogène cellulaire, phénomène qu'on appelle souvent "l'insertion promotrice". Un virus, ou plusieurs virus et/ou des cancérogènes chimiques pourraient agir ensemble par l'intermédiaire des oncogènes. Cela est maintenant à l'étude, et l'on pourrait bientôt voir apparaître une explication unifiée et cohérente des théories apparemment disparates de la cancérogenèse qui ont été basées sur des observations épidémiologiques, expérimentales, chimiques et virologiques.

Modifications précancéreuses dans le foie humain

La cirrhose elle-même est un état précancéreux: elle persiste généralement longtemps, elle est macronodulaire, et associée à la présence du virus HB. On a observé de rares nodules hyperplasiques ou autonomes (Tezuka & Sawai, 1983) et on a rapporté de rares cas de modifications enzymatiques, semblables à celles observées au cours de la cancérogenèse chimique expérimentale (Uchida et coll., 1981). On a suggéré que la dysplasie des cellules hépatiques était un état précancéreux (Anthony et coll., 1973), mais cela a été à la fois confirmé et démenti depuis.

PATHOLOGIE DU CANCER PRIMITIF DU FOIE

Les aspects macroscopiques, le mode de dissémination et l'évolution naturelle du cancer primitif du foie sont maintenant bien connus. Le Tableau 7 résume les données sur le diagnostic de laboratoire, les syndromes paranéoplasiques et les marqueurs tumoraux. Les aspects histologiques ont été passés en revue par un groupe international réuni par l'Organisation Mondiale de la Santé en 1978: on est parvenu à une définition claire, qui était bien nécessaire, des différents types de tumeurs qui peuvent survenir dans le foie, définition essentielle pour la recherche épidémiologique, clinique et fondamentale (Organisation Mondiale de la Santé, 1978). La classification de l'OMS est toujours valable, mais quelques modifications sont devenues nécessaires, principalement en ce qui concerne la reconnaissance progressive de ce qu'on appelle les types à bon prognostic.

Tableau 7. Diagnostic de laboratoire, manifestations paranéoplasiques et marqueurs tumoraux du cancer primitif du foie

---

Diagnostic de laboratoire:

Phosphatases alcalines ⬆
Gamma-glutamyl transpeptidase ⬆
Alpha-foetoprotéine > 1000 ng/ml

Syndromes paranéoplasiques et marqueurs tumoraux

Hypoglycémie
Hypercalcémie
Erythrocytose
Dysfibrinogénémie
Protéine liant la vitamine B12
Hypercholestérolémie
Gonadotrophine chorionique humaine
Proline hydroxylase
Porphyrie cutanée tardive
Ostéoarthropathie pulmonaire hypertrophique

La principale contribution du groupe OMS a été la séparation claire du cancer primitif du foie et de l'épithélioma cholangiocellulaire et la recommandation que tous les sous-types histologiques du cancer primitif du foie (trabéculaire, pseudoglandulaire, compact, squirrheux, pléomorphe, à cellules claires) soient considérés comme des variants morphologiques d'une seule et unique maladie. Il faut reconnaître maintenant qu'il existe en fait des exceptions à cette règle.

On a largement affirmé que les épithéliomas à cellules claires ont un meilleur pronostic que la moyenne de tous les autres sous-types (Lai et coll., 1979).

Le nom d'épithélioma fibrolamellaire est maintenant admis pour le variant qui avait été décrit auparavant comme compact ou squirrheux. C'est une tumeur que l'on rencontre chez les adolescents et les jeunes adultes des deux sexes; elle est communément associée à une hypercalcémie et/ou à des taux élevés de la protéine qui fixe la vitamine B12 et comporte un bon pronostic

(Berman et coll., 1980; Craig et coll., 1980). Le taux de croissance faible permet la résection chirurgicale d'une masse généralement isolée. Il n'est pas encore certain à l'heure actuelle que cette tumeur soit véritablement d'origine hépato-cellulaire et il se peut qu'elle dérive d'une cellule endocrine du foie.

Le cancer primitif du foie encapsulé ou à minima a été décrit à l'origine au Japon (Okuda et coll., 1977), mais il se rencontre aussi dans certaines régions d'Asie du Sud-Est. Il est souvent petit, généralement moins de 5,0 cm, et il est entouré d'une capsule fibreuse qui semble le contenir. On peut le détecter par différentes méthodes d'imagerie, et par le dosage de l'alpha-foetoprotéine dans le sang. Un taux important de guérisons a été obtenu par résection chirurgicale.

D'autres observations morphologiques qui restaient encore inexpliquées en 1978 ont maintenant été mieux étudiées. La présence de corps de Mallory dans les cellules tumorales de patients non-alcooliques a été confirmée: elle résulte probablement d'une perturbation du métabolisme des filaments intermédiaires. L'hétérogénéité de ce qu'on appelle les corps globuleux hyalins a été démontrée par immuno-histologie: ils peuvent représenter de l'albumine, de l'alpha-1-antitrypsine, de l'alpha-foetoprotéine, de l'antigène carcino-embryonnaire, de la gonadotrophine chorionique humaine, de l'isoferritine, etc.

Finalement, on a observé la régression spontanée de quelques cas bien définis de cancers primitifs du foie (Gottfried et coll., 1982), sans que l'on ait pu en déceler la raison.

CONCLUSIONS

Il est difficile de présenter en quelques pages, même sous forme de résumé, l'énorme masse de connaissances qui a émergé durant ces 10 dernières années dans le domaine du cancer primitif du foie. Beaucoup de questions restent encore sans réponse, mais les perspectives sont prometteuses. Ce fléau mortel et sans merci qui frappe les pays en voie de développement va pouvoir être éliminé, ou du moins son incidence va pouvoir être réduite de notre vivant. S'il en est ainsi, cela représentera un succès presque sans parallèle, et auquel les scientifiques Africains auront contribué de façon unique et éclatante.

REFERENCES

Alexander, J.J., Van der Merwe, C.F., Saunders, R.M., McElligott, S.E. & Desmyter, J. (1982) A comparison between in vitro experiments with a hepatoma cell line and in vivo studies. Hepatology, 2, 92-96

Anthony, P.P., Vogel, C.L. & Barker, L.F. (1973) Liver cell dysplasia: a premalignant condition. J. clin. Pathol., 26, 217-223

Arthur, M.J.P., Hall, A.J. & Wright, R. (1984) Hepatitis B, hepatocellular carcinoma and strategies for prevention. Lancet, 1, 607-610

Bassendine, M.F. (1983) Hepatitis B virus and liver cell carcinoma. Recent Adv. Histopathol., 12, 137-146

Beasley, R.P., Hwang, L.Y., Lin, C.C. & Chien, C.S. (1981) Hepatocellular carcinoma and hepatitis B virus. A prospective study of 22707 men in Taiwan. Lancet, 2, 1129-1133

Beasley, R.P., Blumberg, B., Popper, H. & Wain-Hobson, S. (1982) Hepatitis B virus and hepatocellular carcinoma. In: Okuda, K. & MacKay, I., eds, Hepatocellular carcinoma (UICC Technical Report Series, Vol. 74, No. 17), Geneva, UICC, pp. 60-93

Berman, M.M., Libbey, N.P. & Foster, J.H. (1980) Hepatocellular carcinoma polygonal cell type with fibrous stroma - an atypical variant with a favorable prognosis. Cancer, 46, 1448-1455

Bréchot, C., Nalpas, B., Courroucé, A.-M., Duhamel, G., Gallard, P., Carnot, F., Tiollais, P. & Berthelot, P. (1982) Evidence that hepatitis B virus has a role in liver-cell carcinoma in alcoholic liver disease. New Engl. J. Med., 306, 1384-1387

Cameron, H.M., Linsell, D.A. & Warwick, G.P., eds (1976) Liver Cell Cancer, Amsterdam, Elsevier

Cancer Research (1976) Symposium: early lesions and the development of epithelial cancer. Cancer Res., 36, 2475-2706

Centre International de Recherche sur le Cancer (1978) IARC Monographs on the Evaluation of the Carcinogenic Risk of Chemicals to Humans, Vol. 17, Some N-Nitroso Compounds, Lyon

Cohen, C., Berson, S.D. & Budgeon, R.B. (1982) Alpha-1-antitrypsin deficiency in Southern African hepatocellular carcinoma patients, an immunoperoxidase and histochemical study. Cancer, 49, 2537-2540

Craig, J.R., Peters, R.L., Edmondson, H.A. & Omata, M. (1980) Fibrolamellar carcinoma of the liver: a tumour of adolescents and young adults with distinctive clinicopathologic features. Cancer, 46, 372-379

Delong, S. (1979) Drinking water and liver cell cancer. Chin. med. J., 92, 748-756

Drucker, J.A., Coursaget, P., Maupas, P., Goudeau, A., Gerety, R.J., Chiron, J.P., Denis, F. & Diop-Mar I. (1979) Hepatitis A infection and primary hepatocellular carcinoma. Biomedicine, 31, 23-25

Enrietto, P.J. & Wyke, J.A. (1983) The pathogenesis of oncogenic avian retroviruses. Adv. Cancer Res., 39, 269-284

Eriksson, S. & Hägerstrand, I. (1974) Cirrhosis and malignant hepatoma in alpha-1-antitrypsin deficiency. Acta Med. Scand., 195, 451-458

Essex, M. & Gutenssohn, N. (1981) A comparison of the pathobiology and epidemiology of cancers associated with viruses in humans and animals. Prog. med. Virol., 27, 114-126

Farber, E. (1981) Chemical carcinogenesis. New Engl. J. Med., 305, 1379-1389

Fausto, N. & Shank, P.R. (1983) Oncogene expression in liver regeneration and hepatocarcinogenesis. Hepatology, 3, 1016-1023

Gottfried, E.B., Steller, R., Paronetto, F. & Lieber, C.S. (1982) Spontaneous regression of hepatocellular carcinoma. Gastroenterology, 82, 770-774

Hamlyn, P. & Sikora, K. (1983) Oncogenes. Lancet, ii, 326-330

Huggins, G.R. & Giuntoli, R.L. (1979) Oral contraceptives and neoplasia. Fertil. Steril., 32, 1-23

Kew, M.C. (1981) Clinical, pathologic and etiologic heterogeneity in hepatocellular carcinoma: evidence from Southern Africa. Hepatology, 1, 366-369

Kew, M.C., Newberne, P.M. & Popper, H. (1982) Other aetiological processes in hepatocellular carcinoma. In: Okuda, K. & MacKay, I., eds, Hepatocellular Carcinoma (UICC Technical Report Series, Vol. 74, Report No. 17), Geneva, UICC, pp. 110-116

Kew, M.C., Rossouw, E., Paterson, A., Hodkinson, J., Whitcutt, M. & Dusheiko, G. (1983) Hepatitis B virus status of black women with hepatocellular carcinoma. Gastroenterology, 84, 693-696

Klatskin, G. (1977) Hepatic tumours: possible relationship to use of oral contraceptives. Gastroenterology, 73, 386-394

Lai, C.L., Wu, P.C., Lam, K.C. & Todd, D. (1979) Histologic prognostic indicators in hepatocellular carcinoma. Cancer, 44, 1677-1683

Lapis, K. & Johannessen, J.V., eds (1979) Liver Carcinogenesis, Washington, DC, Hemisphere Publishing Co.

Lee, F.I. (1966) Cirrhosis and hepatoma in alcoholics. Gut, 7, 77-85

Leevy, C.M., Chen, T., Luisada-Opper, A., Kanagasundarum, V. & Zetterman, R. (1976) Liver disease of the alcoholic: role of immunologic abnormalities in pathogenesis, recognition and treatment. Prog. Liver Dis., 5, 516-530

Ludwig, J. (1983) Drug effects on the liver. A tabular compilation of drugs and drug-related hepatic diseases. Dig. Dis. Sci., 24, 785-796

MacSween, R.N.M. (1974) A clinico-pathological review of 100 cases of primary malignant tumours of the liver. J. clin. pathol., 27, 669-682

Maupas, P. & Melnick, J.L. (1981) Hepatitis B infection and primary liver cancer. Prog. med. Virol., 27, 1-5

Mettlin, C. & Natarajan, N. (1981) Studies on the role of oral contraceptive use in the etiology of benign and malignant liver tumours. J. surg. Oncol., 18, 73-85

Munoz, N. & Linsell, A. (1982) Epidemiology of primary liver cancer. In: Correa, P. & Haenszel, W., eds, Epidemiology of Cancer of the Digestive Tract, The Hague, Nijhoff, pp. 161-195

Neuberger, J., Portmann, B., Nunnerley, H.B., Laws, J.W., Davis, M. & Williams, R. (1980) Oral contraceptive associated liver tumours: occurrence of malignancy and difficulties in diagnosis. Lancet, 1, 273-276

Obata, H., Hayashi, N., Motoike, Y., Hisamitsu, T., Okuda, H., Kobayashi, S. & Nishioka, K. (1980) A prospective study on the development of hepatocellular carcinoma from liver cirrhosis with persistent hepatitis B virus infection. Int. J. Cancer, 25, 741-747

Okuda, K. (1982) Membraneous obstruction of the inferior vena cava: etiology and relation to hepatocellular carcinoma. Gastroenterology, 82, 376-379

Okuda, K. & Peters, R.L., eds (1976) Hepatocellular carcinoma, New York, Wiley

Okuda, K. & MacKay, I. (1982) Hepatocellular Carcinoma (UICC Technical Report Series, Vol. 74, Report No. 17), Geneva, UICC

Okuda, K., Musha, H., Nakajima, Y., Kubo, Y., Shimokawa, Y., Nagasaki, Y., Sawe, Y., Jinnouchi, S., Kaneko, T., Obata, H., Hisamitsu, T., Motoike, Y., Okasaki, N., Kajiro, M., Sakamoto, K. & Nakashima, T. (1977) Clinicopathologic features of encapsulated hepatocellular carcinoma. A study of 26 cases. Cancer, 40, 1240-1245

Onyemelukwe, C.G., Nirodi, C. & West, C.E. (1980) Aflatoxin B_1 in hepatocellular carcinoma. Trop. geog. Med., 32, 237-242

Organisation Mondiale de la Santé (1978) types histologiques des tumeurs du foie, des voies biliaires et du pancréas (Classification Histologique Internationale des Tumeurs No. 20), Genève

Palmer, P.E. & Wolfe, H.J. (1976) Alpha-1-antitrypsin deposition in primary hepatic carcinomas. Arch. Pathol. lab. Med., 100, 232-236

Pitot, H.C. (1982) The natural history of neoplastic development: the relation of experimental models to human cancer. Cancer, 49, 1296-1304

Popper, H., Shih, J.W.K., Gerin, J.L., Wong, D.C., Hoyer, B.H., London, W.T., Sly, D.L. & Purcell, R.H. (1981) Woodchuck hepatitis and hepatocellular carcinoma: correlation of histologic with virologic observations. Hepatology, 2, 91-98

Purtilo, D.T. & Gottlieb, L.S. (1973) Cirrhosis and hepatoma occurring at Boston City Hospital (1917-1968) Cancer, 32, 458-462

Remmer, H., Bolt, H.M., Bannasch, P. & Popper, H., eds (1978) Primary Liver Tumours, Lancaster, MTP Press

Robertson, M. (1983) Oncogenes and multistep carcinogenesis. Br. med. J., 287, 1084-1086

Rooks, J.B., Ory, H.W., Ishak, K.G., Strauss, L.T., Greenspan, J.R., Hill, A.P. & Tyler, C.W. Jr (1979) Epidemiology of hepatocellular adenoma. The role of oral contraceptive use. J. Am. med. Assoc., 242, 644-648

Saracci, R. & Repetto, F. (1980) Time trends of primary liver cancer: indication of increased incidence in selected cancer registry populations. J. natl Cancer Inst., 65, 241-247

Shafritz, D.A. & Kew, M.C. (1981) Identification of integrated hepatitis B virus sequences in human hepatocellular carcinoma. Hepatology, 1, 1-8

Shafritz, D.A., Shouval, D., Sherman, H.I., Hadziyannis, S.J. & Kew, M.C. (1981) Integration of hepatitis B virus DNA into the genome of liver cells in chronic liver disease and hepatocellular carcinoma: Studies in percutaneous liver biopsies and post-mortem tissue specimens. New Engl. J. Med., 305, 1067-1073

Sharp, H.L. (1982) Alpha-1-antitrypsin: an ignored protein in understanding liver disease. Sem. Liver Dis., 2, 314-328

Simson, I.W. (1982) Membraneous obstruction of the inferior vena cava and hepatocellular carcinoma in South Africa. Gastroenterology, 82, 171-178

Szmuness, W. (1978) Hepatocellular carcinoma and the hepatitis B virus: evidence for a causal association. Prog. med. Virol., 24, 40-69

Tabor, E., Trichopoulos, D., Manousos, D., Zavitsanos, X., Drucker, J.A. & Gerety, R.J. (1980) Absence of an association between past infection with hepatitis A virus and hepatocellular carcinoma. Int. J. Epidemiol., 9, 221-223

Tezuka, F. & Sawai, T. (1983) Hyperplasia of small hepatic cells in the precancerous condition of cirrhotic livers. Tokohu J. exp. Med., 139, 171-177

Tong, M.J., Sun, S.-C., Schaeffer, B.T., Chang, N.-K., Lo, K.-J. & Peters, R.L. (1971) Hepatitis-associated antigen and hepatocellular carcinoma in Taiwan. Ann. intern. Med., 75, 687-691

Tong, M.J., Weiner, J.M., Ashcavai, M.W. & Vyas, G.N. (1979)
    Evidence for clustering of hepatitis B virus infection in
    families of patients with primary hepatocellular carcinoma.
    Cancer, 44, 2338-2342

Uchida, T., Miyata, H. & Shikata, T. (1981) Human hepatocellular
    carcinoma and putative precancerous disorders. Arch. Pathol.
    lab. Med., 105, 180-186

US Department of Health, Education, and Welfare (1978) Oncology
    Overview. Selected Abstracts on Aflatoxin and Other Myco-
    toxin Carcinogenesis, Springfield, National Technical
    Information Service, International Cancer Research Data Bank

Vogel, C.L., Anthony, P.P., Mody, N. & Barker, L.F. (1970) Hepa-
    titis-associated antigen in Ugandan patients with hepato-
    cellular carcinoma. Lancet, 2, 621-624

Waterhouse, J., Muir, C., Shanmugaratnam, K. & Powell, J. (1982)
    Cancer Incidence in Five Continents, Vol. IV, Lyon, Inter-
    national Agency for Research on Cancer

Weinberg, A.G. & Finegold, M.J. (1983) Primary hepatic tumours
    of childhood. Hum. Pathology, 14, 512-537

Welsh, J.D., Brown, J.D., Arnold, K., Matthews, H.M. & Prince,
    A.M. (1976) Hepatitis B surface antigen, malaria titres and
    primary liver cancer in South Vietnam. Gastroenterology,
    70, 392-396

Wogan, G.N. (1976) Aflatoxins and their relationship to hepato-
    cellular carcinoma. In: Okuda, K. & Peters, R.L., eds,
    Hepatocellular Carcinoma, New York, Wiley, pp. 25-41

Wyke, J.A. (1981) Oncogenic viruses. J. Pathol., 135, 39-85

LIVER CARCINOGENESIS IN TROPICAL AFRICA

A.O. Uwaifo & E.A. Bababunmi

Department of Biochemistry
University of Ibadan
Ibadan, Nigeria

RESUME

La pathologie géographique du cancer primitif du foie (CPF) a été essentiellement anecdotique jusqu'à ce que l'on introduise l'enregistrement systématique des cas de cancer; mais il est maintenant clair que l'Afrique sub-saharienne est une région de haute incidence. L'étiologie de la maladie est multifactorielle. Les agents étiologiques possibles comprennent le virus de l'hépatite B et un certain nombre de cancérogènes chimiques, parmi lesquels les aflatoxines et les composés N-nitrosés apparaissent comme les plus importants. Les plantes et les infusions médicinales utilisées dans les tropiques contiennent également des composés tels que les furocoumarines qui sont mutagènes et/ou cancérogènes.

Une forme modifiée du test Salmonella typhimurium de Ames a été utilisée pour étudier la mutagénicité des aflatoxines B_1 et M_1 et de la palmotoxine B_0, co-métabolite de l'aflatoxine B_1, et pour étudier également la mutagénicité de la chamuvaritine et de la chamuvarine, qui sont toutes deux des benzodihydrochalcones issues des racines de Uvaria chamae, utilisées à des fins médicinales en Afrique de l'Ouest. Le même test a été utilisé pour étudier la mutagénicité d'un certain nombre de furocoumarines isolées à partir de plantes médicinales nigérianes. Ces composés ont également été testés avec et sans photoactivation dans des cellules V79 de Hamster Chinois et des cellules C3H 10T1/2. Des tests de transformation cellulaire ont aussi été réalisés avec ces mêmes composés et avec le 8-méthoxypsoralène.

SUMMARY

The geographical pathology of hepatocellular carcinoma (HCC)
was essentially anecdotal until systematic cancer registration
was introduced, but it is now clear that sub-Saharan Africa is a
high-incidence area. The disease is multifactorial in etiology,
the possible etiological agents including hepatitis B virus and a
number of chemical carcinogens, among which the most important
appear to be the aflatoxins and N-nitroso compounds. Medicinal
plants and herbal teas used in the tropics also contain compounds
such as furocoumarins that are mutagenic and/or carcinogenic.

A modified form of the Ames Salmonella typhimurium assay was
used to study the mutagenicity of aflatoxins B_1 and M_1 and palmotoxin B_0, a co-metabolite of aflatoxin B_1, and also of chamuvaritin and chamuvarin, two benzyldihydrochalcones derived from the
roots of Uvaria chamae, which are used for medicinal purposes in
West Africa. The mutagenicity of a number of furocoumarins
isolated from Nigerian medicinal plants was studied by means of
the same assay as well as with Chinese hamster V79 cells and C3H
10T1/2 cells; in the last two systems the studies were carried
out both with and without photoactivation. The same compounds,
and 8-methoxypsoralen, were also investigated by means of cell
transformation studies.

GEOGRAPHICAL PATHOLOGY OF LIVER CANCER

The geographical pathology of liver cancer, like that of
many other types of cancer, was essentially anecdotal until
systematic population-based cancer registration was introduced.
Present-day knowledge of the incidence and geographical spread of
liver cancer is based on data or incidence rates gathered from
cancer registries located in both developed and developing
countries of the world. Although data obtained from outside
major capital cities in Africa are based on proportional rates,
which are subject to a multitude of biases in the selection of
material, the picture of incidence and geographical spread that
has emerged from data obtained from these registries is fairly
accurate.

It is now very clear that sub-Saharan Africa and some Asian countries, such as China, Malaysia, Indonesia, the Philippines and Singapore, are high-incidence areas. Incidence among the indigenous peoples of sub-Saharan Africa varies markedly from country to country in that vast area, generally decreasing as one proceeds northwards. For instance, whereas the age-adjusted incidence rate for males in Mozambique, as reported by Prates (1961) and more recently by Purchase and Goncalves (1971) and Van Rensburg et al. (1974), is about 100 per 100 000, it is much lower in North African countries such as Morocco, Egypt and the Sudan (Oettle, 1964). In South-east Asia, a high frequency of this cancer has been reported among the Chinese not only in China itself but also in Singapore (Shanmugaratnam, 1961), Malaysia (Marsden, 1958), Indonesia (Kouwenaar, 1951) and the Philippines (Vedder, 1927). This high frequency is also found in Chinese communities living in Vancouver, Canada (Strong et al., 1949), San Francisco, USA (Wilbur et al., 1944) and New York (Gustafson, 1937). These reports on overseas Chinese communities seem to suggest an ethnic predisposition for this form of cancer, but this is not supported by reports on incidence in other ethnic communities of African, Asian or Japanese descent who migrated to low-incidence countries (Kennaway, 1944; Shanmugaratnam, 1961). These immigrant communities have tended to acquire the incidence pattern of their adopted countries. On the other hand, Europeans who migrate from low-incidence to high-incidence areas such as Africa have tended to retain their low rates (Higginson, 1963). A plausible explanation for this difference is that, while Europeans have usually managed to take most of their European environment with them to their new homes, the African and Asian communities have usually adopted the totally different life-styles peculiar to their adopted countries. The Chinese, however, like the Europeans, tend to take with them their own particular life-style to the country to which they have migrated. This explains the retention of a high incidence of the disease among Chinese communities in different countries of the world.

It is now also equally clear that areas of relatively low incidence are located in the Indian subcontinent (Gharpure, 1948; Mahju, 1958; Reddy & Rao, 1962; Sudarsanam et al., 1963; Jussawalla et al., 1968), Latin America (Higginson, 1970), North America (Dorn & Cutler, 1959; Griswold et al., 1955) and Europe (Clemmesen, 1965; Doll et al., 1970; Tuyns & Obradovic, 1975; Trichopoulos et al., 1975). The Middle East is also a low-incidence area (Steinitz, 1965; Habibi, 1965). Fortunately, the data from cancer registries in low-incidence countries are

accurate and based mainly on incidence rates, and therefore free
of the biases associated with proportional rates.

POSSIBLE ETIOLOGICAL AGENTS

The picture of hepatocellular carcinoma (HCC) that is beginning to emerge from the study of the epidemiology of this cancer
is that it is multifactorial in etiology. From data on the
incidence of HCC in sub-Saharan Africa and the tendency of immigrant African and Japanese communities to assume the incidence
rate of their new country or area of abode and the retention by
Europeans of their low incidence rates in high-incidence areas
such as Africa, it is apparent that environmental factors
peculiar to the indigenous, non-urbanized, non-industrialized
habitat of the high-incidence countries are responsible for this
high incidence. The environmental factors identified as relevant
to the geographical distribution of this liver disease include
biological factors, such as cirrhosis of the liver, viral hepatitis, malnutrition, parasitic infections, and chemical factors
such as aflatoxin B_1 and other mycotoxins, toxic substances in
plants used as foodstuffs and medicine, N-nitroso compounds and
pesticides. A few of the factors in the above list have been
identified as definite etiological agents in studies in different
laboratories, including viral agents, such as hepatitis B virus
(HBV), aflatoxin B_1 and other mycotoxins, and N-nitroso
compounds, while the others are chemical agents which are mutagenic and/or carcinogenic but have not been directly implicated
in the etiology of this type of cancer.

HEPATITIS B VIRUS

Since the initial observation in the 1950s by workers in
West and East Africa that HCC was usually preceded by viral
hepatitis, a large body of evidence has been accumulated from
numerous field and laboratory studies in many countries to
support a positive correlation between infection by HBV and HCC
(Beasley & Linn, 1978; Obata et al., 1980; Bréchot et al., 1980;
Blumberg & London, 1980). The evidence which strongly supports
the hypothesis that persistent infection with HBV is necessary
for the development of HCC has been recently reviewed by London
(1983) and is further reviewed and referenced by many speakers at
this Symposium.

The existence of HCC associated with a virus similar to HBV in the woodchuck (Marmota monax) also supports the hypothesis that HBV infection preceds HCC (Summers et al., 1978; Snyder et al., 1982). It is not clear at present, however, how the role of HBV is related to that of other etiological factors. There are also many unanswered questions as to HBV's specific role in the initiation, promotion, progression and expression of HCC.

CHEMICAL CARCINOGENS

The number of possible carcinogens that might contribute to the total carcinogenic burden for the liver is potentially very large. In many instances these chemicals or their precursors, as in the case of the nitrosamines, are widely distributed in the environment so that possibilities of exposure, which is usually of a long-term low-level pattern, are wide-spread. The exposure pattern makes it particularly difficult, however, to establish with certainty a cause-and-effect relationship for individual chemicals. The situation is further complicated by the long latency period and low frequency of the disease in the general population, so that the sensitivity of field epidemiological studies on exposed populations is necessarily limited. For the above reasons, heavy reliance on evidence of carcinogenicity in experimental animals, coupled with estimates of the extent to which human populations are exposed to specific carcinogens, are used in making assessments of the public health risks posed by chemical carcinogens.

Aflatoxins

A large number of publications have appeared since the discovery of aflatoxins in 1960, reflecting the enormous amount of work that has been done on the toxicity, mutagenicity, carcinogenicity and other biological and biochemical effects of these substances. Chemically, aflatoxins are heterocyclic dihydrofuro-furan compounds and are of two types: aflatoxin B_1 and its derivatives and aflatoxin G_1, and its derivatives. A total of 13 naturally occurring derivatives of aflatoxin B_1 have been structurally identified, and in some instances studied for their biological effects. Aflatoxins are metabolic products of a few strains of Aspergillus flavus and A. parasiticus, which grow on virtually all types of food in warm humid environments (Bababunmi et al., 1978). It is therefore not surprising that aflatoxins contaminate most foodstuffs in tropical and subtropical regions of the world (Bababunmi et al., 1978) where the warm and humid conditions exist that are necessary for the growth of the fungi which produce the toxins. This explains the wide-spread ingestion of these toxins with food in these areas. Aflatoxins have been reported to be hepatocarcinogenic in a wide range of laboratory animals, including rats (Wogan & Newberne, 1967), mice (Vesselinovich et al., 1972), marmosets (Lin et al., 1974), ferrets (Butler, 1969), ducks (Carnaghan, 1965), rainbow trout (Cameron et al., 1976) salmon (Wales & Sinhuber, 1972), guppy (Sato et al., 1973) and rhesus monkeys (Gopalan et al., 1972; Adamson et al., 1973). Also, their ingestion together with food has been shown to correlate positively with the incidence of HCC in countries like Kenya, Swaziland, Thailand and Mozambique (Van Rensburg et al., 1974; Peers & Linsell, 1973; Peers et al., 1976; Shank et al., 1972a,b,c). Aflatoxins have also been identified in foodstuffs consumed in Nigeria (Bababunmi et al., 1978) and in urine samples taken from Nigerians, including both normal individuals and patients with liver diseases (Bababunmi et al., 1976).

N-Nitroso Compounds

Other chemical carcinogens probably involved in the etiology of HCC are the nitrosamines and nitrosamides. All such N-nitroso compounds have a nitroso group linked to a secondary or tertiary nitrogen atom. Until recently, they were generally regarded as synthetic chemical carcinogens and an environmental hazard only to people involved in their laboratory or industrial use. There is evidence, however, that nitrosamines may be formed de novo in food from precursors such as nitrites, secondary, tertiary and quarternary amines, and other nitrosatable chemicals present in it.

The commonest and most widely distributed nitrosamine, N-nitrosodimethylamine, has been identified in many alcoholic beverages widely consumed in Nigeria (Bababunmi et al., 1978). Since it has been shown to induce malignant tumours in the liver and other organs (Magee & Barnes, 1967), its presence in these beverages indicates that it may be involved in the etiology of HCC in Nigeria. In a more global context, the available evidence suggests that human populations may absorb over long periods of time variable amounts of N-nitroso compounds either directly from the environment or after their formation in the gut. In view of the pleotropic carcinogenicity and potency of various members of this group of chemicals in experimental animals, they constitute a potential carcinogenic risk of considerable magnitude. It is, however, not possible at the moment to assess exactly their role in the etiology of HCC.

Other mutagenic and/or carcinogenic chemicals

Many other chemicals with which human populations may come into contact in the tropics and subtropics have been shown to be mutagenic and/or carcinogenic and are likely, therefore, to contribute to the overall carcinogenic exposure load on the liver of people living in these areas. The extent of the contribution made by these chemicals and their modulating effects on the mutagenic and/or carcinogenic potential of chemicals already implicated in the incidence of HCC is not yet known. The chemicals concerned are found in medicinal plants and herbal teas taken in the tropics (e.g., furocoumarins, pyrrolizidine alkaloids, safrole, capsaicin, cutechin, etc.), food pyrolysis products present in smoked fish and meat preparations (Emerole et al., 1982), organochlorine pesticide residues in food, e.g., DDT and dieldrin, and other pesticide residues.

MUTAGENICITY STUDIES ON MYCOTOXINS AND TOXIC PHYTOCHEMICALS

Aflatoxins and Palmotoxin

Of the mycotoxins, aflatoxins have been the most widely studied for mutagenicity and/or carcinogenicity. The mutagenicity assay systems in which aflatoxins have been studied include the Ames bacterial assay system (Ames et al., 1975; Wong & Hsieh, 1976; Uwaifo et al., 1979; Uwaifo & Bababunmi, 1979; Norpoth et al., 1979; Wheeler et al., 1981; Baker et al., 1980; Decloitre & Hamon, 1980); Chinese hamster V79 cells (Krahn & Heidelberger, 1977; Uwaifo et al., 1983; Langenbach et al., 1978); mouse embryo C3H/10T1/2 cells (Billings et al., 1983; Uwaifo et al., 1983); and the Neurospora crassa adenine-3 (ad-3) test system (Ong, 1970).

A modified form of the Ames Salmonella typhimurium assay system was used to study the mutagenicity of aflatoxins B_1 and M_1 and palmotoxin B_0 (Uwaifo et al., 1979). Palmotoxin B_0 is produced as a cometabolite of aflatoxin B_1 by Aspergillus flavus in a culture medium of palm soup (Bassir & Adekunle, 1968). The procedure for the maintenance and storage of stock cultures of

various tester strains of <u>S. typhimurium</u> was as stipulated by
Ames <u>et al.</u> (1975). The results are shown in Figures 1 and 2.

FIG. 1   REVERTANT COLONIES INDUCED BY 0.5 g OF AFLATOXIN B_1
AND PALMOTOXIN B_0 ACTIVATED BY DIFFERENT AMOUNTS
OF S-9 PREPARATION

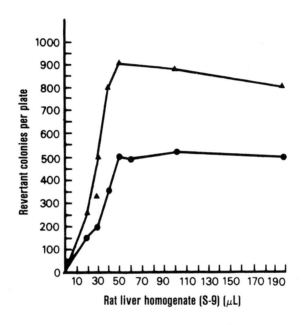

In Figure 1 it should be observed that 50 μl of S-9 preparation is required for optimum activation of aflatoxin B_1 and
palmotoxin B_0. The similarity of the profiles of the curves for
the two toxins may be a reflection of their similar chemical
structures.

In Figure 2, it should also be noticed that optimum
induction of mutagenicity by aflatoxin B_1 and M_1 occurs with
about the same number of μg of toxin per plate. This again may
be a reflection of their similar chemical structures.

FIG. 2 REVERTANT COLONIES INDUCED BY DIFFERENT AMOUNTS OF
AFLATOXINS B_1 AND M_1 ACTIVATED BY $50\mu l$ OF S-9 PREPARATION

Mutagenicity potency is the reciprocal of μg of toxin per plate
which induces 100 revertants of tester strain

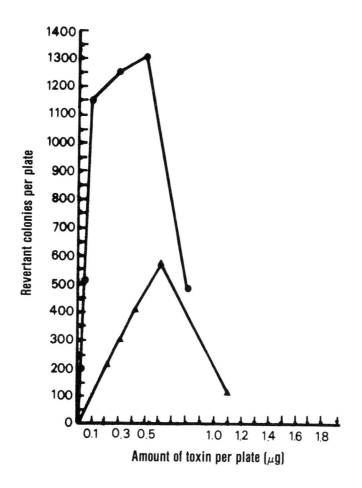

Chamuvaritin and Chamuvarin

Chamuvaritin and chamuvarin are two benzyldihydrochalcones isolated by Okorie (1977) from the roots of Uvaria chamae, a small tree which grows in the tropical rain forests of West Africa. Decoctions of the roots and bark of this plant are drunk for purgative and febrifugal purposes by people living in this region (Daziel, 1948).

Chamuvaritin and chamuvarin were isolated as described in Okorie's original paper (Okorie, 1977), and their mutagenicities were assayed by the Ames S. typhimurium assay system. The methods used were basically the same as those for aflatoxins. The results obtained are shown in Table 1 and Figures 3 and 4. If the mutagenicity of aflatoxin B_1 is assigned a value of 100, that of chamuvaritin is 1.4.

Table 1. Mutagenicity of chamuvaritin and chamuvarin in the Ames test[a]

Compound	Strain of S. typhimurium													
	TA92 MA		TA94 MA		TA98 MA		TA100 MA		TA1535 MA		TA1537 MA		TA1538 MA	
	+	−	+	−	+	−	+	−	+	−	+	−	+	−
Chamuvaritin	−	−	−	−	−	++	−	−	−	−	−	−	+	−
Chamuvarin	−	−	−	−	−	−	−	−	−	−	−	−	−	−

[a] The filter paper disc-spot test was used. Sterile 6-mm filter paper discs to which 20 µl (500 µg) of chamuvaritin and chamuvarin were applied were placed in the centre of petri dishes containing: (i) minimal medium (Vogel-Bonner medium E) thin overlay of top agar; (ii) 0.1 ml 24-h culture of each tester strain; and (iii) 0.5 ml of rat liver homogenate for microsomal activated plates. + +: significant mutagenicity; +: slight mutagenicity; −: no mutagenicity. Spontaneous revertants: TA92, 60 ± 15; TA94, 25 ± 10; TA98, 47 ± 7; TA100, 130 ± 40; TA1535, 20 ± 5; TA1537, 7 ± 3; TA1538, 25 ± 5. MA: microsomal activation.

FIG. 3   REVERTANTS OF TA98 INDUCED BY 0.1 mg CHAMUVARIN
IN 0.1 ml AQUEOUS ETHANOL SOLUTION WITH DIFFERENT AMOUNTS
OF RAT LIVER HOMOGENATE

Half the volume of rat liver homogenate (S-9) indicated in the
figure was used.

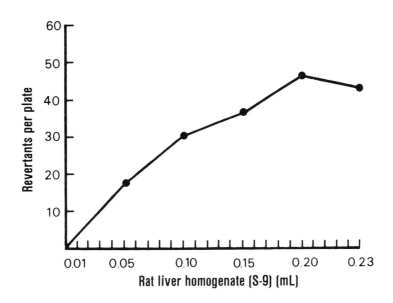

Furocoumarins

Furocoumarins are widely distributed both in nature and
elsewhere in the environment. Our studies (Uwaifo &
Heidelberger, 1983; Uwaifo et al., 1983) have, however, been
confined to those found in nature in general and in medicinal
plants in particular. Our interest in plant furocoumarins is
based on the premise that it is this group that is likely to add
to the carcinogenic and/or mutagenic pressure on people living in
the tropics and consequently more likely to affect the incidence
of HCC in those regions.

FIG. 4 REVERSION OF THE HISTIDINE MUTANT OF SALMONELLA TYPHIMURIUM TA98 BY DIFFERENT CONCENTRATIONS OF CHAMUVARITIN

Each plot of revertants per plate is the mean of counts taken in 5 plates after subtraction of a background count of 47.

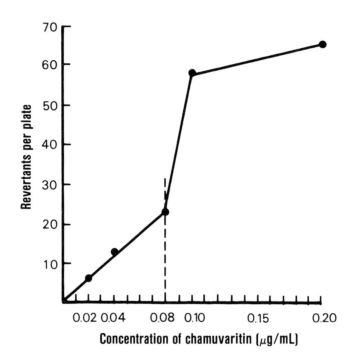

Concentration of chamuvaritin (μg/mL)

The mutagenicity of furocoumarins has been studied by means of three different assay systems, namely the Ames bacterial test system, Chinese hamster V79 cells and C3H10T1/2 cells. In the mammalian cell systems, assays were carried out both under photo-activation by long-wavelength ultraviolet light (black light) and in the absence of such photoactivation, because of the known photosensitizing capacity of furocoumarins.

The mutagenicity of the furocoumarins xanthotoxin, imperatorin, heraclenin, marmesin, chalepin and oxypeucedanin isolated
from the Nigerian medicinal plants Afraeqle paniculata and
Clausena anisata has been studied.   In the Ames test, the
furocoumarins were screened on a number of tester strains of S.
typhimurium selected such that different types of mutation, such
as frameshift and base-pair substitution mutation, were covered.
The assay was essentially the same as that used for the aflatoxins.   The results obtained are shown in Table 2 and Figures 5
and 6.   It should be observed from the data that marmesin is the
most mutagenic of all the furocoumarins screened.

Table 2. Mutagenicity of furocoumarins in the Ames test[a]

Furocoumarin	Plant source	Strain of S. typhimurium											
		TA92 MA		TA94 MA		TA97 MA		TA98 MA		TA100 MA		TA102 MA	
		+	−	+	−	+	−	+	−	+	−	+	−
Chalepin	Clausen anisata	−	−	−	−	..	+	−	+	−	+	−	−
Heraclenin	A. paniculata	−	−	−	−	−	−	−	−	−	−	−	−
Imperatorin	A. paniculata	+	+	−	−	+	+	+	+	++	++	−	−
Marmesin	A. paniculata	+	+	−	−	++	++	++	++	++	++	−	−
Oxypeucedanin	Clausena anisata	−	−	−	−	−	−	−	−	−	−	−	−
Xanthotoxin	A. paniculata	−	−	−	−	−	−	−	−	−	−	−	−

[a] The procedure was essentially the same as that used for the aflatoxins
    (see Table 1)
    ++ significant mutagenicity;   + slight mutagenicity;   − no mutagenicity.
    MA: microsomal activation

FIG. 5. MUTAGENICITY OF IMPERATORIN

Rat liver homogenate was not used in these assays since activation was found not to be necessary in preliminary experiments

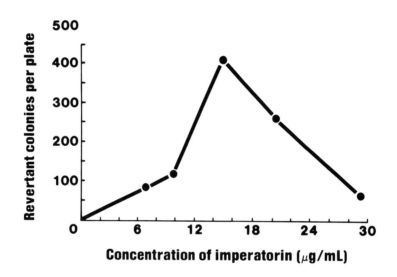

Concentration of imperatorin (μg/mL)

In the assay with Chinese hamster V79 cells, the procedure used was essentially that described by Peterson et al. (1979), in which N-methyl-N-nitro-N-nitrosoguanidine is used as a control. The results are shown in Table 3. All compounds were carried in dimethylsulfoxide (DMSO).

When mutagenicity was determined in the assay using C3H/10T1/2 cells, mutation frequency was calculated as described by Landolph et al. (1980). The results are shown in Table 4. With this assay no mutation at the ouabain locus was observed for any of the furocoumarins, with or without photoactivation except aflatoxin B_1 which, without photoactivation, induced observable mutation. This mutation was, however, reversed by benzoflavone (BF). Only the results obtained with aflatoxin B_1 are therefore shown in Table 4.

Table 3. Mutagenicity of furocoumarins in Chinese hamster V79 cells with and without photoactivation[a]

Treatment		Survival[b]		AzG[c] Mutants/10^5 survivors	
		-BL	+BL	-BL	+BL
AFB_1	(0.5 µg/ml)	0.95	0.92	1.5 ± 0.4[d]	2.3 ± 0.5[d]
AFB_1	(1.0 µg/ml)	0.94	0.82	1.5 ± 0.3	2.6 ± 0.8
AFB_1	(1.5 µg/ml)	0.92	0.74	1.4 ± 0.6	2.7 ± 0.5
AFB_1	(2.5 µg/ml)	0.88	0.72	1.3 ± 0.7	2.9 ± 1.2
AFB_1	(5.0 µg/ml)	0.85	0.70	2.4 ± 1.6	4.5 ± 1.3
DMSO	0.5%	1.00	1.00	1.4 ± 0.6	1.4 ± 0.5
MAR	0.25 (µg/ml)	0.98	0.98	1.6 ± 0.7	1.6 ± 0.3
MAR	0.5 (µg/ml)	0.65	0.66	1.1 ± 1.0	1.7 ± 0.5
MAR	1.0 (µg/ml)	0.27	0.17	1.1 ± 0.6	2.0 ± 0.5
MAR	1.5 (µg/ml)	0.05	0.03	1.9 ± 0.8	2.4 ± 0.4
DMSO	0.5%	1.00	1.00	1.2 ± 0.6	1.3 ± 0.5
MOP	(2.0 µg/ml)	0.80	0.78	0.9 ± 0.3	1.9 ± 0.0
MOP	(5.0 µg/ml)	0.80	0.32	1.1 ± 0.3	6.3 ± 0.4
MOP	(8.0 µg/ml)	0.80	0.29	1.4 ± 0.4	8.8 ± 0.6
MOP	(10.0 µg/ml)	0.77	0.12	2.9 ± 0.5	19.2 ± 0.9
DMSO	0.5%	1.00	1.00	1.2 ± 0.6	1.3 ± 0.5
CHAL	(1.0 µg/ml)	0.58	0.94	0.5 ± 0.3	0.9 ± 0.3
CHAL	(1.5 µg/ml)	0.49	0.86	0.9 ± 0.3	0.9 ± 0.3
CHAL	(2.5 µg/ml)	0.47	0.85	0.7 ± 0.7	1.9 ± 0.6
CHAL	(5.0 µg/ml)	0.42	0.63	1.1 ± 0.8	3.8 ± 0.4
DMSO	(0.5 µg/ml)	1.00	1.00	1.5 ± 0.5	0.9 ± 0.4
IMP	(2.0 µg/ml)	0.82	0.55	2.3 ± 0.5	14.9 ± 0.9
IMP	(5.0 µg/ml)	0.81	0.35	4.3 ± 0.6	15.7 ± 0.9
IMP	(8.0 µg/ml)	0.80	0.20	4.5 ± 0.5	17.7 ± 0.8
IMP	(10.0 µg/ml)	0.78	0.15	7.8 ± 0.7	20.9 ± 1.0
DMSO	0.5%	1.00	1.00	1.4 ± 0.4	1.5 ± 0.4
MNNG[e]	(0.5 µg/ml)	0.32	–	5.7 ± 0.4[f]	–

[a] Black light (BL) long wavelength ultraviolet

[b] Survival relative to DMSO controls. Absolute survival (plating efficiency) of V79 cells in DMSO controls was 0.41 ± 0.3.

[c] AzG = Mutants selected in medium containing azaguanine

[d] Mean mutation frequency (3 experiments) $\pm$ standard deviation.

[e] Cells were treated with MNNG as previously described by Peterson et al. (1979)

[f] Mean mutation frequency (15 experiments) $\pm$ standard deviation

AFB_1 = aflatoxin B_1; DMSO = dimethylsulfoxide; MAR = marmesin; MOP = methoxypsoralen; CHAL = chalepin; IMP = imperatorin; MNNG = N-methyl-N-nitro-N-nitrosoguanidine

FIG. 6. MUTAGENICITY OF MARMESIN

Rat liver homogenate was not used in these assays since activation was found not to be necessary in preliminary experiments

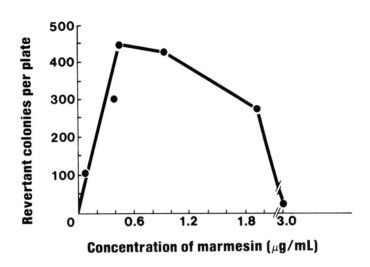

CELL TRANSFORMATION STUDIES

Cells in culture were first used for studying the carcinogenicity of chemicals by Berwald and Sachs (1963). Since the discovery of this in vitro system and its subsequent quantification (Berwald & Sachs, 1965), the number of cell systems used has grown by leaps and bounds. Consequently, today, the long list includes systems derived from a wide range of mammalian species including man (Chen & Heidelberger, 1969; Marquardt et al., 1974; Reznikoff et al., 1973a,b; DiPaolo et al., 1972; Kakunaga, 1973, 1977; Freeman et al., 1975; Rhim et al., 1974; Rasheed et al., 1976; Mishra & Di Mayorca, 1974; Styles, 1977; Evans & DiPaolo, 1975). The method provides a simplified model system that is free from the nutritional, physiological and immunological complexities of in vivo carcinogenicity assay systems, and can therefore be used to identify and study mechanisms at the cellular and molecular levels. In essence, the method is based on the phenotypic changes induced by chemical

Table 4. Mutagenicity of Aflatoxin B_1 with C3H/10T1/2 cells

Treatment	Plating efficiency[a]	Ouabain-resistant mutants/10^5 survivors
Dimethylsulfoxide (0.5%)	0.22	5 ± 1[b]
BF (0.5 µg/ml)	0.25	6 ± 2[b]
AFB_1 (0.1 µg/ml)	0.18	13 ± 8[b]
AFB_1 (0.5 µg/ml)	0.12	14 ± 5[b]
AFB_1 (1.0 µg/ml)	0.09	33 ± 21[b]
AFB_1 (1.0 µg/ml)+BF (0.5 µg/ml)	0.16	6 ± 1[b]
AFB_1 (2.5 µg/ml)	0.07	67 ± 45[b]
AFB_1 (2.5 g/ml)+BF (0.5 µg/ml)	0.12	12[c]
AFB_1 (5.0 µg/ml)	0.02	115[c]
AFB^1 (5.0 µg/ml)+BF (0.5 µg/ml)	0.11	9[c]
N-Methyl-N-nitro-N-nitroso-guanidine (1 µg/ml)	0.15	176 ± 53

[a] Mean absolute plating efficiency of cells reseeded for selection

[b] Mean mutation on frequency $\pm$ standard deviation

[c] Values given are statistical calculations and indicate that no colonies were present in any of the dishes in that group. Actual mutation frequency is lower than this value.

BF = benzoflavone

treatment, but the ultimate criterion is that the treated cells must have undergone transformation such that they are tumorigenic in appropriate hosts.

Such transformation of cells in culture is comparable in most respects to carcinogenesis in whole animals, and at the same time more rapid and less expensive. There is also every reason to believe that the same cellular and molecular mechanisms are involved in both cell transformation and in vivo carcinogenesis. Positive results for a suspected chemical carcinogen in the in vitro cell transformation test are therefore a strong indication of in vivo carcinogenicity.

Aflatoxins

The ability of aflatoxins to transform cells in culture has been widely reported in the literature. Cells in which transformation by aflatoxin B_1 has been reported include Syrian hamster cells (Pienta et al., 1977), guinea-pig cells (Evans & DiPaolo, 1975), 3T3 cells (DiPaolo et al., 1972), mouse embryo C3H/10T1/2 cells (Uwaifo et al., 1983; Billings et al., 1983). The procedure for the assay with C3H/10T1/2 cells is essentially that described by Reznikoff et al. (1973a,b), and the results obtained for aflatoxin B_1 are shown in Tables 5 and 6. Methylcholanthrene was used as a control.

Table 5.   Transformation of C3H/10T1/2 cells by aflatoxin B1 [a]

Treatment	No. of experiments	PE[b]	No. of dishes with type III foci/No. of treated dishes[c]	Fraction of dishes with type III foci[c]
Dimethylsulfoxide (0.5%)	5	0.25	0/124	0
MCA (1.0 µg/ml)	5	0.23	58/115	0.50
AFB$_1$ (0.1 µg/ml)	1	0.22	0/16	0
AFB$_1$ (0.1 µg/ml)[d]	1	0.20	0/17	0
AFB$_1$ (0.5 µg/ml)	2	0.22	0/28	0
AFB$_1$ (1.0 µg/ml)	4	0.15	5/66	0.08
AFB$_1$ (1.0 µg/ml)[d]	1	0.19	1/14	0.07
AFB$_1$ (2.0 µg/ml)	1	0.04	2/20	0.10
AFB$_1$ (2.5 µg/ml)	2	0.07	1/39	0.03
AFB$_1$ (5.0 µg/ml)	2	0.05	0/25	0
BF (0.5 µg/ml)	2	0.17	0/34	0
AFB$_1$ (1.0 µg/ml) + BF (0.5 µg/ml)[e]	3	0.21	4/58	0.07
AFB$_1$ (2.0 µg/ml) + BF (0.05 µg/ml)[e]	1	0.16	3/20	0.15
AFB$_1$ (2.5 µg/ml) + BF (0.5 µg/ml)[e]	1	0.18	1/13	0.08
MCA (1.0 µg/ml) + BF (0.5 µg/ml)[e]	1	0.19	2/20	0.10

[a] MCA = methylcholanthrene;   AFB$_1$ = aflatoxin B$_1$;   BF = benzoflavone

[b] PE= mean absolute plating efficiency

[c] Type III foci are identified on the basis of criteria established by Reznikoff et al. (1973) and are indicative of transformation. Background transformation frequency in control dishes is approximately 0.001 type III focus/dish (unpublished data).

[d] Incubation with AFB$_1$ for 72 hrs one day after seeding

[e] Incubation with AFB$_1$ + BF or MCA + BF for 48 hrs one day after seeding

Table 6. Transformation of C3H/10T1/2 cells by aflatoxin B[1] and furocoumarins with and without photoactivation[a]

Compound	No. of experiments	Concentration (mg/ml)	Survival[b]		Transformation (No. of foci/ No. of dishes scored)				Computed partition coefficient (octanol/ water) (Log P)	No. of dishes with Type II and Type III foci	
					Type II[c]		Type III[c]				
			-BL	+BL	-BL	+BL	-BL	+BL		-BL	+BL
AFB[1]	3	1.0	0.97	0.79	1/40	6/34	2/40	3/34	0.82	3	9
		1.5	0.88	0.75	0/39	0/39	0.39	0/39		0	0
		3.0	0.86	0.70	0/36	0/40	0/36	0/40		0	0
MOP	3	1.0	1.00	0.34	0/37	2/27	0/37	0/27	1.30	0	2
		1.5	1.10	0.10	0/40	3/50	0/40	0/50		0	3
		2.5	1.00	0.03	0/46	3/27	0/46	0/27		0	3
IMP	3	1.0	1.00	0.78	0/36	0/38	0/36	0/38	3.10	0	0
		2.5	1.00	0.70	0/38	0/40	0/30	0/30		0	0
		5.0	0.93	0.56	0/41	0/41	0/41	14/41		0	14
MAR	3	0.25	0.30	0.32	0/58	0/60	0/58	0/60	0.67	0	0
		0.5	0.14	0.17	0/44	0/37	0/44	0/37		0	0
		1.0	0.03	0.05	0/42	0/36	0/42	0/36		0	0
CHAL	3	1.0	0.88	0.82	0/27	0/50	0/27	0/50	2.93	0	0
		2.5	0.42	0.40	0/28	0/35	0/28	0/35		0	0
		5.0	0.30	0.27	0/30	0/30	0/30	0/30		0	0
MCA[d]	15	1.0	1.00	-	83/208	-	125/208	-	-	208	-

[a] Black light (BL) long-wavelength ultraviolet

[b] Relative to controls. Absolute survival (plating efficiency) of C3H/10T1/2 cells in controls was 0.29 ± 0.03

[c] Type II and type III foci are identified on the basis of criteria established by Reznikoff et al. (1973) and are indicative of transformation

[d] Cells were treated with MCA for 48 hrs one day after seeding

AFB[1] = aflatoxin B[1]; MOP – methoxypsoralen; IMP – imperatorin; MAR – marmesin; CHAL – chalepin; MCA = methylcholanthrene

Furocoumarins

Transformation of cells in culture by furocoumarins with ultraviolet light activation has been reported by relatively few workers. The transformation assay of ß-methoxypsoralen (methoxsalen) (International Agency for Research on Cancer, 1980) showed that transformation occurred in various cell systems. Uwaifo et al. (1983) dealt specifically with the transforming ability of four furocoumarins (imperatorin, marmesin, chalepin, and ß-methoxypsoralen) isolated from two Nigerian medicinal plants and aflatoxin B[1]. The procedure followed in the transformation assay by Uwaifo et al. (1983) was essentially the same as that described for aflatoxin B[1]. The results are shown in Table 6. It should be observed that only aflatoxin B[1] and imperatorin were able to induce transformation in C3H/10T1/2 cells. It should also be observed that although IMP has the highest log P and the highest number of dishes with types II and III foci, CHAL which comes second in descending order of log P values was unable to induce any observable transformation whereas aflatoxin B_1 which was third was able to do so. It is therefore apparent that lipid solubility of the compounds is not necessarily a critical factor in the ability of furocoumarins to induce transformation.

PROSPECTS FOR FUTURE RESEARCH

It is well established that aflatoxin and hepatitis B virus play important roles in the initiation of liver carcinogenesis but the contribution of tumour promoting agents to the expression of the 'initiated' cells needs further study. Investigations with 12-0-tetradecanoylphorbol-13-acetate (TPA), identified as the co-carcinogenic principle in croton oil, have in recent years provided valuable information on tumour promotion. Other novel and chemically different tumour promoters will undoubtedly provide new information on their mechanism of action and role in the etiology of liver carcinogenesis. Recently, well characterized diterpenes have been isolated from plant sources other than Croton tiglium or C. flavens. For example, a novel furanoid diterpene, penduliflawo-rosin, from the medicinal plant Croton penduliflorus, has been isolated, purified and characterized at the University of Ibadan (Adesogan, 1981). The promoting potential of this diterpene is yet to be investigated.

ACKNOWLEDGEMENTS

All 12 tester strains of Salmonella typhimurium used in our laboratory were the generous gift of Professor B. Ames of the University of California, Berkeley, CA, USA. Furocoumarins were kindly provided by Dr E.A. Adesogan and Dr D.A. Okorie of the Department of Chemistry, University of Ibadan, Ibadan, Nigeria.

REFERENCES

Adamson, R.H., Correa, P. & Dalgard, D.W. (1973) Occurrence of a primary liver carcinoma in a Rhesus monkey fed aflatoxin B_1. J. natl Cancer Inst., 50, 549-553

Adesogan, E.A. (1981) J. chem. Soc. (Lond), Perkin I, 1151-1158

Ames, B.N., McCann, J. & Yamasaki, E. (1975) Methods for detecting carcinogens and mutagens with the Salmonella mammalian-microsome mutagenicity test. Mutat. Res., 31, 347-364

Bababunmi, E.A. (1976) Excretion of aflatoxin in the urine of normal individuals and patients with liver disease in Ibadan (Nigeria). In: Proc. 3rd Int. Symp. DePca, New York, pp. 1729-1736

Bababunmi, E.A., Uwaifo, A.O. & Bassir, O. (1978) Hepato-carcinogens in Nigerian foodstuffs. Wld Rev. Nutr. Diet, 28, 188-209

Baker, R.S.U., Bonin, A.M., Stupans, I. & Holder, G.M. (1980) Comparison of rat and guinea pig as sources of the S9 fraction in the salmonella/mammalian microsome mutagenicity test. Mutation Res., 71, 43-52

Bassir, O. & Adekunle, A.A. (1968) FEBS Lett., 2, 23-25

Beasley, R.P. & Lin, C.C. (1978) Hepatoma risk among HBsAg carriers. Am. J. Epidemiol., 108, 247

Berwald, Y. & Sachs, L. (1963) In vitro cell transformation with chemical carcinogens. Nature (London), 200, 1182-1184

Berwald, Y. & Sachs, L. (1965) In vitro transformation of normal cells to tumor cells by carcinogenic hydrocarbons. J. natl Cancer Inst., 35, 641-661

Billings, P.C., Uwaifo, A.O. & Heidelberger, C. (1983) Influence of benzoflavone on aflatoxin B_1-induced cytotoxicity, mutation and transformation of C3H/10T1/2 cells. Cancer Res., 43, 2659-2663

Blumberg, B.S. & London, W.T. (1980) Hepatitis B virus and primary hepatocellular carcinoma: Relationship of 'icrons' to cancer. In: Viruses in Naturally Occurring Cancers, Cold Spring Harbor Conferences on Cell Proliferation, Vol. 7, Cold Spring Harbor, Cold Spring Harbor Laboratory, pp. 401-421

Bréchot, C., Pourcel, C., Louise, A., Rain, B. & Tiollais, P. (1980)   Presence of integrated hepatitis B virus DNA sequences in cellular DNA of human hepatocellular carcinoma. Nature (London), 286, 533-535

Butler, W.H. (1969) Aflatoxicosis in laboratory animals.   In: Goldblatt, L.A., ed., Aflatoxin: Scientific Background, Control and Implications, New York, Academic Press, pp. 223-236

Cameron, H.M., Linsell, D.A. & Warwick, G.P. (1976) Liver Cell Cancer, New York, Elsevier Scientific Publ. Co., p. 130

Carnaghan, R.B.A. (1965) Hepatic tumours in ducks fed a low level of toxic groundnut meal. Nature (London), 208, 308

Chen, T.T. & Heidelberger, C. (1969) Quantitative studies on the malignant transformation of mouse prostate cells by carcinogenic hydrocarbons in vitro. Int. J. Cancer, 4, 166-178

Clemmesen, J. (1965) Statistical Studies in Malignant Neoplasms, Copenhagen, Munksgaard, p. 543

Daziel, J.M. (1948) In: The Useful Plants of West Tropical Africa, 2nd ed., London, Crown Agents, p. 7

Decloitre, F. & Hammon, G. (1980) Species-dependent effects of dietary lindane and/or zineb on the activation of aflatoxin B_1 into mutagenic derivatives. Mutat. Res., 79, 185-192

Di Paolo, J.A., Takano, K. & Popescu, N.C. (1972) Quantitation of chemically induced neoplastic transformation of BALB/3T3 cloned cell lines. Cancer Res., 32, 2686-2695

Doll, R., Muir, C. & Waterhouse, J. eds (1970) Cancer Incidence in Five Continents, II, New York, Springer-Verlag

Dorn, H.F. & Cutler, S.J. (1959) Public Health Monograph, No. 56

Emerole, G.O., Uwaifo, A.O., Thabrew, M.I. & Bababunmi, E.A. (1980) The presence of aflatoxin and some polycyclic aromatic hydrocarbons in human foods. Cancer Lett., 15, 123-129

Evans, C.H. & Di Paolo, J.A. (1975) Neoplastic transformation of guinea pig fetal cells in culture induced by chemical carcinogens. Cancer Res., 35, 1035-1044

Freeman, A.E., Igel, H.J. & Price, P.J. (1975) In vitro transformation of rat embryo cells: correlations with the known tumorigenic activities of chemicals in rodents. In Vitro, II, 107-115

Gharpure, P.V. (1948) Indian Med. Gaz, 83, 5-6

Gopalan, C., Tulpule, P.G. & Krishnamurthi, D. (1972) Induction of hepatic carcinoma with aflatoxin in the Rhesus monkey. Food Cosmet. Toxicol., 10, 519-521

Griswold, M.H., Wilder, C.S., Cutler, S.J. & Polack, E.S. (1955) Cancer in Connecticut 1935-1951. Connecticut State Department of Health, Hartford, Conn., p. 141

Gustafson, E.G. (1937) Ann. Intern. Med., 11, 889-900

Habibi, A. (1965) Cancer in Iran. A survey of the most common cases. J. natl Cancer Inst., 34, 553-569

Heidelberger, C., Mondal, S., Peterson, A.R. (1978) Initiation and promotion in cell cultures. In: Slaga, T.J., Sivak, A. & Boutwell, R.K., eds, Carcinogenesis, Vol. 2, New York, Raven, pp. 197-202

Higginson, J. (1963) The geographical pathology of primary liver cancer. Cancer Res., 23, 1624-1633

Higginson, J. (1970) The epidemiology of primary carcinoma of the liver. In: Pack, G.T. & Islami, A.H., eds, Recent Results in Cancer Research, No. 26, Tumours of the Liver, New York, Springer-Verlag, pp. 38-52

IARC (1980) Methoxsalen, Monographs on the Evaluation of the Carcinogenic Risk of Chemicals to Humans, 24, 101-124

Jussawalla, D.T., Haenzel, W., Deshpande, V.A. & Nateker, M.V. (1968) Cancer incidence in greater Bombay: Assessment of the cancer risk by age. Br. J. Cancer, 22, 623-636

Kakunaga, T. (1973) A quantitative system for assay of malignant transformation by chemical carcinogens using a clone derived from BALB/3T3. Int. J. Cancer, 12, 463-473

Kakunaga, T. (1977) The transformation of human diploid cells by chemical carcinogens. In: Hiatt, H.H., Watson, J.D. & Winsten, J.A., eds, Origins of Human Cancer, Cold Spring Harbor, Cold Spring Harbor Laboratory, pp. 1537-1548

Kennaway, E.L. (1944) Cancer of the liver in the negro in Africa and in America. Cancer Res., 4, 571-577

Kouwenaar, W. (1951) Doc. Neerl. Indones. Morbis. Trop., 3, 357-367

Krahn, D.F. & Heidelberger, C. (1977) Liver homogenate-mediated mutagenesis in Chinese hamster V79 cells by polycyclic aromatic hydrocarbons and aflatoxins. Mutat. Res., 46, 27-44

Langenbach, R., Freed, H.J. & Huberman, E. (1978) Liver cell-mediated mutagenesis of mammalian cells by liver carcinogens. Proc. natl Acad. Sci. USA, 75, 2864-2867

Landolph, J.R., Telfer, N. & Heidelberger, C. (1980) Further evidence that ouabain-resistant variants induced by chemical carcinogens in transformable C3H/10T1/2 C18 mouse fibroblasts are mutants. Mutat. Res., 72, 295-310

Lin, J.J., Liu, C. & Svoboda, D.J. (1974) Long term effects of aflatoxin B_1 and viral hepatitis on marmoset liver. Lab. Invest., 30, 267-278

London, W.T. (1983) Hepatitis B virus and primary hepatocellular carcinoma. In: Klein, G., ed., Advances in Viral Oncology, 3, New York, Raven Press, pp. 325-341

Magee, P.N. & Barnes, J.M. (1967) Carcinogenic nitroso compounds. Adv. Cancer Res., 10, 163-246

Mahju, M.Y. (1958) Medicus, 16, 168-178

Marquardt, H., Sodergren, D.E., Sims, P. & Grover, P.L. (1974) Malignant transformation _in vitro_ of mouse fibroblasts by 7,12-dimethylbenz(a)anthracene and 7-hydroxymethylbenz(a)-anthracene and by their K-region derivatives. Int. J. Cancer, 13, 304-310

Marsden, A.T.H. (1958) The geographical pathology of cancer in Malaya. Br. J. Cancer, 12, 161-176

Mishra, N.K. & Di Mayorca, G. (1974) In vitro malignant trans-formation of cells by chemical carcinogens. Biochem. Biophys. Acta, 355, 205-219

Norpoth, K., Grossmeier, R., Bosenberg, H., Themann, H. & Fleischer, M. (1979) Mutagenicity of aflatoxin B_1, acti-vated by S-9 fractions of human, rat, mouse, rabbit and monkey liver, towards S. typhimurium TA98. Int. Arch. Occup. Environ. Health, 42, 333-339

Obata, H., Hayashi, N. & Motoike, Y., Hisamitsu, T., Okuda, H., Kobayashi, S. & Nishioka, K. (1980) A prospective study on the development of hepatocellular carcinoma from liver cirrhosis with persistent hepatitis B virus infection. Int. J. Cancer, 25, 741-747

Oettle, A.G. (1964) Cancer in Africa, especially in regions south of the Sahara. J. natl Cancer Inst., 33, 383-439

Okorie, D.A. (1977) Phytochem., 16, 1591-1594

Ong, T. (1970) Mutagenicity of aflatoxins in Neurospora crassa. Mutat. Res., 9, 615-618

Peers, F.G. & Linsell, C.A. (1973) Dietary aflatoxins and liver cancer - A population based study in Kenya. Brit. J. Cancer, 27, 473-484

Peers, F.G., Gilman, G.A. & Linsell, C.A. (1976) Dietary afla-toxins and human liver cancer. A study in Swaziland. Int. J. Cancer, 17, 167-176

Peterson, A.R., Peterson, H. & Heidelberger, C. (1979) Onco-
    genesis, mutagenesis, DNA damage, and cytotoxicity in
    cultured mammalian cells treated with alkylating agents.
    Cancer Res., 39, 131-138

Pienta, R.J., Poiley, J.A. & Lebherz, W.B., III (1977) Morpho-
    logical transformation of early passage golden Syrian
    hamster embryo cells derived from cryopreserved primary
    cultures as a reliable in vitro bioassay for identifying
    diverse carcinogens. Int. J. Cancer, 19, 642-655

Prates, M.D. (1961) Cancer and cirrhosis of the liver in the
    Portuguese East African with special reference to the
    specific age and sex rates in Lourenco Marques. Acta Unio
    Int. Contra. Cancr., 17, 718-739

Purchase, I.F.H. & Goncalves, T. (1971) Preliminary results from
    food analyses in the Inhambane area. In: Purchase, I.F.H.,
    ed., Mycotoxins in Human Health, London, Macmillan, pp.
    263-269

Rasheed, S., Freeman, A.E., Gardner, M.B. & Huebner, R.J. (1976)
    Acceleration of transformation of rat embryo cells by a type
    C virus. J. Virol., 18, 776-782

Reddy, D.G. & Rao, K.S. (1962) Primary carcinoma of the liver
    among South Indians. J. Indian Med. Assoc., 39, 1-6

Reznikoff, C.A., Brankow, D.W. & Heidelberger, C. (1973a)
    Establishment and characterization of a cloned line of C3H
    mouse embryo cells sensitive to postconfluence inhibition of
    division. Cancer Res., 33, 3231-3238

Reznikoff, C.A., Bertram, J.S. & Heidelberger, C. (1973b) Quan-
    titative and qualitative studies of chemical transformation
    of cloned C3H mouse embryo cells sensitive to postconfluence
    inhibition of cell division. Cancer Res., 33, 3239-3249

Rhim, J.S., Park, D.K., Weisburger, E.K. & Weisburger, J.A.
    (1974) Evaluation of an in vitro assay system for carcino-
    gens based on a prior infection of rodent cells with non-
    transforming RNA tumor virus. J. natl Cancer Inst., 52,
    1167-1173

Sato, S., Matsushima, T., Tanako, N., Sugimura, T. & Takashima, F. (1973) Hepatic tumors in the guppy (Lebistes reticulatus) induced by aflatoxin B_1, dimethylnitrosamine and 2-acetylaminofluorene. J. natl Cancer Inst., 50, 765-778

Shank, R.C., Bhamarapravati, N., Gordon, J.E. & Wogan, G.N. (1972a) Dietary aflatoxins and human liver cancer. IV. Incidence of primary liver cancer in two municipal populations of Thailand. Food cosmet. Toxicol., 10, 171-179

Shank, R.C., Gordon, G.E., Wogan, G.N., Nondasuta, A. & Subhamani, B. (1972b) Dietary aflatoxins and human liver cancer. III. Field survey of rural Thai families for ingested aflatoxins. Food cosmet. Toxicol., 10, 71-84

Shank, R.C., Wogan, G.N., Gibson, J.B. & Nondasuta, A. (1972c) Dietary aflatoxins and human liver cancer. II. Aflatoxins in market foods and foodstuffs of Thailand and Hong Kong. Food cosmet. Toxicol., 10, 61-69

Shanmugaratnam, K. (1961) Liver cancer and cirrhosis in Singapore. Acta Un. Int. Cancr., 17, 898-902

Snyder, R.L., Tyler, G. & Summers, J. (1982) Chronic hepatitis and hepatocellular carcinoma associated with woodchuck virus. Am. J. Pathol., 197, 422-426

Steinitz, R. (1965) Israel Cancer Registry: Malignant neoplasms in four-year period 1960-1963. Jerusalem, Ministry of Health, Division of Chronic Disease and Rehabilitation, in cooperation with Israel Cancer Association, pp. 1-191

Strong, G.F., Fitts, H.H. & MacPhee, J. (1949) Ann. Intern. Med., 30, 791-798

Styles, J.A. (1977) A method for detecting carcinogenic organic chemicals using mammalian cells in culture. Br. J. Cancer, 36, 558-563

Sudarsanam, D., Kutumbiah, P., Samuel, I. & Gault, E. (1963) Primary carcinoma of the liver. A study of 25 cases proved at postmortem examination. Indian J. Pathol. Bacteriol., 6, 8-18

Summers, J., Smolec, J.M. & Snyder, R.L. (1978) A virus similar to human hepatitis B virus associated with hepatitis and hepatoma in woodchucks. Proc. natl Acad. Sci., 75, 4533-4537

Trichopoulos, D., Violaki, M., Sparros, L. & Xirouchaki, E. (1975) Epidemiology of hepatitis B and primary hepatic carcinoma. Lancet, II, 1038-1039

Tuyns, A.J. & Obradovic, M. (1975) Brief communication: Unexpected high incidence of primary liver cancer in Geneva, Switzerland. J. natl Cancer Inst., 54, 61-64

Uwaifo, A.O., Emerole, G.O., Bababunmi, E.A. & Bassir, O. (1979) Comparative mutagenicity of palmotoxin Bo and aflatoxins B_1 and M_1. J. environ. Pathol. Toxicol., 2, 1099-1108

Uwaifo, A.O. & Bababunmi, E.A. (1979) The reduced mutagenicity of aflatoxin B_1 due to hydroxylation: observations on five Salmonella typhimurium tester strains. Cancer Lett., 7, 221-225

Uwaifo, A.O., Billings, P.C. & Heidelberger, C. (1983) Mutation of Chinese hamster V79 cells and transformation and mutation of mouse fibroblast C3H/10T1/2 clone 8 cells by aflatoxin B_1 and four other furocoumarins isolated from two Nigerian medicinal plants. Cancer Res., 43, 1054-1058

Uwaifo, A.O. & Heidelberger, C. (1983) Photobiological activity of marmesin (5-hydroxyisopropyl-4-5-dihydrofurocoumarin) in Chinese hamster V79 cells. Photochem. Photobiol., 38, 395-398

Van Rensburg, S.J., Van der Watt, J.J., Purchase, I.F.H., Coutinho, L.P. & Markham, R. (1974) Primary liver cancer rate and aflatoxin intake in a high cancer area. S. Afr. Med. J., 48, 2508a-2508d

Vedder, E.B. (1927) J. Am. med. Assoc., 88, 1627-1629

Vesselinovitch, S.D., Mihailovich, N., Wogan, G.N., Lombard, L.S. & Rao, K.V.N. (1972) Aflatoxin B_1, a hepatocarcinogen in the infant mouse. Cancer Res., 32, 2289-2291

Wales, J.H. & Sinnhuber, R.O. (1972) Brief communication: Hepa-
    tomas induced by aflatoxin in the sockeye salmon
    (Oncorhynchus nerka). J. natl Cancer Inst., 48, 1529-1530

Wheeler, L., Halula, M. & Demeo, M. (1981) A comparison of
    aflatoxin B_1-induced cytotoxicity, mutagenicity and prophage
    induction in Salmonella typhimurium mutagen tester strains
    TA1535, TA1538, TA98 and TA100. Mutat. Res., 83, 39-48

Wilbur, D.L., Wood, D.A. & Willet, F.M. (1944) Ann. Intern.
    Med., 20, 453-485

Wogan, G.N. & Newberne, P.M. (1967) Dose-response
    characteristics of aflatoxin B_1 carcinogenesis in the rat.
    Cancer Res., 27, 2370-2376

Wong, J.J. & Hsieh, D.P. (1976) Mutagenicity of aflatoxins
    related to their metabolism and carcinogenic potential.
    Proc. natl Acad. Sci. USA, 73, 2241-2244

ETIOLOGY OF HEPATOCELLULAR CARCINOMA IN AFRICA

C.L.M. Olweny

Harare, Zimbabwe

RESUME

Parmi les facteurs étiologiques du cancer primitif du foie (CPF) survenant en Afrique figurent le virus de l'hépatite B (HBV), l'aflatoxine et probablement la malnutrition. La preuve de l'association du virus HB et du CPF est essentiellement épidémiologique et comprend: (a) la répartition géographique similaire des porteurs chroniques de l'antigène de surface de l'hépatite B (AgHBs) et du CPF; (b) la prévalence accrue des marqueurs d'HBV dans le sérum des patients présentant un CPF par rapport au reste de la population et (c) l'observation selon laquelle l'infection par l'HBV précède le développement de la tumeur et selon laquelle l'infection augmente de plus de 200 fois le risque de CPF.

Les résultats obtenus au laboratoire ont révélé que l'ADN du virus HB est intégré dans le génome cellulaire des patients présentant un CPF. Un programme de vaccination réalisé au Sénégal a montré que le vaccin contre l'hépatite B réduisait l'infection HBV et on peut espérer qu'il entraînera également une diminution des CPF.

Des études menées en Afrique de l'Est ont démontré une corrélation entre la contamination par l'aflatoxine et la prolifération du CPF. Le rôle possible de la malnutrition et/ou de l'alcool est également discuté.

SUMMARY

The important factors in the causation of hepatocellular carcinoma (HCC) in Africa include hepatitis B virus (HBV), aflatoxin and possibly malnutrition. The evidence in support of an association of HBV with HCC is mainly epidemiological and includes: (a) the similarity between the geographical distribution of chronic carriers of hepatitis B surface antigen (HBsAg) and that of HCC; (b) the increased prevalence of HBV markers in the serum of patients with HCC when compared with the general population; and (c) the observation that HBV infection precedes the general development of the tumour and that HBV infection increases the risk of HCC over 200-fold.

Laboratory evidence has shown that HBV DNA is integrated in the host tissue in patients with HCC. A vaccination programme in Senegal showed that hepatitis B vaccine reduced HBV infection and it is hoped that it will eventually lead to a reduction in HCC.

Studies in East Africa have shown a correlation between aflatoxin contamination and the incidence of HCC. The possible roles of malnutrition and/or alcohol are discussed.

INTRODUCTION

African hepatocellular carcinoma (HCC) is characterized by: (a) occurrence at a young age with peak age of onset in the third decade of life; (b) the rapid downhill course with most untreated patients dying within 3 months of diagnosis; (c) the association in most cases with posthepatitic macronodular cirrhosis. This is in contrast to HCC seen in Europe or North America where: (a) the peak age of onset is in the fifth or sixth decade; (b) the tumour appears to grow slowly; (c) the tumour is associated with postalcoholic micronodular cirrhosis.

The etiology of HCC remains uncertain although many possibilities have been suggested, including hepatitis B virus (HBV), hepatotoxins, malnutrition, parasites, haemochromatosis, industrial chemicals and hormones. In Africa, the most important factors in the causation of HCC appear to be HBV, aflatoxin and possibly malnutrition.

HEPATITIS B VIRUS AND HEPATOCELLULAR CARCINOMA

There is a wealth of evidence – principally epidemiological, clinical and experimental – incriminating HBV in the causation of HCC. The epidemiological evidence includes:

(a)   The observation of a similarity between the geographical distribution of chronic carriers of hepatitis B surface antigen (HBsAg) and HCC.

(b)   The increased prevalence of HBV markers in the serum of patients with HCC when compared with the general population (Vogel et al., 1970; Bagshawe et al., 1971).

(c)   The observation that HBV infection precedes the development of the tumour (Beasley et al., 1981).

The most convincing evidence has come from the retrospective study in Taiwan of 22 707 Chinese men followed up for a total of 75 000 man-years. Of these individuals, 3454 (15.2%) were HBsAg-positive. Of the 307 deaths, 41 were due to HCC and 19 to cirrhosis. HCC and cirrhosis thus accounted for 19.5% of deaths and were the commonest cause of death, followed by accidents (11.4%) and ischaemic heart disease (10.7%). Of the deaths due to HCC and cirrhosis, 40 out of 41 were in the group of 3454 who were HBsAg-positive, while only one occurred in the remaining 19 253 who were HBsAg-negative, giving a relative risk of over 200 (Beasley et al., 1981).

The experimental evidence in the main consists of the detection of HBV markers such as HBsAg or viral DNA sequences in tumour tissue. These DNA sequences were originally considered to be non-integrated but more recently the presence of HBV DNA sequences integrated in cellular DNA of human HCC has been reported by several workers (Edman et al., 1980; Chakraborti et al., 1980; Bréchot et al., 1980). It has now been reported that all patients with HCC have integrated HBV DNA (Shafritz et al., 1981; Bréchot et al., 1981).

Integration of HBV DNA in a malignant cell does not necessarily imply that the virus is oncogenic. However, viral transformation is usually associated with integration of viral sequences into host chromosomal DNA. The successful propagation of a human cell line (PLC/PRF/5; Alexander cells) derived from a male patient with HCC from Mozambique has facilitated the study

of HBV and its association with HCC. Alexander cell lines
produce HBsAg identical to that isolated from HBV carriers; they
carry at least 6 HBV genomes per cell integrated into the high-
molecular-weight host DNA and injection of these cells into nude
mice induces the growth of HBsAg-positive tumours (Alexander et
al., 1976).

Another source of evidence comes from observations on woodchucks (or ground hogs, Marmota monax), a small American rodent.
The woodchuck carries a hepatitis virus which is serologically
related to human HBV and which is also integrated into the DNA of
woodchuck HCC tissue (Werner et al., 1979).

However, the final proof that HBV is causatively related to
HCC can only be obtained by intervention. In epidemiology the
best proof of an etiological link between a viral infection and a
tumour would be a decrease in the incidence or actual elimination
of the tumour resulting from successful intervention against the
virus, as has been observed in rodents, birds and primates
following the use of viral vaccines or specific antisera (Heubner
et al., 1976). A vaccination programme was started in 1978 in
Senegal, where HBV infection is endemic and HCC is prevalent
(Goudeau, 1982). Children under 2 years of age were randomly
allocated to groups receiving either hepatitis B (HB) vaccine
(HEVAC B^O) or diphtheria, tetanus, poliomyelitis vaccine (IDA-
DPT^O), both from the Institut Pasteur. Immunization with HB
vaccine was safe and induced development of antibody to HBsAg
(anti-HB) in over 95% of previously seronegative recipients.
After 2 years of follow-up a decrease of 85% in the prevalence of
the HBsAg carrier state in the HB vaccine group as compared with
the control group was observed. Continued surveillance of these
vaccinated children is necessary to determine whether there will
be an observable decline in the prevalence of HCC.

AFLATOXIN

Aflatoxins are a group of compounds produced by the mould
Aspergillus flavus which grows readily on nuts and grains in warm
and humid conditions. A single dose of aflatoxin B_1 is sufficient to induce liver cancer in rats (Newberne & Butler, 1969).
A significant correlation between the location of homes of liver
cancer patients and the distribution of groundnut cultivation in
the West Nile District of Uganda was demonstrated by Korobkin and
Williams. Subsequently Alpert, working on stored foods in

Uganda, concluded that aflatoxin exposure may account for the varying incidence of liver cancer in Uganda (Alpert et al., 1971). In a study carried out in the Muranga District of Kenya, a statistically significant association between levels of ingested aflatoxin and liver cancer was observed (Peers & Linsell, 1973). If aflatoxin does play a role in the pathogenesis of liver cancer, the mechanism of carcinogenesis has yet to be explained. Aflatoxin is also known to be an immuno-suppressive agent (Savel et al., 1970). It is possible that, in Africa, HBV is the initiator and aflatoxin is one of several possible promoters leading to the development of HCC. The final proof of an association between HCC and aflatoxin will depend on intervention. If better food storage that avoids contamination can be achieved, and if this reduced the incidence of HCC in an endemic area, this would certainly be proof of a causal relationship. The FAO/WHO study in Swaziland is therefore of great interest to those interested in aflatoxin and its relationship to HCC.

MALNUTRITION

Foy found that baboons fed on pyridoxine-deficient diets containing no recognizable hepatotoxic substances developed hepatic nodules with histological features of malignancy (Foy et al., 1970). The serum of these animals was positive for alpha-fetoprotein (Foy et al., 1974), and in man this would be strong presumptive evidence of HCC. It is possible that lack of certain essential foods may potentiate the effects of more potent carcinogens. Thus it has been suggested that, in certain experimental animals, protein restriction may potentiate the effect of afla-toxin (Madhavan & Gopalan, 1968). Since protein-energy malnu-trition is rampant in most parts of Africa, it is tempting to speculate on the possible role of kwashiorkor in the development of HCC. However, studies by Cook and Hutt in Uganda failed to demonstrate any evidence of chronic liver disease in children who had recovered from kwashiorkor (Cook & Hutt, 1967) and no direct relationship has been shown to exist between childhood malnutri-tion and subsequent development of HCC. Malnutrition may just be one of the multiple co-factors necessary to promote the proli-feration of cells already transformed, perhaps by HBV.

REFERENCES

Alexander, J.J., Beym, E., Geddes, E. & Lecatsas, G.G. (1976) South Afr. med. J., 50, 2124-2128

Alpert, M.E., Hutt, M.S.R., Wogan, G.N. & Davidson, C.S. (1971) Association between aflatoxin content of food and hepatoma frequency in Uganda. Cancer, 28, 253-260

Bagshawe, A.F., Parker, A.M. & Jindani, A. (1971) Hepatitis associated antigen in liver disease in Kenya. Br. med. J., 1, 88-89

Beasley, R.P., Hwang, L., Lin, C. & Chien, C. (1981) Hepato-cellular carcinoma and hepatitis B virus: a prospective study of 22 707 men in Taiwan. Lancet, 2, 1129-1133

Bréchot, C., Pourcel, C., Louise, A., Rain, B. & Tiollais, P. (1980) Presence of integrated hepatitis B virus DNA sequences in cellular DNA of human hepatocellular carcinoma. Nature, 286, 533-535

Bréchot, C., Hadchouel, M., Scotto, J., Fonck, M., Potet, F., Vyas, G.N. & Tiollais, P. (1981) State of hepatitis B virus DNA in hepatocytes of patients with hepatitis B surface antigen positive and antigen negative liver disease. Proc. natl Acad. Sci. USA, 78, 3906-3910

Chakraborti, P.R., Ruis-Oparo, N., Shouval, D. & Shafritz, D.A. (1980) Identification of integrated hepatitis B virus DNA and expression of viral RNA in an HBsAg producing human hepatocellular carcinoma cell line. Nature, 286, 531-533

Cook, G.C. & Hutt, M.S.R. (1967) The liver after kwashiorkor. Br. med. J. , 3, 454-457

Edman, J.C., Gray, P., Valenzuela, P., Rall, L.B. & Rutter, W.J. (1980) Integration of hepatitis B virus sequences and their expression in a human hepatoma cell. Nature, 286, 535-538

Foy, H., Kondi, A., Linsell, C.A., Parker, A.M. & Sizaret, P. (1970) The alpha$_1$-fetoprotein test in hepatocellular carcinoma. Lancet, 1, 411

Foy, H., Kondi, A., Davies, J.N.P., Anderson, B., Parker, A., Preston, J. & Peers, F.G. (1974) Histologic changes in livers of pyridoxine-deprived baboons - Relation to alpha$_1$ fetoprotein and liver cancer in Africa. J. natl Cancer Inst., 53, 1295-1311

Goudeau, A. (1982) Prevention of hepatocellular carcinoma by active immunization against hepatitis B. Br. med. J., 285, 1044-1045

Huebner, R.J., Gilden, R.V., Lane, W.T., Toni, R., Trimmer, R.W. & Hill, P.R. (1976) Suppression of murine type-C RNA virogenes by type-specific oncornavirus vaccines: Prospects for prevention of cancer. Proc. natl Acad. Sci. USA, 73, 620-624

Madhavan, T.V. & Gopalan, C. (1968) The effect of dietary protein on carcinogenesis of aflatoxin. Arch. Pathol., 85, 133-137

Newberne, P.M. & Butler, W.H. (1969) Acute and chronic effects of aflatoxin on the liver of domestic and laboratory animals: a review. Cancer Res., 29, 236-250

Peers, F.G. & Linsell, C.A. (1973) Dietary aflatoxins and liver cancer - A population based study in Kenya. Br. J. Cancer, 27, 473-484

Savel, M. (1970) Proc. Soc. exp. Med. Biol., 143, 1112

Shafritz, D.A., Shouval, D., Sherman, H.I., Hadziyannis, S.J. & Kew, M.C. (1981) Integration of hepatitis virus DNA into the genome of liver cells in chronic liver disease and hepatocellular carcinoma. New Engl. J. Med., 305, 1067-1073

Vogel, C.L., Antony, P.P., Mody, N. & Barker, L.F. (1970) Hepatitis associated antigen in Uganda patients with hepatocellular carcinoma. Lancet, 2, 621-624

Werner, B.G., Smolec, J.M., Snydes, R. & Summer, J. (1979) Serological relationship of woodchuck hepatitis virus to hepatitis B virus. J. Virol., 32, 314-322

EPIDÉMIOLOGIE DU CANCER PRIMITIF DU FOIE AU SÉNÉGAL

P. Touré

Institut du Cancer
Dakar

RESUME

Le cancer primitif du foie représente la tumeur maligne la plus fréquente au Sénégal. L'incidence est évaluée à 22,3 pour 100 000 chez l'homme et 8,3 pour 100 000 chez la femme. Cette estimation repose sur une série de 228 cas enregistrés de 1969 à 1971 dans les laboratoires d'Anatomie Pathologique de Dakar.

La répartition ethnique de ces cas suggère une nette prédominance dans les ethnies d'origine soudano-sahélienne (Ouolofs et Sérères) par rapport aux ethnies métissées (Peulhs) ou d'origine berbère (Maures). Cette constatation se vérifie même lorsque ces différentes ethnies cohabitent dans la même région, ce qui est le cas dans la vallée du fleuve Sénégal.

Du point de vue étiologique, l'accent est mis sur l'hépatite virale, dont une étude épidémiologique précise est faite. La prévention de l'hépatite B est évoquée et l'expérience de la vaccination au Sénégal décrite.

SUMMARY

Hepatocellular carcinoma is the most common malignant tumour in Senegal, the incidence being estimated at 22.3 per 100 000 among men and 8.3 per 100 000 among women. This estimate was made on the basis of a series of 228 cases registered between 1969 and 1971 at the Pathological Anatomy Laboratories in Dakar.

The ethnic distribution of these cases indicates a clear predominance among Sudano-Sahelian groups (Wolofs and Sérers) in comparison with groups of mixed race (Peulhs) or of Berber origin (Moors). This difference holds true even when the different

ethnic groups live in the same region, as in the valley of the
Senegal River.

An epidemiological study indicates a hepatitis viral
etiology. The prevention of hepatitis B is described and the
results given of a vaccination programme in Senegal.

INTRODUCTION

Le cancer primitif du foie compte parmi les cancers les plus
communs dans les régions OMS de l'Asie du Sud-Est et du
Pacifique-Occidental et représente probablement la plus fréquente
des tumeurs malignes en Afrique sub-saharienne, particulièrement
dans le Sud-Est. Des données épidémiologiques récentes fournies
par des études cas-témoins et des études de cohortes, ainsi que
certaines enquêtes de laboratoire indiquent qu'il existe un
rapport étiologique homogène et spécifique entre le virus de
l'hépatite B (HBV) et le cancer primitif du foie (CPF). Ceci est
d'un intérêt capital, car on entrevoit pour la première fois la
possibilité de prévenir un cancer humain grâce à la vaccination.

Nous allons ici faire la synthèse des études qui ont permis
d'évaluer l'incidence du cancer primitif du foie au Sénégal, et
comparer les résultats à ceux obtenus pour différents pays
d'Afrique. Nous allons également discuter, à partir des études
publiées, la distribution de ces cancers en fonction des facteurs
ethniques et raciaux, de l'âge et du sexe. Puis nous évoquerons
les études montrant la relation entre le virus de l'hépatite B et
le cancer primitif du foie, et l'étude réalisée chez les femmes
enceintes et les jeunes enfants, qui permet de préciser les modalités de transmission du virus HB, et d'envisager une prévention
vaccinale.

INCIDENCE DU CANCER PRIMITIF DU FOIE

Au Sénégal, malgré l'insuffisance et la répartition inégale
des moyens diagnostiques, il ressort des nombreuses études cliniques, épidémiologiques et anatomo-pathologiques consacrées aux
cancers, que le CPF est de loin le cancer le plus fréquent.
Quenum et coll. (1973) ont entrepris de 1969 à 1971 une mesure de
l'incidence en enregistrant tous les cas diagnostiqués dans les
laboratoires d'anatomie pathologique de Dakar: celui du Centre
Hospitalo-Universitaire (Dr C. Quenum), celui de l'Institut

Pasteur (Dr Sarrat) et celui de l'Hôpital Principal (Dr Meydat, puis Dr Varieras). Ce registre hospitalier établi avec l'aide du Centre International de Recherche sur le Cancer (CIRC) a permis de recenser 4164 cancers. Parmi ceux-ci, seuls 1893 ont été retenus pour la mesure de l'incidence. Ces cas se rapportaient à des résidents de la province du Cap-Vert (700 000 habitants), région Ouest du Sénégal constituée et organisée autour de la capitale Dakar. Elle compte à elle seule 2678 lits d'hôpitaux (38 lits pour 100 000 habitants) et 217 médecins (3,1 pour 100 000 habitants), ce qui correspond à une couverture sanitaire satisfaisante. Les taux d'incidence obtenus sont de 22,3 pour 100 000 habitants pour le sexe masculin et de 8,3 pour 100 000 habitants pour le sexe féminin. Les taux standardisés figurent au Tableau 1 ainsi que ceux obtenus de la même façon dans plusieurs autres régions d'Afrique (Doll et coll., 1970), auxquels ils peuvent être comparés. Pour le sexe masculin le taux de 22,3 pour 100 000 habitants est proche des taux observés à Durban (20,0), en Afrique du Sud; il n'est pas aussi élevé que ceux de Bulawayo (31,2) ni de Maputo (106,7). Par contre, il est plus élevé qu'à Johannesburg (13,7), à Ibadan (7,8) et à Kampala (5,8). Pour le sexe féminin, les taux sont basés sur des nombres moins élevés et sont donc plus difficiles à interpréter. Le taux de 8,3 pour 100 000 habitants se situe au-dessous des taux de Maputo et de Bulawayo mais au-dessus des autres.

Les taux d'incidence retrouvés à Dakar doivent être considérés comme des taux minimaux pour de nombreuses raisons: il est peu probable que tous les malades de la région atteints de cancer du foie aient été hospitalisés, car nombre d'entre eux reçoivent dans leur village un traitement traditionnel. A l'inverse, il arrive que des malades à un stade avancé de leur cancer ne puissent pas être admis dans les services hospitaliers déjà surencombrés. Selon Quenum et coll. (1973), les taux d'incidence seraient très voisins de 30 pour 100 000 pour le sexe masculin et de 12 pour 100 000 pour le sexe féminin, estimations qui n'ont rien de déraisonnable et qui sont vraisemblablement encore au-dessous de la réalité. Sankale (1974) quant à lui, estime l'incidence à 70 pour 100 000 habitants. Ces données permettent de confirmer que la région du Cap-Vert se situe, avec les régions de Maputo (Mozambique) et de Bulawayo (Zimbabwe), parmi les trois régions du monde où l'incidence du CPF dépasse largement 20 pour 100 000 chez l'homme et 8 pour 100 000 chez la femme.

Tableau 1. Taux d'incidence de CPF dans divers pays d'Afrique (d'après Doll et coll., 1970; et Quenum et coll., 1973)

	KAMPALA (Ouganda)	IBADAN (Nigeria)	MAPUTO (Mozambique)	BULAWAYO (Zimbabwe)	JOHANNESBURG (Af. Sud)	DURBAN (Natal, Bantous, Af. Sud)	DAKAR (Cap-Vert, Sénégal)
Années d'enquête	1954-1960	1960-65	1950-60	1963-67	1953-55	1964-66	1969-71
	7	6	5	5	3	3	3
Nombre de cas							
M	45	108	264	100	113	140	173
F	10	26	61	14	25	21	55
Taux d'incidence annuelle pour 100 000 hts							
M	5,8	7,8	106,7	31,2	13,7	20,0	22,3
F	2,1	2,9	30,0	18,3	5,6	4,7	8,3

Si l'on compare l'incidence des cancers du foie dans la région du Cap-Vert à celle observée dans les autres régions du Sénégal, il apparait que la fréquence relative de CPF est plus élevée dans la région de Thiès et un peu moins élevée dans la région de Diourbel et beaucoup moins élevée dans les autres régions du pays. Le groupe ethnique Ouolof est plus atteint que les groupes Soudaniens (Bambara, Sarakolé) et peut-être Sérères et Casamançais chez les hommes. Les Toucouleurs paraissent relativement plus épargnés que les autres et les Maures beaucoup plus encore. Toutes ces données semblent indiquer, outre des différences entre Sénégalais, des variations suivant les régions et suivant les ethnies.

FACTEURS ETHNIQUES ET RACIAUX

L'idée d'une prédisposition raciale évoquée au Sénégal depuis 1962 par Payet et coll. (1975) semble corroborée par les constatations faites au Nord du pays, de part et d'autre du fleuve Sénégal. Sur chacune des rives du fleuve, il apparaît que les populations Maures de race blanche présentent infiniment moins de cancers primitifs du foie que les Noirs Africains vivant dans les mêmes régions. Cela paraît d'autant plus troublant que les deux types de populations, noire et blanche, vivent dans des cadres écologiques et sociaux absolument identiques.

Le Tableau 2 montre de façon indiscutable la grande fréquence de CPF chez les Noirs Sénégalais vivant dans cette région, en opposition avec sa rareté chez les Maures.

Tableau 2. Répartition des CPF aux confins Sénégalo-Mauritaniens (Hôpital de Saint-Louis)

Année	Nombre total des cancers	Nombre total des CPF	CPF (Maures)
1970	85	26	0
1971	90	43	0
1972	116	64	0

Il était intéressant de vérifier si cette différence coinci-"dait avec une différence de portage de l'antigène HBs dans les deux populations. Les résultats figurent au Tableau 3. La différence n'est pas significative.

Tableau 3. Sujets AgHBs positifs chez les Maures et les Noirs Africains

	Nombre de sujets	Nombre de sujets AgHBs +	% AgHBs +
Maures	81	3	3,7
Noirs Africains	369	23	6,2

NS

En fait, parmi les Maures AgHBs-positifs, 2 sur 3 sont métissés au vu de l'examen clinique et de leurs marqueurs génétiques
déterminés par l'étude allotypique des groupes Gm. Il reste,
après élimination des sujets métissés (Tableau 4) un seul sujet
Maure AgHBs positif sur 81. La différence est significative
(p<0,02).

Tableau 4.   Sujets AgHBs-positifs (après élimination des
Métissés)

	Nombre de sujets	Nombre de sujets AgHBs +	% AgHBs +
Maures	81	1	1,2
Noirs Africains	369	23	6,2

p<0,02

Le comportement des deux populations vis-à-vis du CPF est
donc parfaitement caractéristique d'une aptitude particulière des
Sénégalais Noirs Africains devant ce type de cancer, et semble
liée à une contamination par le virus HB.

AGE - SEXE

A Dakar le CPF se développe aux environs de 36 ans pour les hommes et 34 pour les femmes. Diop et coll. (1981) ont étudié la répartition de 2 000 CPF en fonction de l'âge, à partir des 857 cas de leur série et des cas provenant des séries de Bourgouin (1967), de Daouda (1979) et de Maupas et coll. (1979) (Tableau 5).

Tableau 5. Répartition de 2 000 CPF en fonction de l'âge (d'après Diop et coll. ,1981))

		< 10	11-20	21-30	31-40	41-50	51-60	61-70	71-80	Total
	Age									
CPF	Nombre de cas	0	96	448	560	497	277	79	43	2000
	%	0	4,8	22,4	28,0	24,8	13,8	3,9	2,1	100
Distribution de la population normale selon l'âge	Nbre x %		32,5	23,0	18,1	10,7	7,8	4,4	2,2	1,4	100

Le cancer primitif du foie est rare chez l'enfant à Dakar. Ainsi Bergeret (1946) sur 147 cas colligés de 1937 à 1945, en trouve un seul chez un enfant de 11 ans. Dans une série de 1 667 cas collectés entre 1951 et 1965, Bourgouin (1967) en relève seulement 5 cas chez des enfants. De leur côté, Quenum & N'Diye (1971) lors d'une enquête couvrant la période de 1956 à 1971 retrouvent 9 cancers du foie chez des enfants, dont 8 cancers primitifs du foie et un hépatoblastome chez un enfant de 2 ans.

La prédominance masculine est notée au Sénégal ainsi que dans les autres pays du monde. Le sex-ratio varie selon les études de 3 à 15. Des résultats cumulés portant sur 3 355 cas donnent un rapport de 4,1 (Tableau 6).

FACTEURS ETIOLOGIQUES

Nous n'évoquerons que les relations entre le virus de l'hépatite B et le cancer primitif du foie. Dès 1956, Payet (Payet et coll., 1967, 1972) avançait l'hypothèse d'une filiation hépatite-cirrhose-cancer primitif du foie. Cette hypothèse, fondée sur des observations cliniques et anatomo-pathologiques réalisées à Dakar, est à l'origine de nombreux travaux effectués ultérieurement au Sénégal avec l'équipe de Maupas de l'Institut de Virologie de Tours (Maupas et coll., 1977; 1979; 1981) en collaboration avec la Faculté de Médecine et de Pharmacie de Dakar. Les études ont montré que la prévalence de l'antigène HBs est d'environ 12%, mais qu'en réalité plus de 90% de la population du Sénégal est contaminée par le virus de l'hépatite B si l'on tient compte de tous les marqueurs de virus.

Tableau 6. Répartition du CPF en fonction du sexe

Auteurs	Années	Nbre total de cas	Hommes		Femmes		Sex-ratio
			Nbre	%	Nbre	%	
Bergeret (1946)	1937-1941	147	138	93,8	9	6,2	15,3
Bourgouin (1967)	1951-1965	1 667	1 302	78,1	365	21,8	3,5
Quenum et coll. (1973)	1969-1971	228	173	75,9	55	24,1	3,1
Michon et coll. (1975)	1972-1974	165	127	77,0	38	23,0	3,5
Maupas et coll. (1979)	1975	291	232	79,7	59	20,3	3,9
Diop et coll. (1981)	1976-1979	857	727	84,8	130	15,2	5,5
TOTAL	1937-1979	3 355	2 699	80,5	656	19,5	4,1

Les résultats des études sur les marqueurs du virus sont mentionnés au Tableau 7.

Tableau 7. Fréquences comparées des marqueurs de HBV chez les sujets atteints de CPF et chez des sujets témoins

Pays	Chercheurs	Nbre de sujets	AgHBs + (%)		Anticorps Anti-HBs + (%)		Anticorps Anti HBc + (%)	
			CPF	Témoins	CPF	Témoins	CPF	Témoins
Sénégal	Prince et coll. (1975)	CPF: 165 Témoins 432	61,2	11,4	18,2	43,2	-	-
	Maupas et coll. (1977)	CPF: 291 Témoins 143	51,9	11,9	16,1	36,4	87,3	25,9
Mozambique	Reys & Soquein (1974)	CPF: 25	52,0	8,4	12,0	42,2	-	-
Afrique du Sud	Kew et coll. (1979)	CPF: 289	61,6	11,3	17	41,7	89	37,5

Il apparaît à l'évidence que l'antigène HBs est beaucoup plus fréquent chez les sujets atteints de CPF. Il en est de même de l'anticorps anti-HBc qui est également un marqueur de l'infection par HBV. Par contre les anticorps anti-HBs qui jouent un rôle protecteur sont moins fréquents chez les sujets atteints de CPF que chez les témoins.

Etude de l'infection HBV chez les femmes enceintes et les jeunes enfants

Une autre étude a été entreprise au Sénégal afin d'évaluer l'incidence de l'infection chez les enfants de 0 à 13 ans et chez les femmes enceintes (Barin et coll. 1981). Elle avait également pour but de définir la population à risque en vue de la vaccination et de préciser le mode de transmission du virus. L'étude transversale de l'infection a permis d'identifier les périodes de contaminations maximales chez l'enfant, les modalités de transmission mère-enfant, et de préciser comment on devient porteur chronique de l'antigène HBs.

Cette étude a été menée dans l'arrondissement de Niakhar dans le département de Fatick (Région de Sine Saloum à 150 kilomètres de Dakar). La population de cet Arrondissement est de 39 213 habitants, répartis à peu près également dans trois communautés rurales, comprenant au total 65 villages. Cette population, à majorité Sérère est très sédentaire.

Marqueurs du virus HB chez l'enfant.- La population étudiée comporte 2 212 enfants âgés de 0 à 13 ans (1 134 garçons et 1 078 filles) dont 1 852 âgés de 0 à 2 ans et 360 de plus de 2 ans. Le Tableau 8 résume les résultats globaux.

Tableau 8. Fréquence des marqueurs du virus HB chez l'enfant de 0 à 13 ans (Barin et coll., 1981)

Age	Nombre	AgHBs		Anticorps Anti-HBs		Anticorps Anti-HBc		Marqueurs HBV (%)
		Nbre	%	Nbre	%	Nbre	%	
<1 mois	398	5	1,3	121	30,4	254	63,8	95,5
1-6 mois	358	12	3,3	41	11,5	145	40,5	55,3
7-12 mois	480	27	5,6	21	4,4	46	9,6	19,6
13-18 mois	292	39	13,4	14	4,8	31	10,6	28,8
19-24 mois	324	55	17,0	34	10,5	33	10,2	37,7
2-3 ans	74	8	10,8	6	8,1	36	48,6	67,5
4-5 ans	44	6	13,6	8	18,2	19	43,2	75,0
6-7 ans	50	16	32,0	13	26,0	11	22,0	80,0
8-9 ans	64	11	17,2	26	40,6	14	21,9	79,7
10-11 ans	94	17	18,1	41	43,6	23	24,5	86,2
12-13 ans	34	4	11,8	20	58,8	7	20,6	91,2
TOTAL	2212	200	9,0	345	15,5	619	27,9	52,6

Ainsi:

- A la naissance, 95,5% des enfants possèdent au moins un marqueur du virus HB, 30,4% possèdent des anticorps anti-HBs et 63,8% possèdent seulement des anticorps anti-HBc.

- Une première 'vague' d'infection se produit à partir de 6 mois et à l'âge de 2 ans, 17% des enfants sont AgHBs-positifs. La prévalence de l'antigène HBs augmente régulièrement pendant les deux premières années de la vie, doublant pratiquement tous les 6 mois. Dans cette tranche d'âge il est à noter que seulement 10,5% des enfants possèdent des anticorps anti-HBs.

- Une deuxième vague d'infection se produit vers 6-7 ans, au moment de l'entrée à l'école: 32% des enfants sont alors AgHBs positifs.

- A l'âge de 13 ans, 91,2% de la population enfantine a été en contact avec le virus et possède au moins un marqueur HBV; 11,8% des enfants sont alors AgHBs-positifs et 58,8% sont anti-corps anti-HBs positifs.

Ces résultats démontrent l'importance de la contamination précoce chez l'enfant dans le portage chronique de l'antigène HBs.

Marqueurs du virus HB chez la femme enceinte et le nouveau-né.-

Etude transversale: La recherche des marqueurs du virus HB a été réalisée chez 765 femmes enceintes âgées de 15 à 40 ans (groupe A), et chez 400 mères et leurs nouveaux-nés (Groupe B).

- Dans le groupe A: 89,3% des femmes possèdent au moins un des marqueurs HBV, 13,3% possèdent l'antigène HBs et 43,5% possèdent des anticorps anti-HBs.

La fréquence des anticorps anti-HBs ne diffère pas signi-ficativement en fonction de l'âge; il en est de même des anti-corps anti-HBc. Par contre, l'antigénémie HBs diminue avec l'âge: 14,5% des femmes de moins de 30 ans sont AgHBs-positives, contre 3,6% seulement des femmes de plus de 30 ans.

- Dans le groupe B: 1,2% seulement de nouveaux-nés sont AgHBs positifs; 9,8% des mères qui possèdent l'AgHBs le trans-mettent à leur enfant. Cette transmission verticale est fonction de la présence de l'antigène HBe ou d'anticorps anti-HBe chez la mère. La recherche des marqueurs HBe chez 20 mères Ag-HBs-positives montre que le risque de transmission de l'antigène HBs est 8 fois plus grand quand la mère est également AgHBe positive que lorsqu'elle est anticorps anti-HBe-positive; 29,8% des nouveaux-nés sont anti-HBs-positifs. La transmission verticale des anticorps anti-HBs se fait dans 71,3% des cas.

Etude longitudinale: Parmi les enfants sur lesquels un pré-lèvement a été effectué à la naissance, 115 ont été suivis pen-dant 3 à 15 mois. L'incidence annuelle de l'antigénémie HBs chez les enfants nés de mère AgHBs- positive est de 26,4%. Ces enfants ont un risque d'infection 5 fois plus élevé que ceux nés de mères Ag-HBs-négatives.

En résumé, cette étude prospective où tous les marqueurs du
virus HB ont été recherchés par des méthodes très sensibles
montre que l'hépatite B est un véritable problème de santé publique: en effet, 13% de la population est Ag-HBs-positive et près
de 90% possède un marqueur d'infection ancienne ou active.

Cette infection survient très tôt dans la vie et à l'âge de
13 ans, la prévalence de l'hépatite B est la même que dans la
population adulte. L'infection se produit de façon massive à
deux moments de la vie: entre 6 et 24 mois, au moment où
l'enfant n'est plus protégé par les anticorps maternels, et
ensuite vers 6-7 ans au moment de l'entrée à l'école. La transmission verticale est démontrée, c'est la conséquence à la fois
d'une transmission transplacentaire (enfant AgHBs positif à la
naissance) et plus fréquemment d'une infection périnatale.

REFERENCES

Barin, F., Perrin, J., Chotard, J., Denis, F., N'Doye, R., Diop
    Mar, I., Chiron, J.P., Coursaget, P., Goudeau, A. & Maupas,
    P. (1981) Cross-sectional and longitudinal epidemiology of
    hepatitis in Senegal. Prog. Med. Virol., 27, 148-162

Bergeret, C. (1946) Le cancer primitif du foie à Dakar. Bull.
    Med. A.O.F., 3, 5

Bourgouin, J.J. (1967) Le Cancer Primitif du Foie à Dakar, Thèse
    de Médecine, Dakar, No. 10

Daouda, S. (1979) Profil radio-isotopique du cancer primitif du
    foie au Sénégal, Thèse de Médecine, Dakar

Diop, B., Denis, F. & Maupas, P. (1981) Epidémiologie du cancer
    primitif du foie au Sénégal. Méd. Afr. Noire, 28, 217-223

Doll, R., Muir, C. & Waterhouse, J., eds (1970) Cancer Incidence
    in Five Continents, Berlin, Springer Verlag

Kew, M.C., Desmyter, J., Bradhouve, A.F. & MacNab, G. (1979)
    Hepatitis B virus infection in Southern African Blacks with
    hepatocellular cancer. J. natl Cancer Inst., 62, 517-520

Maupas, P., Coursaget, P., Gaudeau, A., Drucker, J., Sankalé, M., Linhard, J. & Dieholt, G. (1977) Hepatitis B virus and primary liver carcinoma: evidences for an affiliation of hepatitis B, cirrhosis and primary liver cancer. Ann. Microbiol., 128, 245-253

Maupas, P., Coursaget, P., Goudeau, M., Drucker, J., Perrin, J., Raynaud, B., Diop Mar, I., Denis, F. & Chiron, J.P. (1979) Cahiers Méd., 5, 563-572

Maupas, P., Diop Mar, I., Denis, F., Chiron, J.P., Barin, F., Perrin, J., Chotard, J., Goudeau, A., Coursaget, P. & Ndoye, R. (1981) Vaccination contre l'hépatite en zone endémique (Sénégal). Med. Afr. Noire, 28, 249-262

Michon, J., Prince, A.M., Szmuness, W., Demaille, J., Diebolt, G., Linhart, J., Quenum, C. & Sankale, M. (1975) Cancer primitif du foie et infection par hépatite B au Sénégal. Comparaison des sujets cancéreux avec deux groupes témoins. Biomed., 23, 263-266

Payet, M., Sankale, M., Pene, P. & Bourgeade, A. (1967) A propos des corrélations entre la cirrhose commune de l'Africain, l'hépatite virale et le cancer primitif du foie. Med. Afr. Noire, 14, 571-572

Payet, M., Saimot, G., Menache, D. et coll. (1972) Antigène, Australie et affections hépatiques chroniques chez l'Africain de l'Ouest. Ann. Méd. int., 23, 175-179

Payet, M., Sankale, M., Saimot, G., Larouze, B. & Brochard, C. (1975) Facteurs étiologiques du cancer primitif du foie. Dans 40ème Congrès Français de Médecine Interne, Dakar, 1-4 Décembre 1975, Paris, Masson

Prince, A.M., Szmuness, W., Michon, J., Demaille, T., Dieholt, G., Linhard, J., Quenum, C. & Sankale, M. (1975) A case-control study of the association between primary liver cancer and hepatitis B infection in Senegal. Int. J. Cancer, 16, 376-383

Quenum, C. & N'Diye (1971) Etude de 175 cas de cancer de l'enfant observés à l'hôpital Le Dentec. Bull. Soc. Afr. Noire langue franç., 16, 94-101

Quenum, C., Tuyns, A., Leblanc, L. & Sankale, M. (1973) Essai
    de détermination de l'incidence du cancer primitif du foie
    dans la région du Cap-Vert. Med. Afr. Noire, 20, 27-35

Reys, L.L. & Soqueiru, O.A. (1974) Detection of Australia anti-
    gen (HBAg) in blood donors and hepatoma patients in Mosambi-
    que. S. Afr. med. J., 48, 267-269

Sankale, M. (1974) L'hépatome malin de l'Africain. Rev. Prat.,
    24, 3023-3035

CANCER PRIMITIF DU FOIE: SITUATION ACTUELLE AU ZAÏRE

M.M.M.A. Mpat

Kinshasa, Zaire

SUMMARY

An analysis is given of all cases of hepatocellular carcinoma notified between 1 January 1980 and 31 December 1983 at two hospitals in Kinshasa (Zaïre).

This cancer occurs most frequently in males between 20 and 49 years of age. It occurs much less often in women and usually at a later age.

The white population of Zaïre is not affected by hepatocellular carcinoma.

RESUME

Les cas de cancer primitif du foie (CPF) enregistrés entre le 1er janvier 1980 et le 31 décembre 1983 dans deux services hospitaliers de Kinshasa (Zaïre) ont été analysés.

Le CPF est prédominant chez les sujets de sexe masculin: chez eux, il se développe avec une fréquence élevée entre 20 et 49 ans. Chez les femmes, le CPF est beaucoup moins fréquent, et survient généralement à un âge plus avancé.

Par contre, la population blanche vivant au Zaïre est épargnée par ce cancer.

INTRODUCTION

Au Zaïre, le cancer primitif du foie (CPF) est certainement le cancer qui entraîne le plus grand nombre de décès chez les sujets de sexe masculin. Cette fréquence anormalement élevée des cancers du foie avait déjà été signalée dès 1919 par Monchet et Gérard.

Le cancer est cependant une maladie beaucoup moins bien connue que les endémies séculaires spécifiques de la pathologie tropicale qui frappent le Zaïre. Le dépistage systématique des cancers y est pour le moment impossible, du fait des énormes investissements financiers que cela exige, de l'insuffisance en nombre du personnel technique, et des difficultés d'accès à des sources d'information fiables.

Face à ces difficultés qui s'opposent à l'obtention de données épidémiologiques statistiquement valables pour les différents cancers observés au Zaïre, nous avons tenté l'étude des cancers primitifs du foie à partir des cas diagnostiqués au cours des consultations de Médecine Interne de deux services hospitaliers de la ville de Kinshasa.

Nous avons cherché à évaluer, non seulement la fréquence du CPF dans le pays, mais aussi ses variations en fonction du type histologique, du sexe, de l'âge et des conditions socio-économiques des patients.

MATERIEL ET METHODES

Nous avons utilisé les registres des services de Médecine Interne et d'Anatomie Pathologique de l'Hôpital Mama Yemo et de la Clinique Ngaliema (Kinshasa). Ces deux services hospitaliers ont des recrutements différents, les malades soignés à la Clinique Ngaliema ayant généralement un niveau socio-économique supérieur à celui des malades de l'Hôpital Mama Yemo. Ont été inclus dans notre série les cas de cancer enregistrés entre le 1er janvier 1980 et le 31 décembre 1983.

RESULTATS

Durant les quatre années d'étude, 217 cas de cancer primitif du foie ont été enregistrés: 182 à l'hôpital Mama Yemo, et 35 à la Clinique Ngaliema.

Les résultats ont été analysés en fonction du sexe et de l'âge des patients:

- à l'hôpital Mama Yemo, 158 cas de CPF ont été enregistrés chez des hommes et 24 chez des femmes. Une seule avait moins de 50 ans (35 ans); toutes les autres avaient plus de 55 ans; la plupart avaient entre 60 et 70 ans.

- à la Clinique Ngaliema, 8 CPF ont été diagnostiqués chez des femmes et 27 chez des hommes. Quatre des femmes atteintes de CPF avaient moins de 51 ans. Les quatre autres avaient plus de 56 ans.

Par contre, dans les deux séries, chez les sujets de sexe masculin, le CPF se manifeste avec une fréquence élevée entre 20 et 49 ans.

Ainsi, au Zaïre, le CPF est donc une maladie qui frappe les jeunes adultes de sexe masculin. Chez les femmes, le CPF est une maladie des personnes âgées. Ce cancer est rare chez les enfants: 10 seulement des sujets atteints avaient moins de 10 ans.

Il est à noter que la population blanche semble épargnée par le CPF, et que la fréquence de ce cancer paraît diminuer chez les Zaïrois en fonction de l'amélioration de leur niveau de vie socio-économique. Ce fait est illustré par les fréquences respectives des cas de CPF observés à l'Hôpital Mama Yemo (hôpital populaire) et la Clinique Ngaliema, fréquentée par une population plus aisée. Les renseignements obtenus sur les résidences des malades atteints de CPF sont venus confirmer cette observation.

DISCUSSION

L'interprétation des données d'incidence du CPF en milieu
zaïrois est particulièrement délicate, car il est difficile de
collecter tous les cas de cancer, et de définir la population
concernée. De plus, des questions se posent quant à la précision
des informations recueillies:

- Comme dans beaucoup de pays africains, la plupart des
sujets âgés ne connaissent pas avec précision leur date de naissance, et la détermination de leur âge pose quelquefois des
problèmes. Mais dans l'ensemble, ces imprécisions n'ont que peu
d'effet sur l'évaluation des taux d'incidence, qui sont évalués
par groupes d'âge de 10 ans.

- La qualité de résident a été réservée, lors de l'étude aux
sujets installés depuis plus d'un an dans la région urbaine de
Kinshasa. Par contre, les dossiers à notre disposition ne nous
ont pas permis de connaître systématiquement l'origine ethnique
des sujets étudiés.

- La Confirmation anatomo-pathologique du diagnostic de CPF
a pu être fournie dans 85% des cas.

Ces résultats ont été comparés à ceux obtenus par Ngala
(1976) lors d'une étude des tumeurs malignes diagnostiquées de
1967 à 1972 dans les cliniques universitaires. Cette étude
montre également une fréquence très élevée des CPF chez les
sujets de sexe masculin: 104 cas de CPF sur 239 cancers.

Chez les femmes, ces cancers sont nettement moins fréquents
(15 cas sur 151 cancers), et viennent après les cancers du col
utérin (63 cas sur 161) et les cancers du sein (35 cas).

Le CPF représente environ 30% des tumeurs solides rencontrées au Zaïre, d'après la série de Ngala. Chez l'homme, il
représente 43,3% de l'ensemble des tumeurs; alors que chez la
femme, il ne représente que 6,2% des cancers. Le CPF est donc 7
fois plus fréquent chez l'homme que chez la femme.

La fréquence des CPF semble en augmentation depuis l'époque
coloniale, comme en témoignent les publications de Monchet et
Gérard, de Thys (1957), de Ngala et notre étude en cours: Thys
(1957) a enregistré 258 CPF en 16 ans, soit une moyenne annuelle
de 18 cas. Dans sa série portant sur 6 ans, Ngala a enregistré

119 cas de CPF, soit une moyenne annuelle de 19 cas. Dans notre étude, la moyenne annuelle est de 39 cas pour l'Hôpital Mama Yemo, et de 8,7 cas pour la Clinique Ngaliema.

Deux hypothèses peuvent rendre compte de l'incidence élevée des cancers primitifs du foie dans les pays africains. L'une implique l'intoxication par les aflatoxines, l'autre l'infection par le virus de l'hépatite B.

Si le rôle étiologique du virus de l'hépatite B se confirme, il est certain que la vaccination représentera la meilleure stratégie de lutte contre le cancer primitif du foie.

REFERENCES

Monchet, R.R. & Gerard, P. (1919) Contribution à l'étude des tumeurs chez les Noirs d'Afrique Centrale. Bull. Soc. Path. Exot., 12, 567-577

Thys, A. (1957) Considérations sur les tumeurs maligne des indigènes du Congo Belge et du Rwanda-Burundi. A propos de 2546 cas. Ann. Soc. belge Med. Trop., 37, 483-514

LE CANCER À MADAGASCAR

J.J. Séraphin

SUMMARY

Available data on cancer rates in Madagascar are given. Cervical cancer is the most common, accounting for 28% of diagnosed tumours and 47% of genital tumours in women. It occurs most often in women of about 40 years of age. Penile cancer represents 5.2% of male tumours but occurs at different rates in various ethnic groups.

Kaposi's sarcoma is rare in Madagascar. Equally hepato-cellular carcinoma occurs at a low incidence in this country and is found most frequently in males over the age of 40 years.

Cancer control programmes and the problems they encounter are also discussed.

RESUME

Les données épidémiologiques disponibles sur les cancers observés à Madagascar sont exposées.

Le cancer du col de l'utérus est le cancer le plus fréquent. Il représente 28% des tumeurs diagnostiquées, et 47% des tumeurs génitales de la femme. Il se développe généralement chez des femmes d'une quarantaine d'années.

Le cancer du pénis représente 5,2% des tumeurs masculines. La fréquence de ce cancer varie avec les ethnies.

Le sarcome de Kaposi est rare à Madagascar. De même, le cancer primitif du foie est peu répandu à Madagascar. Il survient le plus souvent chez des sujets de sexe masculin, âgés de plus de quarante ans.

Les stratégies de lutte contre le cancer, ainsi que les différents problèmes auxquels elles se heurtent sont discutés.

A Madagascar, comme dans tous les pays en voie de développement, l'importance de la maladie cancéreuse n'est pas bien connue et de toute façon, le cancer ne constitue pas une des priorités de la Santé Publique. L'insuffisance des moyens de diagnostic (Laboratoires d'Anatomie-Pathologie et de Virologie) et des structures de recherche, ainsi que l'insuffisance en personnel spécialisé ne permettent pas de connaître de façon précise la situation en ce domaine.

Néanmoins, ce bref aperçu essaiera de situer les données nosologiques et épidémiologiques et d'envisager les moyens disponibles pour entreprendre le traitement et la lutte contre le cancer.

En 25 ans (de 1954 à 1978), le laboratoire de l'Institut Pasteur de Madagascar (seul laboratoire équipé de l'Ile pour les examens anatomo pathologiques) a observé 9 538 tumeurs malignes chez les Malgaches, réparties inégalement entre hommes (4 109 ou 43,08%) et femmes (5 429 ou 56,91%):

- chez les hommes, la fréquence des tumeurs malignes augmente avec l'âge;

- chez les femmes, il existe un pic de fréquence très net pour la période 41-50 ans.

Le Tableau 1 montre la place prépondérante chez les Malgaches des tumeurs malignes du col, deux fois plus nombreuses que celles du sein. Puis viennent les tumeurs de la peau. Les tumeurs malignes du tube digestif, en particulier, celles du foie se situent au 3ème rang; celles du rhino-pharynx au 5ème rang.

Il est à noter que le classement des tumeurs malignes est différent dans la population européenne de Madagascar.

Tableau 1. Classement des tumeurs malignes à Madagascar (1954-1978)

Maladies	No. des T.M.		Malgaches		Européens	
	No.	Rang	No.	Rang	No.	Rang
Col utérin	1 732	1	1 534	1	100	3
Autres tumeurs de la peau	1 504	2	1 126	2	227	1
Tube digestif, foie, pancreas, péritoine	1 160	3	952	3	92	4
Sein	877	4	705	4	101	2
Bouche, nasopharynx	799	5	675	5	58	5
Lympho-réticulo-sarcomes	597	6	545	6	20	8
Tissu conjonctif	555	7	505	7	16	10
Tumeurs de l'ovaire	508	8	477	8	14	12
Mélanoblastomes cutanés	450	9	416	9	18	9
Corps utérin	283	11	252	11	15	11
Autres tumeurs génitales de la femme	286	10	260	10	13	13
Os	270	12	241	12	12	14
Ganglions lymphatiques	231	13	183	16	23	17
Oeil	228	14	203	13	10	15
Corps tyroïde	206	15	192	14	4	–
Prostate	202	16	181	15	5	–
Larynx, poumons, médiastins	157	17	105	18	37	6
Maladie de Hodgkin	137	18	115	17	7	–
Rein	114	19	103	19	7	–

EPIDEMIOLOGIE DE CERTAINS CANCERS ASSOCIES AUX VIRUS
A MADAGASCAR

Quelques études ont été réalisées par Brygoo & Coulanges sur certains cancers à Madagascar. Dans le cadre de ce symposium sur les cancers associés au virus en Afrique, les études portant sur le cancer du pénis, le cancer du col utérin, le sarcome de Kaposi et le cancer primitif du foie présentent un intérêt particulier.

Cancer du pénis

De 1970 à 1978, 209 cas de cancer du pénis ont été recensés chez les Malgaches, ce qui représente 44,2% des tumeurs génitales de l'homme, soit 5,2% du total des tumeurs masculines. Dans 54% des cas le cancer apparaît avant l'âge de 51 ans (Tableau 2).

Tableau 2.   Répartition des cancers du pénis en fonction de l'âge

Classe d'âge	Nombre de cas
10 à 20 ans	1
21 à 30 ans	16
31 à 40 ans	33
41 à 50 ans	63
51 à 60 ans	52
61 à 70 ans	34
plus de 70 ans	10
Total	209

Dans cette étude, les auteurs ont remarqué la fréquence anormalement élevée du cancer du pénis dans le sud de l'Ile et plus spécialement chez les Antandroy (une ethnie du sud). Soixante six pour cent des malades atteints de cancers du pénis viennent de la province de Tuléar (sud de l'Ile).

L'origine ethnique des malades a pu être précisée dans 147 cas: 65% d'entre eux sont des Antandroy, alors que ceux-ci ne représentent que 5% de la population de l'Ile. Des études récentes portant sur 19 cas de cancer du pénis dans le sud de l'Ile (Fort-Dauphin - Manambaro) ont pu montrer que:

- les sujets malades n'étaient pas circoncis (16 cas sur 19)
- ils étaient tous polygames
- 7 sur 19 avaient une sérologie positive pour la syphilis.

Cancer du col utérin

En 25 ans, 1 534 cancers du col utérin ont été diagnostiqués chez les femmes Malgaches. Ce cancer représente 28% des tumeurs malignes vues dans le Laboratoire.

Les différences suivant les groupes ethniques sont très minimes. Le cancer du col représente 47% des tumeurs génitales survenant chez les femmes Malgaches, alors que le cancer du sein ne représente que 20% des tumeurs génitales de la femme. Le cancer du col frappe surtout les femmes Malgaches autour de la quarantaine. La mortalité par cancer du col serait en moyenne de 10 à 15 décès pour 100 000 habitants soit 800 à 1 200 décès par an pour Madagascar. Ces cancers sont généralement diagnostiqués à un stade très avancé.

Sarcome de Kaposi

De 1956 à 1977, 52 cas de sarcome de Kaposi ont été diagnostiqués, dont 48 chez des Malgaches. Ce sarcome est donc rare chez les Malgaches: il représente 0,52% des tumeurs malignes diagnostiquées.

Il survient généralement chez des sujets jeunes (20-29 ans) avec une prédominance masculine significative (43 hommes pour 5 femmes). Le facteur climatique ou géographique ne joue aucun rôle, car ces malades proviennent de toutes les provinces de l'Ile. Il n'y a pas de prédominance d'une ethnie.

Dans 82,6% des cas, le cancer est localisé au niveau des membres. Les manifestations cliniques sont essentiellement cutanées; 3 cas localisations ganglionnaires ont été observés. Les lésions se présentent sous forme de tumeurs bourgeonnantes avec ou sans lésion inflammatoire, ou de nodules dermo-hypoder-miques. L'évolution est lente avec des poussées successives et une tendance des lésions à devenir symétriques. Elles peuvent s'ulcérer, entraînant des amputations.

Cancer primitif du foie

En 1958, une étude détaillée des cancers primitifs du foie (CPF) a été réalisée à Madagascar par Brygoo. Ces cancers représentaient alors 4,5% des cancers des sujets de sexe masculin et 0,39% des cancers de la femme. Les études menées de 1954 à 1978 ont dénombré 192 cancers primitifs du foie chez les Malgaches, dont 168 chez des hommes et 24 chez des femmes. Le CPF est donc 7 fois plus fréquent chez l'homme que chez la femme.

La répartition par classes d'âge a montré que 64,5% des cas surviennent après 41 ans (Tableau 3), contrairement aux pays où ce cancer est très fréquent (50% à 30 ans). Le cancer du foie est peu répandu et survient après la 4ème décade de la vie.

Tableau 3. Répartition par classes d'âge

Age	Cas	
	H	F
avant 20 ans	8	
de 21 - 30 ans	17	1
de 31 - 40 ans	38	4
de 41 - 50 ans	46	5
de 51 - 60 ans	37	9
de 61 - 70 ans	15	4
plus de 70 ans	7	1

Du point de vue anatomo-pathologique, il s'agit de tumeurs de type hépato-cellulaire.

Plus de la moitié des cas (55,5%) proviennent de la Province de Tuléar, dans le sud de l'Ile, zone à climat tropical sec ou semi-aride. L'affection semble rare sur les Hauts-Plateaux, la Côte-Est (zone tropicale humide).

LA LUTTE CONTRE LE CANCER

A Madagascar, le diagnostic et le traitement du cancer se heurtent à de nombreux problèmes tels que l'insuffisance du nombre de laboratoires d'Anatomie-Pathologie) tous les deux à Antananarivo), l'insuffisance en nombre du personnel qualifié, la difficulté des évacuations sanitaires des malades provenant des régions rurales. Les difficultés de communication (mauvaise infrastructure routière) entraînent un dépistage tardif des cancers qui sont vus à des stades très avancés.

Quelques mesures pourraient aider à faire avancer nos connaissances sur le cancer à Madagascar: médecins et chirurgiens devraient prendre l'habitude de donner des renseignements cliniques complets et précis sur les pièces opératoires adressées au Laboratoire. La réaction de registres du cancer dans les principaux hôpitaux paraît souhaitable.

La Ligue Malgache contre le Cancer, organisme non gouvernemental, mène une action d'information du public et a créé un centre de dépistage actif dans la capitale. Ces actions sont malheureusement limitées.

L'information du public par les médias ,la diffusion des messages de sensibilisation pourraient contribuer à lutter contre le cancer. En effet, un diagnostic précoce et une prophylaxie appropriée pourraient faire diminuer cette cause de morbidité et de mortalité, certainement sous-estimée, que constitue le cancer à Madagascar.

PROFILE OF LIVER DISEASE IN EGYPTIAN INFANTS AND CHILDREN

A.K. Khattab

Ain Shams University
Cairo, Egypt

RESUME

Les causes de maladies hépatiques ont été étudiées rétrospectivement dans un groupe de 200 nourrissons hospitalisés dans le département de Pédiatrie de l'Université Ain Shams, au Caire, durant la période 1977-1981, et prospectivement chez 50 enfants traités en ambulatoire à la Clinique d'Hépatologie Pédiatrique d'Octobre 1982 à Mars 1983. La principale cause d'hépatopathie dans les deux groupes était l'hépatite, suivie par la malnutrition avec carence en protéines et en calories chez les nourrissons et la bilharziose chez les enfants. Des méthodes de prévention sont suggérées.

SUMMARY

The causes of hepatopathies were studied retrospectively in a group of 200 infants who were inpatients at the Paediatric Department of Ain Shams University, Cairo, over the period 1977-1981, and prospectively in 50 children who were outpatients of the Paediatric Hepatology Clinic over the period October 1982-March 1983. The main cause of hepatopathy in both groups was hepatitis, followed by protein-calorie malnutrition in infants and bilharziasis in children. Suggestions are made as to methods of prevention.

***

Liver-disease in the paediatric age-group differs in its pattern from that seen in adults. As an example, the metabolic and inherited liver conditions are more commonly seen in children than in adults. Conversely, bilharzial liver complications and sequelae are more commonly seen in adolescents and adults than in young children.

The aim of this paper is to study the pattern of liver disease as seen in Egyptian infants and children so as to bring out the different systemic diseases that might involve the liver in this age-group.

MATERIALS AND METHODS

Two groups of patients were selected. For the retrospective study on infants, 200 inpatients of the Paediatric Department of Ain Shams University, Cairo, seen during the years 1977-1981, were selected. For the prospective study, the group consisted of 50 children who were outpatients of the Paediatric Hepatology Clinic of the same hospital, and were seen during the period October 1982-March 1983.

For every case in the study, the following was done:

1. Complete history, with particular emphasis on the diet, history of jaundice, bilharziasis, etc.

2. Clinical examination, including in particular jaundice, pallor, signs of vitamin deficiency, haemorrhages and a thorough examination of the liver.

3. Investigations, including examination of urine and stools, blood picture, liver function tests and especially plasma proteins (total and fractions), enzyme studies, prothrombin time, alkaline phosphatase, serological studies of hepatitis, and in selected cases alpha-fetoprotein. In special cases ultrasonography and liver biopsy were performed.

RESULTS

These are shown in Tables 1 and 2 and Figures 1 and 2.

Table 1. Incidence of various causes of hepatomegaly among 200 Egyptian infants in Ain Shams University Hospital during the 5 years 1977-1981

Type of disorder	1977	1978	1979	1980	1981	Total	%
Inflammatory, e.g., hepatitis	10	6	20	18	30	84	42
Nutritional, e.g., protein-calorie malnutrition	10	8	20	16	8	62	31
Haematological, e.g., thalassaemia and leukaemia	2	4	4	6	12	28	14
Metabolic, e.g., glycogen storage disease, muco-polysaccharidosis	–	2	4	2	2	10	5
Miscellaneous, e.g., Venoocclusive disease	1	–	2	1	1	5	
Cystic fibrosis	1	–	–	1	–	2	8
Biliary atresia	–	1	1	2	1	5	
Chronic passive congestion	1	–	1	1	1	4	
Total	25	21	52	47	55	200	100

Table 2.   Causes of hepatomegaly in 50 Egyptian children

Etiological group	Number	%
Inflammatory	25	50
Bilharzial	8	16
Miscellaneous	7	14
Haematological	3	6
Neoplastic	3	6
Nutritional	2	4
Metabolic	2	4

Fig. 1.   Incidence of various types of hepatomegaly among 200 Egyptian infants in Ain Shams University Hospital during the 5 years 1977-1981

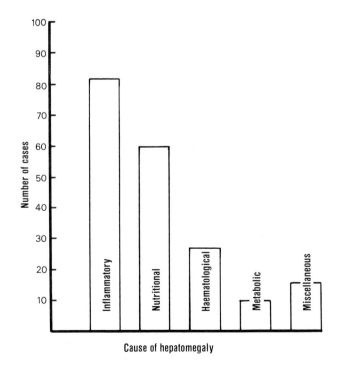

Fig. 2.   Incidence of various causes of hepatomegaly
in 50 Egyptian children

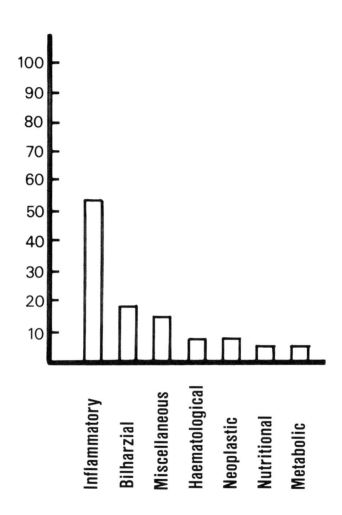

CONCLUSIONS

Inflammatory disorders are the commonest cause of hepatomegaly in both infants (42%) and children (50%), followed in
infants by nutritional disorders (31%) and in children by
bilharzia (16%).   Heamatological and miscellaneous causes are
also significant.

Since hepatitis is the commonest cause of hepatopathy in both infancy and childhood, proper hygiene, prophylaxis against hepatitis and proper management of the acute form of the disease are essential. Nutritional hepatopathy can be prevented by combating protein-calorie malnutrition. The control of bilharzia is also essential.

PATTERNS OF CHILDHOOD HEPATITIS IN THE NIGERIAN AFRICAN

A.O.K. Johnson, F.D. Akinbami, N. Ekambi & O.O. Akinyinka

Department of Paediatrics
University College Hospital
Ibadan, Nigeria

H.A. Odelola

Department of Virology
University College Hospital
Ibadan, Nigeria

RESUME

On a suivi pendant 6 ans 133 enfants âgés de quelques
semaines à 14 ans, atteints d'hépatite, la plupart du temps aiguë
à la phase ictérique. Le pic d'incidence de la maladie se situe
chez les nourrissons. Chez ceux-ci, l'hépatite doit être distin-
guée de l'obstruction congénitale des voies biliaires. Les
enfants plus âgés présentaient, à divers degrés, les manifestations habituelles de léthargie, d'anorexie et de souplesse à la
palpation de la région hépatique. Une fille et un garçon de 13
et 14 ans ont présenté une hépatite chronique active. Ils ont
reçu un traitement stéroïdien. Les tests sérologiques ont révélé
que 55% environ des enfants possèdaient des anticorps dirigés
contre le virus de l'hépatite A (HAV), mais seulement 4% avaient
des IgM spécifiques anti-HAV, alors que 15% possèdaient l'antigène de surface de l'hépatite B (AgHBs) et 23% des anticorps
dirigés contre l'antigène central (anticorps anti-HBc). La
plupart des enfants atteints d'hépatite aiguë ont obtenu une
guérison complète sur le plan clinique et biochimique; 2 ont
cependant gardé une antigénémie HBs persistante et 3 sont morts
d'hépatite fulminante.

Ces résultats montrent que l'exposition au virus de l'hépatite A semble prévalente chez les enfants Nigérians, et qu'elle survient probablement tôt dans la vie, mais que les infections par le virus de l'hépatite B, et peut-être d'autres virus hépatotropiques, ne sont pas rares. Il est nécessaire de surveiller et de suivre ces enfants à long terme. Il a déjà été montré que le cancer primitif du foie, prévalant chez les jeunes adultes de ce pays, peut-être lié à la persistance de l'AgHBs pendant de nombreuses années.

La nécessité d'un vaccin efficace contre l'hépatite B ne saurait être soulignée avec trop d'insistance.

SUMMARY

A total of 133 children aged between less than a month to 14 years presenting consecutively with hepatitis were prospectively studied over a 6-year period. Most cases were acute and presented at the icteric phase. The peak incidence was in very young infants whose illness had to be differentiated from congenital biliary tract obstruction. The older children exhibited the usual manifestations of lethargy, anorexia and tenderness over the liver area to varying degrees. There were 2 cases of chronic active hepatitis in children aged 13 and 14 years, one a female and the other a male. Their illness was controlled with steroid therapy. The serum biochemistry was characteristic in all cases. Serological tests revealed that about 55% of the children had antibody to hepatitis A virus but only 4% demonstrated HAV-specific IgM, while 15% had hepatitis B surface antigen (HBsAg) and 23% demonstrated antibody to core antigen (HBcAg). While most of the children with acute hepatitis made a full clinical and biochemical recovery, 2 have persistent HBs antigenaemia. There were 3 deaths in children who had fulminant hepatitis.

Our results show that exposure to hepatitis A virus appears to be prevalent in Nigerian children and probably occurs quite early in life, and infections with hepatitis B virus and perhaps other hepatotropic viruses are also not uncommon. The surveillance of such children and long-term follow-up are necessary. There is already compelling evidence to indicate that hepatocellular carcinoma, prevalent among young adults in our environment, may be related to hepatitis B antigenaemia persisting over several years.

The need for an effective vaccine against hepatitis B virus infection cannot, therefore, be over-emphasized.

INTRODUCTION

In the developed parts of the world, infection with the hepatitis viruses is not very common in children because of the high standard of hygiene. Even so, the incidence of hepatitis in such areas is often under-estimated, due partly to the fact that most anicteric cases are missed. In the developing countries, under-estimation of the incidence of hepatitis is more marked as few such countries make hepatitis a notifiable disease. Furthermore, the common features of the prodromal phase, such as anorexia and generalized aches and pains, may also be found in conditions like malaria and haemoglobinopathies which are prevalent in such environments. Reports on the natural history of hepatitis in childhood in Africans are therefore uncommon.

Epidemiological studies on viral hepatitis by our centre have shown a prevalence rate of between 4.2% and 15% for the hepatitis B surface antigen and 53% for the anti-hepatitis A virus (Francis, 1975; Johnson et al., 1982). Infection with hepatitis B virus in childhood cannot therefore be considered rare (Williams & Williams, 1972). It was therefore decided to study children with clinical hepatitis to determine the pattern, course and outcome of the infection in Nigerian children.

MATERIALS AND METHODS

All children presenting at the University College Hospital (UCH), Ibadan, with non-haemolytic jaundice were ultimately assessed at the Paediatric Gastroenterology Clinic. A detailed history was taken and the clinical findings on presentation were documented. Initial investigations included full blood count, haemoglobin electrophoresis, liver-function tests, and prothrombin time. Patients' sera were separated within 4 hours of venepuncture and stored at -20°C until tested. A total of 82 sera were tested for antibody to hepatitis A virus using the HAVAB radioimmunoassay (RIA) test kit supplied commercially by Abbot Laboratories (North Chicago, IL, USA). The hepatitis A-specific IgM test was then performed on all samples positive for antibody to hepatitis A virus (anti-HAV) using the modified RIA technique described by Busher et al. (1984). Briefly, a

polyvinyl plate was coated with antihuman IgM (Seward Laboratories) and test serum added. Any specific IgM was detected by
successively adding HAV antigen and ^{125}I-labelled anti-HAV. The
sera were also tested for hepatitis B surface antigen (HBsAg) by
the reversed passive haemaglutination (RPHA) test and counter-
immunoelectrophoresis (CIE), and for antibody to hepatitis B core
antigen (anti-HBc) using CIE and an RIA test kit (CORAB from
Abbot Laboratories). Blood sera, mostly from the younger
children, were subjected to the erythrocyte peroxide haemolysis
test (PHT), as described by Lubin et al. (1971) and tested for
alpha-foetoprotein (AFP) by an immunoelectrophoretic kit method
(SP Test Mochida), and for alpha-1-antitrypsin by an enzymatic
assay method. Percutaneous liver biopsy for histology was done
in all infants whose diagnosis was indefinite, and in all children whose illness persisted beyond 2 months. Blood was also
taken from the mothers of the 21 neonates in this study for
screening for hepatitis B surface antigen.

RESULTS

A total of 133 children (M:F = 63:70) were studied, of whom
39 were below one year of age; the ages of the others are
presented in the histogram (Fig. 1).

Presenting clinical features

These are shown in Table 1. All the children presented
during the icteric phase and apart from jaundice, other major
clinical features included fever, lethargy or weakness and
anorexia. Of the 133 children, 103 (77%) had hepatomegaly, with
tenderness in 79 (59%), while 53 (40%) had splenomegaly. Changes
in sensorium occurred in 5 children and included drowsiness in 3
children and stupor in 2. Pruritus and mild ascites occurred in
one of the cases of chronic active hepatitis, while bleeding
diathesis also involving the gastrointestinal tract occurred in
one of the cases which presented with fulminant hepatitis. Among
the infants, anorexia and failure to thrive (small for age) were
the major features apart from jaundice. Three of these infants
were preterm at birth.

Fig. 1. Age distribution of childhood hepatitis in Ibadan

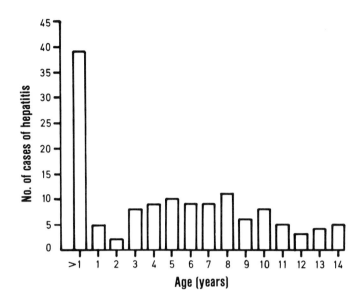

Haematological and serum biochemistry

The blood haematocrit varied between 31 and 40%. Three cases with packed cell volume (PCV) less than 30% had sickle-cell anaemia (SCA) as well. The total mean white blood count (excluding the three cases with SCA) was $9800/mm^3$, while the mean count in those with SCA was $18\ 525/mm^3$. The genotype was determined in 79 cases and was AA in 28, AS in 48 and SS in 3. The total serum bilirubin varied between 4.4 and 17.1 mg/100 ml in the majority of cases. The serum transaminases were variably raised in all cases. The SGPT was above 200 units in the cases with chronic (active) hepatitis, in whom the serum immunoglobulins were also elevated. The liver histology in the majority of acute cases showed a variable inflammatory reaction with mononuclear cells in portal areas but with no fibrosis. Focal necrosis with clear or balloon cells and acidophilic bodies were also often present. The liver in the chronic active cases showed swollen hepatocytes with ballooning deformation and intracanalicular cholestasis, piecemeal necrosis and bridging of portal tracts.

Table 1. Presenting features in 133 cases of childhood hepatitis in Ibadan

Presenting feature	No. of patients	Proportion (%)
Jaundice	133	100
Fever	121	91
Weakness/lethargy	121	91
Hepatomegaly	103	77
Anorexia	89	67
Abdominal tenderness	79	59
Splenomegaly	53	40
Abdominal pain	49	37
Nausea/vomiting	40	30
Joint pain	15	–
Pallor	12	–
Changes in sensorium	5	–
Abdominal distension	2	–
Ascites	1	–
Pruritis	1	–
Bleeding diathesis	1	–

Serology

Of the 82 sera tested for hepatitis markers, 44 (53.7%) showed antibody to hepatitis A virus, only 4 of which showed HAV-specific IgM. Twelve showed HBs antigenaemia and 17 had antibody to the core antigen (Table 2). Only one of the 2 cases of chronic active hepatitis was associated with HBs antigenaemia, and this has persisted on retesting 6 months after initial presentation. Three of the 21 sera of the mothers tested showed positive HBs antigenaemia. Serum alpha-foetoprotein (AFP) was tested for in 73 patients, but only 5 were positive (AFP > 10 mg/ml). The serum alpha-1-antitrypsin levels tested by an enzymatic assay method were within normal limits in the 57 cases tested.

Table 2. Childhood hepatitis in Ibadan: results of serological tests

No. of specimens tested	Hepatitis A markers		Hepatitis B markers	
	anti-HAV	IgM-HAV	HBsAg	Anti-HBc
82	44 (53.7%)	4 (4.9%)	12 (14.6%)	17 (20.7%)

Course and outcome

Of the 133 children, 128 had acute illness which resolved clinically and biochemically within 4-6 weeks. Most of these cases were managed symptomatically on an outpatient basis. Two of the children have persistent HBs antigenaemia 2-5 months after initial presentation. There were 3 deaths in children admitted in a drowsy or stuporous state with fulminant hepatitis; all died within 48 hours of admission without any significant change in their sensorium. The 2 cases of chronic active hepatitis have now been followed up for 6 and 9 months respectively, during which time there have been 2 readmissions due to acute exacerbations associated with cessation of steroid therapy.

DISCUSSION

All the children in this study presented in the icteric phase, which is not unusual. The non-specific symptoms of the prodromal phase were often put down to malaria or some virus infection. The children only entered hospital when jaundice appeared, so that most were seen when they were already improving. Since serum antibodies to hepatitis A virus (anti-HAV) appear in the serum within 1-4 weeks after exposure to the virus, and high antibody titres may persist for a long time thereafter, neither the demonstration of HAV, nor indeed of anti-HAV, indicate on-going acute infection, for which IgM-HAV is more specific. Only 4% of the children in this study demonstrated this specificity, so that it is evident that more than 50% of the children in our environment have already been exposed to HAV.

HBsAg, on the other hand, appears during the course of infection with HBV. It may appear only transiently or may persist for a variable period (Lubin et al., 1971). Only about 15% of the children in the study showed HBs antigenaemia, and in only 2 did this persist beyond the acute illness. These were in addition to one of the children with chronic active hepatitis, whose serum also demonstrated HBsAg. The incidence of antibody to the core antigen (anti-HBc) in this study was higher than that for HBsAg. This may reflect the replication of the virus in the nuclei of liver cells before HBsAg becomes detectable in the serum (Krugman, 1975). The prevalence of HBs antigenaemia appears to be on the increase in our environment. Francis (1975) quoted a figure of 4.2% in an epidemiological study of 715 children, as compared with about 15% in this study. This may, of course, be due to improved methods of detection of this marker and increased exposure. As we have previously pointed out (Johnson et al., 1980), it is not difficult to distinguish neonatal hepatitis from congenital biliary tract obstruction when the child presents early.

The results of the erythrocyte peroxide haemolysis test and the serum alpha-foetoprotein estimations, as well as liver histology, were very useful in differentiating neonatal hepatitis from congenital biliary tract obstruction. The specific course of neonatal hepatitis is often not found (Danks et al., 1977), and in only 3 cases of neonatal hepatitis could vertical transmission of hepatitis B virus have been the source of the infection in the neonate. The congenital transmission of hepatitis B antigen has previously been reported from our centre (Ayoola et al., 1981). Chronic hepatitis is relatively uncommon in children. However, the features of both chronic persistent and chronic active hepatitis (CAH) are well documented. One of the cases of CAH in this study was a male, who had a HBsAg-positive illness of acute onset, while the other, a girl, had a HBsAg-negative CAH. Chronicity is believed likely to develop in HBsAg-positive illnesses when there are no antibodies, and where there is persistence of high titres of antibody to core antigen (anti-HBc) and presence of antigen without the antibody in the host (Sherlock, 1976). This also facilitates the vertical transmission of hepatitis B (Okada et al., 1976). With only 2 cases of chronic (active) hepatitis in this study, not many conclusions can be drawn. However it is well recognized that CAH is a serious disease and that its course may span several years. It is characterized by repeated bouts of exacerbations and may eventually stabilize, go on to cirrhosis, or death may result from progressive liver failure.   CAH is believed to be second only to fulminant hepatitis as the most frequent cause of death from hepatitis in children.

The number of HBsAg-positive cases is few in most published series of CAH (Alagille et al., 1973; Dubois & Silverman, 1974), with the sole exception of the report of Meyer et al. (1975), where detailed seroimmunological studies were done.   It is thus likely that, with the use of more sensitive serological techniques, more HBsAg-positive CAH may be found.   It is noteworthy that other etiological factors for CAH, such as immunological deficiencies, drug reactions to methyl dopa (Goldstein et al., 1973) and isoniazid (Maddrey & Boitnott, 1973), reported in adults, have not been documented in children.   Hepatitis B virus infection thus remains the major factor adversely affecting prognosis in hepatitis in childhood.   There is now also compelling evidence of a causal relationship between hepatitis B virus infection and hepatocellular carcinoma (Ayoola et al., 1984), one of the commonest neoplasia in young adults in Ibadan.   We have recently managed 2 cases of hepatocellular carcinoma in children aged 12 and 14, and the only serum that could be tested was HBsAg-positive.   Thus there is a need for concerted national and international efforts to stem the increasing prevalence of hepatitis B virus infection.   It is hoped that the recently released vaccine against hepatitis B will be found to be effective, and will be made available to the population at risk.

REFERENCES

Alagille, D., Gaucher, M. & Herovin, V. (1973) Chronic hepatitis in children. Acta Pediat. Scand., 62, 556-570

Ayoola, E.A., Ogunbode, O. & Odelola, H.A. (1981) Congenital transmission of hepatitis B antigen in Nigerians. Arch. Virol., 67, 97-99

Ayoola, E.A., Francis, T.A. & Adelaja, A. (1984) The relationship between hepatitis B virus infection and primary liver cancer in the Nigerian African. East Afr. med. J. (in press)

Busher, G.L., Skidmore, S.J., McKendrick, M.W. & Geddes, A.M. (1984) Sporadic non A, non B hepatitis in Birmingham. J. infect. Dis. (in press)

Danks, D.M., Campbell, P.E., Jack, I. et al. (1977) Studies of the aetiology of neonatal hepatitis and biliary atresia. Arch. Dis. Child., 52, 360-367

Dubois, R.S. & Silverman, A. (1974) Treatment of chronic active hepatitis in children. Postgrad. med. J., 50, 386-391

Francis, T.I. (1975) Epidemiology of viral hepatitis B in the tropics. Bull. N.Y. Acad. Med., 51, 501-507

Goldstein, G.B., Lam, K.C. & Mistilis, S.P. (1973) Drug induced active chronic hepatitis. Am. J. dig. Dis., 18, 177-184

Johnson, A.O.K., Nottidge, V.A., Ojo, C.O., Junaid, T.A., Akingbehin, N.A. & Atta, E.B. (1980) Conjugated hyperbili-rubinaemia in Nigerian infants. Afr. J. Med. med. Sci., 9, 117-127

Johnson, A., Sodeinde, O., Odelola, H.A. & Ayoola, E.A. (1984) Survey of hepatitis A and B infections in childhood in Ibadan. In: Ijaiya, K., ed., Proceedings of the 2nd Regional Paediatrics Congress for Africa and the XIIIth Annual Conference of the Paediatric Association of Nigeria, Kaduna 1982 (in press)

Krugman, S. (1975) Viral hepatitis: recent developments and prospects for prevention. J. Pediat., 87, 1067-1077

Lubin, B.H., Bachner, R.L., Schwartz, E., Shohet, S.B. & Nathan, D.G. (1971) The red cell peroxide haemolysis test in the differential diagnosis of obstructive jaundice in the new-born period. Paediatrics, 48, 562-565

Maddrey, W.C. & Boitnott, J.K. (1973) Isoniazid hepatitis. Ann. intern. Med., 79, 1-12

Meyer, K.H., Baumann, W., Arnold, W. & Freudenberg, J. (1975) Immunological aspects in chronic active hepatitis in children. In: Liver Diseases in Children (Colloques de l'Institut National de la Santé et de la Recherche Médicale, No. 49), Paris, INSERM, pp. 15-25

Okada, K., Kaniyama, I., Inomata, M., Emi, M., Miyakawa, Y. & Mayumi, M. (1976) e Antigen and anti-e in the serum of asymptomatic carrier mothers as indicators of positive and negative transmission of hepatitis B virus to their infants. New Engl. J. Med., 294, 746-759

Sherlock, S. (1976) Predicting progression of acute type B hepatitis to chronicity. Lancet, 2, 354-356

Williams, A.O. & Williams, A.I.O. (1972) Hepatitis in Nigerian children. East Afr. med. J.

HEPATOCELLULAR CARCINOMA IN THE ALCOHOLIC

C.M. Leevy, Y. Sameshima, G. MCNeil,
N. Kanaqasundaram & T. Chen

The Liver Institute
University of Medicine and Dentistry of New Jersey
Newark, New Jersey, USA

RESUME

On a étudié la conversion de l'hépatite alcoolique en cirrhose et le développement éventuel d'un cancer primitif du foie (CPF) par une série de biopsies effectuées chez des patients alcooliques ne présentant pas de complications. La toxicité de l'éthanol, la carence alimentaire et les anomalies immunologiques chez un individu prédisposé génétiquement peuvent rendre compte de cette séquence qui peut être accélérée par le virus de l'hépatite B et d'autres agents toxiques. Le déficit immunitaire chez les alcooliques dénutris et présentant une maladie de foie diminue la réponse au vaccin contre l'hépatite B et peut contribuer au développement du CPF. Les fractions antigéniques des corps de Mallory semblent contribuer directement à la cytotoxicité et à la fibrose observées chez les alcooliques, et peuvent agir comme des proto-oncogènes. Les anticorps monoclonaux spécifiques des corps de Mallory vont heureusement pouvoir faciliter le diagnostic et le traitement. Les études de la synthèse de l'ADN et du collagène par la perfusion _in vitro_ de biopsies hépatiques percutanées fournissent des informations sur les lésions qui précèdent le CPF. L'abstinence, un régime et un traitement anabolisant permettent la réparation des lésions hépatiques et la correction des anomalies immunologiques, qui toutes deux peuvent contribuer au développement du CPF chez les alcooliques atteints de cirrhose.

SUMMARY

The conversion of alcoholic hepatitis into cirrhosis and the eventual development of hepatocellular carcinoma (HCC) has been documented by serial biopsies in patients with uncomplicated alcoholism.   Ethanol   toxicity,   nutritional   deficiency   and immunological abnormalities in a genetically predisposed indivi- dual appear to account for this sequence which can be accelerated by the hepatitis B virus and other noxious agents.   Immune deficiency in malnourished alcoholics with liver disease dimi- nishes response to the hepatitis B vaccine and may contribute to the development of HCC.   Antigenic moieties in Mallory bodies appear to contribute directly to cytotoxicity and fibrosis in alcoholics, and may act like proto-oncogens.   Available Mallory- body-specific monoclonal antibodies will hopefully facilitate diagnosis and treatment.   Studies of DNA and collagen synthesis by _in vitro_ perfusion of percutaneous liver biopsies provide information on precursor lesions of HCC.   Abstinence, nutrient therapy and drug-induced anabolism lead to repair of liver damage and correction of immunological abnormalities, both of which may contribute to development of HCC in alcoholics with cirrhosis.

INTRODUCTION

Hepatocellular carcinoma (HCC) has been reported in 3-30% of selected alcoholic patients with cirrhosis (Leevy et al., 1964; Lee, 1966; Norredam, 1979; Faivre et al., 1979).   Until recently, it was assumed that cancer of the liver, like that of the oeso- phagus and pancreas, in alcoholics occurred because of ethanol toxicity, nutritional deficiency and immunological abnormalities, with or without other etiological factors, in a genetically susceptible person (Fig. 1).   This hypothesis has been put in question by results of studies of hepatitis B virus (HBV) sequences, using molecular hybridization in HCC tissue from alcoholics.   Unlike observations by Shafritz and Kew (1981) who only found HBV DNA integrated into the host genome of HBV surface antigen (HBsAg) carriers, Bréchot et al. (1982) found integration in the absence of serological markers for HBV in 7 alcoholics and 12 non-alcoholics with HCC.   These observations may indicate that HBV is needed for the alcoholic to develop HCC, but more probably represent a technical error.   This paper: (a) re-examines natural history studies which indicate that uncomplicated alcoho- lism leads to HCC;   (b) records recent observations on the role of altered immunoreactivity in the genesis of liver injury in alcoholics; and (c) summarizes clinical methods of evaluating and reducing the oncogenic potential of alcoholism.

FIG. 1. FACTORS CONTRIBUTING TO HCC IN ALCOHOLISM

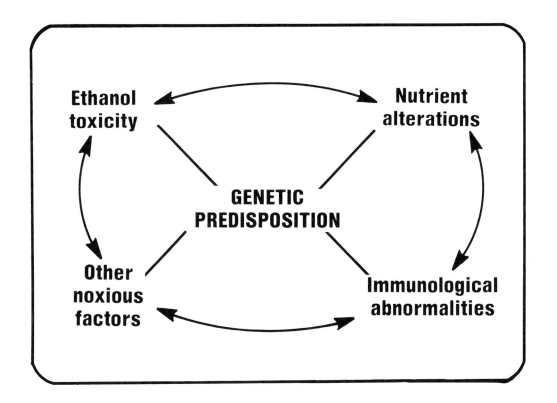

NATURAL HISTORY STUDIES

Retrospective studies were conducted in 100 patients with HCC on biopsy or autopsy at the New Jersey Medical School to determine: (1) whether alcoholism alone (ethanol intake plus dietary deficiency) causes or predisposes to HCC; (2) whether alcoholism enhances the carcinogenic effect of viruses, aflatoxin or other noxious agents. One-half of the patients had uncomplicated alcoholism and cirrhosis, the remainder had viral B hepatitis with or without alcoholism (Fig. 2). In our experience, drug addicts who develop hepatitis B infections are also often alcoholics, and alcoholics increasingly use parenteral drugs. These findings are interpreted as evidence that chronic alcohol abuse and HBV infections may independently or together serve as etiological factors for HCC. It is likely that alcoholism also increases the carcinogenicity of a variety of chemicals, as reflected in the four-fold increase in the number and the change in the cell type of liver cancer in rats when alcohol is added to vinyl chloride (Radike et al., 1977). Alternatively, alcoholism and a noxious agent may induce independent neoplasms in susceptible subjects, as exemplified by the report by Tamburro (1978) on an alcoholic exposed to vinyl chloride who developed both HCC and angiosarcoma. The use of decision-analysis techniques (Leevy et al., 1983) led to the conclusion that onset of unexplained liver failure and weight loss in subjects who had stopped drinking might be due to development of a neoplasm. An increase in the serum alpha-fetoprotein was a sensitive and specific indicator of HCC in the abstinent alcoholic with inactive cirrhosis. Imaging techniques, particularly using tagged alpha-fetoprotein (Kim et al., 1981), also increase diagnostic accuracy.

Sequential percutaneous biopsies in over 3000 alcoholics showed that alcoholic hepatitis is the morphological precursor of chronic liver disease. Serial histological studies in 7 patients showed conversion of alcoholic hepatitis to cirrhosis and eventual development of HCC with continued alcoholism (Fig. 3). Each of these patients had persisting Mallory bodies (MB), a pinkish, structureless material in haematoxylin-eosin-stained liver sections. There was initially an accumulation of neutrophils around the Mallory body; subsequently, chronic lymphocyte infiltration was observed. Electron microscopy revealed a cytoplasmic fibrillar substance consisting of bodies of filaments in parallel arrays and clusters of randomly oriented fibrils (Goldenberg & Pavia, 1982) or large, sharply circumscribed hyalin globular bodies (Keeley et al., 1972). Mallory bodies of the first type have also been found in HCC associated with viral B hepatitis in the absence of alcoholism, as well as in a number of commonly acquired hepatic disorders, including primary biliary cirrhosis (Gerber et al., 1973), Indian childhood cirrhosis (Nayak et al., 1969), drug-induced hepatitis (Paliard et al., 1978), liver damage in diabetes (Falchuk et al., 1980), after prolonged hyperalimentation (Craig et al., 1979), and following ileojejunal bypass (Peters et al., 1975) - none of which have been associated with HCC to date. The relationship of Mallory bodies to HCC has been best studied in those lesions produced by administration of griseofulvin to mice (Denk et al., 1975) or N-nitrosodiethylamine to rats (Borenfreund & Bendich, 1978).

FIG. 2. ETIOLOGICAL FACTORS IN PATIENTS WITH HCC AND CIRRHOSIS
AT THE NEW JERSEY MEDICAL SCHOOL

HBV, hepatitis B virus

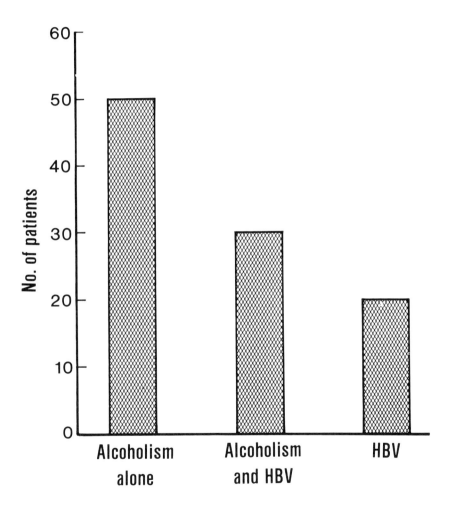

FIG. 3.   SERIAL HISTOLOGICAL STUDIES IN CHRONIC ALCOHOLICS WHO DEVELOPED HCC

MB, Mallory bodies;   F, fibrosis;   A, fat;   R, regeneration;   B, bile stasis;   I, inflammation;   N, necrosis;   O, other

	F	A	R	B	I	N	O
INITIAL PERIOD: Alcoholic hepatitis	0	2	2	2	2	2	M.B.
After 6 mos. Ts	0	0	0	0	0	0	0
2 YEARS LATER: Alcoholic hepatitis with fibrosis	1	2	2	2	2	2	M.B.
After 6 mos. Ts-Cirrhosis	2	1	3	1	2	1	M.B.
4 YEARS LATER: Cirrhosis	3	1	3	2	2	1	M.B.
6 YEARS LATER: Hepatocellular carcinoma	3	1	4	3	2	1	M.B. CANCER

ROLE OF ALTERED IMMUNOREACTIVITY

Studies of alcoholics with hepatitis, cirrhosis or HCC demonstrate both a decrease and an increase in immunoreactivity, either of which may contribute to the development of the cancer. Reduction in immunoreactivity is reflected in a decrease in circulating and liver total T-cells (Leevy et al., 1981a), and a change in the ratio of helper (OKT-4) to suppressor (OKT-8) T-cell subsets (Fig. 4).   Such patients have a diminished or total lack of ability to develop hepatitis B antibodies following administration of hepatitis B vaccine (Mendenhall et al., 1983), perhaps contributing to the development of HCC in the alcoholic with viral B hepatitis infection.   Since non-alcoholics with chronic malnutrition respond to the vaccine, a specific deficit or alteration of intermediary metabolism may be responsible. Thus, vitamin B6, essential for antibody formation (Baker & Frank, 1969), is the second most frequent vitamin deficiency in alcoholics, and plays an important role in ethanol-induced liver injury (Leevy, 1962; Ning et al., 1966; Kakuma et al., 1981). Studies now underway in our laboratory are designed to determine the relationship of such ethanol-induced alterations to immune deficiency.

FIG. 4. PERIPHERAL BLOOD T-LYMPHOCYTE SUBSETS IN ALCOHOLICS WITH LIVER INJURY

OKT-4, helper T-cells;   OKT-8, suppressor t-cells

	CONTROLS	ALCOHOLIC HEPATITIS, CHRONIC	ALCOHOLIC HEPATITIS, ACUTE
OKT-4	50	40	20
OKT-8	30	20	40
OKT-4 / OKT-8	1.8	0.5	0.5

Autologous liver added to lymphocytes from patients with alcoholic hepatitis produces an increase in replication and macrophage migration inhibitory factor (MIF) production equivalent to that seen in schistosomiasis or chronic active hepatitis (Sorrell & Leevy, 1972). When membranes, microsomes, mitochondria and nuclei are added to lymphocytes, there is no stimulation; however, addition of purified isolates of Mallory bodies produces identical results (Zetterman et al., 1976). In a series of experiments at the University of Medicine and Dentistry of New Jersey, it has been found that lymphocytes sensitized to Mallory bodies are cytotoxic (Kakumu & Leevy, 1977), and elaborate fibrogenic (Chen et al., 1973), chemotactic (Kanagasundaram et al., 1980), cholestatic (Marbett et al., 1984) and transfer (Kanagasundaram & Leevy, 1975) factors in alcoholic hepatitis. These observations have led to the postulate that the antigenic moiety in Mallory bodies plays a key role in the development of alcoholic hepatitis, cirrhosis and/or HCC (Fig. 5). In this schema necrosis, inflammation and fibrosis are attributed to cell-mediated and humoral immunity; Mallory bodies may also act like proto-oncogenes, since injections of their cultured isolates from N-nitrosodiethylamine-treated rats produce HCC.

FIG. 5. ROLE OF MALLORY BODIES IN DEVELOPMENT OF HEPATITIS,
CIRRHOSIS AND NEOPLASIA

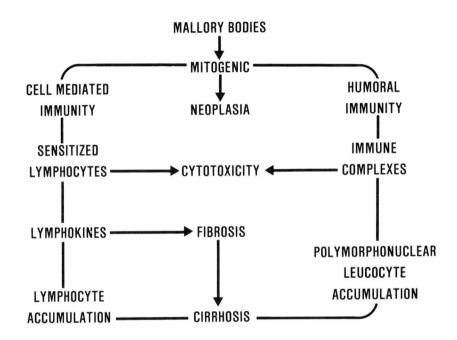

Efforts are underway to identify the antigenic moiety in Mallory bodies as the first step in determining its chemical composition and towards its use in the diagnosis and treatment of alcohol-related hepatic disorders. Using immune hemagglutination tests, it was possible to identify a Mallory body antigen and antibody (Kanagasundaram et al., 1977); however other workers found it difficult to reproduce these findings (Kehl et al., 1981). This is attributable to: (a) differences in specificity of Mallory-body isolates and the antiserum; (b) failure to use sufficient amounts of purified immunologically active Mallory-body antigen in the test; and (c) the relative insolubility of Mallory-body isolates and the fragility of the antigen. An attempt has been made to produce Mallory-body-specific monoclonal antibodies and thereby eliminate these problems. If obtained, they would: (1) facilitate development of sensitive and specific serological immunoassays; (2) allow exploration of the possibility that there are multiple antigenic sites in Mallory bodies responsible for various immune reactions; and (3) provide an additional marker of preneoplasia, reflecting both hepatocellular regeneration and potential neoplasia.

Using standard techniques, McGee and his co-workers (1982) produced three monoclonal antibodies using denatured isolates of Mallory bodies in Freund's complete adjuvant: (a) anti-JMB-1, which can be detected in low concentration in normal hepatocytes, bile ducts and in other organs; (b) anti-JMB-2, which reacts with Mallory-body or non-Mallory-body-containing hepatocytes and intermediate filaments in a variety of other organs; and (c) anti-JMB-3, which reacts with mesenchymal cells in sinusoids and fibrous septa of cirrhotic liver, but not with Mallory bodies themselves (McGee et al., 1982). At the New Jersey Medical School, two monoclonal antibodies, namely anti-NMB-1 and anti-NMB-2, have been produced using non-denatured isolates of Mallory bodies. Binding of anti-anti-NMB-1, an IgM immunoglobulin, is limited to Mallory bodies. In contrast, anti-NMB-2, an IgG$_1$ immunoglobulin, binds to Mallory bodies, plasma membranes and filamentous structures of liver, spleen, kidney, intestine and glandular structures of skin. It does not react with smooth muscle, skeletal muscle or epidermal prekeratin. Anti-NMB-2, but not anti-NMB-1, binds to membrane and filamentous structures in ethanol-treated rabbit liver cells (Sameshima et al., 1984).

CLINICAL EVALUATION AND TREATMENT

A major problem in treatment of liver injury has been that of evaluating the effects of available methods of treatment. In the alcoholic, it is desirable to detect precursor lesions of cirrhosis and HCC. This may best be achieved by evaluating hepatic DNA and collagen synthesis in percutaneous liver biopsies. It is now possible to obtain this information by in vitro perfusion techniques (McNeil et al., 1984a,b). Two 5-mm portions of a fresh biopsy are put into capillary pipettes filled with enriched plasma. A small needle is inserted into one side of each biopsy section to allow perfusion with tritiated thymidine (6 Ci/mmole) and tritiated proline (specific activity, 25-50 Ci/mmole) in an acrylic chamber with control of oxygenation, temperature and pH, for 2 hours. The perfusate is collected by suction, utilizing peristaltic pumps. Autoradiographs are developed, stained and DNA or collagen synthesis expressed as the number of labelled cells per 10 000 hepatocytes.

These studies indicate that liver regeneration and fibrogenesis are interrelated. During healing phases, there is predominantly replication of mesenchymal cells and ductular cells, with lesser degrees of hepatocyte hyperplasia. Marked hepatocyte hyperplasia is associated with or followed by HCC (Fig. 6). There is an increase in collagen deposition with fibrosis and lobular distortion in cirrhosis, which is reactivated with development of neoplasia (Fig. 7).

FIG. 6. AUTORADIOGRAPH SHOWING INCREASED INCORPORATION
OF TRITIATED THYMIDINE INTO DNA IN HEPATOCYTES
IN PATIENT WITH INACTIVE ALCOHOLIC CIRRHOSIS,
A FINDING OFTEN FOLLOWED BY HCC

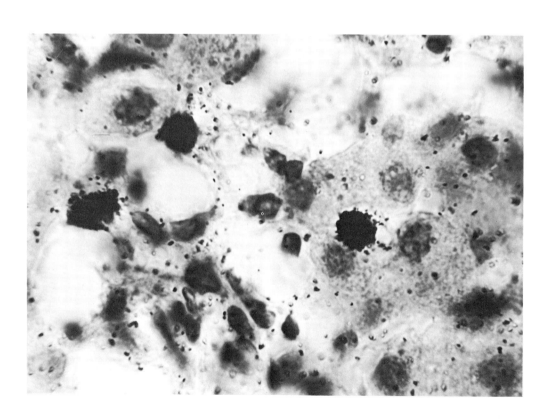

FIG. 7.   AUTORADIOGRAPH SHOWING INCREASED INCORPORATION
OF TRITIATED PROLINE INTO COLLAGEN IN ALCOHOLIC CIRRHOSIS,
OFTEN PRESENT IN AREA SURROUNDING HCC

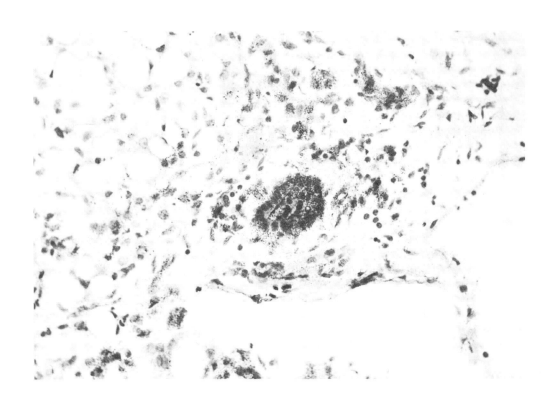

Whether alcoholism is a primary or associated event in the
development of HCC, the important first objective is to interrupt
alcoholism, despite lack of correlation between the amount, duration or type of alcohol and development of liver injury (Leevy et
al., 1981b). Studies of compliance indicate that it is independent of sex, age, ethnic background, religion or education. In
contrast, there is a good correlation with patient-physician
interrelationships. Thus, in our experience, less than 30% of
alcoholics seen periodically for a medical ailment will adhere to
a programme of abstinence. On the other hand, follow-up by a
concerned physician and associates on a weekly to daily basis as
a part of prospective controlled trials has led to a compliance
rate of 80-95% (Fig. 8).

FIG. 8.   COMPLIANCE WITH PROGRAMME FOR ABSTINENCE IN ALCOHOLICS
WITH LIVER INJURY

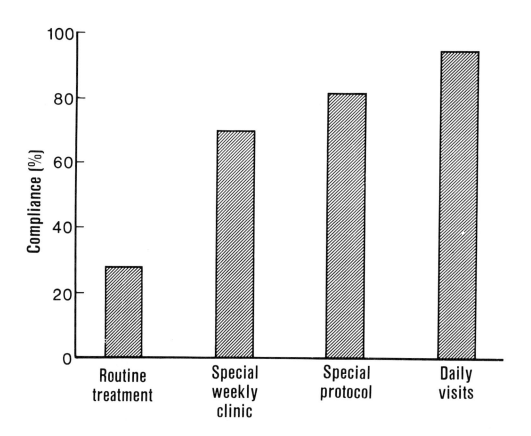

Once alcoholism is interrupted, it is possible to repair
liver damage. This is usually readily accomplished by a balanced
diet with supplements of vitamins and minerals (Leevy et al.,
1970); in patients refractory to this regimen, anabolism may be
induced by androgenic anabolic steroids which evoke increments of
RNA and DNA synthesis (Jabbari & Leevy, 1967) and significant
improvement in both quality of life and longevity. Recent
experimental studies indicate that administration of 16, 16-di-
methylprostaglandin, which has been found to be increased in
malignant tissue, also facilitates regeneration and inhibits
fibrogenesis. Such measures may restore normal immunological
reactivity as measured by phytohaemaglutinin (PHA) response and

percentage of peripheral blood lymphocytes (Fig. 9), thus simultaneously interrupting progression of liver disease and decreasing susceptibility to chronic injury from other agents, both of which should diminish the incidence of HCC in the alcoholic.

FIG. 9.   INFLUENCE OF NUTRITIONAL THERAPY WITH CORRECTION OF PROTEIN, VITAMIN AND MINERAL DEFICITS ON IMMUNOLOGICAL STATUS OF PATIENT WITH ALCOHOLIC HEPATITIS AND CIRRHOSIS

PHA, phytohaemagglutinin

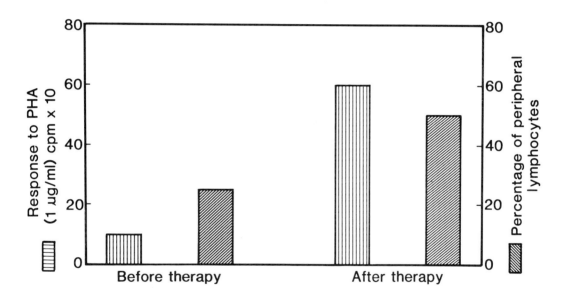

REFERENCES

Baker, H. & Frank, O. (1969) Clinical Vitaminology, Methods and Interpretation, New York, John Wiley, Interscience

Bréchot, C., Nalpas, B., Couroucé, A.-M., Duhamel, G., Callard, P., Carnot, F., Tiollais, P. & Berthelot, P. (1982) Evidence that hepatitis B virus has a role in liver-cell carcinoma in alcoholic liver disease. New Engl. J. Med., 306, 1384-1387

Borenfreund, E. & Bendich, A. (1978) In vitro demonstration of Mallory body formation in liver cells from rats fed diethylnitrosamine. Lab. Invest., 8, 295-303

Chen, T., Zetterman, R.K. & Leevy, C.M. (1973) Sensitized lymphocytes and hepatic fibrosis. Gastroenterology, 65, 532

Craig, R.M., Neumann, T., Jeejeeboy, K.N. & Yokoo, H. (1980) Severe hepatocellular reaction resembling alcoholic hepatitis with cirrhosis after massive small bowel resection and total parenteral nutrition. Gastroenterology, 79, 131-137

Denk, H., Gschnait, F. & Wolff, K. (1975) Hepatocellular hyalin (Mallory bodies) in long term griseofulvin-treated mice. A new experimental model for the study of hyalin formation. Lab. Invest., 32, 773-776

Faivre, J., Milan, C., Bugnon, P., Legoux, J.L., Martin, F. & Klepping, C. (1979) Primary liver cancer in Cote d'Or (Burgundy). Results of three years systematic registration in a well defined French population. Biomedicine, 31, 150-152

Falchuk, K.R., Fiske, S.C., Haggit, R.C., Federman, M. & Trey, C. (1980) Pericentral hepatic fibrosis and intracellular hyalin in diabetes mellitus. Gastroenterology, 78, 535-541

Gerber, M.A., Orr, W., Denk, H., Schaffner, F. & Popper, H. (1973) Hepatocellular hyalin in cholestasis and cirrhosis: its diagnostic significance. Gastroenterology, 64, 89-98

Goldenberg, D.M. & Pavia, R. (1982) In vivo horizontal oncogenesis by a human tumor in nude mice. Proc. natl Acad. Sci. USA, 79, 2389-2392

Jabbari, M. & Leevy, C.M. (1967) Protein anabolism and fatty liver of the alcoholic. Medicine, 46, 131-139

Kakumu, S. & Leevy, C.M. (1977) Lymphocyte cytotoxicity in alcoholic hepatitis. Gastroenterology, 72, 594-597

Kakumu, S., Leevy, C.M., Frank, O. & Baker, H. (1981) Protection of pyridoxal 5-phosphate against toxicity of acetaldehyde to hepatocytes. Proc. Soc. exp. Biol. Med., 168, 325-329

Kanagasundaram, N. & Leevy, C.M. (1975) Transfer factor: its occurrence and significance in alcoholic hepatitis. Gastroenterology, 69, 813

Kanagasundaram, N., Kakumu, S., Chen, T. & Leevy, C.M. (1977) Alcoholic hyalin antigen (AHAg) and its antibody (AHAb) in alcoholic hepatitis. Gastroenterology, 73, 1368-1373

Kanagasundaram, N., Dhingra, R. & Leevy, C.M. (1980) Alcoholic hyalin and neutrophil accumulation in acute liver injury of the alcoholic. Clin. Res., 28, 545A

Keeley, A.F., Iseri, O.A. & Gottlieb, L.S. (1972) Ultrastructure of hyaline cytoplasmic inclusions in a human hepatoma: relationship to Mallory's alcoholic hyaline. Gastroenterology, 62, 280-293

Kehl, A., Schober, A., Junge, U. & Winckler, K. (1981) Solidphase radioimmunoassay for detection of an alcoholic hyalin antigen (AHAg) and antibody (AHAb) (anti AH). Clin. exp. Immunol., 43, 215-221

Kim, E.E., De Land, F.H., Salyer, J.R., Benett, S.J. & Goldenberg, D.M. (1981) Radioimmunodetection of various human carcinomata with radiolabelled antibodies to tumour-associated antigens. In: Medical Radionuclide Imaging 1980, Vienna, International Atomic Energy Agency, pp. 511-518

Lee, F. (1966) Cirrhosis and hepatoma in alcoholics. Gut, 7, 77-85

Leevy, C.M. (1962) Medical pioneers. J. natl med. Assoc., 54, 73

Leevy, C.M., Gellen, R. & Ning, M. (1964) Primary liver cancer in cirrhosis of the alcoholic. Ann. N.Y. Acad. Sci., 114, 1026-1040

Leevy, C.M., Thomson, A.D. & Baker, H. (1970) Vitamins and liver injury. Am. J. clin. Nutr., 23, 493-499

Leevy, C.M., Kanagasundaram, N. & Chen, T. (1981a) Immunologic aspects of liver disease of the alcoholic. Res. Adv. Alcohol drug Prob., 6 , 255-280

Leevy, C.M., Kanagasundaram, N. & Smith, F. (1981b) Treatment of liver disease of the alcoholic: A composite approach. Semin. liver dis., 1, 254-266

Leevy, C.M., Levitt, E. & Jordan, T. (1983) Decision analysis - its use in instruction and patient care. In: Hurst, W., ed., Teaching Internal Medicine, Atlanta, Emory University Press

Marbett, U., Shefer, S. & Leevy, C.M. (1984) Studies of the influence of immunological and serological factors from patients with cholestasis due to alcoholic or viral hepatitis on biliary function in the rat (in press)

McGee, J.O'D., Morton, J.A., Barbatis, B., Bradley, J.F., Fleming, K.A., Yoate, A.M. & Burns, J. (1982) Monoclonal antibodies to Mallory bodies - intermediate filaments and HLA (Class 1) antigens in human liver disease. In: McMichael, A.J. & Fabre, J.W., eds, Antibodies in Clinical Medicine, New York, Academic Press

McNeil, G.E., Habba, S.F. & Leevy, C.M. (1984a) A perfusion technique for in vitro evaluation of hepatic DNA synthesis in man. Clin. Res. (in press)

McNeil, G.E., Habba, S.F. & Leevy, C.M. (1984b) Evaluation of hepatic collagen synthesis in man by an in vitro perfusion technique. Gastroenterology (in press)

Mendenhall, C. et al. (1983) Survival after steroid treatment for alcoholic hepatitis. Hepatology, 3, 850

Nayak, N.C., Sagreiya, K. & Ramalingaswami, V. (1969) Indian childhood cirrhosis: the nature and significance of cytoplasmic hyalin of hepatocytes. Arch. Pathol., 88, 631-637

Ning, M., Baker, H. & Leevy, C.M. (1966) Reduction of glutamic pyruvic transaminase in pyridoxine deficiency in liver disease. Proc. Soc. exp. Biol. Med., 121, 27-30

Norredam, J. (1979) Primary carcinoma of the liver. <u>Acta Pathol. Microbiol. Scand.</u>, <u>87</u>, 227-236

Paliard, P., Vitrey, D., Fournier, G., Balhadjali, L. & Berger, F. (1978) Perhexaline maleate induced hepatitis. <u>Digestion</u>, <u>17</u>, 419-427

Peters, R.L., Gay, T. & Reynolds, T.B. (1975) Post jejunoileal bypass hepatic disease: its similarity to alcoholic hepatic disease. <u>Am. J. clin. Pathol.</u>, <u>63</u>, 318-331

Radike, M.J., Stemmer, K.L. & Brown, P.G. (1977) Effect of ethanol and vinyl chloride on the induction of liver tumors: preliminary report. <u>Environ. Health Perspect.</u>, <u>21</u>, 153-155

Sameshima, Y., Kanagasundaram, N., Lubit, B., Thaler, H. & Leevy, C.M. (1984) Identification and reactivity of NMB-1, a Mallory body-specific antigen. <u>Gastroenterology</u> (in press)

Shafritz, D.A. & Kew, M.C. (1981) Identification of integrated hepatitis B virus DNA sequences in human hepatocellular carcinomas. <u>Hepatology</u>, <u>1</u>, 1-8

Sorrell, M. & Leevy, C.M. (1972) Lymphocyte transformation and alcoholic liver injury. <u>Gastroenterology</u>, <u>63</u>, 1020-1025

Tamburro, C.H. (1978) Health effects of vinyl chloride. <u>Texas Rep. Biol. Med.</u>, <u>37</u>, 126-144

Zetterman, R.K., Luisada-Opper, A. & Leevy, C.M. (1976) Alcoholic hepatitis and cell mediated immunologic response to alcoholic hyalin. <u>Gastroenterology</u>, <u>70</u>, 382-384

LIVER CANCER AND MYCOTOXINS

A. Linsell

Nairobi, Kenya

RESUME

Les preuves expérimentales et épidémiologiques du rôle potentiel des aflatoxines dans l'étiologie du cancer primitif du foie sont discutées. Comme ces mycotoxines présentent également un risque de toxicité aiguë, des mesures préventives devraient être prises sans délai dans les zones rurales où le risque de contamination des récoltes est élevé. Toutes les études effectuées dans le but d'évaluer les effets de telles mesures préventives sur l'incidence des maladies hépatiques devraient associer une évaluation de l'hépatite B au contrôle des mycotoxines.

SUMMARY

The evidence from laboratory and epidemiological studies for the potential role of the aflatoxins in the causation of hepato-cellular carcinoma is discussed. As these mycotoxins also present acute health hazards, it is recommended that preventive measures should be undertaken without delay in rural areas where there is a high risk of crop contamination. The monitoring of mycotoxin control should be linked with the evaluation of hepa-titis B infection in any studies assessing the effects of such preventive measures on the incidence of liver disease.

INTRODUCTION

It is now recognized that hepatocellular carcinoma (HCC) is among the most frequent of human cancers and particularly so on the continent of Africa. A significant association between chronic liver disease, more specifically cirrhosis, and HCC has led many to suggest that either alcoholism or viral hepatitis were the main etiological factors. Alcoholism has not been associated with the HCC occurring in areas of high incidence in Africa or the Far East, but the incrimination of viral liver disease has been shown to be fully justified wherever the cancer occurs. The evidence, discussed elsewhere in this publication, for the hepatitis B virus (HBV) being the major and necessary factor in the etiology is now overwhelming and attention is therefore being concentrated at the moment on the production and use of vaccines for the primary prevention of this cancer. However, all carriers of HBV, and it is estimated that world-wide there are over 200 million of them, do not progress to HCC. Other factors or circumstances must be involved. This cancer, like all cancers, has a complex causation, and so far we can only speculate on the interplay between the various factors with which the evolution of HCC has been associated. Therefore, whilst the use of vaccines for hepatitis B infection and the evaluation of immunization in the prevention of HCC should be strongly supported, it is worth-while reviewing the possible role of the mycotoxins in the etiology of HCC. This is particularly so as they represent a more general health hazard in addition to being naturally occurring carcinogens.

ROLE OF AFLATOXINS IN LIVER CANCER

Many chemicals, both naturally occurring and synthetic, have been shown to produce HCC in animal experiments but man is exposed to only a few of these potential carcinogens. Mycotoxins are produced by fungi on cereals and other foods which have been harvested and stored under hot, humid conditions. It is clear from recent reviews (Munoz & Linsell, 1982; International Union Against Cancer, 1982) that, of the mycotoxins, the aflatoxins are still the only members of this group of toxins considered to be a probable cause of HCC in man, either independently or in association with HBV infection. Aflatoxin B_1 has been the most frequently studied, both in the laboratory and as a human hazard. It is the most potent toxic and carcinogenic member of the aflatoxins in laboratory experiments. There is considerable variation in the susceptibility of different animals to aflatoxin under experimental conditions, but it is a very potent liver carcinogen in many, including monkeys. The animal most frequently used in laboratory trials has been the rat, and a dose of one part per billion produced liver tumours in 10% of the animals. HCC was reported in all rats surviving an experiment lasting 18 months using a feed containing 100 parts per billion. Between these two extremes, the response of the rat to the carcinogenic effect of aflatoxin was dose-related. Tumours were even reported after a single dose of aflatoxin and subsequent normal feeds. Female rats are more resistant than males to both the toxic and carcinogenic effects, and this difference is observed even at low doses. HCC is certainly more common in males in most parts of the world, as indeed are other associated factors, e.g., cirrhosis and, in some countries, the carrier state of HBV infection. The laboratory evidence for the carcinogenicity of aflatoxins is therefore convincing and places these compounds among the most potent of known chemical carcinogens (International Agency for Research on Cancer, 1976).

Man is certainly exposed to aflatoxin, since the contamination of maize, peanuts, rice and other foodstuffs by toxin-producing fungi has been reported world-wide, particularly in hot, humid climates. Epidemics of acute aflatoxicosis have been reported both in Kenya and in India, where over 100 deaths were attributed to exceptional high levels of aflatoxin on contaminated cereals (Krishnamachari et al., 1975). However, given the laboratory demonstration of the extreme carcinogenic potency of aflatoxin, it is the continuous exposure to smaller doses, not acutely toxic, which remains a major concern. Field studies in Africa and Asia to assess the association between aflatoxin contamination and the incidence of HCC have been undertaken (Linsell et al., 1977). Food ready for ingestion from areas with a varying risk of contamination was analysed for aflatoxin and the results compared with the incidence rates of HCC. These studies were greatly facilitated by the development of the alpha-feto-protein test as a diagnostic aid for HCC, as they had often to be carried out in areas where medical services were limited. Although evidence of a positive association between the levels of aflatoxin and the rates of HCC was found, many epidemiological criteria were not satisfied. The basic problem is that the evidence of chemical carcinogenicity in man must often remain indrect as, unlike a virus infection, no biological stigmata which can be measured years after exposure have been identified.

ELIMINATION OF AFLATOXINS

The acute and chronic hazards of aflatoxin are primarily a problem in developing countries, where agriculture is based on subsistence farming. The measures needed to eliminate mycotoxin contamination of food, mainly improved methods of harvesting and

storage, will also reduce food losses from insect and rodent
damage. The crop husbandry improvements needed do not require
sophisticated machinery or large capital outlays, so that they
should be attractive to agriculturists in developing countries.
However, the impact on the risk for HCC would be difficult to
assess and would require a long period of observation under
almost experimental conditions.

The laboratory and field evidence of the health hazards of
aflatoxin, including the carcinogenic risk, was examined in
detail in 1979 by a WHO committee and guidelines have been
published (World Health Organization, 1979). Because of the
acute hazard of aflatoxicosis and the potential role of the
aflatoxins in the high incidence of HCC in many developing
countries, these guidelines should be implemented without delay.
Field trials of immunization against HBV infection are now
underway and these should be linked with monitoring the effects
of aflatoxin control in order to assess whether a global campaign
for the elimination of HCC is possible.

The primary goal is prevention and the scientific evidence
is sufficient to justify action without waiting for further
research refinements.

REFERENCES

International Agency for Research on Cancer (1976) IARC Mono-
    graphs on the Evaluation of the Carcinogenic Risk of
    Chemicals to Humans, Vol. 10, Some Naturally Occurring
    Substances, Lyon, pp. 51-72

International Union Against Cancer (1982) Okuda, K. & Mackay,
    J., eds, Hepatocellular carcinoma (Workshop on the Biology
    of Human cancer), No. 17, Geneva

Krishnamachari, K.A.V.R., Bhat, R.V., Nagarajan, V. & Tilak,
    T.B.G. (1975) Hepatitis due to aflatoxicosis - an outbreak
    in Western India, Lancet, 1, 1061-1063

Linsell, C.A. & Peers, F.G. (1977) Field studies on liver cell cancer. In: Hiatt, H.H., Watson, J.D. & Watson, J.A., eds, Origins of Human Cancer, Cold Spring Harbor, NY, Cold Spring Harbor Laboratory, pp. 549-556

Munoz, N. & Linsell, C.A. (1982) Epidemiology of primary liver cancer. In: Correa, P. & Haenszel, W., eds, Epidemiology of Cancer of the Digestive Tract, The Hague, Martinus Nijhoff, pp. 161-195

World Health Organization (1979) Mycotoxins (Environmental Health Criteria No. 11), Geneva

Reprinted from: VIRUS-ASSOCIATED CANCERS IN AFRICA
LES CANCERS ASSOCIÉS AUX VIRUS EN AFRIQUE
(IARC Scientific Publications No. 63 OAU/STRC Scientific Publications No. 1)
A. OLUFEMI WILLIAMS, GREGORY T. O'CONOR,
GUY B. DE-THE & COUAVI A. JOHNSON, eds
Lyon, International Agency for Research on Cancer, 1984

SYNERGISM BETWEEN HEPATITIS B VIRUS AND AFLATOXIN IN HEPATOCELLULAR CARCINOMA

E.A. Ayoola

Liver Unit,
University College Hospital,
Ibadan, Nigeria

RESUME

Les études épidémiologiques ont montré que les facteurs de l'environnement jouent un rôle important dans le développement du cancer primitif du foie (CPF). Parmi ces facteurs figurent le virus de l'hépatite B (HBV), les cancérogènes chimiques, et les parasites. Les données disponibles ont démontré de façon convaincante qu'il existe une relation causale entre le CPF et l'infection HBV, dont le rôle exact n'a cependant pas encore été déterminé. De même, les études sur le terrain ont montré l'importance de la contamination des denrées alimentaires par l'aflatoxine dans les régions où l'incidence de CPF est élevée. Cependant, le rôle exact de cette mycotoxine est encore l'objet de débats. L'hypothèse selon laquelle l'aflatoxine et l'HBV pourraient agir de façon réciproque et synergique est contestée par ceux qui postulent que l'aflatoxine ne fait que supprimer l'immunité cellulaire, permettant ainsi la persistance d'HBV dans le foie. L'évaluation critique des études réalisées aussi bien chez les humains que chez les animaux suggère que le CPF résulte de l'interaction, chez un hôte génétiquement sensible, de facteurs initiateurs (facteurs génotoxiques), et promoteurs (facteurs épigénétiques). Ainsi, l'infection HBV pourrait, dès le plus jeune âge, déclencher le processus de cancérisation, en attaquant l'ADN cellulaire; par la suite, l'aflatoxine, ou d'autres facteurs promoteurs tels que l'alcool ou les nitrosamines, pourraient transformer les cellules initiées (de stade I) en cellules de stade III, qui pourraient à leur tour être 'attaquées' par des facteurs 'activateurs', produisant alors des clones de cellules malignes, indépendantes du promoteur.

La susceptibilité génétique détermine la capacité de l'individu à activer l'aflatoxine B (AFB) en métabolites actifs tels
que l'AFB-époxyde, et son aptitude à détoxifier cet époxyde par
conjugaison avec le glutathion. La quantité de substrat (AFB) et
l'activité des systèmes enzymatiques déterminent un équilibre
critique entre ces deux réactions. Il est possible que dans
chaque population, il existe des sous-groupes d'individus chez
qui le rapport activation/détoxification soit génétiquement
altéré.

Le développement du CPF pourrait être le résultat de l'interaction de facteurs génétiques, initiateurs (HBV), promoteurs
(aflatoxine, nitrosamines) et activateurs (alcool, tabac, HBV,
mutation du gène codant pour le récepteur des chalones). Cette
hypothèse, basée sur des observations effectuées chez les humains
et chez les animaux, peut expliquer les variations dans la
distribution du CPF selon les zones géographiques, le sexe,
l'ethnie, et le niveau socio-économique.

SUMMARY

Epidemiological data have suggested that environmental
factors play a major role in hepatocellular carcinoma (HCC).
Such factors include hepatitis B virus (HBV), infection, chemical
carcinogens and parasites. The available data provide compelling
evidence of the causative association of HBV with HCC but its
exact role has not been defined. Similarly, field studies have
indicated the importance of aflatoxin contamination of foodstuffs
in areas with high prevalence rates of HCC. The precise role of
this mycotoxin has been the subject of debate. The hypothesis
that aflatoxin and HBV can interact and cause HCC synergistically
has been challenged by those who postulate that aflatoxin merely
suppresses cell-mediated immunity, thereby permiting persistence
of HBV in the liver.

A critical evaluation of the available data from both human and animal studies suggests that HCC results from the interaction of (genotoxic) initiating and (epigenetic) promoting factors in a genetically susceptible host. Specifically, it is suggested that HBV infection initiates a carcinogenic process early in life by its attack on cellular DNA; that thereafter aflatoxin or other promoting factors, such as alcohol or nitrosamines, convert the initiated altered cells (stage-I cells) into stage-III cells, which may be 'attacked' by other 'activating' factors to produce clones of promoter-independent HCC cells.

Genetic susceptibility determines the ability to convert aflatoxin B (AFB) into active metabolites such as AFB-epoxide, and to detoxify AFB-epoxide by glutathione conjugation. A critical balance is maintained by the amount of substrate (AFB) and the activity of the enzyme systems. It is suggested that a subgroup of each population concerned may be genetically conditioned to alter this activation/detoxification ratio.

It is postulated that HCC development is the outcome of the interaction between genetic, initiating (HBV), promoting (afla-toxin, nitrosamines) and activating (alcohol, smoking, mutation of chalone receptor gene, HBV) factors. This theory is supported by observations in animal and human populations and can explain the geographic, sex-related, socioeconomic and ethnic variation in the pattern of HCC in the world.

INTRODUCTION

Hepatocellular carcinoma (HCC) is one of the most common cancers in the world. It is particularly prevalent in tropical Africa and the Far East. Although some progress has been made in the last decade, the actual mechanisms involved in the pathogenesis of HCC remain obscure. It is generally accepted, however, that it may be the cumulative result of several factors including hepatitis B virus (HBV) infection, immunological and hormonal influences, and hepatocarcinogenic toxins such as mycotoxins (Table 1).

Table 1. Etiological factors in HCC

Chronic HBV infection

Mycotoxins (aflatoxins)

Liver cirrhosis (alcohol, etc.)

Chemicals (nitrosamines)

Hormones (steroids?)

Genetic factors

Other (parasites, drugs, malnutrition?)

THE ROLE OF HEPATITIS B VIRUS

The role of HBV infection in the etiology of chronic liver diseases including HCC has been the subject of debate for many years. The various observations were competently reviewed by Zuckerman and Dunne (1974). The relationship betweeen HCC and HBV is implicit in the world-wide epidemiological data which show a highly significant excess of HBV markers in patients with HCC when compared with normal controls. The evidence is further reinforced by the common geographical distribution of high incidence of this cancer and the high prevalence of HBV carrier status in sub-Saharan Africa, China and South-east Asia (Williams, 1975; Szmuness, 1978). Additional observations which support the causal relationship are summarized in Table 2.

Table 2. Evidence for etiological role of HBV in HCC

Geographical distribution

High incidence of HBV markers

High risk of HCC in HBV carriers

HBsAg in cytoplasm of non-tumorous hepatocytes

HBV-specific DNA in HCC tissue

Secretion of HBsAg by HCC cell lines

Integration of viral DNA into host DNA

Woodchuck virus induces HCC in animal models
 (Peking ducks)

Compelling as these observations appear to be, they are not conclusive proof that HBV is unique as a factor in the genesis of HCC. In some geographical areas, the incidence rates of HBV infection and HCC do not coincide (Skinhoj et al., 1978). This and other reports indicate that some HCC cases are not HBV-related. Furthermore, in animal studies, the tumours caused in woodchucks by hepatotropic viruses differ in some ways from human HCC. In chimpanzees infected with HBV no cancer has yet been reported.

Despite these observations, and whatever the exact pathway of HCC transformation, available evidence suggests that HBV may be the initiator of a chain of cellular events which lead to the development of liver cirrhosis and cancer. It is equally evident that other factors do influence persistence of HBV infection and the development of HCC.

THE ROLE OF AFLATOXINS

In the pathogenesis of HCC toxic factors which are present in the daily diet of populations with a high prevalence of the disease must be considered important. One such factor is afla-toxin, a mycotoxin produced by a widely distributed fungus (Aspergillus flavus). A common contaminant of grains, aflatoxin is a potent carcinogen in many animals. Evidence of its carcino-genic activity in man is supported by field studies, which have documented a high correlation between high aflatoxin consumption and high prevalence rates of HCC (Peers & Linsell, 1973; Nwokolo & Okonkwo, 1978).

However, it has been observed that, in some parts of the world, such as Greece, a high prevalence of HCC is not necessar-ily associated with a high degree of aflatoxin contamination of foodstuffs (Trichopoulos, 1981). Questions have therefore been raised about the exact role of aflatoxin in the pathogenesis of HCC. Lutwick (1979) hypothesized that aflatoxin may not be a primary carcinogen but rather an immunosuppressive agent that produces an increase in the number of HBV carriers. This hypo-thesis is contradicted by the results of the study in Kenya, which revealed similar prevalence rates of HBV markers in areas of high and low aflatoxin contamination (Bagshawe et al., 1975). Comparative data from Mozambique (a high aflatoxin area) and the USA (a low aflatoxin area) indicate that the annual HBV-negative HCC rate is about 30 times higher in the former than the latter (Lutwick, 1979).

THE ROLE OF OTHER FACTORS

It is clear that HBV and aflatoxin do not have a unique role in hepatocarcinogenesis and that other factors do play a contri-butory role. The age of exposure to carcinogens, and genetic, hormonal and immunological factors must play individual roles in order to explain the observed intraethnic and socioeconomic variations. For example, in Nigeria, the prevalence rates of HBV carriers are nearly identical in males and females, yet HCC occurs 5 times more frequently in the male than in the female, an observation that can best be explained by sex-related factors. Alcohol and smoking have been incriminated in the carcinogenesis in some parts of the world (Goudeau et al., 1981; Trichopoulos, 1980).

SYNERGISM BETWEEN FACTORS

As a result of the pioneering work of Friedwald and Rous (1944), the concept of two-stage carcinogenesis, i.e., initiation followed by promotion, has become generally accepted. Although the mechanisms involved in promotion are only now in process of being clarified, the enhancing effects on a carcinogen of another administered chemical are usually regarded as evidence of promotion (Pitot et al., 1980). Thus the sequential administration of aflatoxin B_1 and N-nitrosodiethylamine (NDEA) has been demonstrated to produce synergistic effects in the development of tumours in animals (Newbern & Connor, 1980).

Initiation

Based on these concepts, an initiating factor must exist in HCC carcinogenesis. Epidemiological data, including the early HBV infection that occurs in areas of high HCC prevalence, would indicate that HBV plays this role. HBV can and does alter DNA in man. Molecular hybridization techniques have confirmed that part or all of the HBV DNA is integrated into host DNA. In this role, HBV acts as a genotoxic initiating factor. Continuous viral replication within the liver cells occurs, and may lead to the proliferation of the altered cells (stage-I cells). A similar state of affairs has been observed in the rat liver after phenobarbitone administration.

It should be noted, however, that HBV may not be unique in its role as an initiator. Other hepatotropic viruses, such as non A, non B hepatitis viruses may also act in this way. Although hepatitis A is not known to replicate in the liver cells, alteration of hepatocytes by this virus has not been conclusively excluded. Chemicals such as aflatoxin may initiate carcinogenesis if and when they modify DNA and when exposure occurs early in life.

Given a situation where cells have been altered by the initiating factor, the altered or initiated (stage-I) cells are held, under normal conditions, in a non-proliferative state by inhibitors referred to as chalones. These are produced by adjacent hepatocytes (Potter, 1980; Lijinsky et al., 1970). This restriction operates until promotion or spontaneous 'escape' takes place.

Promotion

In an area of high mycotoxin contamination, aflatoxin acts
as an epigenetic promoting factor which, through its metabolites,
is capable of inhibiting intracellular communication and thereby
blocking the transmission of growth and differentiation signals
to the stage-I cells. These cells, with appropriate genetic
alteration, may therefore proliferate with consequent progression
to cancer formation.

Under certain conditions, it is possible that aflatoxin may
act as a genotoxic promotion factor, combining both genetic modification and intercellular blockade. Aflatoxin (AFB_1) requires
activation by conversion into metabolites such as AFB_1-8, 9
epoxide in order to exert its biological activity. This metabolite does interact with cellular macromolecules, including DNA
(Lijinsky et al., 1970). AFB_1 binds human liver and the level of
DNA binding with AFB_1 has been correlated with carcinogenesis
(Degan & Newman, 1981; Lutz, 1979).

It has been established that the degree of AFB_1 binding
varies from one species to another and from one individual to
another (Booth et al., 1981). The rates of inactivation of AFB_1
and its metabolites vary from one species to another and may
influence the degree of carcinogenesis. In vivo regulation of
AFB_1 activation and detoxification, which is mainly by glutathione conjugation, may be genetically determined in man.

GENETIC POLYMORPHISM

The rates of inactivation of some drugs are known to show
genetic polymorphism. -In the metabolism of isoniazid, slow
inactivators have been described and are defined as being homozygous for a recessive gene believed to lead to a lack of the
relevant hepatic enzyme needed for isonicotinic acid hydrazide
(INH) metabolism. 'Rapid inactivators' are normal homozygous or
heterozygous. The racial differences in the rates of INH inactivation are shown in Table 3 (Thompson & Thompson, 1973). About
80% of Africans are 'slow inactivators' of INH. A similar
genetic polymorphism has been shown in the metabolism of debrisoquin (Woolhouse et al., 1979). A critical evaluation of the
data suggests that a high prevalence of HCC exists where there is
a high incidence of INH slow inactivators. Extending this comparison, it may reasonably be speculated that genetic polymorphism

occurs in populations where dietary aflatoxin has to be metabolized, and that 'slow inactivators' of AFB_1 metabolites are both genetically determined and more predisposed to the carcinogenic effects of AFB_1.

Table 3. Prevalence of hepatocellular carcinoma and differences in speed of isoniazide inactivation[a]

Group	HCC prevalence	Slow inactivators (%)
North American Whites (USA, Canada)	Low	55.0
American Blacks	Low	52.5
Eskimos	Very low	5.0
Latin Americans	Low	33.0
Africans	High	80.0

[a] Source: Thompson & Thompson (1978)

THE UNIFYING HYPOTHESIS

Based on the above mentioned observations, it can be postulated that hepatitis B virus initiates carcinogenesis very early in life, and that aflatoxin, the metabolism of which is genetically controlled, promotes the transformation of altered cells to cancer cells, with or without the assistance of additional factors such as alcohol, smoking and liver cirrhosis. Table 4 summarizes the possible sequence of events.

Table 4. Proposed sequence of events in pathogenesis of HCC

Event 1: Initiation

(a) Occurs between 0-10 years
(b) HBV alters DNA - Stage-I cells
(c) Restriction of proliferation by chalones
(d) Spontaneous mutation (rarely)
(e) AFB_1 can initiate

Event 2: Promotion

(a) Occurs between 5-25 years
(b) AFB_1 attacks membrane
(c) Blockade of intercellular communication by AFB metabolites
(d) Replication of stage-I cells
(e) Production of stage-II cells
(f) Alteration of DNA (AFB_1) - stage-III cells
(g) Escape from inhibiting controls - stage-IV cells (HCC)

Event 3: Activation

(a) Destruction of 'normal' cells:
        hepatotoxins (alcohol)
        immune system
(b) Emergence of stage-IV HCC cells

The hypothesis can explain the geographical variation in HCC prevalence, and its association with aflatoxin and HBV in certain areas, if it is recognized that other agents such as nitrosamines can act as promoters and that initiation can be induced by non B viruses.

It is postulated that, in the majority of HCC patients, HBV acts synergistically with aflatoxin to produce HCC in the genetically susceptible populations.

Based on the proposed hypothesis, the prevention strategy must take into consideration all the probable causal agents operating in areas of high prevalence. A comprehensive scheme is

summarized in Table 5. Identification of susceptible subpopulations may permit the early detection and treatment of HCC. In
view of the prevalence and mortality rates due to HCC, no effort
should be spared in reviewing current knowledge of its pathogenesis, diagnosis and prevention.

Table 5. Strategy for prevention of HCC

---

1.   Early prevention of HBV infection:

      - active/passive immunization

2.   Reduction of aflatoxin contamination:

      - improved farming and foodstuff storage techniques
      - monitoring of aflatoxin consumption in susceptible
         populations

3.   Reduction of exposure to activating factors:

      - prevention of alcohol abuse
      - prevention of hepatotropic virus infections
      - prevention of liver cirrhosis

4.   Definition of susceptible subpopulations:

      - study of genetic polymorphism in handling of aflatoxins
      - application of genetic markers, e.g., HLA

REFERENCES

Bagshawe, A.F., Gacengi, D.M., Cameron, C.H., Dorman, J. & Dane, D.S. (1975) Hepatitis B surface antigen and liver cancer: A population based study in Kenya. Br. J. Cancer, 31, 581-584

Booth, S.C., Bosenberg, H., Garner, R.C., Hertzog, P.J. & Nitpoth, K. (1981) The activation of aflatoxin B_1 in liver slices and in bacterial mutagenicity assays using liver from different species including man. Carcinogenesis, 2, 1063-1068

Degan, G.H. & Newman, H.G. (1981) Differences in B_1 susceptibility of rat and mouse are correlated with the capability to inactivate aflatoxin B_1 epoxide. Carcinogenesis, 2, 299-306

Friedwald, W.F. & Rous, P. (1944) The initiating and promoting elements in tumour production. An analysis of the effects of tar, benzpyrene and methylcholanthrene on rabbit skin. J. exp. Med., 80, 101-126

Goudeau, A., Maupas, P., Dubois, F., Coursaget, P. & Bougnoux, P. (1981) Hepatitis B infection in alcoholic liver disease and primary hepatocellular carcinoma in France. Prog. med. Virol., 27, 26-34

Lijinsky, W., Lee, K.Y. & Galegher, C.H. (1970) Interaction of aflatoxins B_1 and G_1 with tissues of the rat. Cancer Res., 30, 2280-2283

Lutwick, L.I. (1979) Relation between aflatoxin, hepatitis B virus and hepatocellular carcinoma. Lancet, 1, 755-757

Lutz, W.K. (1979) In vivo covalent binding of organic chemicals to DNA as a quantitative indicator in the process of chemical carcinogenesis. Mutat. Res., 65, 289-356

Newbern, P.M. & Connor, M. (1980) Effects of sequential exposure to aflatoxin B_1 and diethylnitrosamine on vascular and stomach tissue and additional target organs in rats. Cancer Res., 40, 4037-4042

Nwokolo, C.W. & Okonkwo, P. (1978) Aflatoxin load of common food in savannah and forest regions of Nigeria. Trans Roy. Soc. trop. Med. Hyg., 72, 329-332

Peers, F.G. & Linsell, C.A. (1973) Dietary aflatoxins and liver cancer: a population based study in Kenya. Br. J. Cancer, 27, 473-484

Pitot, H.C., Goldsworthy, T., Campbell, H.A. & Poland, S. (1980) Quantitative evaluation of the promotion by 2,3,7,8-tetrachlorodibenzodiethylnitrosamines. Cancer Res., 40, 3616-3620

Potter, V.R. (1980) Initiation and promotion in cancer formation. The importance of studies on intercellular communication. Yale J. Biol. Med., 53, 367-384

Skinhoj, P., Hanssen, J.P.H., Nielsen, M.H. & Middlesen, F. (1978) Occurrence of cirrhosis and primary liver cancer in an eskimo population hyperendemically infected with hepatitis B virus. Am. J. Epidemiol., 108, 121-125

Szmuness, W. (1978) Hepatocellular carcinoma and hepatitis B virus: evidence for causal association. Prog. med. Virol., 24, 40-44

Thompson, J.S. & Thompson, M.W. (1973) Genetics in Medicine, 2nd ed., Philadelphia, W.S. Saunders, pp. 125-126

Trichopoulos, D. (1981) The causes of primary hepatocellular carcinoma in Greece. Prog. med. Virol., 27, 14-25

Williams, A.O. (1975) Hepatitis B surface antigen and liver cell carcinoma. Am. J. med. Sci., 270, 53-56

Woolhouse, N.M., Andoh, B., Mahgoub, A., Sloan, T.P., Idle, J.R. & Smith, R.L. (1979) Debrisoquin hydroxylation polymorphism among Ghanaians and caucasians. Clin Pharmacol. Ther., 26, 584-591

Zuckermann, A.J. & Dunne, A. (1974) Hepatitis, hepatocarcinogens and hepatoma. Gazz. Sanit., 23, 3-11

HEPATITIS B VIRUS SEROLOGICAL MARKERS IN AFRICANS WITH LIVER CIRRHOSIS AND HEPATOCELLULAR CARCINOMA

P. Coursaget, J.P. Chiron, J.L. Barres & F. Barin

Institut de Virologie de Tours
Tours, France

P. Cottey, E. Tortey, B. Yvonnet, B. Diop, S. MBoup & I. Diop-Mar

Faculté de Médecine et de Pharmacie de Dakar
Dakar-Fann, Senegal

P. Kocheleff & J. Perrin

Faculté de Médecine
Bujumbura, Burundi

B. Duflo

Ecole de Médecine et de Pharmacie
Bamako, Mali

RESUME

On a prélevé des échantillons de sérum sur 221 Noirs Africains originaires du Sénégal, du Burundi et du Mali, hospitalisés pour cirrhose, et sur 453 sujets souffrant de cancer primitif du foie (CPF). La population témoin était composée de 6 655 adultes appartenant à différents groupes de population de ces mêmes pays.

Les marqueurs sériques du virus de l'hépatite B (HBV) tels que: l'AgHBs, l'AgHBc, les anticorps anti-HBs, anti-HBc et anti-HBe ont été déterminés par des tests radioimmunologiques. Les alpha-foetoprotéines et les complexes entre l'AgHBs et les IgM ont été déterminés par des tests ELISA.

L'AgHBs a été mis en évidence chez 11,8 à 17,6% des témoins chez 63,3% des patients souffrant de cirrhose et chez 62,7% des patients atteints de CPF.

Les preuves de la réplication d' HBV chez les patients atteints de cirrhose et de CPF diminuent en fonction de leur âge.

On observe une augmentation significative de la fréquence des complexes AgHBs/IgM lorsque l'on passe du stade du portage chronique de l'AgHBs (13,9%) au stade de la cirrhose (29,9%) et enfin au stade du CPF (33,7%).

SUMMARY

Serum samples were collected at the time of hospitalization from 221 black Africans suffering from cirrhosis and 453 suffering from hepatocellular carcinoma (HCC). These patients came from Senegal, Burundi and Mali, and 6655 adults from different population groups in these countries were used as controls.

Hepatitis B virus (HBV) serum markers, including hepatitis B surface antigen (HBsAg), anti-HBs, antibody to hepatitis B core antigen (anti-HBc), HBeAg and anti-HBe, were determined by radioimmunoassay, while alpha-fetoprotein and complexes between HBsAg and IgM were detected by ELISA tests.

HBsAg was detected in 11.8-17.6% of controls as opposed to 63.3% of patients suffering from cirrhosis and 62.7% of patients suffering from HCC. There was less evidence for HBV replication in cirrhosis and HCC in older patients. A significant increase in the frequency of HBsAg/IgM complexes was found in passing from the HBsAg chronic carrier state (13.9%) to cirrhosis (29.9%) and finally to HCC (33.7%).

INTRODUCTION

In many countries of Africa and Asia, hepatitis B infection occurs mainly during infancy and up to 90% of the adult population show evidence of past or present infection (Barin et al., 1981; Oon et al., 1983). Moreover, 10-15% of the adult population are hepatitis B surface antigen (HBsAg) chronic carriers. In such countries, hepatocellular carcinoma (HCC) is one of the commonest cancers and there is evidence to incriminate hepatitis B virus (HBV) as the etiological agent of both liver cirrhosis (LC) and HCC (Kew et al., 1976; Chien et al., 1981; Coursaget et al., 1981). Conclusive epidemiological evidence has come from prospective studies of HBsAg carriers and non-carriers (Beasley et al., 1981; Lo et al., 1982; Heyward et al., 1982). Beasley et al. (1981), in a study performed in Taiwan, estimated that HBV carries had over 200 times the risk of HCC as compared with non-carriers.

In the present study, we looked for HBV markers, including the newly described HBsAg/IgM complexes (Palla et al., 1981), in patients with LC or HCC from 3 African countries, namely Senegal, Mali and Burundi.

MATERIALS AND METHODS

Detection of HBV serum markers

HBsAg was detected by radioimmunoassay (Ausria II, Abbott Laboratories, North Chicago, IL, USA) in all sera except in those from Senegalese soldiers, where it was detected by an ELISA test (Behring, Oslo, Norway). Anti-HBs, antibody to HBV core antigen (anti-HBc), HBeAg and anti-HBe were searched for by radio-immunoassays (AUSAB, CORAB, Abbott HBe, Abbot Laboratories). An ELISA test kindly provided by Institut Pasteur Production (Marnes-la-Coquette, France) was used to detect alpha-fetoprotein (AFP). HBsAg/IgM complexes were detected by a previously described ELISA test (Coursaget et al., 1983). The complexes were bound to anti-IgM fixed in the wells of microplates. After incubation and washing, peroxidase-conjugated antibodies to HBsAg were added. Fixation was demonstrated by addition of hydrogen peroxide.

Populations

The control groups were black Africans from different population groups from Senegal, Mali and Burundi considered as representative of the general population and made up as follows: soldiers from Senegal (4568), country dwellers from Senegal (188), Mali (176) and Burundi (543); pregnant women from Senegal (884) and from Burundi (406); and finally patients hospitalized at Bujumbura Hospital (Burundi) for non-liver diseases (296). All were adults.

Sera were also collected from 221 patients with LC and 453 patients with HCC. The male/female sex ratio was 1.5 in LC patients and 4.3 in HCC patients. The age of LC patients varied from 8 to 80 years with a mean of 38 years, and that of HCC patients varied from 15 to 80 years with a mean of 44.6 years (Fig. 1).

FIG. 1. AGE DISTRIBUTION OF PATIENTS SUFFERING FROM LIVER CIRRHOSIS (▨) AND HEPATOCELLULAR CARCINOMA (■)

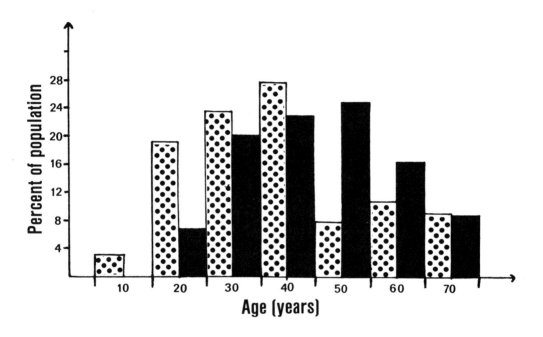

HBV infection in control groups from Senegal, Mali and Burundi

The distribution of HBV markers in the control groups (Figs 2 & 3) brings out the extent of hepatitis B endemicity in Senegal, Mali and Burundi, since 12-16% of them were positive for HBsAg. A higher prevalence rate was observed in Senegal and Mali than in Burundi, where a very low percentage (4%) was found in pregnant women. As found in other parts of the world (Sobeslavsky, 1980), there were differences between males and females. Thus in Senegal, HBsAg was detected in 13% of pregnant women and in 16.2% of soldiers. The total HBV infection rate in these population groups (Fig. 3) showed that more than 90% of adults had a marker of past or present infection in Senegal and Mali, but only about 75% in Burundi. Moreover, the proportion of individuals with anti-HBc alone was very low in Burundi (4-6%) as compared to Senegal (28%) and Mali (36%).

FIG. 2.   HBsAg IN DIFFERENT POPULATION GROUPS FROM SENEGAL, MALI AND BURUNDI

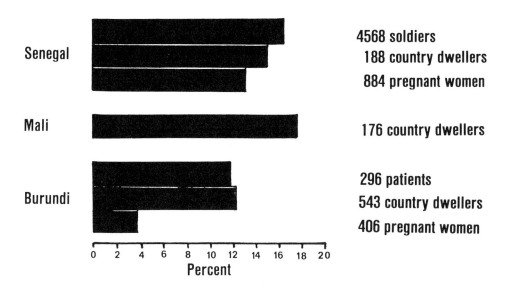

Senegal   4568 soldiers
           188 country dwellers
           884 pregnant women

Mali   176 country dwellers

Burundi   296 patients
           543 country dwellers
           406 pregnant women

0 2 4 6 8 10 12 14 16 18 20
Percent

HBV infection in liver cirrhosis and hepatocellular carcinoma

HBV infection is highly prevalent in LC and HCC patients: All had at least one HBV serum marker of present or past infection (Fig. 4). The frequency of HBsAg detection was very similar in patients suffering from LC as compared with HCC namely 63.3 and 62.7% respectively. The distribution of HBV markers in patients suffering from HCC according to the country of collection was similar (Fig. 5). There was, however, only a small proportion (2.0%) of HCC patients with anti-HBc alone in Burundi, something that was also observed in the control groups from that country.

FIG. 3. HBV INFECTION RATE AND ANTI-HBcAg ALONE
IN DIFFERENT POPULATION GROUPS FROM SENEGAL, MALI AND BURUNDI

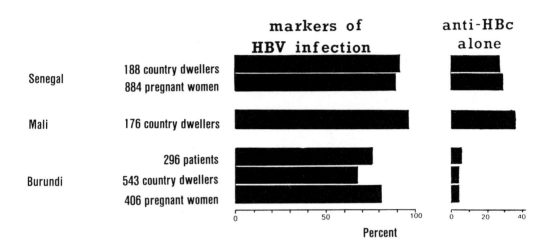

FIG. 4. HBV SERUM MARKERS IN PATIENTS SUFFERING FROM LC AND HCC

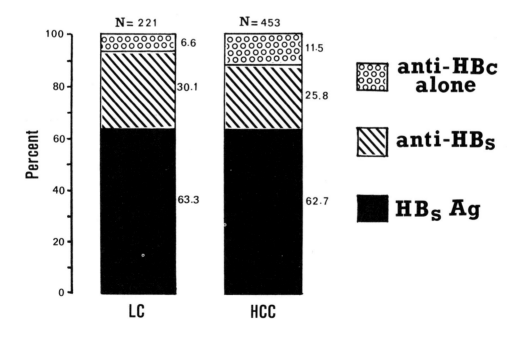

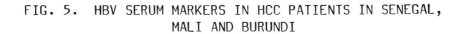

FIG. 5.   HBV SERUM MARKERS IN HCC PATIENTS IN SENEGAL,
MALI AND BURUNDI

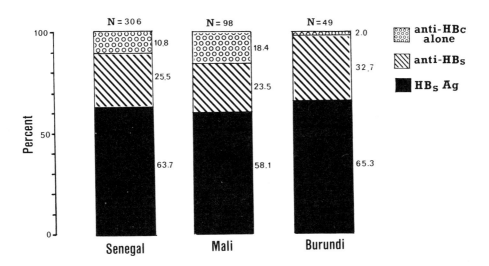

HBeAg.   HBeAg detection was performed in HBsAg-positive LC and
HCC patients and in HBsAg-positive soldiers and pregnant women
from Senegal and Burundi. HBeAg was found in 13% of HBsAg-
positive soldiers and in 18.6% of the HBeAg-positive pregnant
women, as against 33% in LC and 25% in HCC patients (Fig. 6).
Moreover, HBeAg was detected in 8.8% of the HBsAg-negative sera
from LC patients and in 1.1% of HBsAg-negative HCC patients.

Anti-HBe.   This was observed in 75% of HBsAg-positive soldiers
(Fig. 7) and in 53 and 60% respectively of LC and HCC patients.
Moreover anti-HBe was detected in 26% of HBsAg-negative sera from
LC patients and in 30% of HCC patients.   These results showed a
higher replication rate of the virus in patients suffering from
LC and HCC, although these subjects are older than the soldiers.
However, no difference was observed between LC and HCC patients
for HBeAg and anti-HBe.

FIG. 6. HBeAg IN HBsAg-POSITIVE SERA FROM SOLDIERS,
PREGNANT WOMEN AND LC AND HCC PATIENTS

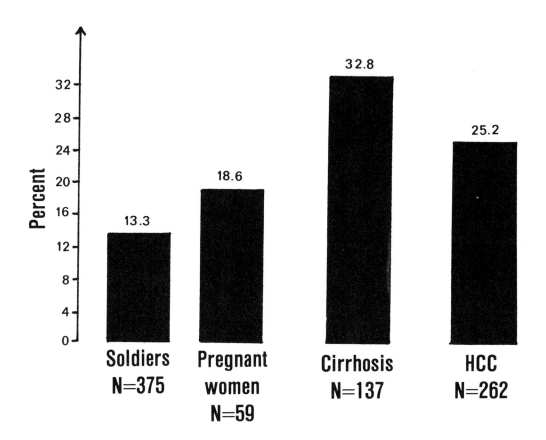

HBsAg/IgM complexes

Complexes between HbsAg and IgM have recently been described
in acute type B hepatitis (Palla et al., 1981) and the results
suggested that sequential serum testing for these complexes was
the best predictor of disease chronicity (Careoda et al., 1982).
Such complexes have also been detected in 14% of healthy HBsAg
carriers from Senegal (Coursaget et al., 1983), showing that, in
some carriers, they persist many years after infection, which
occurs early in life in Senegal.

FIG. 7.   ANTI-HBe IN HBsAg-POSITIVE SERA FROM SOLDIERS, AND LC
AND HCC PATIENTS

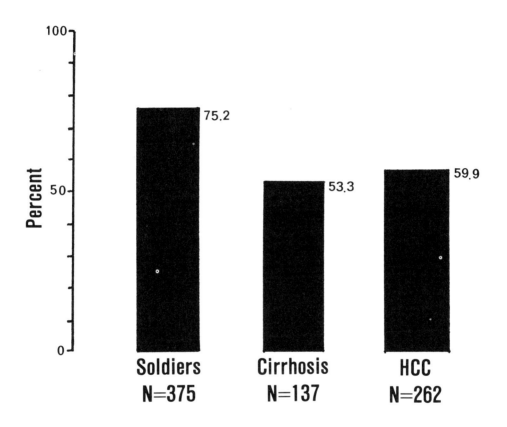

We also looked for such complexes between HBsAg and IgM in HBsAg-positive patients suffering from LC and HCC in order to determine whether they had any prognostic value in these diseases. Such complexes have been found in 30% of HBsAg-positive LC patients and in 34% of HBsAg-positive HCC patients (Fig. 8). They have also been detected in 3% of HBsAg-negative patients suffering from LC or HCC.

FIG. 8. HBsAg/IgM COMPLEXES IN HBsAg-POSITIVE SERA
FROM SOLDIERS, AND LC AND HCC PATIENTS

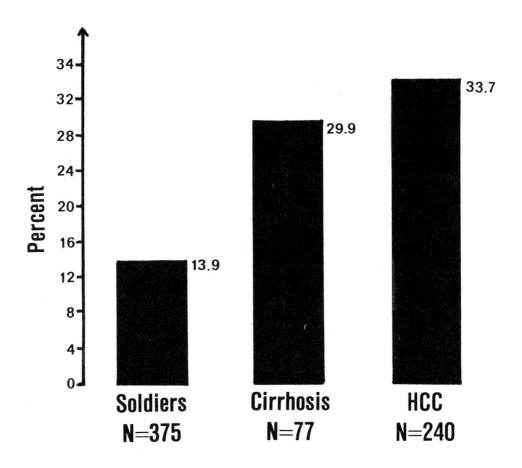

In HBsAg-positive patients, the relationship between HBeAg
and HBsAg/IgM complexes was studied, as it was observed in acute
type B hepatitis. In HBeAg-positive sera, HBsAg/IgM complexes
were detected in similar proportions among soldiers, and LC and
HCC patients (48-55%). However, a dramatically increased proportion of HBsAg/IgM complexes was observed in anti-HBe-positive
patients with LC (22%) or HCC (27%) as compared to anti-HBe-
positive soldiers (5%) (Fig. 9).

FIG. 9. HBsAg/IgM COMPLEXES IN HBsAg-POSITIVE SERA
FROM SOLDIERS, AND LC AND HCC PATIENTS,
AS A FUNCTION OF THE PRESENCE OF HBeAg OR ANTI-HBe

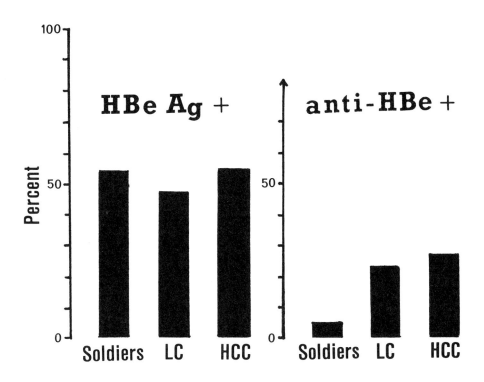

We were surprised to find a variation in the frequency of
such HBsAg/IgM complexes in patients suffering from LC or HCC in
relation to periods of blood collection (Fig. 10): such complexes were twice as frequent in the batch of samples collected
during the last two years. These results indicate that the
complexes disappeared with time and the numerous freeze-thaw
cycles necessary in testing for all HBV markers. We have therefore compared the results for the detection of these complexes
between HBsAg and IgM only for sera collected at the same period
of time (1982-1983) in Senegal, namely HBsAg-positive sera from
375 soldiers, 32 patients with LC and 86 HCC patients. In these
populations an increase in the number of HBsAg/IgM complexes

COURSAGET ET AL.

detected was observed in the sequence chronic carrier, LC, HCC in both HBeAg and anti-HBe subjects (Fig. 11). Thus HBsAg/IgM complexes constitute a valuable serum marker that could help in identifying those HBsAg carriers in whom LC or HCC will develop.

FIG. 10. HBsAg/IgM COMPLEXES IN HBsAg-POSITIVE SERA FROM LC AND HCC PATIENTS IN RELATION TO PERIOD OF BLOOD SAMPLING (⊞, 1975-1981; ■, 1982-1983)

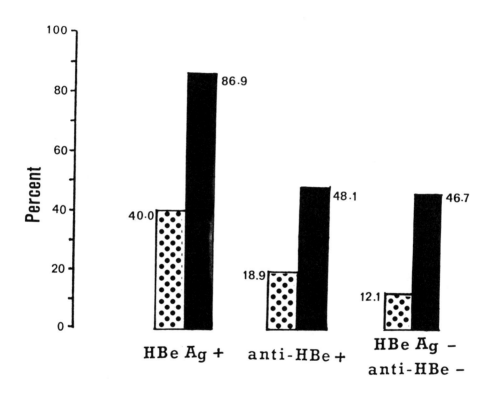

FIG. 11. HBsAg/IgM COMPLEXES IN HBsAg-POSITIVE SERA
FROM SOLDIERS, LC AND HCC PATIENTS COLLECTED 2 YEARS PREVIOUSLY

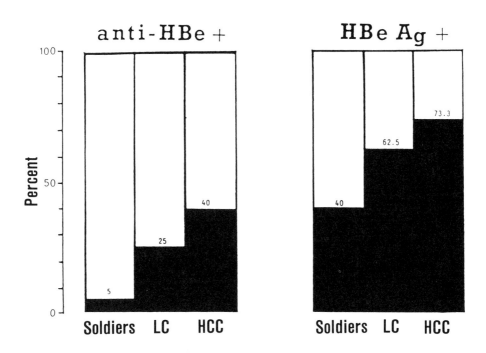

Comparison of alpha fetoprotein, anti-HBe and HBsAg/IgM complexes

It has been reported that, in the sequence leading from
chronic hepatitis to LC and HCC, the prevalence of anti-HBe
(Heyward et al., 1982) and AFP levels increased (Leblanc et al.,
1973). In our study, only AFP levels and HBsAg/IgM complexes
have been found to increase in the sequence leading from chronic
carrier state to HCC (Fig. 12).

HBV markers and age of patients suffering from HCC

In a previous study, we observed a decrease in HBV replication markers with advancing age in patients suffering from HCC
(Coursaget et al., 1981). These results are confirmed (Fig. 13)
in the present study for HBsAg. No change in AFP, however, was
observed with advancing age. A change in the frequency of

FIG. 12. COMPARISON OF LEVELS OF AFP, ANTI-HBe AND HBsAg/IgM
COMPLEXES IN HBsAg-POSITIVE SERA COLLECTED 2 YEARS PREVIOUSLY
FROM SOLDIERS (1), LC (2) AND HCC (3) PATIENTS

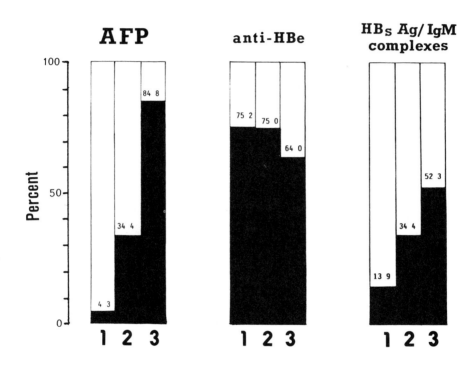

detection of HBeAg and anti-HBe was also observed with advancing
age, but not for HBsAg/IgM complexes (Fig. 14).

CONCLUSIONS

     The results obtained demonstrate the importance of HBV
infection in tropical Africa and its close association with LC
and HCC, the commonest cancer in Africa. Increased levels of two
serum markers, namely AFP and HBsAg/IgM complexes, are detected
during the sequence leading from the HBsAg carrier state to LC
and HCC and could thus be used in identifying the HBsAg subjects
in which these two liver diseases will develop.

FIG. 13.   AGE DISTRIBUTION OF HBsAg (■) AND HIGH LEVELS
OF AFP (⊡) (> 400 IU/ml) IN PATIENTS SUFFERING FROM HCC

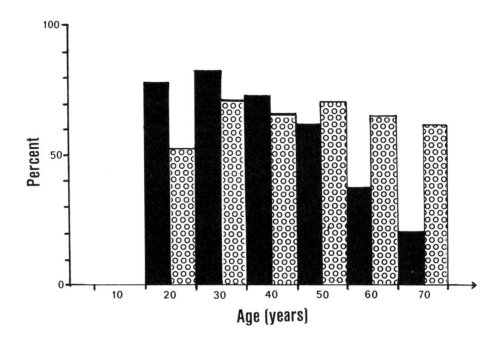

FIG. 14.   HBeAg (■), ANTI-HBe (▨) AND HBsAg/IgM COMPLEXES (⊡)
           IN HCC PATIENTS AS A FUNCTION OF AGE

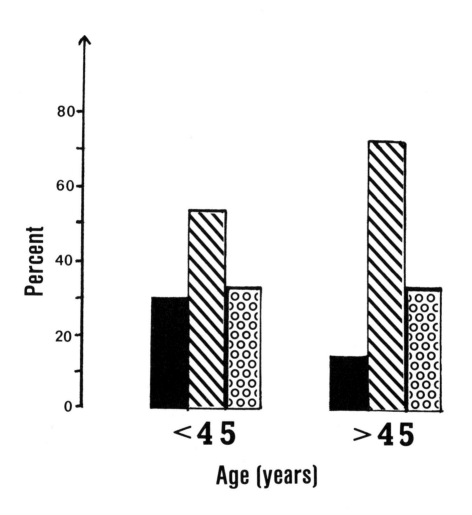

REFERENCES

Barin, F., Perrin, J., Chotard, J., Denis, F., N'Doye, R., Diop-Mar, I., Chiron, J.P., Coursaget, P., Goudeau, A. & Maupas, P. (1981) Cross-sectional and longitudinal epidemiology of hepatitis B in Senegal. Prog. med. Virol., 27, 148-162

Beasley, R.P., Hwang, L.Y., Lin, C.C. & Chien, C.S. (1981) Hepatocellular carcinoma and hepatitis B virus: A prospective study in 22707 men in Taiwan. Lancet, 2, 1129-1132

Careoda, F., De Branchis, R., D'Arminio Monforte, A., Vecchi, M., Rossi, E., Primignani, M., Palla, M. & Dioguardi, N. (1982) Persistence of circulating HBsAg/IgM complexes in acute viral hepatitis type B: an early marker of chronic evolution. Lancet, 2, 358-360

Chien, M.C., Tong, M.J., Lo, K.J., Lee, J.K., Millich, D.R., Vyas, G.N. & Murphy, B.L. (1981) Hepatitis B viral markers in patients with primary hepatocellular carcinoma in Taiwan. J. natl Cancer Inst., 66, 475-479

Coursaget, P., Maupas, P., Goudeau, A., Chiron, J.P., Raynaud, B., Drucker, J., Barin, F., Denis, F., Diop-Mar, I. & Diop, B. (1981) A case-control study of hepatitis B virus serologic markers in Senegalese patients suffering from primary hepatocellular carcinoma. Prog. med. Virol., 27, 49-59

Coursaget, P., Barres, J.L., Yvonnet, B., Petat, E., MBoup, S., Bocande, J.E., Diop-Mar, I. & Chiron, J.P. (1983) Circulating HBsAg/IgM complexes in chronic BsAg carriers. Ann. Virol. (Inst. Pasteur), 134E, 569-572

Heyward, W.L., Bender, T.R., Lanier, A.P., Francis, D.P., McMahon, B.J. & Maynard, J.E. (1982) Serological markers of hepatitis B virus and alpha-foetoprotein levels preceding primary hepatocellular carcinoma in Alaskan Eskimos. Lancet, 2, 889-891

Kew, M.C., Desmyter, J., Bradburne, A.F. & Macnab, G.M. (1979) Hepatitis B virus infection in southern African Blacks with hepatocellular cancer. J. natl Cancer Inst., 62, 517-520

Leblanc, L., Tuyns, A.J. & Masseyeff, R. (1973) Screening for primary liver cancer. Relationship between the time of appearance of alpha-fetoprotein in the serum and clinical symptoms in nine cases. Digestion, 8, 8-14

Lo, K.J., Tong, M.J., Chien, M.C., Tsai, Y.T., Liaw, Y.F., Yang, K.C., Chian, H., Liu, H.C. & Lee, S.D. (1982) The natural course of hepatitis B surface antigen-positive chronic active hepatitis in Taiwan. J. infect. Dis., 146, 205-210

Oon, C.J., Chan, L., Ha, C.S., Ngoh, G.C., Tai, G.K., Lim, C., Keow, L.G., Wan, O.Y., Hock, O.S., Leong, T.K., Tsakok, M. & Boon, W.H. (1983) Immune status of various populations to hepatitis B virus in Singapore and a strategy for its prevention and immunoprophylaxis. Dev. biol. Standard, 54, 295-305

Palla, M., Toti, M., Recchia, S., Rizzi, R. & Bonino, F. (1981) Complexes between IgM and HBsAg in serum of HbsAg carriers. Ital. J. Gastroenterol., 13, 223

Sobeslavsky, O. (1980) Prevalence of markers of hepatitis B virus infection in various countries: a WHO collaborative study. Bull. World Health Organ., 58, 621-628

INFECTION PAR LE VIRUS DE L'HÉPATITE B EN TUNISIE

N. El Goulli, P. Coursaget & J.P.Chiron

Institut de Virologie de Tours
2 bis Boulevard Tonnelé
37000 Tours, France

R. Kastally & H. Ben Khaliffa

Hôpital Habib Thameur
Tunis

M. Chouchi

Centre d'Utilisation du Rein Artificiel de Tunis (CURAT)
Tunis

SUMMARY

Recent reports show that the frequency of HBsAg varies around 4 to 6% in most Mediterranean and Middle East countries. Those areas are therefore considered as areas of intermediate endemicity for hepatitis B virus (HBV) infection.

The purpose of this study is to investigate the HBV global situation in Tunisia, by means of third generation testing methods.

Blood samples were obtained from 3 distinct population groups from Tunis:

- blood donors, consisting of young male adults
- staff members and patients from 4 haemodialysis units
- patients with either acute hepatitis or liver cirrhosis

They were tested for HBsAg, anti-HBs and anti-HBc by radio-immunoassay tests.

HBsAg was detected in 6.5% of the young male adults, and approximately 60% had either anti-HBs or anti-HBc antibodies.

Haemodialysis staff members and patients respectively displayed 9.1% and 19.5% of HBsAg positivity, but an increase of HBsAg positivity and of all HBV serum markers in relation to the amount of time spent in dialysis units was shown among the patients. After 3 years of dialysis sessions, none remained seronegative.

HBsAg was detected in approximately two-thirds of the patients with acute hepatitis or liver cirrhosis, and all cirrhosis patients had at least one HBV serum marker.

These global results stress the importance of HBV infection in Tunisia. Immunization against hepatitis B virus therefore has to be considered. Nevertheless, the immunization strategy must take into account the epidemiological and economic characteristics of the country.

RESUME

Des études récentes ont montré que la fréquence de l'antigène HBs varie de 4 à 6% dans la majeure partie des pays du pourtour de la Méditerranée et du Moyen-Orient. Ces régions sont considérées comme des zones d'endémie intermédiaire pour l'infection par le virus de l'hépatite B (HBV). Pour préciser la situation en Tunisie, nous avons recherché les marqueurs de l'infection HBV. La présence de l'AgHBs, et des anticorps anti-HBs et anti-HBc a été recherchée par des techniques radio-immunologiques, dans le sérum de trois groupes de sujets:

- des jeunes adultes de sexe masculin
- les membres du personnel et les malades hémodialysés de quatre centres d'hémodialyse,
- des malades atteints d'hépatite aiguë ou de cirrhose du foie.

L'AgHBs a été détecté chez 6,5% des jeunes gens et approximativement 60% ne possédaient pas d'anticorps anti-HBs ni anti-HBc.

Respectivement 9,1% et 19,5% des membres des centres d'hémodialyse et des sujets hémodialysés possèdaient l'antigène HBs.
Mais chez les patients, la présence de l'antigène HBs et des
autres marqueurs sériques d'HBV augmentait en fonction du temps
écoulé depuis la première dialyse. Après trois ans en dialyse,
aucun n'était séronégatif.

L'AgHBs a été détecté chez environ un tiers des patients
souffrant d'hépatite aiguë ou de cirrhose du foie. Tous les
patients cirrhotiques possédaient au moins un marqueur sérique
d'HBV.

Ces résultats soulignent l'importance de l'infection HBV en
Tunisie. L'immunisation contre le virus HB doit donc être envi-
sagée. Cependant, la stratégie de cette immunisation devra tenir
compte des réalités économiques et épidémiologiques du pays.

INTRODUCTION

Des études récentes ont montré que la fréquence de l'antigène
HBs (AgHBs) varie de 4 à 6% dans la majeure partie des pays du
pourtour de la Méditerranée et du Moyen-Orient, comme l'Italie
(Giusti et coll., 1981), la Grèce (Hadziyannis, 1975), l'Egypte
(Sobeslavsky, 1980), le Koweit (El Mekki & Al Nakib, 1983), et
l'Arabie Saoudite (Basalamah & Serebour, 1982).

Ces régions sont considérées comme des zones d'endémie intermédiaire, par opposition aux zones de faible endémie comme
l'Europe et l'Amérique où la prévalence de l'AgHBs est inférieure
à 1%, et aux zones de forte endémie comme l'Afrique et l'Asie où
on observe des prévalences supérieures à 10% (Sobeslavsky, 1980).

Le but de cette étude est de préciser la fréquence des infections par le virus de l'hépatite B (HBV) dans différents groupes
de population en Tunisie, à l'aide de méthodes sensibles de
détection des marqueurs sériques du virus de l'hépatite B.

MATERIEL ET METHODES

Les marqueurs sériques d'infection par le virus de l'hépatite B ont été recherchés dans le sérum de 272 sujets tunisiens qui se répartissent ainsi:

- 124 adultes de sexe masculin dont 60 prisonniers et 64 militaires, âgés de 18 à 35 ans. Ce groupe a servi de population témoin.

- 115 sujets provenant de 4 centres d'hémodialyse de Tunis, dont 33 membres du personnel et 82 hémodialysés. L'âge des hémodialysés varie entre 14 et 60 ans.

- 33 sujets présentant une pathologie hépatique, dont 16 hépatites aigües et 17 cirrhoses du foie. La moyenne d'âge est de 34 ans pour les sujets présentant une hépatite aiguë et de 51 ans pour les sujets atteints de cirrhose.

L'antigène HBs et les anticorps anti-HBs et anti-HBc ont été recherchés par méthode radioimmunologique (Austria II[o], Ausab[o], Corab[o], Lab. Abbot). De plus, les sujets présentant une hépatite aiguë ont fait l'objet de la recherche d'IgM dirigées contre le virus de l'hépatite A (IgM anti-HAV) (hepanostika anti-HAV-IgM[o], laboratoires Organon-Teknika), d'IgM anti-cytomégalovirus (anti-CMV) (Enzygnost-cytomEgalie[o], lab. Behring) et d'anticorps hétérophiles associés à une mononucléose infectieuse (Rythrotex[o], laboratoires I.C.L. Scientific).

RESULTATS

Population adulte de sexe masculin (Population témoin)

L'antigène HBs a été détecté chez 6,5% des 124 sujets. Les anticorps anti-HBs ont été retrouvés chez 48,4% et les anticorps anti-HBc seuls chez 9,7% des sujets. Ainsi, 2/3 des sujets présentent au moins un marqueur sérique d'infection présente ou ancienne par le virus de l'hépatite B (Fig. 1)

Ces résultats montrent la fréquence importante des infections par le virus de l'hépatite B en Tunisie.

Centres d'hémodialyse

  Membres du personnel.- L'AgHBs a été détecté chez 9,1% des 33 membres du personnel d'hémodialyse. Ce taux est supérieur à celui qui est observé dans la population témoin (Fig. 2). De plus, 66,7% des sujets possèdent, soit des anticorps anti-HBs, soit des anticorps anti-HBc seuls.

FIG. 1. MARQUEURS SERIQUES D'INFECTION
PAR LE VIRUS DE L'HEPATITE B
DANS DES GROUPES DE POPULATION D'ADULTES EN TUNISIE

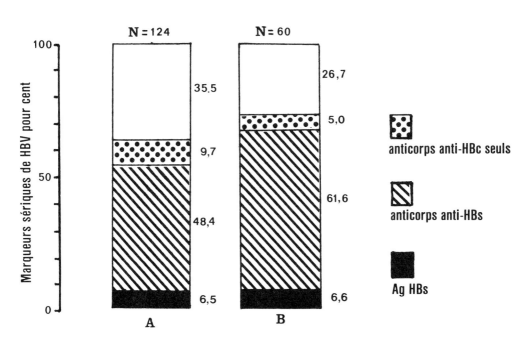

A=présente étude

B=Saffar et coll.

FIG. 2. MARQUEURS SERIQUES D'INFECTION PAR LE VIRUS HB
CHEZ LES MEMBRES DU PERSONNEL ET LES PATIENTS DE 4 CENTRES
D'HEMODIALYSE DE TUNIS

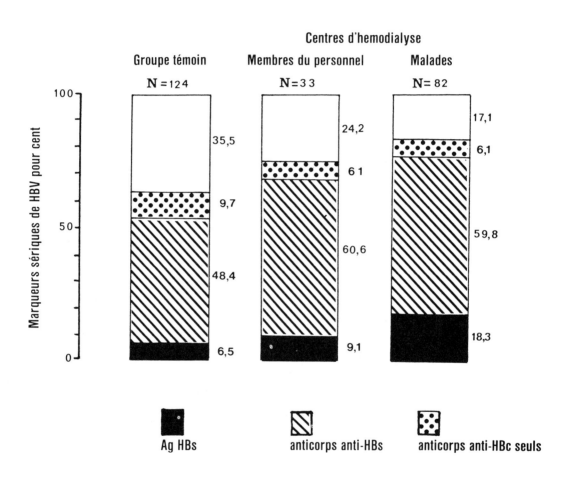

Hémodialysés.- L'AgHBs a été détecté chez 18,3% des sujets hémodialysés. Ce chiffre est trois fois plus élevé que celui que l'on observe dans la population témoin. De plus, 84% des sujets possèdent au moins un marqueur d'infection par HBV (Fig. 2).

Nous avons étudié le pourcentage des marqueurs de l'infection HBV en fonction de la date de première dialyse. Il s'avère que 13,3% des sujets dialysés depuis moins d'un an sont porteurs de l'Ag HBs. Seulement 27% sont séronégatifs.

Au-delà d'un an de dialyse, 27,8% des sujets sont porteurs de l'AgHBs, et au-delà de 3 ans de dialyse, tous les sujets possèdent au moins un marqueur d'infection HBV (Fig. 3).

FIG. 3. MARQUEURS SERIQUES D'HBV CHEZ DES HEMODIALYSES EN FONCTION DE LA DATE DE PREMIERE DIALYSE

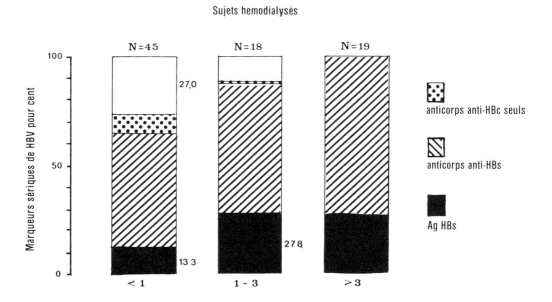

Une recherche du sous-type de l'AgHBs a été effectuée chez 7 sujets hémodialysés par Mme Courouce (CNTS, Paris). L'antigène HBs est du sous-type ayw$_3$ chez tous ces sujets.

Ces résultats montrent qu'en Tunisie, tout comme dans les pays de faible endémie, les membres du personnel et les patients des centres d'hémodialyse sont soumis à un risque particulier d'infection par le virus HB, bien que ces infections soient relativement fréquentes dans la population témoin.

Hépatites aiguës et cirrhoses

Hépatites aiguës.- Des IgM anti-HAV ont été décelées chez un des 16 malades atteints d'hépatite aiguë (6,25%).

Ce sujet, âgé de 20 ans, était également porteur de l'AgHBs. L'intensité des signes cliniques est probablement due à la sur-infection par le virus de l'hépatite A d'un sujet porteur chronique du virus de l'hépatite B.

L'antigène HBs a été retrouvé chez 10 sujets (62,5%), en l'absence de marqueurs d'infection par d'autres virus que celui de l'hépatite B. Il s'agissait d'hépatites virales aiguës de type B (Fig. 4).

Une recherche du sous-type de l'antigène HBs a été effectuée par Mme Courouce (CNTS, Paris) chez 6 des sujets présentant une hépatite AgHBs-positive.

Le sous-type ayw^2 a été détecté chez tous ces sujets. Les anticorps anti-CMV n'ont été retrouvés chez aucun des 16 sujets, et la recherche d'une infection aiguë par le virus d'Epstein-Barr (EBV) s'est également révélée négative dans tous les cas.

Soit, sur 16 hépatites aiguës survenues chez des adultes,

1 hépatite aiguë de type A	= 6,25%
10 hépatites aiguës de type B	= 62,50%
5 hépatites aiguës ni A, ni B, ni CMV, ni EBV soit non-A, non-B par exclusion	= 31,25%

Cirrhoses

Onze des 17 sujets atteints de cirrhose sont porteurs de l'Ag HBs (64,7%); 17,6% présentent des anticorps anti-HBs et 17,6% des anticorps anti-HBc seuls. Tous les sujets possèdent au moins un marqueur d'infection par le virus de l'hépatite B (Fig. 4).

FIG. 4.   MARQUEURS SERIQUES D'INFECTION PAR LE VIRUS HB
CHEZ DES MALADES ATTEINTS D'HEPATITE AIGUE OU DE CIRRHOSE

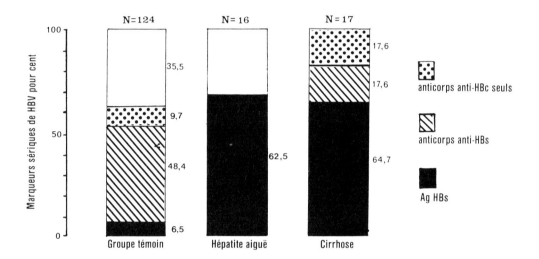

Ces résultats sont très proches de ceux qui ont été observés par Saffar et coll. (1983) et par Meknini et coll. (1982) chez des sujets atteints de cirrhose en Tunisie.

Les résultats combinés de ces 3 études portant sur 144 sujets atteints de cirrhose et comparés à un groupe témoin de 184 personnes sont regroupés dans la Figure 5.

On remarque que l'AgHBs est présent chez 53,5% des malades atteints de cirrhose contre 6,5% des sujets de la population témoin. Seulement 10% des sujets atteints de cirrhose sont exempts de marqueurs sériques d'infection HBV.

Ces résultats soulignent la gravité des infections par le virus de l'hépatite B en Tunisie, et leur rôle important dans les cirrhoses.

DISCUSSION

Les résultats obtenus montrent la fréquence importante des infections par le virus de l'hépatite B en Tunisie: près de 65% des sujets adultes de sexe masculin possèdent au moins un marqueur d'infection par ce virus, et 6,6% sont porteurs chroniques de l'AgHBs.

Ces résultats sont très similaires à ceux qui ont été observés dans une étude réalisée par Saffar et coll. (1983). Il s'agissait d'une population témoin de 60 personnes appariées pour l'âge et le sexe avec un groupe de sujets tunisiens atteints de cirrhose. Cette population comprenait 1/3 de femmes, et les âges variaient entre 32 et 53 ans. Cette étude a montré que 6,6% des sujets étaient porteurs de l'AgHBs et 73,2% possédaient au moins un marqueur sérique d'infection par l'HBV (Fig. 1). Ces chiffres, légèrement plus élevés que ceux observés dans notre étude, sont probablement liés à l'âge plus avancé de ces sujets.

Parallèlement, l'existence de sujets à haut risque d'infection HBV a été mise en évidence dans les centres d'hémodialyse. En effet, 9.1% des membres du personnel et 18,3% des hémodialysés sont porteurs de l'Ag HBs. De plus, tous les sujets hémodialysés depuis plus de 3 ans possèdent au moins un marqueur d'infection HBV. On note que le sous-type de l'AgHBs retrouvé chez les hémodialysés (ayw^3) est différent de celui que l'on observe dans la population générale (ayw^2).

FIG. 5.   MARQUEURS SERIQUES D'INFECTION PAR LE VIRUS HB
          CHEZ DES SUJETS ATTEINTS DE CIRRHOSE:
SYNTHESE DES RESULTATS DE 3 ETUDES EFFECTUEES EN TUNISIE

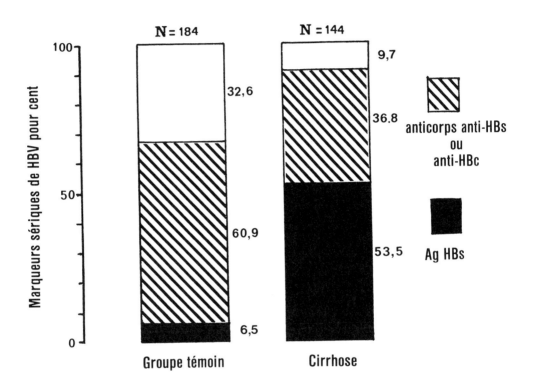

    La coexistence d'une forte proportion d'infections dans la
population générale et de groupes à très haut risque d'infection
semble être la caractéristique des pays d'endémie intermédiaire.

    La recherche de l'agent étiologique des hépatites aiguës dans
la population générale montre qu'une grande proportion des hépatites aiguës survenant chez l'adulte sont de type B (62,5%).
Ceci s'explique par le fait qu'en Tunisie, 1/3 des sujets adultes
n'ont pas été infectés par le virus de l'hépatite B, et sont soumis au risque de contamination par des sujets porteurs de l'AgHBs
(6% de la population adulte).

L'AgHBs a été détecté chez 64,7% des sujets présentant une cirrhose. Ce résultat montre qu'il existe en tunisie une étroite corrélation entre l'infection par le virus de l'hépatite B et le développement d'une cirrhose. De plus, Zaffrani et coll. (1981) ont montré que, dans les cirrhoses AgHBs-négatives survenant chez des sujets ayant séjourné plus de 20 ans en Afrique du Nord, l'AgHBs est détecté dans le cytoplasme des hépatocytes dans les 2/3 des cas. Ce résultat montre que la presque totalité des cirrhoses est probablement due à une infection chronique par le virus de l'hépatite B.

L'ensemble de ces résultats montre l'importance des infections dues au virus de l'hépatite B en Tunisie et la gravité de leurs conséquences. Un programme de vaccination contre le virus de l'hépatite B doit par conséquent être envisagé en Tunisie. Celui-ci doit tenir compte des réalités économiques et épidémiologiques du pays.

La vaccination doit être appliquée aux sujets à haut risque d'infection: en Tunisie, il s'agit des membres du personnel hospitalier et de certains malades (polytransfusés) d'une part, et des enfants nés de mère porteuse de l'AgHBs d'autre part. Pour les adultes à très haut risque d'infection, le protocole de vaccination doit prévoir la recherche préalable de l'AgHBs et des anticorps anti-HBs. Seuls seront vaccinés les sujets pour lesquels ces recherches auront été négatives, suivant un protocole de 3 injections à 1 mois d'intervalle et un rappel un an après. L'éradication à long terme des porteurs chroniques de l'Ag HBs dans la population générale implique la mise en place d'un programme de détection des mères porteuses de l'AgHBs et la vaccination de leurs enfants dès la naissance.

REFERENCES

Basalamah, H. & Serebour, F. (1982) Materno-foetal transmission of hepatitis B: 30 case studies of mother-infant pairs in Saudi Arabia. Dans: W. Szmunes et al., eds, Viral Hepatitis, Philadelphia, Franklin Institute Press, p. 671

El Mekki, A. & Al Nakib, W. (1983)   The seroepidemiology of enteroviruses, measles, mumps, varicella, hepatitis A and B among Arab nationalities in Kuwait.   Dans: Troisième Conférence Internationale sur l'Impact des Maladies à Virus sur le Développement des Pays du Moyen-Orient et de l'Afrique, Koweit, 19-27 mars 1983, p. 121

Giusti, G., Galanti, B., Gaeta, G.B., Piccinino, F. & Ruggiero, G. (1981) Hbs Ag carriers among blood donors in Italy: a retrospective survey of data from 189 blood banks. Hepato-gastroenterol., 28, 96-98

Hadziyannis, S.J. (1975)   Non-parenteral transmission of viral hepatitis in Greece. Am. J. Med. Sci., 270, 313-318

Meknini, B., Ayed, K., Elkhil, K., Gorgi, Y., Trigui, A. & Boujnah, A. (1982) Relations du virus HB avec la cirrhose 'dite méditerranéenne'. Gastroenterol. Clin. Biol., 6, 14A

Saffar, H., Said, S., Harbi, A., Maalel, K., Gaumer, B., Jemmali, M., Gaudebout, C., Dazza, M.C., Coulaud, J.P. & Larouze, B. (1983) Hepatitis B virus and adult cirrhosis: a case control study in Central Tunisia. Ann. Trop. Med. Parasi-tol., 77, 223-225

Sobeslavsky, O. (1980) Prevalence of markers of hepatitis B virus infection in various countries: A WHO collaborative study. WHO Bull., 58, 621-628

Zafrani, E.S., Kaabar, N., Potet, F. & Benhamou, J.P. (1981) L'infection chronique par le virus B est-elle la cause unique de la cirrhose observée en Afrique du Nord? Gastroenterol. Clin. Biol., 5, 1192-1193

SPECTRUM OF HEPATITIS B VIRUS INFECTION IN ETHIOPIA

L. Gebreselassie

Central Laboratory and Research Institute
Virology Section
Addis Ababa, Ethiopia

RESUME

Durant la période 1981-1984, on a trouvé que 304 sujets éthiopiens atteints d'hépatite B aiguë ou chronique étaient porteurs de l'antigène de surface du virus de l'hépatite B (AgHBs), à la Section de Virologie du Laboratoire Central de l'Institut de Recherche d'Addis Abeba. D'après le spectre de l'infection par le virus de l'hépatite B (HBV), les 304 patients ont pu être classés en 5 groupes.

Le premier groupe comprend la grande majorité des patients (260/304, soit 85%) et est caractérisé par la disparition rapide de l'AgHBs et par la guérison rapide. Dans ce groupe, l'hépatite B représente une infection spontanément limitée. Le second groupe comprend 10% des patients (30/304), identifiés comme des porteurs chroniques asymptomatiques de l'AgHBs; les tests hépatiques de ces sujets étaient généralement normaux deux mois et demi après le début de l'infection, mais l'AgHBs a persisté chez ces patients pendant plus de 6 mois. Le troisième groupe, qui représente 5% des patients (14/304), comprend ceux qui sont infectés de façon chronique par le virus HB et qui souffrent de maladie maligne du foie, le plus souvent de cancer primitif du foie (CPF). Les marqueurs spécifiques détectés chez ces sujets atteints de CPF sont l'AgHBs et l' alpha-foetoprotéine. La plupart des patients de ce groupe sont comparativement plus âgés (55 ans ou plus).

Le quatrième groupe consiste en un sous-groupe de patients du premier groupe, qui ont été simultanément infectés par l'agent delta, ainsi que le prouvent les anticorps anti-delta rencontrés

chez 2,7% des patients (3/111). Le cinquième groupe est constitué de sujets de sexe masculin, jeunes (entre 21 et 30 ans)
représentant 40% des patients (122/304). Le ratio hommes:femmes
est supérieur à 3:1.

SUMMARY

A total of 304 Ethiopian patients with acute or chronic
hepatitis B have been found to be positive for hepatitis B
surface antigen (HBsAg) at the Virology Section of the Central
Laboratory and Research Institute in Addis Ababa over the period
1981-1984. On the basis of the spectrum of hepatitis B virus
(HBV) infection, the 304 patients could be divided into 5 groups.

The first group includes the vast majority of the patients,
i.e., up to 85% (260/304) and is characterized by rapid clearance
of HBsAg and by rapid recovery from infection. In this group of
patients, hepatitis B was a self-limiting infection. The second
group comprises the 10% (30/304) of patients identified as asymptomatic chronic carriers of HBsAg; liver function tests on these
patients were usually normal after two and a half months from the
onset of infection, but HBsAg persisted in the patients for more
than 6 months. The third group, which accounts for 5% (14/304)
of patients includes those chronically infected by HBV and
suffering from some form of malignant liver disease, mainly
hepatocellular carcinoma (HCC). The specific markers detected in
those patients with HCC were HBsAg and alpha-fetoprotein. Most
of the patients in this group were comparatively old (55 years
and above). The fourth group consists of a subgroup of patients
of the first group with self-limiting hepatitis B, who were
simultaneously infected by the delta agent, as shown by the
detection of anti-delta antibody in 2.7% (3/111) of the patients.
The fifth group is constituted by the young males between the
ages of 21 and 30 years, accounting for 40% (122/304) of
patients. The male-to-female ratio was greater than 3:1.

INTRODUCTION

The discovery of the so-called Australia antigen by Blumberg
et al. (1965), now called the hepatitis B virus surface antigen
(HBsAg), has led to major advances in hepatitis B research.
Hepatitis B virus (HBV), which is the causative agent of hepatitis B, has now been fully described.

HBV is a remarkably succesful virus, as shown by the number of people found to be infected with it. As many as 200 000 000 persons world wide, or approximately 5% of the earth's population, have chronic HBV infection (Dienstag, 1980). The virus-host relationship appears to be much more complex than in other viral diseases, and the spectrum of host responses, both immunological and clinical, is unusually wide, ranging from fulminant hepatitis to asymptomatic carriage of the virus and finally to no response at all. Both overt and asymptomatic infections are ubiquitous and their frequency rates in many parts of the world are unusually high. The other end of the spectrum of infection by HBV - the development of chronic liver diseases in the form of chronic active hepatitis (CAH), cirrhosis and hepatocellular carcinoma (HCC) - is a common experience in many tropical countries throughout the world (Szmuness, 1975). Chronic liver diseases, although a major problem in Ethiopia, have not yet been fully described, particularly from the point of view of the role played by HBV in the pathogenesis of malignant liver diseases in general.

The present investigation, which is based on a retrospective study, was initiated in an attempt to study the spectrum of HBV infection, and the differences in response to it, and to understand the role of HBV in the causation of chronic liver diseases in Ethiopia.

STUDY POPULATION AND METHODS

A total of 304 patients (236 males and 68 females) identified as positive for HBsAg at the Virology Section of the Ethiopian Central Laboratory and Research Institute, were studied from the point of view of their response to infection by HBV. All 304 patients were tested for HBsAg, but only 111 of the patients with self-limiting HBV infection were also tested for delta antigen and anti-delta antibody.

Immunoelectroosmophoresis (IEOP), as described by Hansson & Johnsson (1971), was first used for the detection of HBsAg in the routine test, which was replaced by Hepanostika (ELISA) kits (Organon Teknika, The Netherlands). A gel diffusion test was used to detect alpha-fetoprotein using anti-alpha-fetoprotein antiserum from Dako, Denmark, in Hyland immunodiffusion plates.

Delta and anti-delta testing was performed in the Department of Clinical Virology of Malmö General Hospital, Sweden, by Dr B.G. Hansson.

RESULTS

The entire study population could be divided into five groups on the basis of the spectrum of HBV infection and of the response to that infection, as indicated in Table 1.

Table 1. Spectrum of HBV infection in different groups of hepatitis B (HB) patients

Total No. of HB patients	Group	No. in group	%	Mean age (years)
304	Self-limiting HB	260	85.5	25
	Asymptomatic chronic carriers of HBsAg	30	9.9	30
	HCC patients	14	4.6	55
111	HB patients with delta infection	3	2.7	25
304	Male	236	77.6	
	Female	68	22.4	

Group I: Self-limiting hepatitis B patients

This group makes up the vast majority of the patients, accounting for up to 85% (260/304). The patients typically showed HBsAg antigenaemia for a short period during the acute stage of the infection, with abnormal liver function tests which, in most cases, returned to normal two and a half months after the disappearance of HBsAg. The mean age of the patients in this group was 25 years.

Group II: Asymptomatic chronic carriers of HBsAg

This pattern of infection by HBV is observed in about 10% (30/304) of the patients and is characterized by the persistence of HBsAg for more than 6 months without obvious symptoms of liver damage. The liver function tests were within the normal range after two and a half months from the onset of infection in most cases. The mean age of the patients in this group was 30 years.

Group III: HCC patients

This group includes patients with malignant liver disease in the form of HCC, and accounts for nearly 5% (14/304) of the entire study population. The feature typical of these patients is chronic carriage of HBsAg for at least 6 months with signs and symptoms of liver disease, as indicated by abnormal liver function tests. Most patients were also positive for alpha-feto-protein, which was present in high concentration in the serum. The presence of this oncofoetal protein has been taken as additional evidence of tumour progression in the liver of these patients. The mean age of the patients in this group was 55 years.

Group IV: Hepatitis B patients with delta infection

Of 111 patients in group I, only 3 (2.7%) were found to be positive for anti-delta antibody. No delta antigen was detected in any of these 111 patients.

Group V: Young males

The susceptibility of young males to infection by HBV has been observed in this study, 77.6% (236/304) of the patients being males and 22.4% (68/304) females. The male-to-female ratio is thus more than 3:1. The highest infection rate was observed in the age-group 21-30 years, as indicated in Figure 1.

FIG. 1.   PREVALENCE OF HBsAg IN HEPATITIS B PATIENTS BY AGE

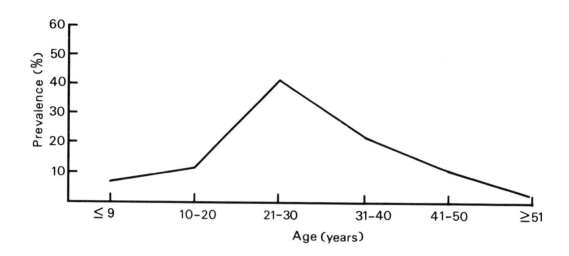

DISCUSSION

The observation in this study that the vast majority of the patients had self-limiting hepatitis B infection is additional evidence that, in most cases, HBV infection does not develop to the chronic state.   On the contrary, those patients with established hepatocellular carcinoma may be unusually susceptible to acute HBV infection and to the development of the persistent carrier state of HBsAg, which is the necessary condition for the neoplastic transformation of the hepatocytes.   The observed high concentration of oncofoetal protein in the serum may be a marker of hepatocytes which have undergone malignant neoplastic transformation.   The role of HBV in causing HCC has been described (Sobeslavsky, 1978).   In those patients with HCC, the development of this cancer could be the result of a persistent infection by HBV of long duration, and the observation of this malignancy in older people in Ethiopia (above the age of 55 years) supports this view.

The significance of infection by the delta agent simultaneously with hepatitis B in the pathogenesis of chronic liver diseases was reported recently (Rizzetto et al., 1977). Delta antigen has been detected in chronically infected patients with HBV while anti-delta seems to be associated with the termination of infection by HBV. The detection of anti-delta antibody in only 3 patients with self-limiting hepatitis B and the absence of the delta antigen in the remaining 108 patients in the same category supports the suggestion that the delta agent requires helper factors from HBV for its replication (Rizzetto et al., 1977). On the other hand, the detection of anti-delta antibody in the 3 patients indicates the presence of this new infective agent in Ethiopia. However, the role of delta agent in the pathogenesis of chronic hepatitis B in Ethiopia has not yet been clarified.

The preponderance of young males between the ages of 21 and 30 years among those infected by HBV has been reported before (Szmuness, 1975; Szmuness et al., 1978). The same pattern has been observed in this study. The mechanism underlying this preponderance is not clear; however, genetic susceptibility, behavioural characteristics, etc., have been suggested (Szmuness et al., 1978) as possible factors affecting such sex differences in response to HBV infection.

CONCLUSIONS

This paper, although far from complete, throws some light on the spectrum of HBV infection in Ethiopia. The observed complexity in the pattern of infection by HBV provides additional evidence to show that HBV infection is unique in terms of its clinical features, pathogenesis, epidemiology and, in general, in the spectrum of host responses to the infection.

ACKNOWLEDGEMENTS

This work was conducted at the Central Laboratory and Research Institute with the help of research funds available from the Institute. I am also grateful to Dr B.G. Hansson for testing the 111 specimens for delta and anti-delta and to Miss Zewditu Amenu for typing the paper.

REFERENCES

Blumberg, B.S., Alter, H.J. & Visnich, S. (1965) A 'new' antigen in leukemia sera. J. Am. med. Assoc., 191, 541-546

Dienstag, J.L. (1980) Toward the control of hepatitis B. New Engl. J. Med., 303, 874-876

Hansson, B.G. & Johnsson, T. (1971) Improved technique for detecting Australia antigen by immunoelectroosmophoresis. Vox Sang. (Basel), 21, 531-539

Rizzetto, M., Canese, M.G., Arico, S., Crivelli, O., Trepo, C., Bonino, F. & Verme, G. (1977) Immunofluorescence detection of a new antigen-antibody system (delta/anti-delta) associated to hepatitis B virus in liver and in serum of HBsAg carriers. Gut, 18, 997-1003

Sobeslavsky, O. (1978) HBV as a global problem. In: Vyas, G.N., Cohen, S.N. & Schmid, R., eds, Proceedings of the 2nd International Symposium on Viral Hepatitis, Philadelphia, Franklin Institute Press, pp. 347-356

Szmuness, W. (1975) Recent advances in the study of the epidemiology of hepatitis B. Am. J. Pathol., 81, 629-649

Szmuness, W., Harley, E.J., Ikram, H. & Stevens, C.E. (1978) Sociodemographic aspects of the epidemiology of hepatitis B. In: Vyas, G.N., Cohen, S.N. & Schmid, R., eds, Proceedings of the 2nd International Symposium on Viral Hepatitis, Philadelphia, Franklin Institute Press, pp. 297-320

L'ANTIGÈNE HBs: MARQUEUR DE LA RELATION ENTRE LE VIRUS DE L'HÉPATITIS B ET LE CANCER PRIMITIF DU FOIE:

SITUATION À BRAZZAVILLE EN 1984

C. M. Gombe

Service de Médecine et Carcinologie
Hôpital Général, B.P. 32
Brazzaville, Congo

SUMMARY

HBs antigen was looked for in three groups of people: patients with hepatocellular carcinoma (HCC), patients with other cancers and healthy subjects. Analysis of the results of this study demonstrates that there is a strong association between HCC and hepatitis B virus, as indicated by the presence of HBs antigen.

RESUME

On a recherché l'antigène HBs dans trois groupes de population: chez des patients atteints de cancer primitif du foie, des malades atteints d'autres cancers et des personnes saines. Les résultats montrent l'existence d'une relation importante entre le cancer primitif du foie et le virus de l'hépatite B, ainsi que l'indique la présence de l'antigène HBs.

INTRODUCTION

En 1980, s'est tenu à Dakar, un colloque international sur le virus de l'hépatite B (HBV) et le cancer primitif du foie (CPF) (Anon., 1981). Au cours de cette réunion, la valeur de plusieurs facteurs épidémiologiques et biologiques en tant que marqueurs de la relation HBV-CPF a été discutée. La signification de la présence de l'antigène HBs, ainsi que d'autres systèmes antigéniques, en particulier HBc et HBe, a été évoquée.

Nous avons déjà montré, d'une part, l'importance des hépatites virales et du taux de portage de l'antigène HBs chez les sujets sains, et d'autre part, la fréquence élevée des cancers primitifs du foie au Congo (Gombe, 1981a,b; Gombe et coll., 1981; Itoua Ngaporo & Gombe, 1981).

Ces faits suggèrent une relation entre les CPF et l'HBV. Aussi nous proposons de commenter ici les résultats des différents dosages d'antigène HBs pratiqués à Brazzaville dans trois groupes de population.

MATERIEL ET METHODES

Au cours de l'étude, on a testé 256 sérums provenant des sujets appartenant à trois groupes de population:

- 120 sérums provenant de sujets donneurs de sang présumés sains, agés de 21 à 50 ans;

- 65 sérums de patients atteints de cancer primitif du foie, hospitalisés à l'Hôpital Général de Brazzaville, agés de 28 à 63 ans, et en majorité de sexe masculin. Le diagnostic de CPF a reçu une confirmation anatomo-pathologique et, dans de nombreux cas, l'alpha-foetoprotéine a pu être dosée.

- 71 sérums de malades atteints de divers autres cancers, dont le diagnostic a également été confirmé par l'examen anatomo-pathologique.

Chez les donneurs de sang la recherche de l'antigène HBs a été effectuée au Centre de Transfusion Sanguine et au Centre d'Immunologie et de Biologie Parasitaires de Lille, par une technique radio-immunologique et par hémagglutination passive. Pour les malades cancéreux, le dosage a été effectué à Brazzaville, dans le Service d'Hématologie et d'Immunologie Générale de l'Hôpital Général de Brazzaville, par la technique d'hémagglutination passive. Le nombre de sérums analysés a été restreint du fait des possibilités limitées du service.

RESULTATS

Les résultats des examens effectués chez les donneurs de sang ont déjà été publiés (Itoua Ngaporo & Gombe, 1981). Onze sérums (soit 9,2%) contenaient l'antigène HBs. Chez les malades atteints de cancer primitif du foie, 48 sérums (soit 73,8%) étaient positifs. Chez les malades atteints d'autres formes de cancer, 2,8% seulement de sérums étaient positifs.

Ces résultats sont résumés dans le Tableau 1.

DISCUSSION

La recherche de l'antigène HBs effectuée antérieurement à Brazzaville avait un double but: d'une part, déterminer le taux de portage de l'AgHBs et de ses sous-types chez les sujets sains (Itoua-Ngaporo & Gombe, 1981; Yala et coll. 1982) et, d'autre part, évaluer le pourcentage de sérums positifs chez les malades atteints de cancer primitif du foie.

Nous avons aussi dans un précédent travail (Gombe, 1981a) montré la place prépondérante des hépatites virales B dans la pathologie hépatique à Brazzaville.

Ces différentes études montrent que dans les pays comme le Sénégal et le Congo, où les CPF sont les cancers les plus fréquents, le taux de portage de l'antigène HBs est élevé (supérieur à 5%) (Anon., 1981; Itoua-Ngaporo & Gombe, 1981). Dans les autres pays, comme les pays européens, où les CPF sont peu fréquents, ce taux est inférieur à 1% (Itoua-Ngaporo & Gombe, 1981). Les taux élevés observés chez des personnes présumées saines peuvent expliquer la présence et la transmission du virus de l'hépatite B.

Une différence significative apparaît lorsque l'on compare les taux de portage de l'antigène HBs des deux populations de malades cancéreux: en effet, 73,8% des sujets atteints de CPF sont porteurs de l'antigène HBs contre 2,8% des sujets atteints d'un autre cancer. Ceci montre que les cancers primitifs du foie se développent avec prédilection chez les sujets antigène HBs-positifs (Michon et coll., 1975). Une étude du même type réalisée à Dakar avec des moyens plus importants a donné des résultats comparables.

Tableau 1. Portage de l'antigène HBs chez des sujets donneurs de sang, chez des sujets atteints de CPF et chez des sujets atteints d'un autre cancer

	Sexe	Ag. HBs +		Ag. HBs −		Total
		Nbre	%	Nbre	%	
Donneurs de sang	Hommes	10		105		115
	Femmes	1		4		5
	Total	11	9.2	109	90.8	120
Sujets atteints de CPF	Hommes	40		7		47
	Femmes	8		10		18
	Total	48	73.8	17	26.2	65
Sujets atteints de cancer (sauf CPF)	Hommes					
	Cancer de la prostate	0		5		)
	Lymphome et L.L.C.[a]	0		6		) 13
	Cancer du colon	0		2		)
	Femmes					
	Cancer du col utérin	1		34		)
	Cancer du sein	0		12		) 58
	Cancer de l'ovaire	1		7		)
	Cancer du corps utérin	0		3		)
	Total	2	2.8	69	97.2	71

[a] L.L.C. = Leucémie lymphoïde chronique

Des études réalisées à Brazzaville, il ressort que plusieurs éléments militent pour une relation de causalité entre le virus HB et les CPF; ce sont:

- la fréquence élevée des hépatites virales B dans la population
- la prédominance des cancers primitifs du foie dans la même population
- le taux très élevé de porteurs de l'antigène HBs chez ces malades
- le faible taux de portage des malades atteints d'autres cancers
- le taux de portage de l'AgHBs élevé chez les sujets présumés sains.

L'antigène HBs apparaît comme un des marqueurs de cette relation entre le virus HB et le CPF.

Aussi, comme cela a été souligné dans une récente réunion de l'OMS (1983) la vaccination contre l'hépatite B représentera probablement la meilleure voie de lutte contre le cancer primitif du foie en Afrique, lorsque les problèmes de purification du vaccin auront été résolus.

REFERENCES

Anon. (1981) Virus de l'hépatite B et cancer primitif du foie (Colloque international, Dakar, 21-24 Avril 1980, 1982). Med. Afr. Noire, 28, 211-262

Gombe, C.M. (1981a) Regards sur les affections hépatiques au Congo. Afr. méd., 20, 279-284

Gombe, C.M. (1981b) Le cancer au Congo: étude épidémiologique. Afr. méd., 20, 593-596

Gombe, C.M., Ntari, B., Nkoua, J.L., Itoua-Ngaporo, A. & Dupont, A. (1981) La ponction-biopsie du foie à l'Hôpital Général de Brazzaville. Résultats à propos de quarante deux cas. Sem. Hôp. Paris, 57, 404-408

Itoua-Ngaporo, A. & Gombe, C.M. (1981) Le portage de l'antigène HBs à Brazzaville. Med. Afr. Noire, 28, 113-114

Michon, J., Prince, A.M., Szmuness, W., Demaille, J., Diebolt, G., Linhard, J., Quenum, C. & Sankale, M. (1975) Cancer primitif du foie et infection par hépatite B au Sénégal. Comparaison des sujets cancéreux avec deux groupes témoins. Biomed., 23, 263-266

Organisation Mondiale de la Santé (1983) Prevention du Cancer du Foie. Rapport d'une réunion de l'OMS (Ser. Rapports Techniques No. 691), Genève, Organisation Mondiale de la Santé

Organisation Mondiale de la Santé (1983) Prevention of Liver Cancer Report of a WHO Meeting (Tech. Rep. Ser., 691), Geneva, World Health Organization

Yala, F., Courouce, A.M., Monjour, L. & Choisy, C. (1982) Enquête préliminaire sur le portage de l'antigène HBs et de la détermination de ses sous-types à Brazzaville. Pathol. Exot. Filiales, 75, 258-261

HÉPATITES VIRALES AIGÜES ET MARQUEURS DU VIRUS HB
DANS LES MALADIES CHRONIQUES DU FOIE
ET DANS LES CANCERS PRIMITIFS DU FOIE

M.F. Sebti

Service de Médecine C
Hôpital Avicenne
Rabat, Maroc

SUMMARY

A clinical and etiological study of 171 cases of acute hepatitis in subjects over 15 years of age showed that 73.7% were of the B type and 25.7% of the non-A, non-B type. A single case of hepatitis A was seen. Hepatitis B and non-A, non-B affect equally young men and women (mean age, 29 and 28, respectively), and infection occurs, for both types of hepatitis, by the parenteral route. More than 90% of cases recovered completely.

The search for markers of hepatitis B virus in subjects with chronic liver diseases has shown that the B virus plays an important role in these diseases in Morocco: 6.7% of controls, 38.5% of cirrhotics and 40.9% of patients with chronic hepatitis were carriers of HBsAg. The anti-hepatitis Bc antibody was present in 53.3% of the control population, in 86.5% of cirrhotics and 90.9% of active chronic hepatitis patients.

Hepatocellular carcinoma is relatively rare in Morocco, representing 5.9% of hepatic tumours and accounting for one hospitalization out of 84. It occurs in older subjects (mean age, 58 years) and more often in men than in women (40:23). The presence of HBsAg was investigated in 46 patients and 379 controls: it was found in 17% of hepatocellular carcinoma patients and 4.7% of controls. Anti-HBc antibodies were present in 76.8% of patients and 53.3% of controls.

RESUME

L'étude clinique et étiologique de 171 cas d'hépatite aiguë chez des sujets de plus de 15 ans a montré que 73,7% de ces hépatites étaient de type B et 25,7% de type Non-A, Non-B (NANB). Un seul cas d'hépatite A a été observé. Les hépatites B et NANB frappent de la même façon les hommes et les femmes jeunes (âges moyens respectifs de 29 et 28 ans) et la contamination se fait dans les 2 types d'hépatite par voie parentérale. La guérison a été obtenue dans plus de 90% des cas.

La recherche des marqueurs du virus HB chez des sujets atteints de maladies chroniques du foie a montré que le virus B joue un rôle important dans ces maladies au Maroc: alors que 6,7% des sujets témoins sont porteurs de l'AgHBs, ce pourcentage passe à 38,5% chez les cirrhotiques et 40,9% chez les sujets atteints d'hépatite chronique. L'anticorps anti-HBc est présent dans 53,3% de la population témoin, dans 86,5% des cirrhoses et 90,9% des hépatites chroniques actives.

Le cancer primitif du foie est relativement rare au Maroc où il constitue 5,9% des tumeurs hépatiques et représente une hospitalisation sur 84. Il survient chez des sujets relativement âgés (moyenne d'âge 58 ans). Il est plus fréquent chez l'homme que chez la femme (40 hommes pour 23 femmes). On a recherché la présence de l'AgHBs dans le sérum de 46 malades et 379 témoins; on l'a retrouvé chez 17% des sujets porteurs de CPF et 4,7% des sujets témoins. Des anticorps anti-HBc étaient présents chez 76,8% des malades et 53,3% des sujets témoins.

INTRODUCTION

Les hépatites virales sont très fréquentes au Maroc. Bénignes dans la majorité des cas, elles peuvent cependant parfois évoluer de façon défavorable.

Ce papier regroupe trois études réalisées à l'hôpital Avicenne de Rabat (Maroc). La première est une étude clinique et étiologique des hépatites virales aiguës observées chez l'adulte. Le mode de contamination, la répartition selon le sexe et l'évolution des hépatites B et des hépatites Non-A, Non-B (NANB) sont analysées.

Dans les deux autres études, on a recherché les marqueurs du virus HB (Ag HBs, anticorps anti-HBs, anticorps anti-HBc), par des méthodes radioimmunologiques, chez des sujets atteints de maladies chroniques du foie (hépatite chronique, cirrhose) et chez les sujets porteurs de cancer primitif du foie (CPF).

MATERIEL ET METHODES

Populations étudiées

1. Caractérisation des hépatites virales

Les caractéristiques des hépatites virales aiguës ont été étudiées chez 171 sujets âgés de plus de 15 ans, hospitalisés à l'hôpital Avicenne à Rabat pour une hépatite aiguë.   Ont été exclus les sujets atteints d'hépatite toxique médicamenteuse.

2. Marqueurs d'HBV dans les maladies chroniques du foie

Les marqueurs du virus ont été étudiés dans trois groupes de sujets:

- un groupe de 52 patients atteints de cirrhose, dont le diagnostic a été confirmé par histologie et par laparoscopie;

- un groupe de 22 patients atteints d'hépatite chronique active (HCA) confirmée histologiquement;

- un groupe de 90 sujets témoins, comprenant des sujets sains, des patients atteints de maladie digestive extra-hépatique, et des patients atteints de maladie extra-hépatique non digestive.

3. Virus HB, cirrhose et CPF

Deux groupes de sujets ont été étudiés:

- un groupe de 63 patients porteurs de CPF, hospitalisés à l'hôpital Avicenne entre 1976 et 1983. Le diagnostic de CPF a été établi sur des critères biologiques (présence d'alpha-foetoprotéine recherchée par radio-immunoessai) et histologiques. Les marqueurs sériques d'HBV ont pu être recherchés chez 46 de ces malades.

- un groupe de 379 sujets témoins (sujets sains, ou malades porteurs de maladies digestives extra-hépatiques ou malades porteurs d'une maladie extra-digestive et extra-hépatique).

Détection des marqueurs sériques du virus HB

L'AgHBs, les anticorps anti-HBs, anti-HBc et les IgM anti-A ont été détectés par des méthodes radio-immunologiques (Kits Abbott: AUSRIA II, AUSAB, CORAB, et antiAIgM).

Analyse statistique des résultats

Elle a été réalisée avec les tests de Student et de Chi^2.

RESULTATS

1. Caractérisation des hépatites virales

L'examen sérologique effectué chez les patients atteints d'hépatite aiguë au tout début de la maladie a permis de les classer en 5 groupes (Tableau 1).

Tableau 1. Distribution des hépatites virales selon le virus en cause, mis en évidence par les marqueurs biologiques

	Ag HBs	Anticorps anti-HBc	Anticorps anti-HBs	IgM anti-A	Total
Hépatite B certaine	+	+	-	-	118
Hépatite B très probable	+	+	+	-	8
Hépatite NANB certaine	-	-	-	-	25
Hépatite NANB probable	-	+	+	-	19
Hépatite A	-	-	-	+	1

Pour l'analyse des résultats, les hépatites virales certaines et probables ont été regroupées, ce qui donne:

Hépatite virales de type B   126 cas (73,7%)
Hépatites virales de type NANB   44 cas (25,7%)
Hépatites virales de type A   1 cas

Il est à noter que l'hépatite virale de type A est extrêmement rare chez les adultes.

L'âge moyen des malades était de 29,3 ans ($\pm$ 8,95) pour l'hépatite B et 28 ans ($\pm$ 9,4) pour l'hépatite NANB.

Parmi les malades atteints d'hépatite B, 44% étaient de sexe masculin, 56% de sexe féminin. Dans le cas des hépatites NANB, 48% des malades étaient des hommes et 52% des femmes.

L'origine de la contamination a été recherchée. Dans le cas de l'hépatite B, la contamination a eu lieu par voie parentérale dans 58,5% des cas; par voie non parentérale dans 8,5% des cas. La voie de contamination n'a pas pu être établie dans 33% des cas.

Dans le cas de l'hépatite NANB, le mode de contamination n'a pas pu être établi dans 40% des cas. Dans les 60% des cas où le mode de contamination a pu être établi, celle-ci s'est effectuée par voie parentérale.

Evolution des hépatites virales.- Après 6 mois, 34 patients ont été perdus de vue (20%). La guérison a été obtenue dans plus de 90% des cas; une évolution anormale a été observée dans 8,8% des cas (Tableau 2).

Tableau 2. Evolution des hépatites virales à 6 mois ou plus

Nombre de cas	Hépatite B	Hépatite NANB
Au moment du diagnostic	126	44
Suivis 6 mois ou plus	97 (77,0%)	39 (88,6%)
Guérison	89 (91,7%)	35 (89,7%)
Absence de guérison	8 (8,2%)	4 (10,3%)

Parmi les 12 sujets présentant une évolution anormale, 5 ont accepté de subir une ponction biopsie du foie (PBF) qui a montré:

- une hépatite chronique persistente: 1 cas
- une hépatite chronique active: 3 cas
- une cirrhose: 1 cas

Il est à noter qu'un patient est devenu porteur chronique de l'Ag HBs.

2. Marqueurs de l'hépatite B dans les maladies chroniques du foie

Les marqueurs de l'hépatite B se retrouvent chez les sujets atteints de maladies chroniques du foie avec une fréquence significativement plus grande que chez les sujets témoins (Tableau 3).

La présence des anticorps anti-HBc et anti-HBs a été recherchée (Tableau 4).

Les sujets atteints d'hépatite chronique active (HCA) et présentant des anticorps anti-HBc sont plus souvent anticorps anti-HBs-négatifs (63%) que les malades souffrant de cirrhose (50%) et que les sujets témoins (23%).

La présence des anticorps anti-HBc a été étudiée en fonction du sexe des malades (Tableau 5).

3. Virus HB, cirrhose et CPF

Les cancers primitifs du foie représentent 5,9% des tumeurs du foie observées à l'hôpital Avicenne.

Parmi les 1 009 personnes hospitalisées à Avicenne en 1981 dans le service de Médecine C, 12 l'ont été pour CPF, ce qui correspond à 1 hospitalisation pour 84. En 1982, 17 sujets ont été hospitalisés pour CPF; durant la même année, 1 416 malades ont été hospitalisés. Le CPF correspondait donc à l'hospitalisation pour 83.

L'âge moyen des 63 malades hospitalisés pour CPF entre 1976 et 1983 était de 58 ans.

Tableau 3. Fréquence de la présence d'anticorps anti-HBc et de la présence de l'AgHBs chez les sujets atteints de maladies chroniques du foie et chez les sujets témoins

	Anti-HBc +							Anti-HBc −	
	Total		AgHBs +		AgHBs −			N	%
	N	%	N	%[1]	N	%[1]			
Témoins: 90	48	53,3	6	12,5	42	87,5		42	46,6
Hépatite chronique active: 22 cas	20	90,9	9	45,0[a]	11	55,0[c]		2	9,1
Cirrhose: 52 cas	45	86,5	20	44,4[a]	25	55,5[b]		7	13,5

N = Nombre de cas; [1] = Pourcentage calculé par rapport au nombre de porteurs de l'anticorps anti-HBc

[a] $p < 0,001$

[b] $p < 0,01$

[c] $p < 0,05$

Tableau 4. Présence des anticorps anti-HBc et anti-HBs

	Anti-HBc +			Anti-HBc −		
	Total	Anti-HBs +	Anti-HBs −	Total	Anti-HBS +	Anti-HBs −
	N	N $\%^1$	N $\%^1$	N	N $\%^2$	N $\%^2$
Témoins: 90	48	37 77,1	11 22,9	42	11 26,2	31 73,8
HCA: 21	19	7 36,8	12 63,2	2	0	2
Cirrhose:52	42	21 50,0	21 50,0	7	3 42,9	4 57,1

N = nombre de cas

[1] Pourcentage calculé par rapport au nombre de sujets présentant des anticorps anti-HBc

[2] Pourcentage calculé par rapport au nombre de sujets ne possédant pas d'anticorps anti-HBc

    Le CPF frappe plus les hommes (40 cas) que les femmes (23 cas). La présence d'une cirrhose a été observée chez 44 sujets porteurs de CPF (70%).

    Les marqueurs sériques du virus HB ont pu être recherchés chez 46 patients (Tableau 6).

Tableau 5.   Présence des anticorps anti-HBc en fonction du sexe
des malades

	Anti-HBc +			Anti-HBc −		
	Total	N	%[1]	Total	N	%[2]
	N %			N %		
Témoins: 90 46 H	48 53,3	30	62,5	42 46,7	16	38,1
44 F		18	37,5		26	61,9
HCA: 22 14 H	20 95,2	13	65,0	2 9,5	1	50,0
8 F		7	35,0		1	50,0
Cirrhose:52 31 H	45 86,5	26	57,8	7 13,5	5	71,4
21 F		19	42,2		2	28,6

N = nombre de cas

[1] Pourcentage en fonction du nombre de sujets porteurs de
l'anticorps anti-HBc

[2] Pourcentage en fonction du nombre de sujets anti-HBc −

Tableau 6. Présence des marqueurs d'HBV chez les sujets atteints
de CPF et chez les sujets témoins

	Nombre de cas	AgHBs +		Anti-HBs +		Anti-HBc +	
		N	%	N	%	N	%
CPF	46	8	17,4[a]	28	60,9	35	76,1
Témoins	379	18	4,7	194	51,1	202	53,3

[a] Différence statistiquement significative

L'AgHBs se retrouve dans 17% des cas de CPF. Cette proportion de CPF associés au virus HB est faible par rapport à celle
observée en Afrique noire.

SHORT COMMUNICATION: PRESENCE OF HBV DNA IN HEPATOCELLULAR CARCINOMA TISSUE

G. Greenfield

Wellcome Virus Research Laboratory
Nairobi, Kenya

RESUME

Les examens réalisés sur des biopsies de patients ayant un cancer primitif du foie ont révélé que 35% d'entre eux avaient des séquences de l'ADN du virus HB intégrées dans leur génomes cellulaires. Cette proportion est considérablement plus élevée que celle qu'on retrouve chez les témoins, mais néanmoins inférieure à ce que l'on attendait.

SUMMARY

Tests on biopsies from HCC patients showed that 35% had integrated sequences of HBV DNA in their cell genomes. This was considerably more than controls but less than had been expected.

INTRODUCTION

There is now strong epidemiological evidence associating hepatitis B virus (HBV) infection with hepatocellular carcinoma (HCC). Other incriminating evidence is the presence of HBV DNA integrated into hepatic cellular DNA in HCC tissue, and the presence of a similar virus in the Grand Mammal, which also develops HCC.

In Kenya, HCC is the third commonest cancer. The general carrier rate for HBV surface antigen (HBsAg) is 10% but among patients with HCC it is 69%. It was therefore decided to look for HBV DNA sequences in Kenyan patients suffering from HCC.

METHODS

A total of 47 percutaneous liver biopsies were performed on inpatients at Kenyatta National Hospital over the period 1983-1984. Each biopsy was divided into 2 halves, one of which was frozen immediately in dry ice, and the other sent for routine histology. The frozen material was kept at -70^{0}C and the controls dispatched in dry ice to the Royal Free Hospital, London.

The frozen samples were analysed for the presence of HBV DNA by blot transfer hybridization using cloned ^{32}PHBV DNA.

RESULTS

Of the 47 cases biopsied, HCC was diagnosed definitely in 20 and probably in 2 cases, while 7 cases had other liver tumours, 7 were normal or with changes indicative of tropical splenomegaly syndrome. Seven had cirrhosis and 4 had obstructive jaundice.

Of the 20 definite HCC cases, HBV DNA sequences were found in 10, of which 5 had only integrated DNA, 3 had only free DNA and 2 had both; thus, 35% of HCC cases had definite integrated sequences of HBV DNA in their cell genomes (the number of sequences varied from 1 to 5). Both the probable cases had integrated DNA.

In contrast, only 2 of the other 25 biopsies had HBV DNA. One case of HBsAg-positive cirrhosis had free HBV DNA and one HBsAg-negative tumour had integrated DNA.

No information is available on other HBV markers in these patients.

DISCUSSION

The presence of integrated HBV DNA sequences in livers with HCC is highly significant, yet we were surprised not to find it in a much larger proportion of cases. In other parts of Africa HBV DNA integrated sequences have been found in almost all HCC tissue. However, these studies were performed on post mortem material, where the exact site of the tumour can be located. Our biopsies were blind and the material sent for DNA analysis may bear little relation to that sent for histology. And yet, with the same technique and material of Chinese origin, higher rates of integration have been found.

HEPATOCELLULAR CARCINOMA: CONTROL

HEPATITIS B VIRUS AND THE CONTROL
OF HEPATOCELLULAR CARCINOMA

B.S. Blumberg

Fox Chase Cancer Center
Philadelphia, PA, USA

RESUME

Il est maintenant bien établi que dans un pourcentage très élevé de cas, le développement du cancer primitif du foie (CPF) est lié à l'infection par le virus de l'hépatite B (HBV). Le CPF est l'un des cancers les plus répandus dans le monde. Dans de vastes régions d'Asie, d'Afrique et d'Océanie, c'est un des cancers les plus courants chez les sujets de sexe masculin. On a estimé globalement, à un million le nombre annuel de décès imputables à cette maladie.

Le virus de l'hépatite B peut être identifié dans plus de 90% des cas de CPF. Dans tous les cas ou dans la plupart d'entre eux, l'ADN du virus de l'hépatite B est intégré à celui de la cellule hôte. Dans certaines régions, les individus porteurs du virus pendant une longue période, en particulier ceux qui ont été contaminés pendant leur jeunesse, ont un risque de développer un cancer du foie près de 200 fois plus élevé que ceux qui n'ont pas eu d'infection chronique. Le groupe de sujets porteurs du virus HB représente la catégorie la plus exposée au cancer.

Le Dr Millman et l'auteur ont introduit un vaccin pouvant prévenir l'infection HBV, vaccin actuellement disponible et utilisé aux Etats-Unis, en Asie et en Afrique. Des programmes de vaccination des nouveaux-nés sont actuellement en voie de planification ou d'exécution dans les régions où l'infection HBV est endémique. On peut espérer que ceci entraînera dans un avenir relativement proche une diminution considérable de la fréquence des porteurs d'HBV et, par la suite, une réduction de la fréquence du CPF. L'efficacité de ces programmes quant à la réduction du pourcentage de porteurs devrait être connue dans quelques

années. Des essais de vaccination de grande envergure réalisés
sur le terrain ont prouvé l'efficacité du vaccin et son innocuité. De nombreuses démarches sont actuellement entreprises
pour réduire son coût. Ceci devrait permettre son usage dans les
régions d'Asie, d'Afrique et de l'Océanie qui en ont le plus
besoin. Un projet financé sur le plan international pourrait
efficacement accélérer l'exécution de ces programmes.

Il existe actuellement dans le monde plusieurs centaines de
millions de porteurs d'HBV dont beaucoup courent un risque élevé
de développer un CPF. La recherche actuellement en cours est
orientée vers des programmes devant permettre de comprendre la
pathogénie du CPF chez ces individus afin de pouvoir prévenir ou
retarder considérablement l'évolution du cancer. Cette recherche
pourrait fournir une forme complémentaire de prévention pour les
populations à haut risque. En cas de succès, elle aurait un
effet immédiat sur la mortalité et la morbidité dues au CPF.

SUMMARY

There is now a substantial body of evidence that, in a very
high percentage of cases, infection with hepatitis B virus (HBV)
is required for the development of hepatocellular carcinoma
(HCC), which is one of the most common cancers in the world. In
vast areas of Asia, Africa and Oceania it is one of the commonest
cancers in males, and it has been estimated that overall there
are as many as 1 million deaths a year from this disease.

HBV can be identified in over 90% of cases of HCC. In most
or all of these the HBV DNA is integrated into the DNA of the
host cell. Individuals who are HBV carriers for a long period,
in certain regions, particularly if infected in their youth, have
about a 200-fold greater risk of developing cancer than those who
have not been chronically infected. This makes the HBV carrier
group the highest known risk category for a common cancer.

A vaccine to prevent infection with HBV has been introduced
and is now available and in use in the United States, Europe,
Asia and Africa. Public health programmes are currently being
planned, or are in progress, for the vaccination of newborn
children in areas where HBV infection is endemic. It is hoped
that in a relatively short time this will considerably decrease
the incidence of HBV carriers and, in due course, markedly

decrease the incidence of HCC.   The effectiveness of these programmes in reducing the carrier rate should be known in a few years.

Extensive field trials with the vaccine have shown that it is highly effective and, based on these initial studies, extremely safe. A variety of steps are now being undertaken to markedly reduce its cost. This should make it possible to use it in the areas of Asia, Africa and Oceania where the greatest need exists. An internationally funded programme could be very effective in speeding the application of the vaccine.

There are now several hundred million carriers of HBV in the world, many of whom are at high risk of developing HCC. Current research is directed towards understanding the pathogenesis of HCC in these individuals with the hope that the development of the cancer can be prevented or markedly delayed. This research could provide a form of secondary prevention for the high-risk population. If successful, it could have an immediate effect in decreasing the incidence of HCC mortality and morbidity.

INTRODUCTION

There is now a convincing body of evidence that it is possible to prevent the transmission of hepatitis B virus (HBV) and a substantial series of investigations which indicate that this, in due course, could lead to the marked reduction and possibly the elimination of hepatocellular carcinoma (HCC).

In this introductory paper (more detailed references are given in Blumberg and London (1982)) I hope to provide an overall view of this problem with a general discussion of the possibilities and actualities of:

(1)   Primary prevention, i.e., prevention of HCC by preventing infection with HBV.

(2)   Secondary prevention, i.e., prevention of HCC in people who are already infected by detecting very early tumours and removing them surgically before they become larger.

(3)   Prevention by delay. This term has been introduced to
      describe the approach in which asymptomatic carriers of
      HBV can be detected and managed so that the onset of
      symptomatic chronic liver disease and HCC can be
      delayed for a sufficiently long period to enable the
      carrier to live out his or her normal life span without
      experiencing the detrimental effects of liver disease
      including cancer.

In the 1950s, Payet, Davis, Steiner and other investigators
in West and East Africa, on the basis of clinical, pathological,
and observational evidence, suggested that hepatitis might be the
cause of hepatocellular carcinoma, a common disease in the areas
in which they worked. At that time it was not possible to test
this hypothesis directly, but after 1967, with the introduction
of relatively simple methods for the detection of HBV in serum
and other secretions and tissues, tests were undertaken.

In 1971, at a meeting on cancer in Africa held in Uganda,
several studies showing a striking association between HBV and
HCC were presented. This appeared to be a turning point in the
development of interest in this association, and the intensity of
the work in the field increased. In 1975 we said (Blumberg et
al., 1975):

"During recent years, there have been parallel developments
in understanding, on the one hand, the pathogenesis of primary
hepatic carcinoma. ... and, on the other, the biology of
Australia antigen ... and the infectious agent hepatitis B virus
(HBV), to which it is intimately related. Recently, the paths of
these developments have begun to converge, and from this it is
possible to design a preliminary strategy which could, if the
interpretations of these data are correct, result in the prevention of many, and perhaps most, cases of one of the most widespread and deadly cancers in humans."

We presented the then available evidence that supported the
statement and concluded by discussing the vaccine we had introduced, and possible prevention strategies.

In the relatively short time since that article appeared,
prevention programmes have begun and there is considerable hope
that the sought-for objectives may be achieved.

EVIDENCE THAT HBV IS NEEDED FOR THE DEVELOPMENT OF HCC

The evidence that persistent infection with HBV is required for the development of HCC has been reviewed in several publications (for example, see London and Blumberg (1983)) and in other papers presented at this Symposium. It now appears that there is reasonable agreement that this hypothesis has been amply supported. For practical purposes, it can be said that HBV is a necessary cause of HCC. This does not rule out the possibility that other external (for example, aflatoxins) and host factors may also be required or play a significant role in pathogenesis.

The evidence supporting the hypothesis will be briefly summarized.

Carriers of HBV are common in the parts of the world where HCC is most common, including such surprising locations as Alaska and Greenland, where HBV and HCC are common in the Eskimo populations. A large number of case-control studies, in which the frequency of the virus in patients with HCC is compared to that in controls, have been completed. In some of these studies, in which the most sensitive methods for the detection of the virus are used, the frequency of virus infection in the cases may approach 100%, i.e., the attributable risk is extremely high.

The virus can be identified by immunofluorescent and other methods in the liver tissue of people with HCC. An interesting feature of this observation, pointed out by Professor Popper and others who have pioneered this work, is that the virus is most abundant in the cells which do not appear to have undergone malignant transformation, i.e., the more normal looking cells surrounding the actual tumour. The anaplastic cells themselves may have no or sparse infection with the whole virus. I shall return to this point later (Thung et al., 1979).

Currently one of the most exciting areas of research is the molecular biology of HBV. The entire base sequence of the virus has been determined and confirmed by several groups. The HBV DNA is integrated into the DNA of the host liver cells in a very large percentage of the cases, and in some studies in all the cases. However there is also integration of HBV DNA in the liver cells of patients without HCC, including those with chronic liver disease, and asymptomatic carriers of HBV. Hence integration per se cannot explain the pathogenesis of the cancer. Integration appears to be clonal in an individual tumour, but the insertion locations of the several copies of HBV DNA are not the same in different tumours (Bréchot et al., 1980).

It is interesting that, although the molecular biology of HBV and HCC is likely to help in the understanding of pathogenesis, it has not as yet made any contribution to prevention or control. It will, however, be of value in the future in the manufacture of vaccine, or for sensitive methods of detection.

Some of the most impressive evidence supporting the HBV-HCC hypothesis is epidemiological. In one of the most convincing studies on cancer etiology, Beasley and his co-workers in Taiwan studied 22 707 male government workers between the ages of 40 and 59. The recruitment into the study population began in November 1975 and was concluded in June 1978. Of these, 3435 men were asymptomatic carriers of HBV and the remainder were not. As of October 1982, 86 cases of HCC had developed in the study population, all but 3 recruited from the group who were carriers at the beginning of the study. The annual incidence for the whole population was 55 per 100 000, but for the carrier group it was 351 per 100 000. In his initial report, Beasley estimated the relative risk for the carrier men to be 223 (Beasley & Lin, 1978). This is probably the highest risk ratio for any known environmental cause for a common cancer. Based on life-table projections, they estimated the life-time risk of death from HCC or cirrhosis for a Chinese male carrier to be between 40% and 50%, a remarkably high value.

Beasley's study established that the association between HBV and HCC was closer than that for any other virus and a site-specific cancer or probably for any environmental factor and a specific cancer. It has also been shown that it is infection with the virus, rather than liver cirrhosis, that is the high-risk factor for cancer. Patients with cirrhosis due to a cause other than HBV have a low risk for HCC, while those with cirrhosis due to HBV have an extremely high one.

Prospective studies similar to Beasley's are now in progress in Eskimos in Alaska, Chinese in Hong Kong and Singapore, and Japanese in Tokyo. Early reports indicate findings similar to his, i.e., a greatly increased risk of HCC in the carriers.

In 1971 (Blumberg et al., 1971) we had proposed, based on the unusual population, clinical and physical characteristics of HBV, that it represented the first member to be found of a new group of infectious agents that we termed 'icrons'. Summers, working at the Institute for Cancer Research, was searching for viruses similar to HBV utilizing his knowledge of the unique molecular characteristics of the virus. He subsequently discovered 2 such viruses (in woodchucks and ducks) (Summers et al., 1980) and another has been identified in California ground squirrels.

The finding of the woodchuck hepatitis virus (WHV) provided another convincing piece of evidence for the hypothesis that HBV and viruses similar to it cause cancer of the liver. Woodchucks (Marmota monax) which develop persistent infection with WHV predictably (80% or more) develop HCC whereas uninfected or transiently infected animals never or rarely do. Another example is seen in ducks found in China (and possibly elsewhere). The duck virus (DHBV) is similar to HBV and WHV and it is also associated with HCC.

It has been shown both indirectly and directly that many of the individuals who go on to develop HCC are infected at a very early age (Larouze et al., 1976). In some parts of the world, particularly Asia, the transmission may be maternal, in others the children may be infected by their sibs or others in the community. In any case, since infection at an early age increases the probability of persistent infection, protection by vaccination in infancy appears to be indicated.

VACCINES

Infectious agents may produce many antibodies in the infected host and/or in experimental animals. Some of these may protect against subsequent infection and others may not; production of an appropriate vaccine requires the identification of the protective antibody. From the very first observations on what was then called Australia antigen, it was obvious that the virus and the antibody against its surface antigen (anti-HBs) rarely occurred together in the same serum. These observations were further supported by the early studies of Okochi and his colleagues (1968), who were able to demonstrate in their first transfusion studies that the patients who had anti-HBs before transfusion, or who developed it after transfusion, had a lower risk of infection with HBV than those who did not have the antibody.

These observations, scanty as they were, were sufficient to stimulate the development of a vaccine. In October 1969, Blumberg and Millman described the methods for extracting surface antigen free from whole virus, using the blood of carriers as the source of the vaccine. This vaccine was based on a unique concept, that viral protein could be extracted directly from human plasma by methods that would make it safe for inoculation in humans and would preserve its antigenicity (Millman, 1984).

Experiments in humans were not undertaken at the time of the vaccine's initial introduction and the value of this kind of vaccine was questioned by some authorities. Later (in 1979) Krugman and his colleagues, who had long experience with the experimental transmission of hepatitis in humans, inoculated children with a preparation of HBV-positive serum which had been boiled for 1 minute. In challenge experiments, the heated serum provided protection against HBV infection. This experiment had the effect of convincing manufacturers and researchers that the Blumberg-Millman vaccine would probably work and the Merck company in the United States, among others, proceeded with the preparation of large batches of it.

In a brilliant field trial, the late Wolf Szmuness demonstrated the safety and effectiveness of the vaccine, using as a study population a high-risk group of male homosexuals in New York City (Szmuness et al., 1980). (Trials in foreign populations were not used at that time for licensure of a vaccine in the United States.) We shall hear more about the trials and the manufacture of the vaccine in other papers presented to the Symposium and I will not elaborate further on it here.

PRIMARY PREVENTION OF HCC

Prevention programmes will be based primarily (but probably not exclusively) on the use of the vaccine. The price of the vaccine is currently very high, expensive even for countries with a large public health budget. It is highly likely that it will decrease as more is required, as more companies and countries begin to manufacture the product, and as new methods of manufacture are developed.

Prevention programmes can be divided into a number of different categories.

Populations with a low prevalence of HBV

Most northern European countries, most of North America and other non-tropical or subtropical areas fit into this category. Vaccination is recommended for people in high-risk groups. These include health-care groups, particularly those with frequent exposure to human blood, travellers, the military, male homosexuals, individuals working on renal dialysis units, and possibly the dialysis patients, drug abusers, and others. Individuals in each of the groups need to balance their risks of developing hepatitis B against any reluctance they may have to use the vaccine.

The field trials have shown that, within the limits of those trials, the vaccine is extremely safe. However, there has been a curious development. Acquired immune deficiency syndrome (AIDS) has, since 1980, occurred with increasing frequency in certain susceptible populations, primarily in the United States. Under some circumstances AIDS can be transmitted by blood. Although there is no evidence that the disease has ever been transmitted by HBV vaccine and the process of manufacture includes several steps which would kill any known virus, some have been reluctant to use the vaccine for fear of the transmission of AIDS. It is likely that, as we learn more about AIDS, this problem will be solved and will not inhibit the use of the vaccine.

Populations of moderate prevalence in which maternal transmission is important

In Japan the frequency of carriers is about 3%. There is evidence that from 30% to 50% of the carriers are a consequence of maternal transmission. Dr Nishioka and his co-workers in Tokyo, and other Japanese workers have for several years been screening expectant mothers for HBsAg. Carriers' mothers are then tested to see if they also have HBeAg. For those that are found to be positive, immunization of the newborn is recommended. The infant is given high titre anti-HBs at birth, and a vaccination programme is started at about 3 months.

In the future more extensive vaccination programmes may be introduced in these populations. This could include all newborns as well as adults who are still susceptible. The extension of the programme to these other groups will probably depend on the availability and cost of the vaccine.

Populations with a high frequency of carriers

These are found in much of China, other regions of Asia and sub-Saharan Africa. Although maternal transmission may occur, it is relatively less important than transmission to the newborn from sibs, other family members, and members of the general community. In these populations universal childhood vaccination (at about 3 months old) is recommended and is being used in some regions. If vaccine becomes more readily available and inexpensive, then susceptible adults may also be vaccinated. In this case, it may be useful to test the population first to determine who is already susceptible. The cost of the testing would then have to be balanced against the potential saving in vaccine cost.

An interesting problem arises in some low-frequency areas which include sizeable populations from high-frequency areas. For example, in the United States there are many immigrants from high-frequency regions of Asia. In Philadelphia we have tested mothers in this population for the presence of HBsAg and HBeAg. An immunization programme for the newborns of the positive mothers is now in progress. In due course, vaccination may also be made available to susceptible adults.

Similarly, the Eskimo and Indian population of Alaska have a high frequency of HBV carriers. A programme is now being planned to immunize all susceptible individuals in this relatively small population (about 60 000) as well as newborns.

Extensive immunization programmes are therefore already in progress and we shall hear more about this later. We can now consider what can be done for the (about) 200 000 000 people in the world who are already carriers.

SECONDARY PREVENTION

Carriers of HBV are at a high risk of developing HCC. Small resectable tumours can be detected by following carriers prospectively with periodic testing for alpha-fetoprotein (AFP) and other foetal proteins such as acidic ferritin. Dr Sun and his co-workers (1980) in China have had extensive experience of mass surveys for persistent elevations of AFP. When elevations are detected, the carriers are brought to hospital for imaging procedures (particularly ultrasound), which can localize even small masses. If a tumour is visualized, surgery is recommended. Using these methods they have reported a significant improvement in survival. In some cases more than one tumour has been detected with continuing surveillance of a patient who has already undergone resection.

We are conducting similar studies on populations of Asian origin residing in Philadelphia. The results from these studies are not yet suitable for analysis; however, during the course of the next few years, the value of this approach should become known. The question of screening of carriers in low-frequency areas is also not yet resolved. Analysis of studies now in progress should allow the identification of carriers who are at particularly high risk of developing tumours earlier than others.

In collaboration with Professor Palmer Beasley we are currently evaluating the role of the iron-binding proteins ferritin and transferrin in predicting the development of cancer in carriers. It is likely that a series of predictors may eventually be identified which could improve the precision of the survey techniques (Lustbader et al., 1983).

A MODEL FOR THE PATHOGENESIS OF HCC

There are certain features of the HBV-HCC relation which require an explanation which is not entirely provided by conventional theory. London and Blumberg (1983) have introduced a model to explain these findings which could lead to interesting and possibly novel approaches to prevention and therapy. I will first briefly review the findings which are explained by the model and then describe the model itself.

HCC is associated with chronic hepatitis and not with acute hepatitis that does not have any chronic component. Hepatitis A virus infection, which does not appear to have a chronic form, is not associated with cancer, and most people who go on to develop the carrier state of HBV and HCC do not experience a preceding acute disease. The 'incubation period' for the development of HCC appears to be very long; people who develop HCC may be infected as early as the first year of their lives, but the disease usually does not appear until very much later, i.e., in the fourth, fifth and sixth decades.

Histological studies of the liver tissues of patients with HCC reveal that the actual anaplastic cells, those which seem to have been malignantly transformed, do not contain large amounts of HBsAg, HBV core antigen (HBcAg), or whole virus, while the surrounding cells which do not appear to have been transformed contain large amounts of the virus and its components. The amount of HBsAg in the serum of patients with HCC is low compared to that in carriers and individuals with other forms of chronic HBV infection. Further, the amount of HBsAg in the serum decreases as the cancer progresses. From the molecular studies it is known that the HBV DNA is integrated into the DNA of the tumour cells. It may also be integrated into the cells which do not show malignant transformation or, in fact, in individuals, such as carriers, who do not have cancer at all. Finally, chronic infection with HBV may cause not only HCC but also various forms of chronic liver disease; that is, the model must explain how the same agent can cause more than one disease.

The model postulates that the livers of mature humans (and those of animals such as woodchucks (Marmota monax) which can be infected with a similar virus) contain two populations of cells. The first, which is initially the much larger component, readily becomes infected with HBV, synthesizes viral proteins and can produce infectious virus. These have been referred to as susceptible or S cells.

The second population of cells, initially very small in number, is relatively resistent to replicative infection with HBV; these are called resistant or R cells. If these cells become infected, integration may occur, but they produce little or no virus.

In individuals chronically infected with HBV, S cells have a shortened survival period. This can be the result of an immune response of the host to viral and cellular antigens expressed on the surface of the virus-infected hepatocytes or because cells which are actively replicating virus are metabolically compromized. The death of the S cells which, in a chronically infected liver would be continuous, stimulates the division of the R cells. Hence there is a continuous process of death, regeneration and, possibly scarring of the liver. The R cells are relatively immune to death from HBV infection, since replication does not occur, and they are at a selective advantage compared to the S cells. The S-cell population gradually decreases, and the R-cell population increases.

Eventually, integration of HBV DNA into the DNA of the host cells may occur. If integration occurs in an S cell, this probably is of little consequence since the S cell will eventually die as a result of the HBV replication. If the integration occurs in an R cell it may lead to a tumour. The R-cell population, because of the continuing death of S cells, is already expanding. Integration of viral DNA may give an advantage to the clone of R cells originating from the cell in which the integration event occurred. As this clone expands, it may, by the process of clonal evolution, develop the characteristics of a malignant neoplasm.

What are the origins of the R and S cells? London (1982) has proposed that R cells are the less mature cells and S cells are fully differentiated hepatocytes. The R cells are the predominant cell form in early foetal life, decreasing in number, but never totally disappearing in the maturing liver. The S cells are the predominant form in the normal mature liver.

According to this scheme, an R cell can divide and yield two R cells or it can divide and differentiate into two mature S cells, or it can give rise to an R cell and a S cell. The more mature S cell, if it can divide at all, will produce only S cells. Since the selective pressure of the HBV infection is applied mainly to the S cells, R cells will gradually accumulate. Integration of HBV DNA into the R-cell genome would hinder further differentiation and ensure that only R cells are produced. This will further increase the rate of expansion of the R-cell component. If the integration of DNA results in the turning on of a cellular gene which alters the cell phenotype in some way that provides a growth advantage, the clone resulting from the transformed R cell will have an even greater growth and selective advantage.

PREVENTION BY DELAY

There are some interesting consequences of this model which will be briefly discussed. It must be emphasized that this section of the paper deals with new possibilities and on-going research and is not applicable to public health practice, as are the primary and secondary means of prevention discussed above.

The driving force in the growth of the cancer is the death of the S cells as a result of the replication of HBV. Hence, if we could devise methods to stop, or even slow down this process, it might be possible to prevent the development of disease during the normal life-span of the individual. If this process could be started early enough before a very large R-cell component had accumulated, then very mild procedures could be used over a long period, rather than severe treatments over a relatively short time, the technique that is generally used in cancer therapy.

Most forms of cancer therapy are directed toward the killing of as many cancer cells as possible. In the process, because cancer cells and normal (particularly developing) cells have much in common, many normal cells are also affected. This places a limit on the agressiveness of cancer therapy. The procedures recommended by this model are directed toward preserving the health of the S cells rather than destroying the infected R cells.

The suggested 'therapies' have a limited goal. It is not necessary to eliminate all the R cells, but only to keep their numbers at a sufficiently low level so that they are not percep- tible to the carrier. Further, it is not even necessary to completely eliminate the HBV infection, which in any case may be very difficult to do if integration has occurred. What is required is to slow down the process to such an extent that the presence of the virus is not perceived by the patient, i.e., to prolong the asymptomatic phase of the carrier state while at the same time significantly altering the risk of chronic hepatitis and HCC.

Another aspect of this form of prevention is that it can be applied very early, although at present it is hard to say how early. We would want to know how to predict which carriers detected in the first few years of life will remain carriers into their adulthood, and methods for doing this should be uncovered with further research. Again, what is proposed is prevention rather than therapy, since we hope to be able to develop a benign form of management that could be used by carriers who are not sick.

What can be done to slow down the process of cancer and liver-disease pathogenesis? The answer to this is not now known, but certain approaches are currently being studied and a few are under investigation in our laboratory, while others will be described.

There is evidence that liver cells with high concentrations of the iron-binding protein ferritin, and possibly high levels of iron as well, are more likely to become infected and to replicate HBV. We are trying to understand this process sufficiently well to see if some management of iron or of iron-binding proteins can favourably alter this process (Blumberg et al., 1981).

A variety of chemicals, many derived from plants, can alter the HBsAg characteristics in a manner which affects their immune reactions. Such materials may have a role in preventing cell infection. There are also materials which may affect HBV replication by altering its enzymes and such chemicals may help to ameliorate infection.

HBV, like other viruses, must enter the cell through specific attachment sites. If these can be affected then invasion of the cells may be controllable. A series of investigations on polymerized serum albumin have indicated a possible role for this material in the process. In addition, superoxide may play a role in liver-cell destruction. The formation of superoxides is related to HBV infection, and may be controllable.

It is hoped that these and similar lines of investigations may eventually lead to the prevention by delay that has been proposed.

CONCLUSIONS

From the proceedings of this Symposium and the material reviewed in this paper it appears that national and international prevention programmes for the control of HBV are in progress, and that more are contemplated. There is every reason to hope that, in due course, this could eventually lead to a considerable decrease in the frequency of HCC.

More experience with these programmes will be needed before a decision can be taken on the best manner to proceed, but it is entirely possible that a campaign to completely eliminate the virus might be eventually considered. This could have considerable consequences for human ecology and for ecology in general (see for example, our (London et al., 1982) discussions of the role of HBV in human sex determination and fertility) which should be considered as the prevention programmes evolve.

The price of HBV vaccine is high but it can be predicted that it will decrease. Even when this does happen, the programmes will be expensive, and they are most needed in areas of the world where public health budgets are low. The programme for the control of HBV may therefore be conducted as an internationally funded world-wide effort, and the character of the sponsors of this Symposium shows the international interest in such a programme.

Infection with HBV leads to considerable loss of life and an enormous toll of illness, not only from HCC but from acute hepatitis, and the life shortening caused by chronic liver disease. It is not, however, the most important medical problem in Africa; bacterial and viral diseases, malaria, bilharzia, filariasis, malnutrition and others exert a terrible toll on this continent, and it would be unfortunate if an anti-HBV campaign detracted from useful work on the control of these diseases. However, although HBV infection may not be the most important disease in Africa, it may, at the moment, be the most important disease for which control appears feasible.

I would like to close on a personal note. I have been involved in field work and research in Africa for nearly 30 years, beginning in Nigeria and including studies in Senegal, Mali, Ethiopia and Uganda. At the time this work was done it often appeared to be esoteric, 'basic' and remote from application. It was always our hope and conviction that it would eventually aid the people among and with whom we were working. It is very gratifying to see that this may now be happening.

ACKNOWLEDGEMENTS

This work was supported by USPHS grants CA-06551, RR-05539 and CA-06927 from the National Institutes of Health and by an appropriation from the Commonwealth of Pennsylvania.

REFERENCES

Beasley, R.P. & Lin, C.C. (1978) Hepatoma risk among HBsAg carriers. Am. J. Epidemiol., 108, 247-248

Blumberg, B.S. & London, W.T. (1982) Hepatitis B virus: Pathogenesis and prevention of primary cancer of the liver. Cancer, 50, 2657-2665

Blumberg, B.S., Millman, I., Sutnick, A.I. & London, W.T. (1971) The nature of Australia antigen and its relation to antigen-antibody complex formation. J. exp. Med., 134, 320-329

Blumberg, B.S., Larouze, B., London, W.T., Werner, B., Hesser, J.E., Millman, I., Saimot, G. & Payet, M. (1975) The relation of infection with the hepatitis B agent to primary hepatic carcinoma. Am. J. Pathol., 81, 669-682

Blumberg, B.S., Lustbader, E.D. & Whitford, P.L. (1981) Changes in serum iron levels due to infection with hepatitis B virus. Proc. natl Acad. Sci. USA, 78, 3222-3224

Bréchot, C., Pourcel, C., Louise, A., Rain, B. & Tiollais, P. (1980) Presence of integrated hepatitis B virus DNA sequences in cellular DNA of human hepatocellular carcinoma. Nature, 286, 533-534

Krugman, S. & Gilei, J.P. (1910) Viral hepatitis. New lights on an old disease. J. Amer. med. Assoc., 212, 1019-1029

Larouze, B., London, W.T., Saimot, G., Werner, B.G., Lustbader, E.D., Payet, M. & Blumberg, B.S. (1976) Host responses to hepatitis B infection in patients with primary hepatic carcinoma and their families. A case/control study in Senegal, West Africa. Lancet, 2, 534-538

London, W.T. & Blumberg, B.S. (1982) A cellular model of the role of hepatitis B virus in the pathogenesis of primary hepatocellular carcinoma. Hepatology, 2

London, W.T. & Blumberg, B.S. (1983) Hepatitis B and related viruses in chronic hepatitis, cirrhosis and hepatocellular carcinoma in man and animals. In: Cohen, S. & Soloway, R.D., eds, Chronic Active Liver Disease, New York, Churchill Livingstone, pp. 147-170

London, W.T., Stevens, R.G., Shofer, F.S., Drew, J.S., Brunhofer, J.E. & Blumberg, B.S. (1982) Effects of hepatitis B virus on the mortality, fertility, and sex ratio of human populations. In: Szmuness, W., Alter, H.J. & Maynard, J.E., Viral Hepatitis, 1981 International Symposium, Philadelphia, Franklin Institute Press, pp. 195-202

Lustbader, E.D., Hann, H.L. & Blumberg, B.S. (1983) Serum ferritin as a predictor of host response to hepatitis B virus infection. Science, 220, 423-425

Millman, I. (1984) The development of the hepatitis B vaccine. In: Millman, I., Blumberg, B.S. & Eisenstein, T., eds, Hepatitis B: The Virus, the Disease and the Vaccine, New York, Plenum Press (in press)

Okochi, K. & Murakami, S. (1968) Observations on Australia antigen in Japanese. Vox Sang., 15, 374-385

Summers, J., Smolec, J.M., Werner, B.G., Kelley, T.J., Tyler, G.V. & Snyder, R.L. (1980) Hepatitis B virus and woodchuck hepatitis virus are members of a novel class of DNA viruses. In: Essex, M., Todaro, G. & zur Hausen, H., eds, Viruses in Naturally Occurring Cancers (Cold Spring Harbor Conferences on Cell Proliferation, Vol. 7), Cold Spring Harbor, NY, Cold Spring Harbor Laboratory, pp. 459-470

Sun, Z., Wang, L., Xia, Q., Chu, Y., Wang, N. & Zhang, Y. (1980) Immunological approach to natural history, early diagnosis and etiology of human primary hepatocellular carcinoma. In: Essex, M., Todaro, G. & zur Hausen, H., eds, Viruses in Naturally Occurring Cancers (Cold Spring Harbor Conferences on Cell Proliferation, Vol. 7), Cold Spring Harbor, NY, Cold Spring Harbor Laboratory, pp. 471-479

Szmuness, W., Stevens, C.E., Harley, E.J., Zang, E.A., Oleszko, W.R., William, D.C., Sadovsky, R., Morrison, J.M. & Kellner, A. (1980) Hepatitis B vaccine. Demonstration of efficacy in a controlled clinical trial in a high risk population in the United States. New Engl. J. Med., 303, 833-841

Thung, S.N., Gerbert, M.A., Sarno, E. & Popper, H. (1979) Distribution of five antigens in hepatocellular carcinoma. Lab. Invest., 41, 101-105

WHO CANCER CONTROL PROGRAMME IN THE AFRICAN REGION

C. Chuwa

World Health Organization
Regional Office for Africa
Brazzaville, Congo

RESUME

Le contrôle des maladies transmissibles, de la malnutrition et des complications péri-natales a constitué la préoccupation majeure des Etats Membres de la Région Africaine de l'OMS. Les mesures prises dans ce sens ont entraîné une diminution régulière des taux de mortalité, en particulier chez les nourrissons et les jeunes enfants. De ce fait, l'espérance de vie a augmenté au point que l'on assiste actuellement à l'apparition des maladies prévalentes dans le monde industriel: celles-ci sont déjà devenues un problème majeur de santé publique en Afrique.

L'épithélioma du col utérin et le cancer primitif du foie sont les formes de cancer les plus fréquentes dans la population de cette Région. Les autres cancers comprennent les cancers du sein, de la peau, de la prostate, de l'oesophage, de l'estomac et de la vessie. Le lymphome de Burkitt constitue le cancer de l'enfance le plus courant. On connaît les facteurs étiologiques de certaines de ces tumeurs, et on peut de ce fait les éliminer par la prévention primaire. L'absence totale de cancers du pénis dans les communautés qui pratiquent la circoncision, et la diminution de l'incidence des épithéliomas spinocellulaires de la peau, grâce à la prévention des ulcères tropicaux par un traitement efficace des plaies et des blessures, en apportent la preuve.

Les priorités du Programme Cancer de l'OMS sont donc la prévention primaire, la détection précoce, et le soulagement de la douleur. Le succès du programme ne sera assuré que si les services fournis peuvent profiter à la majorité de la population.

SUMMARY

The control of communicable diseases, malnutrition and birth complications has been the main preoccupation of the Member States of the African Region of WHO. As a result of these control measures, death rates, particularly among infants and young children, have continued to decline. This has increased life expectancy to the extent that we are now witnessing the emergence of the diseases prevalent in the industrial world: they have already become a major public health problem in Africa.

Carcinoma of the cervix and hepatocellular carcinoma are the commonest forms of cancer afflicting the people of this Region. Others include cancers of the breast, skin, prostate, oesophagus, stomach and bladder. Burkitt's lymphoma is the commonest child-hood malignancy. The causal factors of some of these tumours are known, and can therefore be eliminated by primary prevention. This is shown by the almost total absence of carcinoma of the penis in those communities that practise male circumcision, and the decrease in the incidence of squamous-cell carcinoma of the skin that resulted from the prevention of tropical ulcer, thanks to effective care of injuries and wounds.

The priorities of the WHO cancer programme are therefore primary prevention, early detection and the provision of adequate pain relief. The success of the programme will depend mainly on whether the services provided will benefit the majority of the population.

INTRODUCTION

The control of communicable diseases, malnutrition and birth complications has been the main concern of the Member States of the African Region of WHO. As a result of these control measures, death rates, particularly among infants and young children, have continued to decline. This trend has given rise to a longer life expectancy to the extent that we are now wit-nessing the emergence of the diseases most prevalent in the industrial world; they are already a major public health pro-blem. This situation is already a matter of great concern to the Member States, as expressed vividly through their several reso-lutions, the latest of which (WHA 35.30), among others, called for the 'development of cancer control measures as an integral part of national health plans' (World Health Organization, 1982).

SITUATION ANALYSIS

Cancer constitutes a series of diseases of multiple etiology, and differing in natural history and treatment modalities.
It is already one of the first three causes of death among the
adult population of Africa. Its effects are now being felt far
beyond homes and neighbourhoods, as it strikes mainly at the age
of optimum contribution to family and nation.

From the few general studies already done in tropical
Africa, carcinoma of the cervix and hepatocellular carcinoma are
the commonest forms of cancer afflicting the people of the
Region. Others include cancers of the breast, skin, prostate,
oesophagus, stomach and bladder, to mention just a few.
Burkitt's lymphoma is the commonest childhood malignancy.
Primary cancer of the lungs is no longer the exclusive scourge of
the industrial world. This disease is present among our adult
population and its incidence is unfortunately rising. With the
alarming increase in tobacco consumption and the introduction of
industry, the Region is now witnessing an increase in this form
of cancer, as well as in those related to occupation.

Following the successful antismoking campaigns in the developed countries, the international tobacco firms have expanded
their operations in Africa and the rest of the Third World, where
they face none of the irksome advertising restrictions and
controls, imposed by their own governments on domestic sales. In
these developing countries, the affluent few are leading their
fellow countrymen towards the practice of cigarette smoking,
which is unfortunately viewed as a symbol of status and modern-
ity. As a result, the consumption of these lethal agents is
rapidly increasing. This is not to mention the quality of most
of the cigarettes in circulation, which is poor in terms of tar
and nicotine content. Figures available from Nigeria indicate
that 19.1% of men and 1.5% of women consume tobacco products. In
Ghana, the prevalence is between 11 and 24%, and here also,
smoking is predominantly a male characteristic. And on average,
the number of cigarettes smoked by every adult Kenyan per annum
rose from 390 in 1965 to 470 in 1973. For Malawi, the figures
were 150 and 200 respectively. These figures may seem modest,
but coming as they do from countries where, barely a century ago,
tobacco consumption was confined to a handful of pipe-smoking
elderly males, point to an imminent catastrophe.

The present trend has been confirmed to some extent by the coordinators of the sub-region I and III cancer-control centres, who in 1983 carried out promotional visits to several African countries and prepared situation analyses on cancer. Efforts to control this disease are being hampered by the lack of awareness of the community of the magnitude of the problem. In addition, the resources needed for primary prevention, early detection and treatment, if available, are confined to a few urban centres with none at all in the areas on the periphery of those centres and the rural areas where the majority of the people live. The shortage of manpower is obvious in all our countries - only 7 oncologists and 6 radiotherapists are providing services in the central hospitals of the capital cities of the Congo, Kenya, Liberia, Nigeria, Senegal, Tanzania, Uganda and Zimbabwe. While radiotherapy services are available in only 6 countries, some form of chemotherapy is used in most of the central hospitals, where cancer surgery is usually performed by general surgeons.

ON-GOING ACTIVITIES

The trend is now towards world-wide prevention and control of disease, the only rational approach to preventing spread to the community. Indeed, the causal factors of some neoplasms are now known and therefore capable of being dealt with by primary prevention. This has stimulated WHO to institute control programmes whose priorities are based on primary prevention and early detection, including effective therapy and pain relief. This is being carried out in collaboration with the Member States through the three sub-regional cancer-control centres which were set up in 1975 at Dakar, Ibadan and Kampala.

Some encouraging trends are being seen, e.g., the almost total absence of carcinoma of the penis in those communities that practise male circumcision, and the decrease in the incidence of squamous-cell carcinoma of the skin, thanks to proper personal hygiene and the care given to injuries and wounds that would have otherwise led to the so-called tropical ulcers.

It is realized, however, that one of the most effective actions that can be taken to prevent the emergence of some of these malignancies is smoking control. To this end, WHO has contacted the Organization of African Unity and the major United Nations agencies based in Africa and requested them to assist in the endeavours to curb cigarette smoking in our continent. In the same spirit, WHO has shared the concern shown by Member States with regard to this problem and actively collaborated with them in organizing the International Conference on Smoking and Health in Developing Countries, which took place in Swaziland in April 1982, and at which the innumerable health hazards arising from the continuous interplay between man and tobacco were high-lighted. The conclusions and recommendations of this Conference have been brought to the attention of the national health autho-rities in the Region. As a follow-up of this Conference, a regional seminar on smoking and health is being organized and will take place at Lusaka, Zambia, in July of this year.

Another example of activity in the area of primary preven-tion, although based on a completely different approach, is the exploration of the feasibility of immunization against hepato-cellular carcinoma. The evidence implicating hepatitis B virus in the etiology of this cancer is based on epidemiological and geographical observations, which have pointed to a strong asso-ciation between hepatitis B infection and this form of neoplasm - one of the commonest forms of cancer afflicting the people of Africa. This evidence is now sufficiently strong to justify the use of a vaccine against this infection as a means of preventing hepatocellular carcinoma. It was agreed at a recent WHO meeting (World Health Organization, 1983) that there is now a unique opportunity, for the first time, of preventing a frequent cancer by immunization. It was considered appropriate that internatio-nal action should be taken to initiate intervention trials on populations in an attempt to break the chain of vertical trans-mission from infected mother to newborn. It is encouraging to note that the United Kingdom Medical Research Council (MRC) proposes to effect studies in the Gambia, in collaboration with the International Agency for Research on Cancer, aimed at evaluating the effectiveness of hepatitis B virus vaccine in the prevention of hepatocellular carcinoma in a high-risk population. Similar studies being carried out elsewhere in Africa, including a WHO-supported project in Zambia. It is believed that these studies will help to determine the potency and safety of this vaccine. Let us also hope that they will also contribute to solving the problem of its price, which for the moment is too high and therefore places it outside the reach of those for whom it is intended.

Health education and information has been recognized as an important part of the efforts aimed at effective prevention and control of disease. WHO is therefore fostering and coordinating the collection of basic epidemiological information on the extent of cancer and its trends in the community. It is also coordinating training activities that will impart expertise and public health skills to those nationals working in the cancer field. To this end a Regional training course on the epidemiology of non-communicable diseases with emphasis on cancer was held in Zambia in 1981 and in Cameroon in November 1983. Participants in these two countries were drawn from all over the Region, 27 attending the first and 33 the second. We are satisfied that, on their return to their countries, participants will be able to contribute more effectively to the programmes for the prevention and control of cancer, mainly through community-based health services and primary health care activities. These training activities were organized in collaboration with IARC.

Further training activities will, it is hoped, be carried out in collaboration with the African Organization for Research and Training in Cancer (AORTC), which was launched during the inaugural meeting held at Lomé in July 1983. This Organization will serve as a forum for the exchange of ideas and expertise among those involved in the field of neoplastic diseases. As such, it will participate in formulating and promoting programmes for research and training in cancer that are realistic and relevant to the continent of Africa. It is therefore hoped that it will soon extend its membership outside the confines of the African Region of WHO to embrace all the OAU Member States.

PLANNED ACTIVITIES

Plans for the future are embodied in the WHO medium-term programme, which is in turn based on the WHO Seventh General Programme of Work. This medium-term programme is geared towards the prevention and control of the preventable cancers, effective treatment of the curable forms, and the provision of pain relief and other cost-effective palliative measures for those suffering from the incurable forms. Its main priorities are therefore prevention, early detection and pain relief. The time has now come for the initiation and consolidation of the national cancer control programmes. This will be stimulated by promoting training programmes geared to the attainment of the public health skills required for the integration of cancer control into community-based health services within the context of primary health care. This will involve the training of all categories of medical workers, including medical auxiliaries, in order to enhance their capabilities for the prevention, early detection and treatment of cancer, as well as research.

Efforts will be made to identify the existing health practices and life-styles that should be reinforced and promoted by health education. Since health education and information must be based on local conditions, WHO will continue to encourage those health workers responsible for informing and motivating the community and its leaders so as to induce them to support and participate in the programmes for the prevention and control of cancer. Among other things, this will help in tackling the problem of delay in reporting to hospital by patients who, in most cases, are seen at an advanced stage of the disease, which is therefore not amenable to treatment.

The main goal is therefore to encourage the efforts for promoting and coordinating activities aimed at the prevention and control of these diseases. This does not necessarily reduce the importance of the concept of centres of excellence, whose main concern has been in the field of curative medicine and surgery. The good work done in these centres should be continued as far as possible. In view, however, of the prevailing social, cultural and economic conditions of the countries of the Region, WHO cancer programmes can only make an effective contribution to the overall concept of health for all by the year 2000 by fostering those methods and strategies that will lead to effective prevention, early detection and the provision of adequate pain relief. The success of these programmes will depend mainly on whether the services provided are able to benefit the majority of the population.

REFERENCES

World Health Organization (1982) WHA 35.30: Resolution of the World Health Assembly: Long-term Planning of International Cooperation in the Field of Cancer, Geneva

World Health Organization (1983) Prevention of liver cancer: Report of a WHO Meeting, Geneva

STRATEGIES FOR PREVENTION AND CONTROL OF HEPATITIS B AND HEPATOCELLULAR CARCINOMA

O. Sobeslavsky

Virus Diseases, World Health Organization
Geneva, Switzerland

RESUME

L'hépatite B représente un grave problème de santé publique dans toutes les parties du monde, et en particulier dans les zones d'hyperendémicité où la majorité des infections surviennent durant l'enfance. Comme cette infection évolue fréquemment vers la chronicité lorsqu'elle survient tôt dans la vie, les taux de prévalence des séquelles à long terme, telles que l'hépatite chronique active et la cirrhose, sont élevées dans ces régions. De plus, les études épidémiologiques, virologiques et de biologie moléculaire effectuées récemment ont montré que l'infection persistante ou ancienne par le virus de l'hépatite B joue un rôle important dans le développement du cancer primitif du foie (CPF).

Bien qu'une action au niveau de l'environnement et l'emploi de l'immunisation passive aient prouvé qu'elles pouvaient réduire les infections par l'hépatite B, la principale méthode de prévention généralisée de l'hépatite B et de ses séquelles chroniques est l'immunisation active. Des vaccins contenant l'antigène de surface (AgHBs) purifié ont été préparés, et se sont révélés hautement immunogènes et efficaces.

En fonction des différents schémas géographiques de prévalence de l'hépatite B et de la disponibilité du vaccin, plusieurs stratégies vaccinales ont été proposées, allant de l'administration limitée du vaccin à son administration généralisée.

On pourrait réserver la vaccination sélective de groupes à haut risque sélectionnés, comprenant les nourrissons nés de mères porteuses de l'antigène HBs, aux zones où la prévalence de l'infection est faible, tandis qu'on pourrait envisager une vaccination massive dans les zones d'endémicité intermédiaire et élevée. Dans ce dernier cas, il sera possible de maîtriser véritablement l'hépatite B lorsque des groupes de population suffisamment importants auront été immunisés avant l'exposition, c'est-à-dire durant les premières années de la vie.

La production de grandes quantités de vaccin bon marché est la condition préalable aux campagnes de vaccination de masse. L'installation dans plusieurs zones d'hyperendémicité, d'unités intégrées orientées vers la production simultanée de vaccin contre l'hépatite B, de réactifs diagnostiques de cette maladie, d'immunoglobulines et d'autres produits thérapeutiques dérivés du plasma, devrait permettre une réduction des coûts et l'optimisation de ces unités de production.

De plus, le transfert continu des technologies modernes vers de tels centres assurerait le maintien des hauts standards technologiques nécessaires pour la production du vaccin contre l'hépatite B.

SUMMARY

Hepatitis B represents a serious public health problem in all parts of the world, and particularly in hyperendemic areas, where the majority of infections occur in childhood. As this infection in early life leads frequently to chronic infection, the prevalence rates of long-term sequelae, such as chronic active hepatitis and cirrhosis, are high. In addition, recent epidemiological, virological and molecular biological studies have provided evidence that persistent or past infection with hepatitis B virus plays an important role in the development of hepatocellular carcinoma (HCC).

Although environmental control and the use of passive immunization have proved useful in reducing hepatitis B infections, the most important method of achieving widespread prevention of hepatitis B and its chronic sequelae is active immunization. Vaccines containing purified hepatitis B surface antigen (HBsAg) have been prepared and shown to be both highly immunogenic and efficacious.

Depending on the different geographical patterns of hepatitis B prevalence and the availability of vaccine, a variety of vaccination strategies have been proposed ranging from limited to large-scale vaccine administration.

Targeted vaccination of selected high-risk groups, including infants of HBsAg-carrier mothers, might be reserved for areas of low prevalence of infection, while large-scale vaccination should be considered for intermediate- and high-endemicity areas. In the latter case, effective control of hepatitis B could be achieved when sufficiently large population groups can be immunized prior to exposure, e.g., during infancy or early childhood.

The prerequisite for large-scale vaccination campaigns is the production of large quantities of low-cost vaccine. The establishment of integrated facilities in several hyperendemic areas for simultaneous production of hepatitis B vaccine, hepatitis B diagnostic reagents, immune globulins and other therapeutic plasma products, could lead to a reduction in their cost and to optimal utilization of production facilities.

In addition, the continuous transfer of modern technology to such centres will ensure that the high technological standards required in the production of hepatitis B vaccine are maintained.

INTRODUCTION

Viral hepatitis is a major public health problem in all parts of the world. The disease exists in three forms, hepatitis A, hepatitis B and hepatitis non-A, non-B.

Tens of millions of people are infected with these viruses each year with an enormous impact on health and national economies. The exact prevalence of viral hepatitis is difficult to estimate because of lack of uniformity in surveillance systems and the high incidence of subclinical infections in some settings. Not only are the basic data often poorly collected but clinical diagnosis is not always supported by laboratory confirmation. Reliable information on the incidence and long-term trends is therefore only available from a few of the more affluent countries. Improved surveillance and diagnostic capabilities are therefore necessary.

Hepatitis B represents a particular problem, especially in hyperendemic areas where the majority of infections occur in childhood. As this infection early in life frequently leads to chronic infection, the prevalence rates of long-term sequelae, such as chronic active hepatitis and cirrhosis, are high. In addition, recent epidemiological, virological and molecular biology studies (showing HBV DNA integration into the hepatocyte genome) have provided evidence that persistent or past infection with hepatitis B virus plays an important role in the development of hepatocellular carcinoma (HCC). It is estimated that this virus is responsible for up to 80% of all HCC, one of the 10 most common tumours of man, particularly in the Far East, South-east Asia and tropical Africa, where the actual incidence of the disease is at least 30 new cases per 100 000 population each year. It is also estimated that at present there are at least 200 million persistent carriers of hepatitis B infection in the world, many of whom risk dying of chronic liver disease damage or HCC.

As mentioned above, on the whole the majority of infections caused by hepatitis B virus (HBV) occur in childhood, including mother-to-infant HBV transmission and establishment of the hepatitis B surface antigen (HBsAg) carrier state. As improvements in the environment and personal hygiene are unlikely to have a major impact on the disease prevalence, the most effective way of combating hepatitis B is likely to be large-scale immunization. Safe and effective vaccines have recently been developed and have been shown to prevent acute and chronic HBV infections and their sequelae.

Aware of this serious health problem and of the knowledge and technologies available for controlling the disease by active immunization, WHO convened in July 1983 a Consultative Group for the Development of a WHO Programme for Viral Hepatitis. The Group made a number of proposals as to the content of the WHO Programme, with particular emphasis on the application of available technology, the improvement and simplification of diagnostic and control measures, and the development of strategies for their application in developing countries. It also concluded that high priority should be given to the coordination of field studies using hepatitis B vaccine. These should include smaller studies to evaluate optimal timing and dosage schedules for infant and childhood immunization, as well as several large-scale trials in areas where both hepatitis B and HCC are common, in order to demonstrate the effect of the vaccine in preventing the latter disease. It would also be desirable to conduct these studies in different parts of the world, e.g., in Africa, South-east Asia and the Western Pacific, since the long-term effectiveness of immunization may vary with factors affecting HBV transmission.

ACTIVE IMMUNIZATION IN PREVENTION OF HEPATITIS B AND HEPATOCELLULAR CARCINOMA

Although environmental control and the use of passive immunization have proved useful in reducing hepatitis B infection and its chronic sequelae, the most important method for achieving widespread prevention of hepatitis B is active immunization. Purified subunit vaccines have been prepared from HBV surface components found in the blood of chronic carriers of HBV. Such vaccines have been shown in several countries to be both immunogenic and highly efficacious.

Nevertheless, strategies for the use of this vaccine must take into consideration the different geographical patterns of hepatitis B prevalence, which may be conveniently divided into three categories of endemicity. In low-endemicity areas, such as North America, Western Europe and Australia, the prevalence of HBsAg in healthy carriers may reach only 0.2-0.5% and anti-HBs 4-6%, while in areas of intermediate endemicity, such as Eastern Europe, the Mediterranean region, the European part of the Soviet Union and the Middle East, the frequency of HBsAg generally varies from 2 to 7 % and anti-HBs from 20 to 55%. In high-prevalence areas, such as some parts of the People's Republic of China, South-east Asia and tropical Africa, rates of HBsAg carriage may be as high as 8-15%. Prevalence of infection, as measured by the presence of anti-HBs, may reach 70-95%. Prevalences of HBsAg of up to 50% have been identified in some isolated Pacific islands.

In countries where hepatitis B is uncommon, infection rarely occurs during childhood. As the overall frequency of infection increases, it appears earlier in life, and in areas of high prevalence, the bulk of infection occurs in infancy and childhood. In countries within a particular geographical region, considerable differences in prevalence may exist among various ethnic and socioeconomic groups. However, prevalence of infection is generally correlated with socioeconomic level.

Depending on the availability of vaccine, a variety of vaccination strategies have been proposed, ranging from limited administration to individuals at high risk of acquiring hepatitis B, to large-scale administration in infancy and early childhood, including infants of HBsAg-carrier mothers.

Targeted vaccination of selected groups might be reserved for areas of low prevalence, while large-scale vaccination should be anticipated for intermediate- and high-endemicity areas. In the latter case, no effective control of hepatitis B will be achieved unless large groups of the population can be immunized prior to exposure, i.e., during infancy and early childhood. Fortunately, immunogenicity studies of available subunit vaccines which have so far been conducted indicate that humoral antibody response in infants and young children is good and that immunization is also effective when vaccine is administered at birth or when given under cover of maternally transferred passive antibodies. There is therefore ample evidence that vaccination alone, or in combination with hepatitis B immune globulin, can provide successful early immunization of infants at risk or prevent the development of the chronic carrier state in infants born to HBsAg-positive mothers.

Decisions regarding prescreening prior to vaccination will differ from country to country, depending on the cost and availability of both reagents and vaccine. Identification and vaccination of medical and paramedical personnel prior to entrance into high-risk situations should be included as part of the vaccination policy.

In the implementation of the above strategies, it is clear that the use of hepatitis B vaccine in hyperendemic areas will have to be considered, which calls for a reduction in its cost and a considerable increase in its availability. A critical requirement in increasing vaccine availability will be the establishment of an alternative to the chimpanzee safety test for certification of lot safety. Also important is the redefinition of vaccination schedules to determine whether simultaneous administration of this vaccine with other vaccines, such as oral poliomyelitis or diphtheria-tetanus-pertussis, will be possible. If the vaccine is to be administered at birth, this procedure can be combined with ocular instillation of silver nitrate.

As mentioned above, global strategies for the prevention of hepatitis B and its chronic sequelae should aim at the production of large quantities of vaccine at low cost in hyperendemic areas. Identification of HBsAg-positive repeat donors and establishment of plasmapheresis facilities on a regional basis in those areas should be an integral part of the hepatitis B prevention programme. It should be noted that, with few exceptions, similar purification procedures are used both in the preparation of HBsAg for production of diagnostic reagents and for the production of vaccine. The establishment in several hyperendemic areas of integrated facilities for simultaneous production of hepatitis B vaccine, hepatitis B diagnostic reagents, immune globulins, and other therapeutic products, by centralizing production, should reduce costs and ensure that the best use is made of available technology.

As with any biological product for human use, the highest technological standards must be maintained in the production of hepatitis B vaccine. There are fortunately several hyperendemic areas in the world where maintenance of such standards is relatively easy, and these areas might well serve as focal points for vaccine development and production programmes aimed at immunization of large numbers of susceptibles.

Some hesitation has been expressed regarding the inherent safety of blood products in general, and hepatitis B vaccine in particular because it is derived from plasma from human HBV carriers. These concerns have led to a call for restraint in the implementation of vaccination programmes until second-generation recombinant DNA vaccines or third-generation synthetic vaccines become available. These vaccines have been thought to be inherently safer and less costly than currently available human-plasma-derived vaccines.

However, such restraint cannot be seriously advocated, since highly efficacious vaccines are currently on hand, and second- and third-generation vaccines will not be available for large-scale use for some years, while there is a pressing need to begin immediate programmes to prevent hepatitis B infection and its chronic sequelae, including HCC. Plasma-derived vaccines are purified preparations subjected to one or more inactivation processes which ensure the highest degree of safety. Also although recombinant DNA vaccines have been postulated to be inherently less expensive and capable of being produced on a larger scale than plasma-derived vaccines, this has yet to be proved, especially when production of plasma-derived vaccine is transferred to centres in hyperendemic regions where donor sources are more plentiful and production costs can be minimized.

Large-scale efforts to control hepatitis B in hyperendemic areas through appropriate demonstration projects utilizing plasma-derived vaccines will in no way impede the advent of second- and third-generation vaccines. Rather, these efforts will serve to define and evaluate the effectiveness of a variety of approaches to large-scale vaccination at an early enough stage to enable newer vaccines to be used immediately and effectively as they become available.

HEPATITIS B VACCINE: CLINICAL EXPERIENCE

F. Tron

Institut Pasteur Production
Marnes-la-Coquette, France

RESUME

Les infections par le virus de l'hépatite B (HBV) se produisent dans le monde entier et on a estimé à plus de 200
millions le nombre de porteurs chroniques de l'antigène de surface du virus (AgHBs). On a associé le portage chronique et
prolongé de l'AgHBs à un risque accru d'hépatite chronique
active, de cirrhose, et de cancer primitif du foie (CPF).

Dans les pays Occidentaux, la prévalence de l'infection HBV
est faible dans la population générale. Seuls certains sous-
groupes, composés pour la plupart de sujets adultes, sont exposés
à une telle infection. Ils comprennent les personnes travaillant
dans les professions de santé, les malades hémodialysés, les
patients transfusés, les toxicomanes et les homosexuels. Par
contre, en Asie et en Afrique tropicale, la prévalence de l'infection HBV est relativement élevée. La transmission se produit
principalement pendant la période périnatale et la petite
enfance. L'infection à un jeune âge aboutit souvent à l'état de
porteur chronique.

Un vaccin contre l'hépatite B a été développé en France, et
il s'est avéré sûr, immunogène et efficace dans la prévention de
l'infection HBV. Une expérience étendue provenant des essais
cliniques permet maintenant de recommander des stratégies de
vaccination en termes de populations-cibles et de protocoles
optimaux.

Ce papier décrit les résultats de la vaccination contre
l'hépatite B et présente en particulier une vue d'ensemble sur
l'expérience de vaccination des nouveaux-nés et des enfants.

SUMMARY

Hepatitis B virus (HBV) infections occur world-wide and more than 200 million people have been estimated to be chronic carriers of HB surface antigen (HBsAg). Long-term chronic carriage of HBsAg has been associated with an increased risk of chronic active hepatitis (CAH), cirrhosis and hepatocellular carcinoma (HCC). In Western countries, the prevalence of HBV infection is low in the general population. Only particular sub-groups, for the most part adults, are at risk of such infections: health care workers, haemodialysis patients, transfusion patients, drug abusers and homosexuals. In Asia and tropical Africa, however, the prevalence of HBV infection is relatively high. Transmission occurs mainly during the perinatal period and infancy. Infection at a young age often results in the chronic carrier state.

A hepatitis B vaccine has been developed in France and has been demonstrated to be safe, immunogenic, and effective in preventing HBV infection. Extensive experience from clinical trials now makes it possible to recommend vaccination strategies in terms of target populations and of optimal schedules. This paper reports the results of hepatitis B vaccination and, in particular, presents an overview of the vaccination experience in newborns and children.

HEPATITIS B VACCINE (HEVAC B PASTEUR)

The vaccine is prepared (Adamowicz et al., 1981) in accordance with the WHO requirements (BS/83.191 Revision 2 Geneva, 6-8 December 1983), by purification of hepatitis B surface antigen (HBsAg) from plasma collected from HBsAg chronic carriers. The vaccine should then be free from both plasma proteins and potentially contaminant viruses, and is highly immunogenic. The different stages in HBsAg purification are summarized in Table 1.

Table 1. Purification and inactivation procedures

Stage No.	Procedure
1	Collection of plasma (ad or ay)
2	5.5% PEG precipitation
3	10% PEG precipitation
4	2 sucrose-gradient zonal (velocity) centrifugations
5	Zonal (velocity) centrifugation in caesium chloride
6	Isopycnic centrifugation in caesium chloride
7	Sterilization with formaldehyde (1/4000)

Plasma is collected from HBsAg-positive but e antigen (HBeAg)-negative asymptomatic blood donors. Upon arrival in the laboratory, each plasma donation is checked for HBsAg titre, absence of HBeAg and syphilis antibodies, and bacterial sterility. Plasma pools are then tested for viral sterility, the absence of detectable HBV (by molecular hybridization) and of detectable retroviruses (by a reverse transcriptase assay).

Plasma pools are then fractionated twice by polyethylene glycol (PEG) precipitation (5.5% and 10% PEG), and subjected to 2 successive velocity centrifugations through sucrose gradients, 2 successive isopycnic, caesium chloride gradient centrifugations (the second being of the flotation type) and several sterilizing filtration steps through 0.22-μm-pore-size filters. HBsAg particles are capsid-free and nucleic-acid-free fragments of the viral envelope and, as such, occupy a unique position in a size-buoyant density diagram. No known virus has physicochemical properties which could allow its co-purification together with HBsAg throughout the entire purification process. The last step in the preparation of the vaccine consists of treating the purified HBsAg preparation with 0.01% formaldehyde for 48 h at 30°C. Numerous tests are performed on the final product. The purity of the sample is ascertained by sodium dodecylsulfate-polyacrylamide gel electrophoresis (SDS-PAGE) analysis and is demonstrated to be > 98%.

The absence of HBV DNA is confirmed by molecular hybridization and the absence of blood-group antigens, HBeAg and hepatitis A virus (HAV) is also confirmed. Monovalent ay and ad antigen suspensions are mixed and checked for bacterial and fungal sterility and the absence of mycoplasma.

Ten human doses of vaccine are injected intravenously into 2 quarantined chimpanzees. Biological examinations (transaminases, HBV serological markers) and repeated liver biopsies are performed. The batch of vaccine is released, after having undergone tests over a period of 6 months, and the final product is distributed, as individual doses (5 μg), in 1-ml syringes.

IMMUNOGENICITY, CLINICAL EFFICACY AND SAFETY IN HEALTHY ADULTS

Immunogenicity and efficacy

Trials carried out on adults of hepatitis B vaccination with 3 injections of 5 μg of vaccine at 1-month intervals have given the following results.

A randomized, placebo-controlled trial was performed in 1979 on the medical staff of a French haemodialysis unit where the prevalence of HBsAg among patients was as high as 40%, and the annual incidence of clinical hepatitis B among the medical staff was 15%. Among the 348 seronegative volunteers who completed the protocol, 164 received 3 injections of 5 μg at 1-month intervals and 184 received corresponding injections of placebo. Of the immune staff members, 94% seroconverted to anti-HBs after 3 injections of the HB vaccine. Figure 1 shows the geometric mean anti-HBs levels (mIU/ml) at different times during the study. The anti-HBs peak was reached at 5 months (560 mIU/ml). When the booster dose was given, the geometric mean anti-HBs level was 300 mIU/ml. Hepatitis B infections were observed in 3.6% of the vaccinated group and in 12.3% of the placebo group ($p < 0.005$). The 6 infections in the vaccinated group all arose within the 63 days following the first injection, whereas the 19 cases in the placebo group arose throughout the 12-month follow-up period. These results clearly demonstrate the efficacity of the vaccine in preventing HBV infection (Crosnier et al., 1981).

FIG. 1. GEOMETRIC MEAN ANTI-HBs TITRES (mUI/ml) (+2SE)
IN 148 HEALTHY ADULTS GIVEN 3 INJECTIONS OF 5 μg OF VACCINE
AT 1-MONTH INTERVALS

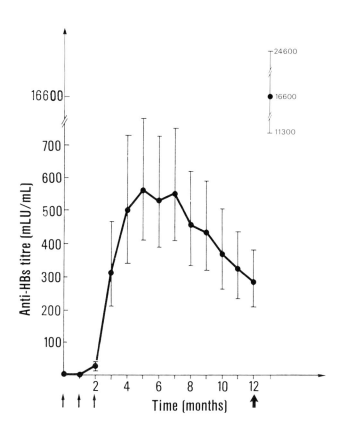

Since this randomized study, a large number of clinical
trials have been conducted in adults;   the results of some of
them are summarized in Table 2.   More than 95% of vaccine recipients produced anti-HBs antibodies 3 months after the first
injection.   When the booster dose was given, more than 99% of
vaccine responders still had anti-HBs antibodies.

Table 2. Clinical trials of hepatitis B vaccine: seroconversion
rate in healthy adults

Country	Author	No. in trial	Percentage seroconversion		
			1 month	2 months	3 months
France	Crosnier et al., 1981	148	18	66	94
France	Goudeau et al., 1982	696	31	73	96
Belgium	Donea-Debroise et al., 1982	150	20	75	86
Italy	Panichi et al., 1983	40	17.5	80	100
Italy	Piazza et al., 1982	96	15.6	53.1	92.7
Greece	Zouboulis-Vafiadis et al., 1983	51	35.3	92.3	100
France	Lotz et al., 1983	338	ND[a]	ND[a]	97.9
Fed. Rep. of Germany	Wildgrube et al., 1984	637	50	89	94
Fed. Rep. of Germany	Frosner et al., 1983	20	40	84	100
Austria	Horad et al., 1984	93	ND[a]	ND[a]	94
	Total	2269	28.4	77.8	95.5

[a] ND, Not done

      These studies have shown that the immune response to HBsAg
in healthy adults was age- and sex-dependent. Females responded
better than males. Although most studies reported identical percentages of seroconversion for both sexes, males had delayed
kinetics of anti-HBs production and lower anti-HBs titres.   In

this connection, it should be remembered that the frequency of chronic HBsAg carriage is higher in males than in females, and that the general level of the immune response to thymodependent antigens is higher in females.

Immunological memory

The vaccination schedule recommends a booster dose 12 months after the first injection, which enables a strong immunological memory to be developed. The booster dose elicited an anamnestic anti-HBs response. Table 3 shows the geometric mean anti-HBs titres observed in 3 major studies. All anti-HBs values were above 3000 mIU/ml one month after the booster. This anamnestic response ensures the long-term persistence of anti-HBs antibodies. The study performed by Goudeau et al. (1983) showed that anti-HBs levels remained stable for 3 years following the booster dose (half the antibody titres remained in the 300-3000 mIU/ml range). Four years after the booster dose, 97.2% of responders still had anti-HBs antibodies.

Table 3. Anamnestic response elicited by a booster injection[a]

Author	Anti-HBs titres (mIU/ml)	
	On administration of the booster	1 month after the booster
Crosnier et al., 1981	290 (148)	16 600 (148)
Goudeau et al., 1983	194 (696)	10 828 (696)
Wildgrube et al., 1984	273.6 (317)	3321.5 (255)

[a] Numbers vaccinated in parentheses

These results demonstrate the immunogenicity of the vaccine, which only contains 5 μg per dose. It must be emphasized that, despite the low amount of HBsAg per dose, the vaccine is immuno-

genic.   This may be the consequence of a manufacturing process
based on purification rather than multiple step inactivation,
since the latter may be deleterious for major epitopes.

Safety

Because the HBsAg is derived from plasma, the major hypothetical side-effects of this vaccine are reactions to blood substances and the transmission of HBV or other blood-borne agents.
Follow-up of vaccine recipients enrolled in clinical trials and
information collected by spontaneous notification during post-
marketing surveillance did not reveal any long-term reactions or
any case of transmission of hepatitis B, non-A, non-B hepatitis
or any other infectious disease (Nutini et al., 1983).

IMMUNOGENICITY AND CLINICAL EFFICACY OF HEPATITIS B VACCINATION IN CHILDREN AND NEWBORNS

Children

The immunogenicity of hepatitis B vaccine was evaluated in
72 seronegative children 1-13 years old (mean 6 years) immunized
according to a protocol of 3 doses of 5 μg given at 1-month
intervals, and a booster dose 12 months later (Picciotto et al.,
1983).   Table 4 shows that at 1, 2 and 3 months respectively,
38.9, 90.3 and 98.6% had seroconverted.   The geometric mean
anti-HBs titres were respectively 70, 320 and 750 mIU/ml.   The
vaccine potency was also evaluated in 342 seronegative Senegalese
children aged 3-24 months and tested at various intervals, starting at 2 months and up to 36 months after the first injection.
The seroconversion rates observed at these times are indicated in
Table 5 (Coursaget et al., 1983).   These studies demonstrated
that the anti-HBs response to HB vaccine in children was very
similar to that observed in healthy adults.   Again, a high rate
of seroconversion and long-term persistance of anti-HBs constitute the major characteristics of the response.

Table 4.   Anti-HBs antibody response in 72 children aged 1-13 years[a]

Response	Time after first injection (months)		
	1	2	3
% seroconversion	38.9	90.3	98.6
Anti-HBs antibodies (mIU/ml)	70	320	750

[a] Source: Picciotto et al., 1983

Table 5. Anti-HBs antibody response to HB vaccine in Senegalese children[a]

Time after first injection (months)	No. tested	No. with anti-HBs	% with anti-HBs
2	342	241	70.5
4	298	280	94.0
12	309	285	92.2
14	74	72	97.3
24	101	97	96.0
36	28	27	96.4

[a] Source: Coursaget et al., 1983

Early infections occur in infants born to HBsAg-positive
mothers, and particularly to mothers with HBeAg. Approximately
90% of the newborns of these mothers become carriers. This perinatal transmission may be reduced by administration of hepatitis
B immunoglobulin (HBIg) at birth (Beasley et al., 1981). However, around 25% of the newborns are not protected against early
onset of the infection, and 20% will be infected later in the
postnatal period (Beasley et al., 1981). These observations have
led to the active immunization of infants born to HBsAg-positive
mothers.

Newborns

A study was carried out in Senegal (Yvonnet et al., 1984) on
the HB vaccination of 60 infants born to unselected mothers.
Each subject received the first dose of HB vaccine on the first
day of life. The second injection was administered at the age of
1 month and the third at the age of 2 months. A booster dose was
given at the age of 12 months. Blood samples were collected from
the children on the day of birth, 1 month after the third injection, on the day that the booster dose was given and 2 months
later. A blood sample was taken from each mother on the day of
delivery. Control groups consisted of children aged 3-24 months
and immunized according to the same schedule.

At 3 months of age, 1 month after the third injection of HB
vaccine, 96.7% of the infants immunized at birth had circulating
anti-HBs antibodies and 90% had positive titres at the age of 1
year. The seroconversion rate and the geometric mean titre were
not different from those observed in children aged 3-24 months.
In addition, Table 6 shows that no differences in the immune
response were observed as between newborns with passively transmitted anti-HBs and newborns with no anti-HBs (geometric mean
titres were 75 and 62 mIU/ml, respectively, at 12 months and 2423
and 2357 mIU/ml 2 months after the booster). Similarly, the
immune response was not affected by the HBV status of the mother
(Table 7).

Table 6. Anti-HBs antibody response to HB vaccine in newborns[a]

Group	Time after first injection (months)	No.	Response				
			Anti-HBs-positive		Titre (mIU/ml)		
			No.	%	Range	Median	Geometric mean
Newborns anti-HBs-positive at birth	0	35	35	100.0	2-22000	34	58
	3	35	35	100.0	3- 4000	109	82
	12	35	30	85.7	0- 2000	115	75
	14	30	28	93.3	0-897000	2577	2423
Newborns anti-HBs-negative at birth	0	25	0	0	-	-	-
	3	25	23	92.0	3- 600	43.5	46
	12	25	24	96.0	4- 1435	101	62
	14	19	18	94.7	35-92000	2436	2357

[a] Source: Yvonnet et al., 1984

Infants born to HBsAg- and HBeAg-positive mothers

Clinical trials were conducted in Taiwan on 38 infants born to HBsAg- and HBeAg-positive mothers; the infants received 3 injections, 5 μg each, at 1-month intervals, starting on the 15th day of life. A total of 29 newborns received no treatment and constituted the control group. Table 8 shows the seroconversion rates, the geometric mean titres and the HBsAg status of the newborns at 6, 10 weeks, 6 and 18 months of age. At 6 months, the geometric mean anti-HBs titre was 506.7 mIU/ml in the vaccinated group. At 18 months of age, 17.6% of children had HBsAg. In contrast, 90% of control-group children were HBsAg-positive. This study therefore demonstrates that hepatitis B vaccine alone reduced maternal-infant transmission of HBV infection by more than 80%.

Table 7. Anti-HBs antibody response to HB vaccine in newborns
according to maternal HBV markers present at delivery

HBV markers present in mothers at delivery	Anti-HBs antibodies in infants at		
	birth	3 months	12 months
Seronegative	0/8	8/8	8/8 (100%)
Anti-HBc alone	0/2	2/2	2/2 (100%)
Anti-HBs alone	3/7	7/7	7/7 (100%)
Anti-HBs and anti-HBc	31/32	32/32	27/32 (84.4%)
HBsAg	1/11	9/11	10/11 (90.9%)
Total	35 (58.3%)	58 (96.7%)	54 (90.0%)

Table 8. Immunogenicity and efficacy of HB vaccination alone and
combined with passive immunization with HBIg in infants born to
HBsAg- and HBeAg-positive mothersa

Procedure	Response	No. of cases/total cases after			
		6 weeks	10 weeks	6 months	18 months
Vaccination alone	HBsAg	3/21 (14.3%)	9/38 (23.7%)	7/38 (18.4%)	3/19 (15.8%)
	Anti-HBs	1/21 (4.8%)	21/38 (55.3%)	30/38 (78.9%)	
	Geometric mean titre (mIU/ml)	60.0	62.5	506.7	
Vaccination + HBIg	HBsAg	1/27 (3.7%)	2/36 (5.6%)	4/37 (10.8%)	3/22 (13.6%)
	Anti-HBs	25/27 (92.6%)	34/36 (94.4%)	33/37 (89.2%)	
	Geometric mean titre (mIU/ml)	56.2	40.0	465.4	

a 90% of control-group children were HBsAg-positive

In addition, 37 infants born to HBsAg- and HBeAg-positive mothers were given 3 injections of 5 μg at 1-month intervals, starting on the 15th day of life and I injection of 100 IU of HBIg at birth. Table 8 shows that, firstly, HBIg administration did not reduce the immune response to HBsAg (geometric mean titre at 6 months: 465 mIU/ml) and, secondly that the HBV infection rate was only 13.6% in this group receiving both active and passive immunization.

NEW PROTOCOLS CURRENTLY UNDER INVESTIGATION

Since the cost of the vaccine limits its use in large-scale immunization programmes, the immunogenicity of new protocols using either a reduced number of 5-μg injections or a lower dose in each of the 3 injections is currently being tested in different countries.

Infants

In Italy (Piazza et al., 1982) a group of 24 seronegative children aged 2-12 years received 2 injections of 5 μg of vaccine at an interval of 2 months. At 1, 2 and 3 months after the first injection, the seroconversion rates were respectively 37.5, 45.8 and 95.8%. The geometric mean anti-HBs titres were 60, 92 and 726 mIU/ml, respectively (Table 9).

Table 9. Anti-HBs antibody response of seronegative children after 2 injections of 5 μg of vaccine at an interval of 2 months

Response	Time after 1st injection (months)		
	1	2	3
% seroconversion	37.5	45.8	95.8
Geometric mean titre of anti-HBs antibodies (mIU/ml)	60	92	726

In Senegal (Coursaget et al., 1983), 72 seronegative children aged 3-24 months were immunized according to the same vaccination schedule. The seroconversion rate 12 months after the
first injection was 93.1% and the geometric mean anti-HBs titre
was 85 mIU/ml. These results are compared with those of the
study on older children in Italy (Table 10).

Table 10. Anti-HBs antibody response of seronegative children
given 2 injections of 5 μg of vaccine at an interval of 2 months

Country	Age	No.	Anti-HBs antibodies	
			%	Geometric mean titre (mIU/ml)
Italy[a]	1-12 years	24	95.8	95.8
Senegal[b]	< 24 months	72	94.6	85[c]

[a] Source: Piazza et al., 1982

[b] Source: Coursaget et al., 1983

[c] Measured 12 months after the first dose of vaccine

Newborns

A study was carried out in Burundi in which 95 newborns were
given 2 injections of 5 μg each, at 2-month intervals. At birth,
64 had passively transmitted anti-HBs antibodies. Four months
after the first injection, 83.9% of the seronegative children had
seroconverted. At the time that the booster dose was given,
82.6% of the children from the vaccinated group had anti-HBs
antibodies (see Perrin, this volume).

CONCLUSIONS

Immunization against hepatitis B is both effective in preventing HBV infections and safe. The major characteristics of the HB vaccine are its immunogenicity and the development of a strong immunological memory which ensures a long-term persistance of anti-HBs antibodies.

Vaccination strategies are now well established for adults at high risk of contracting hepatitis B. Recent data obtained from countries with a high incidence of hepatitis B have made it possible to determine the best protocols for children and new-borns.

Vaccination is immunogenic in newborns irrespective of their HBV marker status prior to immunization and of the HBV status of the mother, and is also immunogenic when combined with HBIg treatment at birth. It is effective in preventing HBV infection and the rate of HBsAg carriage is reduced by as much as 94% when the vaccine is associated with HBIg at birth.

Large-scale vaccination programmes against hepatitis B should be carried out in African and Asian countries. However, the cost of the vaccine limits its use. New protocols, using lower doses, are currently being studied and preliminary results suggest that they are as immunogenic as 'full-dose' protocols. Lower-dose protocols will allow use of the vaccine in extensive vaccination programmes and decrease the incidence of chronic HBsAg carriage, and consequently of CAH and HCC.

REFERENCES

Adamowicz, P., Gerfaux, G., Platel, Muller, L., Vacher, B., Mazert, M.-C. & Prunet, P. (1981) Large scale production of an hepatitis B vaccine. In: Maupas, P. & Guesry, P., eds, Hepatitis B Vaccine (INSERM Symposium No. 18), Amsterdam, Elsevier-North Holland, pp. 37-49

Beasley, R.P., Hwang, L.Y., Lin, C.C., Stevens, C.E., Wang, K.Y., Sun, T.S., Hsieh, F.J. & Szmuness, W. (1981) Hepatitis B immune globulin (HBIg) efficacy in the interruption of peri-natal transmission of hepatitis B virus carrier state. Lancet, 2, 388-393

Coursaget, P., Chiron, J.-P., Barin, F., Goudeau, A., Yvonnet, B., Denis, F., Lorrea, P., N'Doye, R. & Diop-Mar, I. (1983) Hepatitis B vaccine: immunization of children and newborns in an endemic area (Senegal). Dev. biol. Stand., 54, 245-257

Crosnier, J., Jungers, P., Courouce, A.M., Laplanche, A., Benhamou, E., Degos, F., Lacour, B., Prunet, P., Cerisier, Y. & Guesry, P. (1981) Randomised placebo-controlled trial of hepatitis B surface antigen vaccine in French haemo-dialysis units: I, medical staff. Lancet, 1, 455-459

Donea-Debroise, B., François-Gérard, C., Sondag-Thull, D. & André, A. (1982) Le vaccin contre l'hépatite B: résultats de l'essai clinique belge réalisé sur 150 volontaires. Rev. méd. Liège, 28, 261-267

Frosner, G.G., Franco, E. & Thomssen, P. (1983) Evaluation of the immunogenicity of different hepatitis B vaccines. In XIX Symposium of the European Society against Virus Diseases, Clermont-Ferrand, 13-15 September 1983

Goudeau, A., Dubois, F., Barin, F., Dubois, M.-C. & Coursaget, P. (1983) Hepatitis B vaccine: clinical trials in high risk settings in France. Dev. biol. Stand., 54, 267-284

Horad, W., Leithner, C., Kemenesi, W. & Pingerra, W. (1984) Zur Wirksamkeit und Sicherheit der Hepatitis B Impfung bei medizinischem Personal und bei Haemodialysispatienten. Wien. klin. Wochenschr., 4, 161-165

Lotz, E., Laguitton, C., Beaumanoir, C., Fauchet, R., Philippe, P., Zourbas, J., Brissot, P. & Bourrel, M. (1983) Préven-tion de l'hépatite B au C.H.R. de Rennes. Bilan d'un an de vaccination. Concours méd., 3, 135-143

Nutini, M.-T., Marie, F.-N., Loucq, C. & Tron, F. (1983) Hepati-tis B vaccine, clinical experience and surveillance. Lancet, 2, 1301

Panichi, G., Pescini, A., Debac, C., Taliani, G. & Pezzella, M. (1983) Vaccinazione anti-epatite B con vaccino HBVax e Hevac B. Risultati dopo le prime tre dosi in due diversi gruppi a rischio. Recent. Prog. Med., 74, 27-35

Piazza, M., Picciotto, L., Guadagnino, V., Orlando, R., Memoli, A.M. & Macchia, V. (1982) Vaccinazione contre l'epatite B. Esperienze nel napoletano. Ann. Sclavo, 24, 661

Picciotto, L., Guadagnino, V., Orlando, R., Villari, R. & Cangiano, F. (1983) Vaccinazione anti-epatite B nel bambino a rischio. In: 22 Congresso della Societa Italiana per lo Studio delle Malattie Infettive Parasitarie, Abano Terme, October 1983

Wildgrube, H.J., Classen, M., von Lohr, R., Kurth, R. & Brede, H.D. (1984) Aktive Immunisierung gegen Virus Hepatitis B. Dtsch med. Wochenschr., 109, 246-250

Yvonnet, B., Coursaget, P., Deniz, F., Digoutte, P., Petat, E., Barin, F., Goudeau, A., Correa, P., Diop-Mar, I. & Chiron, J.P. (1984) Immune response to hepatitis B vaccination at birth. Pediatrics (in press)

Zouboulis-Vafiadis, I.J., Galankis, N.I., Daikos, G.K., Psalidaki, E.E. & Hadziyannis, S.J. (1983) Active immunisation of hospital personnel against hepatitis B. In: 13th International Congress of Chemotherapy, Vienna, 28 August-2 September 1983

HEPATITIS B VACCINE IN DEVELOPING COUNTRIES: PROBLEMS AND PROSPECTS

E.A. Ayoola

Liver Unit,
University College Hospital,
Ibadan, Nigeria

RESUME

Les vaccins contre l'hépatite B sont hautement immunogènes. Pour déterminer l'efficacité de la vaccination lorsqu'on utilise des doses faibles et la voie intradermique, 197 enfants Nigérians ont reçu 3 doses mensuelles du vaccin Hevac B. Quatre vingt seize d'entre eux ont reçu 2 μg de vaccin par voie sous-cutanée, et 101 ont reçu 2 μg par voie intradermique. Un mois après la fin du protocole, 82,3% des enfants du premier groupe et 74,3% des enfants du second groupe ont développé des anticorps anti-HBs sans effets secondaires. Dans la seconde partie de l'étude, 50 porteurs chroniques de l'AgHBs ont été vaccinés. Par rapport aux témoins porteurs de l'AgHBs et traités avec un placebo, aucun effet sur la disparition de l'AgHBs ou la production d'anticorps anti-HBs n'a pu être démontré. Les immun-complexes observés n'étaient pas dus au vaccin Hevac B. Aucun effet secondaire n'a été noté. La vaccination de rappel de 50 sujets qui n'avaient pas répondu initialement a entraîné l'apparition de taux significatifs d'anticorps anti-HBs chez 20 d'entre eux (40%). Aucun des 'non-répondeurs' n'a développé de signes cliniques ou virologiques de l'infection HBV. On peut conclure que la vaccination avec de faibles doses est efficace, et que la voie intradermique peut être utile dans les pays en voie de développement.

SUMMARY

Hepatitis B vaccines are highly immunogenic. To determine the efficacy of low doses and of the intradermal route of vaccination, 197 Nigerian children were given 3 monthly doses of Hevac B. Of these, 96 had 2 μg subcutaneously and 101 had 2 μg intradermally. One month after completing the schedule, 82.3% and 74.3% of the respective groups had become anti-HBs positive without adverse side-effects. In the second part of the study, 50 chronic HBsAg carriers were vaccinated. Compared to placebo-treated carriers, no effect was demonstrated with regard to HBsAg clearance or anti-HBs production. Immune complexes were not attributable to Hevac B. No untoward effects were noted. Booster vaccination of 50 initial non-responders resulted in the development of significant levels of anti-HBs in 20 (40%) of the recipients. None of the 'non-responders' developed clinical or virological evidence of HBV infection. It is concluded that low-dose vaccination is effective and that the intradermal route may be useful in developing countries.

INTRODUCTION

It is estimated that there are 200 million chronic carriers of hepatitis B surface antigen (HBsAg) in the world. The majority of these carriers are found among the population of tropical Africa and South-East Asia where hepatitis B virus (HBV) infection occurs mainly during the perinatal period and infancy (Tabor & Gerety, 1979). In these areas, the majority of the adults show evidence of chronic or past infections.

Available epidemiological and virological data have supported the existence of a causal relationship between HBV infection and hepatocellular carcinoma (HCC), both of which are highly prevalent in tropical countries (Maupas & Melnick, 1981). In view of this pattern, and to prevent the development of chronic liver diseases, a high proportion of the susceptible populations need to be protected early in life.

Recent studies have indicated that effective prophylaxis is likely to depend on active immunization using the relatively new vaccines (Maupas et al., 1981; Szmuness et al., 1980). Although the vaccines have been shown to be safe and highly immunogenic, a number of practical problems need to be evaluated in order to permit successful and effective vaccination programmes in developing countries.

Firstly, the sophisticated technology involved in the production of currently available vaccines makes them very expensive. Limited resources in the developing countries must necessarily restrict expenditure on the provision of vaccines.

Secondly, a complicated vaccination procedure will require the commitment of skilled personnel, who are in short supply in most countries. A simple but efficient procedure is therefore a necessity.

Before firm recommendations are made, additional question which require assessment include the need for prevaccination blood tests to determine the HBV marker status of individuals; the need for obligatory cold storage of vaccines; the most efficient route of administration and dose schedule; and the need to evaluate further 'non-responders' to standard dose schedules.

A study commenced in Janary 1979 was designed to answer some of these questions, and some of the results obtained are reported here.

MATERIALS AND METHODS

Study population

Between January 1979 and May 1982, about 3 000 healthy volunteers were tested for HBV markers. They included civil servants, medical students, nursing and medical staff, mothers attending antenatal clinics, school children, and babies attending infant welfare clinics in and around Ibadan city in Nigeria.

From this population volunteers were selected if they were negative for HBV markers. Informed consent was obtained from participants, or from one of the parents.

Hepatitis B vaccine

The vaccine used in this study was Hevac B (Pasteur Institute) prepared as previously described (Adamowicz et al., 1981). The subcutaneous (s.c.) vaccines with subtypes ad and ay contained 5 μg and 2 μg of antigen protein per millilitre (ml) respectively. The intradermal vaccine was prepared without aluminium hydroxide (Al(OH)$_3$) adjuvant and contained 2 g per ml.

Protocol 1

A total of 208 participants were randomly allocated to two groups (A and B) and included those who had participated in the first phase of the trials reported elsewhere. Group A (102) received three s.c. injections of 2 μg 1 month apart. Group B were similarly treated with 2 μg vaccine intradermally.

Blood samples were obtained for HBV markers and serum alanine aminotransferase (ALT) immediately before the first injection (T0) and monthly thereafter for 7 months (T1-T7) and 12 months later (T12). Untoward effects were documented by means of questionnaires and clinical examinations at each visit.

Protocol 2: Vaccination of carriers of HBsAg

A total of 100 Nigerian males (aged 5-30 years) who were positive for HBsAg on two occasions 6 months apart and who were otherwise healthy, were randomly assigned to two groups (C and D). Group C had 3 s.c. injections (2 μg) of vaccine, 1 month apart while group D had placebo by the same schedule of injections. Blood samples were obtained as in Protocol 1. Randomly selected samples were tested for immune complexes.

Protocol 3: Further vaccination of non-responders

A group of 50 recipients (aged 5-45 years) who had failed to response to 3 consecutive doses (2 μg) of Hevac B vaccine were randomly divided into 2 groups (groups E and F). Group E (24 recipients) were given a booster dose of vaccine 1 month after the third dose (T3). Group F received levamisole (2.5 mg per kg per day) orally for 3 days in each week for 4 weeks before receiving the booster vaccination at T3. In addition to testing for HBV markers, and estimating serum immunoglobulins and albumin, E-rosette-forming cells were counted before and after treatment in both groups. Skin anergy was assessed by skin tests using PPD and Candida antigens.

Laboratory methods

HBV markers were detected by radioimmunoassay (RIA) using commercial kits (AUSRIA, AUSAB, CORAB) for HBsAg, anti-HBs and anti-HBc respectively (Abbott Laboratories, North Chicago, IL, USA). Anti-HBs response was defined as an increase of anti-HBs (AUSAB Ru) from less to greater than 2.1 in the absence of anti-HBc or HBsAg. Anti-HBs was estimated and expressed in milli international units (mIU) using a standard curve for conversion (Hollinger et al., 1982). Circulating immune complexes were detected using the Clq method (Zubler et al., 1976). Statistical analysis was performed using the chi-square and the Student t tests.

RESULTS

For protocol 1, a total of 197 children received the three doses scheduled. Of the remaining 11 lost to follow-up, 5 had 1 injection each and 6 had 2 injections.

Safety

No significant side-effects were noted in any of the participants in this study. The most common minor complaint was sore arm (21 of the 197 recipients).

Efficacy

Table 1 summarizes the immunogenic response to the 2 g dose of vaccine. The differences in seroconversion rates at various stages were not significant. The geometric mean titres at T3 were 162.5 mIU/ml and 102.4 MIU/ml in groups A and B respectively. At T12, the values were 114.4 and 89.5 mIu/ml, respectively.

Table 1. Seroconversion rates in recipients of subcutaneous (Group A) and intradermal (Group B) vaccines

Group	No. studied	No. (%) positive for anti-HBs at:			
		T1	T2	T3	T6
A	96	39 (40.6)	57 (59.4)	79 (82.3)	78 (81.3)
B	101	35 (34.7)	50 (49.5)	75 (74.3)	73 (72.3)
Both	197	74 (37.6)	107 (54.3)	154 (78.2)	151 (76.6)

Vaccination of chronic carriers

All chronic carriers retained HBsAg until T3, when 4 recipients in group C and 2 in group D became HBsAg-negative. These 6 recipients were positive for anti-HBc.   At T6, 3 carriers in Group C and 1 carrier in Group D developed anti-HBs positivity. Circulating immune complexes were detected in 5 (10%) of these 100 recipients at T0 (3 and 2 in the respective groups), and in 8 (16%) during the follow-up period.   This included 3 recipients of placebo.   None had evidence of immune complex diseases.

Vaccination of non-responders

The response to booster vaccination with or without levamisole immunopotentiation is summarized in Table 2.   No case of agranulocytosis or other side-effects of levamisole was detected. For the duration of the follow-up, no member of these two groups (E and F) developed jaundice or virological evidence of HBV infection.   None had skin anergy.   Serum albumin, immunoglobulins and the E-rosette-forming cells were within normal ranges before during and after vaccination, in all the recipients.

Table 2. Anti-HBs response to booster vaccination with (Group E) and without (Group F) levamisole immunopotentiation

Group	No.	No. (%) positive for anti-HBs at:			Mean anti-HB-s at T6
		T4	T5	T6	
E	25	14 (56)	14 (53)	13 (42)	104.4 mIU/ml
F	25	6 (24)	5 (20)	5 (20)	62.6 mIU/ml
p		< 0.01	< 0.01	< 0.05	< 0.05

DISCUSSION

The safety and efficacy of even relatively low doses of hepatitis B vaccine are further confirmed in this study. It has been reported that about 95 - 97% of vaccinated populations become anti-HBs-positive when given a 5 g dose of Hevac B (Maupas et al., 1981). This indicates, as might be anticipated, that the larger dose is slightly more effective than the smaller one. In view of the cost of vaccines, and the fact that the 'non-responders' appear to be protected against HBV infection even when anti-HBs levels are not considered adequate for positivity, the difference is less significant.

Administration of the vaccine by the intradermal route is shown by this study to be equally as effective and efficient as subcutaneous vaccination. However, the stability of this vaccine which contains no adjuvant needs to be evaluated. Fresh preparations were used in the study reported here. If the efficiency of this route were to be confirmed, it would permit the use of a dermal injection system that might encourage rapid vaccination of large populations. In addition, less skilled personnel could be trained as vaccinators, using dermal applicators, as was done for vaccination against tuberculosis.

Earlier studies excluded individuals positive for HBV markers from vaccination, possibly for two reasons, namely to ensure that vaccines were not wasted, and to avoid the theoretical possibility of immune complexing. The present study indicates that vaccination of HBV carriers does not present a hazard. Similarly, Maupas et al. (1981) have shown that previously immune persons could also be safely vaccinated. The decision to prescreen vaccine recipients must therefore by an economic one, based on cost-benefit analysis in each defined population. Vaccination appears not to modify appreciably the HBV status of recipients who are chronic carriers.

In view of the reluctance of tropical populations to permit venepuncture, and the difficulty and cost of virological tests in developing countries, it is reasonable to suggest that prescreening of children for vaccination may be unnecessary.

What should be done about 'non-responders'? Unless blood tests are performed after completion of the vaccination schedule, this group will be unidentifiable. Findings in the present study suggest that the majority of 'non-responders' are protected by booster doses of vaccine, even if they fail to mount recognisable levels of anti-HBV antibodies - at least during the follow-up period of our study. Firm conclusions must await a larger number of cases and longer follow-up.

It is concluded that available vaccines are safe and highly immunogenic. The relatively high cost may be considerably reduced, if lower doses are used. The intradermal route of vaccination is efficient and may be more useful in developing countries. 'Non-responders' respond to booster vaccination, and in any case appear to be protected against HBV infections.

REFERENCES

Adamowicz, P.H., Gerfaux, G., Platel, A., Muller, L., Vacher, B., Mazert, M.C. & Prunet, P. (1981) Large scale production of a hepatitis B vaccine. In: Maupas, P. & Guesry, P., eds, Hepatitis B Vaccine (INSERM Symposium No. 18), Amsterdam, Elsevier-North Holland, pp. 37-49

Hollinger, F.B., Adam, I., Heiberg, D. & Melnick, J.L. (1982) Response to hepatitis B vaccine in a young adult population. In: Szmuness, W., Alter, H.J. & Maynard, J.E., eds., Viral Hepatitis, Philadelphia, The Franklin Institute Press, pp. 451-466

Maupas, P., Chiron, J.P., Barin, F., Coursaget, P., Goudeau, A., Perrin, J., Denis, F. & Diop-Mar, I. (1981) Efficacy of hepatitis B vaccine in prevention of early HBsAg carrier state in children: Controlled trial in an endemic area (Senegal). Lancet, 1, 289-292

Maupas, P. & Melnick, J.L. (1981) Hepatitis B infection and primary liver cancer. Prog. med. Virol., 27, 1-5

Szmuness, W., Stevens, C.E., Harley, E.J., Zang, E.A., Oleszko, W.R., William, D.C., Sadousky, R., Morrison, J.M. & Kellner, A. (1980) Hepatitis B vaccine: Demonstration of efficacy in a controlled clinical trial in a high risk population in the United States. New Engl. J. Med., 202, 883-841

Tabor, E. & Gerety, R.J. (1979) Hepatitis B virus infection in infants and toddlers in Nigeria: The need for early intervention. J. Pediatr., 95, 647-650

Zubler, R.H., Lange, G., Lambert, P.H. & Miescher, P.A. (1976) Detection of immune complexes in unheated sera by a modified ^{125}I-Clq binding test. J. Immunol., 116, 232-235

VACCINATION DU NOUVEAU-NÉ CONTRE L'HÉPATITE B AU BURUNDI

J. Perrin & F. Ntareme

Faculté de Médecine
B.P. 1020
Bujumbura, Burundi

P. Coursaget & J.-P. Chiron

Laboratoire de Microbiologie-Immunologie
Faculté des Sciences Pharmaceutiques
37032 Tours, France

SUMMARY

Vaccination against hepatitis B is carried out at birth in the Bujumbura Hospital in Burundi. The vaccination protocol comprises only two injections, the first being given during the first 48 hours after birth and the second two months later. A booster is given at the age of one year. The results of this vaccination programme are compared with those obtained in a control population. At the time of the booster, 82% of vaccinated subjects had anti-HBs antibodies, compared with 3% of control subjects. Six months after the second injection, all vaccinated subjects had anti-HBs antibodies.

RESUME

A l'hôpital de Bujumbura (Burundi), la vaccination contre l'hépatite B est réalisée à la naissance.

Le protocole de vaccination comprend deux injections seulement, pratiquées à deux mois d'intervalle, la première étant

faite dans les premières 48 heures de la vie. Un rappel est
effectué à l'âge d'un an. Les résultats de cette vaccination sont
comparés à ceux d'un groupe témoin non vacciné.

Au moment du rappel, 82% des sujets vaccinés présentent des
anticorps anti-HBs contre 3% des sujets témoins. Six mois après
le rappel, tous les sujets vaccinés possèdent des anticorps
anti-HBs.

INTRODUCTION

Au Burundi, l'infection par le virus de l'hépatite B (HBV)
représente un problème important de santé publique, puisque la
fréquence de l'antigène HBs dans la population est de 11% et que
76% de celle-ci possède au moins l'un des marqueurs sériques
d'HBV. Par ailleurs, 57% des cancers primitifs du foie sont antigène HBs-positifs (Kocheleff et coll., 1984), et donc, comme dans
d'autres pays d'Afrique tropicale (Coursaget et coll., 1981),
le cancer primitif du foie (CPF) apparaît essentiellement lié au
virus de l'hépatite B.

La vaccination contre l'hépatite B est ainsi justifiée au
Burundi. Cette vaccination a été appliquée pour la première fois
chez l'homme en 1975 (Maupas et coll., 1976). Le vaccin, constitué par l'antigène de surface HBs du virus de l'hépatite B (Barin
et coll., 1978; Maupas et coll., 1981b), a fait la preuve de son
innocuité, de son pouvoir immunogène et de son efficacité, d'une
part en France, dans les populations à risque (Maupas et coll.,
1981c; Crosnier et coll., 1981a & b), d'autre part en Afrique, au
Sénégal, où un essai contrôlé de vaccination chez l'enfant de
moins de deux ans a commencé dès 1978 (Maupas et coll., 1981a &
d; Diop Mar et coll., 1982). Au cours de cette dernière étude,
l'immunisation active du nouveau-né par vaccination spécifique,
par trois injections de vaccin à un mois d'intervalle, a été
prouvée (Barin et coll., 1982).

L'infection par le virus de l'hépatite B survenant très tôt
en zone d'endémie (Barin et coll., 1981), il est en effet
essentiel de réaliser une prévention la plus précoce possible,
donc dès la naissance. Au Burundi, nous avons mis en place un
protocole original de vaccination du nouveau-né, comprenant
seulement deux injections à 2 deux mois d'intervalle, afin que la
prévention soit plus simple et moins coûteuse.

MATERIEL ET METHODES

Vaccin

Le vaccin contre l'hépatite B utilisé est le vaccin Hevac B (Institut Pasteur); il s'agit d'un vaccin bivalent (ad et ay), contenant 5 μg d'antigène HBs, inactivé par le formaldéhyde, et adjuvé par l'hydroxyde d'aluminium.

Protocole de vaccination HB et contrôles (Fig. 1)

- Le protocole de vaccination adopté est le suivant:

    - vaccination dès la naissance, la première injection de vaccin étant réalisée dans les premières 48 heures de la vie.

    - deux injections seulement ont été pratiquées, à deux mois d'intervalle (T0 et T2), avec un rappel à un an (T12).

- Un prélèvement sanguin a été réalisé chez l'enfant à:

    - T0: dans les 48 heures qui suivent la naissance, lors de la 1ère injection; un prélèvement a également été effectué chez la mère afin de connaître le statut sérologique vis-à-vis du virus de l'hépatite B, non seulement de l'enfant mais aussi de la mère.

    - T4: à 4 mois, pour étudier la réponse immunitaire post-vaccinale deux mois après la 2ème injection.

    - T12: à 12 mois, au moment du rappel.

    - T18: 6 mois après l'injection de rappel.

FIG. 1. PROTOCOLE DE VACCINATION DU NOUVEAU-NE CONTRE L'HEPATITE B AU BURUNDI

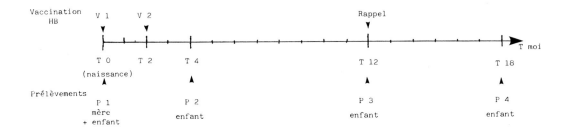

Groupe témoin

Un groupe témoin a été constitué, avec randomisation à l'échelle individuelle. Les enfants du groupe témoin ont reçu à la naissance une vaccination par BCG à la place de la vaccination contre l'hépatite B.

Les deux groupes, vacciné HB et témoin, ont bénéficié de toutes les vaccinations incluses dans le Programme Elargi de Vaccination de l'OMS (Diphtérie - Tétanos - Coqueluche - Polio à 2, 3 et 4 mois, et rappel à 12 mois; BCG à 6 mois pour le groupe vacciné HB; Rougeole à 9 mois).

Des prélèvements sanguins ont été pratiqués dans le groupe témoin à 0, 4 et 12 mois (T0, T4 et T12).

Marqueurs sériques d'HBV

Les marqueurs sériques du virus de l'hépatite B ont été recherchés par méthode radio-immunologique (Laboratoire Abbott):

- antigène HBs: AUSRIA$^{\circ}$

- anticorps anti-HBs: AUSAB$^{\circ}$; le titre des anticorps anti-HBs est exprimé en unités radio-immunologiques (URI).

- anticorps anti-HBc: CORAB[o].

Population étudiée

- L'étude de la transmission mère-enfant des marqueurs sériques du virus de l'hépatite B a porté sur 383 couples
  mère-enfant.

- Les résultats de la vaccination concernent 168 enfants
  contrôlés à 4 mois (T4), 88 vaccinés HB et 80 témoins; 84
  enfants contrôlés à 12 mois (T12), 45 vaccinés HB et 39
  témoins; par ailleurs, 21 enfants vaccinés HB ont été
  contrôlés à 18 mois (T18).

RESULTATS

Transmission mère-enfant des marqueurs d'HBV (Tableau 1)

- parmi les mères antigène HBs-positives (4% des cas seulement), aucune n'a transmis l'antigène HBs à son enfant.

- par contre, la transmission mère-enfant est importante en
ce qui concerne les anticorps:

- les anticorps anti-HBs, fréquents chez la mère (72%
  des cas) ont été transmis dans 90% des cas; ainsi,
  près de 65% des nouveau-nés possèdaient des anticorps anti-HBs.

- les anticorps anti-HBc ont presque toujours été
  transmis (99% des cas), et, ainsi, 70% des nouveau-
  nés possèdaient des anticorps anti-HBc.

- seulement 25% des enfants ne possèdaient aucun
  marqueur d'HBV à la naissance.

Tableau 1. Répartition des marqueurs sériques du virus de l'hépatite B chez 383 mères et enfants.

	MERES N=383		ENFANTS N=383		TRANSMISSION %
HBs AG +	15	(3,9%)	0	(0,0%)	0
Anti-HBs +	276	(72,1%)	248	(64,8%)	90
Anti-HBc +	271	(70,8%)	267	(69,7%)	99
Aucun marqueur	74	(19,3%)	95	(24,8%)	-

Résultats de la vaccination

Innocuité: Comme lors d'études précédentes, le vaccin s'est révélé d'une innocuité totale: aucune réaction locale ou générale n'a été observée.

Résultats 4 mois après la 1ère injection: Les résultats à T4 ont été analysés en fonction du statut sérologique à la naissance (Tableau 2).

Sujets anti-HBs-négatifs à T0: Parmi les 26 sujets vaccinés contre l'hépatite B, 23 sont devenus anti-HBs-positifs à T4, soit 88%. Par contre, 3 témoins seulement sont devenus anti-HBs-positifs. La différence est très significative (p < 10^{-7}).

Sujets anti-HBs-positifs à titre faible ($\leq$ 512 URI ou 125 mUI/ml à T0): Parmi les 24 sujets vaccinés HB, 23 sont restés anti-HBs-positifs à T4, soit 96%. Par contre, 18% seulement des témoins ont conservé leurs anticorps anti-HBs. La différence est également significative ($p<10^{-4}$).

Chez les sujets anti-HBs-positifs à titre élevé (> 512 URI à T0), on ne note pas de différence entre les vaccinés HB et les témoins: tous les sujets restent anti-HBs-positifs à T4.

Tableau 2. Résultats à T4 en fonction du statut sérologique à T0.

Statut sérologique à T 0	Nombre de subjets testés	Sujets anti-HBs + à T 4	
		N	(%)
groupe vacciné HB			
anti-HBs -	26*	23	(88,5)
anti-HBs + $\leq$512 URI	24	23	(95,8)
anti-HBs + >512 URI	38	38	(100,0)
groupe témoin			
anti-HBs -	27**	3	(11,1)
anti-HBs + $\leq$512 URI	11	2	(18,2)
anti-HBs + >512 URI	42	42	(100,0)

* : 17 séro-négatifs et 9 anti-HBc + seul
**: 21 séro-négatifs et 6 anti-HBc + seul

PERRIN ET AL.

Si on ne tient pas compte du statut sérologique initial,
à 4 mois (T4), 95% des sujets vaccinés sont anti-HBs-
positifs, contre 59% des sujets témoins; la différence
est significative ($p < 10^{-8}$). (Tableau 3).

Résultats 12 mois après la 1ère injection: La différence
entre les sujets vaccinés HB et témoins est très significative ($p < 10^{-9}$), 82% des sujets vaccinés étant anti-HBs-
positifs contre seulement 3% des témoins (Tableau 3).

Tableau 3. Resultats globaux à T 4 et à T 12.

	T 4			T 12		
	Nombre de sujets testés	Sujets anti-HBs +		Nombre de sujets testés	Sujets anti-HBs	
		N	(%)		N	(%)
Groupe vacciné HB	88	84	(95,5)	45	37	(82,2)
Groupe témoin	80	47	(58,8)	39	1	(2,6)

Résultats 18 mois après la 1ère injection: Actuellement, 21
sujets vaccinés HB ont été prélevés à T18:   ils sont tous
anti-HBs-positifs.

Efficacité: A T12, deux enfants du groupe témoin étaient
antigène HBs-positifs;   aucun ne l'était dans le groupe
vacciné HB.

DISCUSSION

Ce protocole de vaccination contre l'hépatite B mis en place au Burundi avait pour but de réaliser une prévention la plus précoce possible avec le moins d'injections possible. La séro-vaccination, recommandée chez les enfants nés de mères antigène HBs-positives (Goudeau, 1982), n'a pas été pratiquée en raison de son coût élevé dans un pays en développement.

L'innocuité du vaccin a été absolue, et ceci, quel que soit le statut sérologique des nouveau-nés ou de leurs mères.

L'immunisation du nouveau-né avec deux injections s'est révélée efficace. Deux mois après la deuxième injection, à T4, les résultats sont très significatifs en ce qui concerne les enfants ne présentant pas d'anticorps anti-HBs ou des anticorps à titre faible à la naissance: 92% des sujets vaccinés HB sont anti-HBs positifs contre 13% des sujets témoins ($p < 10^{-9}$). Par contre, parmi les sujets anti-HBs-positifs à titre élevé, on ne note pas de différence entre les sujets vaccinés HB et les témoins. La décroissance des anticorps d'origine maternelle n'est en effet pas suffisante au bout de 4 mois, quand on part d'un titre élevé d'anticorps, pour que les témoins se négativent. A T12, les anticorps passivement transmis ayant disparu; on constate dans ce même groupe une différence significative: tous les témoins se sont négativés, tandis que 76% des sujets vaccinés HB ont des anticorps anti-HBs ($p < 10^{-5}$).

Les résultats ne sont donc vraiment interprétables qu'à T12: la différence est alors très nette entre les vaccinés HB, dont 82% ont des anticorps anti-HBs, et les témoins, dont 3% seulement possèdent ces mêmes anticorps. Il apparaît donc que les anticorps d'origine maternelle n'interfèrent pas avec l'immunisation active du nouveau-né.

Après l'injection de rappel, les résultats sont excellents: 100% des sujets vaccinés contre l'hépatite B sont protégés.

Au point de vue de l'efficacité sur la diminution du portage chronique de l'antigène HBs, la différence entre les deux groupes ne peut pas être significative, en raison du faible échantillon d'enfants et du pourcentage peu élevé de mères antigène HBs posi-tives.

En conclusion, ce protocole de vaccination permettra une prévention plus facile et moins coûteuse de l'hépatite B et, à plus
long terme, du cancer primitif du foie, 80% des CPF étant attri-
buables au virus de l'hépatite B (Organisation Mondiale de la
Santé, 1983).

REFERENCES

Barin, F., Andre, M., Goudeau, A., Coursaget, P. & Maupas, P.
    (1978) Large-scale purification of hepatitis B surface
    antigen (HBs Ag). Ann. Microbiol. (Inst. Pasteur), 129 B,
    87-100

Barin, F., Perrin, J., Chotard, J., Denis, F., N'Doye, R., Diop
    Mar, I., Chiron, J.P., Coursaget, P., Goudeau, A. & Maupas,
    P. (1981) Cross-sectional and longitudinal epidemiology of
    hepatitis in Senegal. Prog. med. Virol., 27, 148-162

Barin, F., Goudeau, A., Denis, F., Yvonnet, B., Chiron, J.P.,
    Coursaget, P. & Diop Mar, I. (1982) Immune response in
    neonates to hepatitis B vaccine. Lancet, i, 251-253

Coursaget, P., Maupas, P., Goudeau, A., Chiron, J.P., Raynaud,
    B., Drucker, J., Barin, F., Denis, F., Diop Mar, I. & Diop,
    B. (1981) A case/control study of hepatitis B virus serologic
    markers in Senegalese patients suffering from primary hepato-
    cellular carcinoma. Prog. med. Virol., 27, 49-59

Crosnier, J., Jungers, P., Courouce, A.M., Laplanche, A.,
    Benhamou, E., Degos, F., Lacour, B., Prunet, P., Cerisier, Y.
    & Guesry, P. (1981a) Randomised placebo-controlled trial of
    hepatitis B surface antigen vaccine in French hemodialysis
    units. I - Medical staff Lancet, i, 455-459

Crosnier, J., Jungers, P., Courouce, A.M., Laplanche, A.,
    Benhamou, E., Degos, F., Lacour, B., Prunet, P., Cerisier, Y.
    & Guesry, P. (1981b) Randomised placebo-controlled trial of
    hepatitis B surface antigen vaccine in French hemodialysis
    units. II - Hemodialysis patients. Lancet, i, 797-800

Diop Mar, I., Yvonnet, B., Denis, F., Perrin, J., N'Doye, R., Chiron, J.P., Barin, F., Coursaget, P. & Goudeau, A. (1982) Essai contrôlé de vaccination contre l'hépatite B du jeune enfant en zone endémique (Sénégal). Méd. Afr. Noire, 29, 687-699

Goudeau, A. (1982) Transmission mère-enfant du virus de l'hépatite B. Perspectives de prévention de l'infection néonatale. Nouv. Presse méd., 11, 3051-3054

Kocheleff, P., Constant, J.L., Carteron, B., Perrin, J., Kabondo, P., Perrin-Bedere, C. & Chiron, J.P. (1984) Recherche sur le cancer primitif du foie au Burundi. Projet FED 4507-062-15-35.

Maupas, P., Goudeau, A., Coursaget, P., Drucker, J. & Bagros, P. (1976) Immunisation against hepatitis B in man. Lancet, i, 1367-1370

Maupas, P., Chiron, J.P., Goudeau, A., Coursaget, P., Perrin, J., Barin, F., Denis, F. & Diop Mar, I. (1981a) Active immunisation against hepatitis B in an area of high endemicity. Part II: Prevention of early infection of the child. Prog. med. Virol., 27, 185-201

Maupas, P., Coursaget, P., Goudeau, A., Barin, F., Chiron, J.P. & Raynaud, B. (1981b) Hepatitis B vaccine: rationals, principles and applications. In: Maupas, P. & Guesry, P., eds, Hepatitis B vaccine. INSERM Symposiun no. 18 - Elsevier North Holland Biomedical Press, pp. 3-11

Maupas, P., Goudeau, A., Dubois, F., Coursaget, P. & Barin, F. (1981c) Potency and efficacy of HB vaccine applied to a high risk population. A five year study. In: Maupas, P. & Guesry, P., eds, Hepatitis B vaccine. INSERM Symposium no. 18 - Elsevier North Holland Biomedical Press, pp. 117-131

Maupas, P., Chiron, J.P., Barin, F., Coursaget, P., Goudeau, A., Perrin, J., Denis, F. & Diop Mar, I. (1981d) Efficacy of hepatitis B vaccine in prevention of early HBs Ag carrier state in children. Controlled trial in an endemic area (Senegal). Lancet, i, 289-292

Organisation Mondiale de la Sante (1983) Prévention du cancer du
    foie. Série de Rapports Techniques, no. 691

IMMUNE RESPONSE TO HEPATITIS B VACCINE IN INFANTS AND NEWBORNS: CONTROL TRIAL IN AN ENDEMIC AREA (SENEGAL)

P. Coursaget, F. Deciron, E. Tortey, F. Barin & J.P. Chiron

Institut de Virologie de Tours
Tours, France

B. Yvonnet, C. Diouf, F. Denis, I. Diop-Mar, P. Correa
& R. N'Doye

Faculté de Médecine et de Pharmacie
Dakar-Fann, Sénégal

RESUME

En 1978, nous avons proposé l'utilisation du vaccin contre l'hépatite B pour empêcher que les enfants ne deviennent porteurs de l'AgHBs de façon précoce. L'immunisation a été effectuée par trois injections de vaccin HB à un mois d'intervalle, suivies d'un rappel un an plus tard. Les enfants du groupe témoin ont été immunisés avec le vaccin DT-Polio selon le même protocole.

La réponse des enfants à la vaccination contre le virus HB a été étudiée en fonction de leurs marqueurs sériques d'HBV avant l'immunisation: 70,5% des enfants séronégatifs ont acquis l'immunité après deux injections de 5 μg chacune et 94% après la troisième injection.

On a démontré l'efficacité du vaccin en comparant les manifestations d'infection HBV un an plus tard chez 309 enfants séronégatifs immunisés par le vaccin contre le virus HB et chez 252 enfants séronégatifs immunisés avec le vaccin DT Polio, et deux ans après la vaccination, chez 101 enfants du premier groupe et 119 du second. L'incidence de l'infection latente (mise en évidence par la présence de l'AgHBs) a été réduite de 80% chez les enfants vaccinés contre l'hépatite B.

Pour éviter la transmission du virus HB aux nouveaux-nés lors
de l'accouchement, par les mères porteuses de l'AgHBs on a étudié
les possibilités d'immunisation à la naissance. Les nouveaux-nés
ont aussi bien répondu à la vaccination que les enfants plus
âgés, ceci indépendamment du statut de leurs mères vis-à-vis
d'HBV. L'incidence des infections latentes (mises en évidence
par la présence de l'AgHBs) a été réduite de 80%.

En Afrique, les équipes préposées à l'immunisation ne peuvent
consacrer qu'un temps limité à chaque communauté rurale. Aussi,
nous avons étudié l'effet immunogène de l'administration de deux
doses de vaccin à deux ou six mois d'intervalle. Tous les enfants ont eu une dose de rappel un an après la première injection. On n'a pas observé de différence entre les protocoles ni
dans le taux de séroconversion, ni au niveau des titres d'anticorps. Ces résultats montrent que deux doses de 5 μg du vaccin
suffisent à induire chez les enfants un degré d'immunité élevé.

Nous avons en outre étudié la réponse à l'administration
simultanée du vaccin contre l'hépatite B et du vaccin DT Polio.
La réponse immune est au moins égale à celle observée après
l'administration séparée de chacun de ces vaccins.

SUMMARY

In 1978 it was suggested that hepatitis B (HB) vaccine should
be used to prevent the early hepatitis B surface antigen (HBsAg)
carrier state in children. Immunization was effected by 3 injections of HB vaccine at one-month intervals followed by a booster
injection after one year. Children in a control group were
immunized with DT-polio vaccine according to the same schedule.
The anti-HBs response of the children to HB vaccination was
studied in relation to their hepatitis B virus (HBV) serum
markers prior to immunization. Of the seronegative children,
70.5% responded to immunization after 2 injections of 5- g doses
of HB vaccine and 94% after the third injection.

The efficacy of the vaccine was demonstrated by comparison of
HB events after one year in 309 seronegative children immunized
with HB vaccine and 252 seronegative children immunized with DT-
polio vaccine, and after two years in 101 and 119 children,
respectively. The incidence of the HBsAg carrier state was
reduced by 80% in susceptible children.

In order to eliminate the perinatal transmission occurring in newborns with HBsAg-positive mothers, a study of immunization at birth has been instituted. A total of 86 newborns responded to the vaccination as well as older children, irrespective of the HBV status of their mothers. After one year, the incidence of the HBsAg carrier state was reduced by 80%.

In Africa, immunization teams have a limited amount of time to devote to each rural community. The immunogenic effect of 2 doses of HB vaccine given at an interval of 2 or 6 months has therefore been investigated. All were given a booster dose one year after the first injection of vaccine. No difference was observed in the seroconversion rate or in the anti-HBs titres as between the two protocols. these results demonstrate that 2 doses of 5 μg of HB vaccine are sufficient to obtain a high immunogenic effect in infants.

In addition, an investigation was carried out on the immune response to HBsAg and tetanus toxoid antigen when administered simultaneously to children as HB vaccine and DT-polio vaccine. The immune response was at least equal to that observed after administration of these vaccines separately.

INTRODUCTION

In Senegal as in tropical Africa and Asia, hepatitis B infection occurs mainly during infancy and 90-95% of the adult population have evidence of past or present infection, as indicated by the presence of serological markers of hepatitis B virus (HBV) (Barin et al., 1981; Szmuness et al., 1973). More-over 10-20% of this population are chronic carriers of the virus and there is much evidence to incriminate HBV as the oncogenic agent of hepatocellular carcinoma (HCC) (Beasley et al., 1981; Heyward et al., 1982).

Since the initial study in 1975 of hepatitis B vaccine in man by Maupas et al. (1976), numerous immunization trials have shown that formalin-inactivated 22 nm hepatitis B surface antigen (HBsAg) subunit vaccines are highly immunogenic. The safety and the protection provided by such vaccines have been demonstrated by controlled trials in several susceptible populations (Crosnier et al., 1981a,b; Szmuness et al., 1980; Francis et al., 1982; Desmyter et al., 1983). In order to prevent the early HBsAg carrier state in children in Senegal, we therefore initiated an

immunization programme against hepatitis B in this country in
1978 (Maupas et al., 1981a,b).

MATERIALS AND METHODS

The programme, entitled Prévention hépatite-hépatome, was
conducted in a rural area of Senegal, located in the centre of
the peanut growing area (Niakhar district in the Department of
Fatick of the Sine-Saloum region) (Maupas et al., 1981c). In
this region, massive infection by HBV occurs at two different
periods of life. A first wave is observed during the breast-
feeding period and a second coincides with the beginning of
schooling at 6-7 years of age, where 75% of the children have at
least one HBV serum marker of HBV infection (Fig. 1). Early
infection results in 15% HBsAg-positive children at 2 years.

FIG. 1. AGE DISTRIBUTION OF HEPATITIS B VIRUS MARKERS
IN CHILDREN

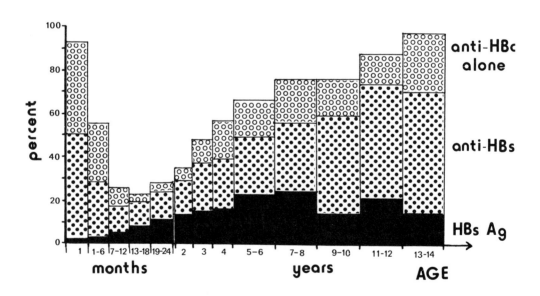

Vaccine

The hepatitis B vaccine used in Senegal is produced by Institut Pasteur, Paris (HEVAC B). The vaccine is composed of purified HBsAg (5 μg/ml), inactivated with formaldehyde. Both subtypes ad and ay are mixed in the final preparation. Aluminium hydroxyde is added as adjuvant (Adamowicz et al., 1981).

Laboratory studies

Each blood sample was investigated for antibody to the HBV surface antigen (anti-HBs), HBsAg and antibody to the HBV core antigen (anti-HBc) by radioimmunoassays (AUSAB, AUSRIA II, CORAB, Abbott Laboratories, North Chicago, IL, USA). Anti-HBs antibody concentration is expressed in mIU/ml calculated according to the method proposed by Hollinger et al. (1982).

Tetanus toxoid antibodies were sought by solid-phase radio-immunoassay adapted from that described by Vulpillat & Carbon (1976).

Protocols

Children aged 3-24 months at the time of the first dose of vaccine

Immunization was effected by means of 3 injections of hepatitis B vaccine (subcutaneously) at one-month intervals followed by a booster injection after one year. Children belonging to the control group were immunized with DT-polio vaccine according to the same schedule.

We also investigated the immune response to HBsAg and tetanus toxoid antigen when administered simultaneously to children as hepatitis B vaccine and DT-polio vaccine (Chiron et al., 1984). One group of children received hepatitis B vaccine, a second group DT-polio vaccine, and a third group was given both vaccines simultaneously but in different arms.

From September 1981 onwards, immunization was effected by means of 2 injections of vaccine at 2 or 6 months interval, followed by a booster injection after one year (Yvonnet et al., 1984).

Newborns

Each newborn received the first dose of hepatitis B vaccine on the day of birth, the second at the age of one month, the third at the age of 2 months and a booster injection at the age of 12 months.

RESULTS

Only transient local reactions were reported after immunization with hepatitis B vaccine, irrespective of the HBV marker status, age and sex of recipients.

Potency

Seronegative children

For the 3-dose protocol (see Table 1), the vaccine potency was determined in infants bled 2, 4, 12, 14, 24 and 36 months after they had received the first dose of HB vaccine. The proportion of anti-HBs individuals reached 94% after the third dose of vaccine, and up to 90% were always positive after 1, 3 and 3 years.

Table 1. Anti-HBs response to hepatitis B vaccine in sero-negative children (3-dose protocol)

Time after first injection (months)	No. tested	No. anti-HBs-positive	% Anti-HBs-positive
2	342	241	70.5
4	298	280	94.0
12	309	285	92.2
14	74	72	97.7
24	101	97	96.0
36	28	27	96.4

The vaccine potency when the two-dose protocol was used (Fig. 2) was determined in 72 infants tested 12 months after the first dose of HB vaccine, 93.1% showing evidence of anti-HBs at that time. The geometric mean anti-HBs titre was 85 mIU/ml. A comparison was made with 111 infants who received the 3 doses at 1 month $\pm$ 1 week intervals. The percentage of anti-HBs-positive infants (94.6%) was about the same and the geometric mean titre was 92 mIU/ml.

FIG. 2. ANTI-HBs IMMUNE RESPONSE AT T12:
COMPARISON OF 2 AND 3-DOSE PROTOCOLS

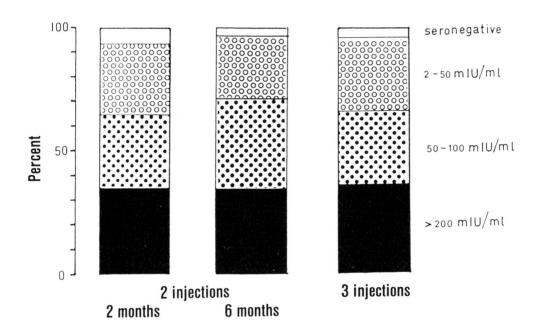

When two doses of vaccine were administered at an interval of 6 months, the potency was determined in 30 infants tested 12 months after the first dose of hepatitis B vaccine, 96.6% of whom had anti-HBs, and the distribution of anti-HBs titre was equivalent to that observed with 2 doses at an interval of 2 months or 3 doses at one-month intervals (Fig. 2).

Children with HBV markers prior to immunization

The anti-HBs response in children who had only anti-HBc prior to immunization was the same as that observed in the seronegative group. Anti-HBs antibodies were present in 91.7% (77/84) after one year and in 95.2% (20/21) after 2 years.

In infants who were HBsAg-positive at the time of the first injection of hepatitis B vaccine, 12.8% (6/47) had developed anti-HBs at T12 and 35.3% (6/17) at T24. The difference was not statistically significant as compared with the natural sero-conversion observed in the control group at T12 (2/21, 9.5%) and T24 (1/12, 8.3%). At the end of the follow-up period (T24), 58.8% of the vaccinated group was still HBsAg-positive as compared to 75.0% of the control group (not significant).

Efficacy

The efficacy of the hepatitis B vaccine was established after 1 and 2 years follow-up (2- and 3-dose protocols) in infants seronegative at the time of the first injection. Of 362 children in the hepatitis B vaccine group, 4 (1.1%) were found to be HBsAg-positive after one year, as compared to 17 out of 252 (6.7%) in the control group ($p < 10^{-3}$), while 2 years after the beginning of the programme 3% of the infants in the vaccine group were found to be HBsAg-positive, as compared to 12.6% in the control group ($p = 0.019$) (Fig. 3).

If all HBV events are taken into account (HBsAg and/or anti-HBc-positive), infection was observed in 2.3% after one year and 4.0% after two years in the vaccinated group, as compared to 10.3% after one year and 20.2% after two years in the control group (Fig. 4).

The efficacy of the vaccine has also been estimated in sero-negative infants and infants who were anti-HBc alone (Fig. 5). HBsAg was detected in 1.3% of the vaccinated children at T12 and in 3.3% at T24, as against 6.5% and 15.4%, respectively, in infants belonging to the control group ($p < 10^{-3}$ and $p = 2.10^{-3}$, respectively). Thus a reduction of 80% in the chronic carrier state was observed after one year and 79% after two years follow-up.

FIG. 3. EFFICACY OF HEPATITIS B VACCINE IN SERONEGATIVE INFANTS:
COMPARISON OF HBsAg CARRIER STATE IN HEPATITIS B VACCINE
GROUP (V) AND CONTROL GROUP (C)

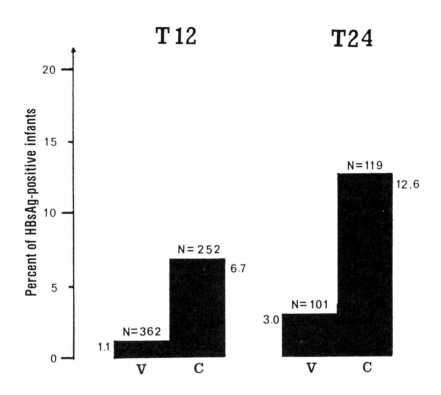

Immunization of newborns

Immunization was carried out and blood samples taken in the
maternity unit of Le Dantec hospital in Dakar (Senegal). Of the
119 infants who entered the study, 94 received the 3 vaccine
doses and 60 the booster injection. At 3 months, 58 of the 60
newborns (96.4%) had circulating anti-HBs in the absence of
HBsAg, as did 54 (90.0%) at 12 months, i.e., at the time of the
booster injection. Two months later (T14), 49 infants were bled
and 46 of them (93.9%) showed evidence of anti-HBs in the

FIG. 4. EFFICACY OF HEPATITIS B VACCINE IN SERONEGATIVE INFANTS:
COMPARISON OF HBV EVENTS IN HEPATITIS B VACCINE GROUP (V)
AND CONTROL GROUP (C)

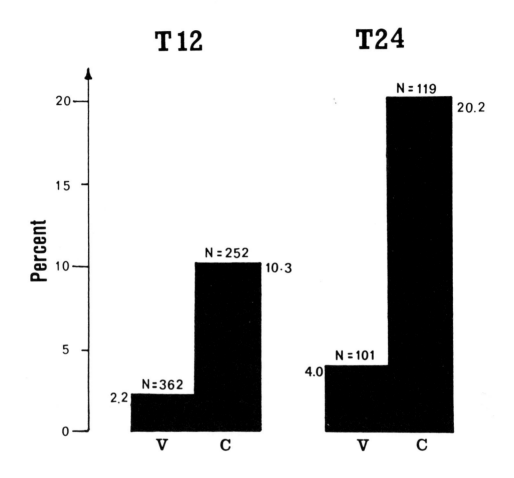

absence of HBsAg. One infant was both HBsAg and anti-HBs-
positive at T3, T12 and T14. The immune response of the children
in relation to the HBV status before immunization is shown in
Table 2.

FIG. 5. EFFICACY OF HEPATITIS B VACCINE IN SERONEGATIVE INFANTS
AND INFANTS WITH ANTI-HBc ALONE: COMPARISON OF HBsAg
CARRIER STATE IN HEPATITIS B VACCINE GROUP (V)
AND CONTROL GROUP (C)

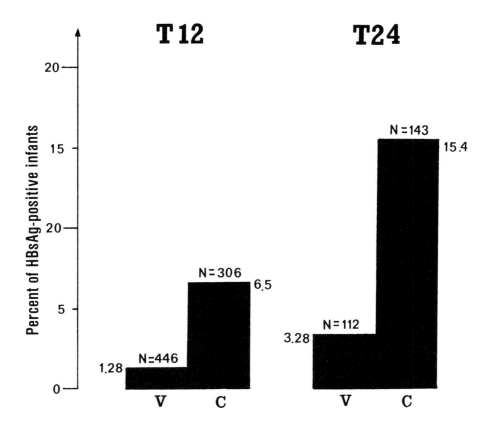

Although this vaccine trial did not include a control group,
the HBV status of immunized neonates has been compared with the
epidemiological data being collected in Senegal; 7.5% of 239
children aged 12 months have been found to be HBsAg-positive. In
comparison, in immunized newborns, only 1.7% were HBsAg-positive
at 12 months (Fig. 6).

Table 2.   Anti-HBs response to hepatitis B vaccine in immunized
newborns

HBV status of newborns	Time	No.	Anti-HBs response	
			% Positive	Geometric mean titre
Anti-HBs-positive at TO	TO	35	100.0	58
	T3	35	100.0	82
	T12	35	85.7	75
	T14	30	93.3	2423
Anti-HBs-negative at TO	TO	25	0.0	–
	T3	25	92.0	46
	T12	25	96.0	62
	T14	19	94.7	2357

Simultaneous administration of hepatitis B and DT-polio vaccines

One month after the second injection of vaccine, 43 infants
from the DT-polio vaccine group and 42 from the DT-polio + hepatitis B vaccine group were investigated for tetanus toxoid antibodies.   All infants had anti-tetanus-toxoid antibody, and no
difference in the geometric mean titre was observed (977 and 1233
mIU/ml). Two months after the third injection of vaccine, 22 and
20 infants were bled, respectively.   At that time, the anti-
tetanus-toxoid geometric mean titre was 1402 mIU/ml in infants
receiving DT-polio vaccine and 3580 mIU/ml in infants receiving
DT-polio + hepatitis B vaccines (p = 0.05).   The hepatitis B
vaccine immune response was investigated only in infants who were
seronegative or anti-HBc alone at the time of the first injection
of vaccine. At the time of the third injection, anti-HBs was
detected in 94% of 50 infants from the hepatitis B vaccine group
and in 97% of 31 infants from the hepatitis B + DT-polio vaccine
group.   Two months after the third injection of the vaccines,
anti-HBs antibodies were detected in 98% of infants from the
hepatitis B vaccine group (64/65) and 93% of infants from the

FIG. 6.   HBsAg (■) AND ANTI-HBs (⊠) IN INFANTS
12 MONTHS OF AGE: COMPARISON BETWEEN INFANTS IMMUNIZED
AT BIRTH AND NON-IMMUNIZED INFANTS

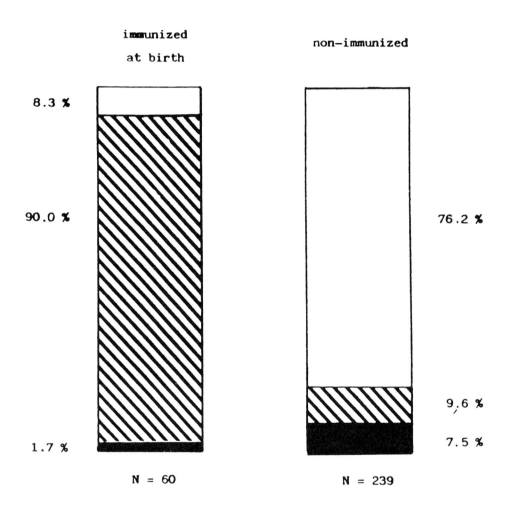

immunized

at birth

non-immunized

8.3 %

90.0 %   76.2 %

                                             9.6 %

1.7 %   7.5 %

N = 60   N = 239

hepatitis B + DT-polio vaccines group (13/14). No difference was
observed in the proportion of high anti-HBs titres (> 200
mIU/ml).   Thus the immune response to HBsAg and tetanus toxoid
antigens observed after immunization of infants with hepatitis B
vaccine and DT-polio vaccine in combination was at least equal to
that observed after administration of these vaccines alone.

CONCLUSIONS

The major features of this trial of hepatitis B immunization conducted in infants and newborns in Senegal may be summarized as follows:

- Vaccination of every child against hepatitis B is safe, irrespective of the HBV marker status prior to immunization, age or sex. Thus mass vaccination campaigns against hepatitis B can be considered in areas of high endemicity, without screening for HBV markers prior to immunization.

- The administration of two 5-μg doses of vaccine at intervals of 2 or 6 months gave results similar to those given by 3 doses at 1-month intervals.

- Hepatitis B vaccine was immunogenic when administered at birth: 90% of the immunized newborns developed an anti-HBs response.

- Active immunization against HBV can be effected in infants with passive immunity due to anti-HBs of maternal origin.

- Hepatitis B vaccine did not significantly reduce the chronic carrier state in recipients who were HBsAg-positive before the first injection of HB vaccine.

- Hepatitis B vaccination reduces the chronic carrier state by 80% in susceptible infants (seronegative or anti-HBc alone).

- Hepatitis B vaccine can be combined with DT-polio vaccine.

Immunization against hepatitis B is thus as essential in African countries as vaccination against tetanus, diphtheria, poliomyelitis and measles. To be feasible, such mass vaccination of the general population requires a vaccine that is available in adequate amounts and at a reasonable price. To this end, the use of a protocol calling for two 5-μg doses will have to be considered.

ACKNOWLEDGEMENTS

This work was inspired and directed by Philippe Maupas until his death on 6 February 1981. The Franco-Senegalese programme Prévention hépatite-hépatome was supported by grant No. 28/77/432, project 223/DH/77, Ministère de la Coopération (France) and Secrétariat d'Etat à la Recherche Scientifique et Technique (Senegal), and by grants Nos 130008, 130028, 130007, 130055, 130060 and 130054 from the Institut National de la Santé et de la Recherche Médicale (France). We should like to emphasize that the trial in Senegal was possible only thanks to the support of the Senegalese Government. We also thank the medical officers and government officials of Dakar and the Sine-Saloum region, the village chiefs and elders, and the population of the Niakhar District for their help and cooperation.

REFERENCES

Adamowicz, P., Gerfaux, G., Platel, A., Muller, A., Vacher, B., Mazert, M.C. & Prunet, P. (1981) Large scale production of a hepatitis B vaccine. In: Maupas, P. & Guesry, P., eds, Hepatitis B Vaccine (INSERM Symposium No. 18), Amsterdam, Elsevier North-Holland, pp. 37-49

Barin, F., Perrin, J., Chotard, J., Denis, F., N'Doye, R., Diop-Mar, I., Chiron, J.P., Coursaget, P., Goudeau, A. & Maupas, P. (1981) Cross-sectional and longitudinal epidemiology of hepatitis B in Senegal. Prog. med. Virol., 27, 148-162

Beasley, R.P., Lin, C.C., Hwang, L.Y. & Chien, C.S. (1981) Hepatocellular carcinoma and hepatitis B virus. A prospective study of 22,707 men in Taiwan. Lancet, 2, 1129-1133

Chiron, J.P., Coursaget, P., Yvonnet, B., Auger, F., Lee Quan, T., Barin, F., Denis, F. & Diop-Mar, I. (1984) Simultaneous administration of hepatitis B and diphtheria/tetanus/polio vaccines. Lancet, 1, 623-624

Crosnier, J., Jungers, P., Couroucé, A.M., Laplanche, A., Benhamou, E., Degos, F., Lacour, B., Prunet, P., Cerisier, Y. & Guesry, P. (1981a) Randomised placebo controlled trial of hepatitis B surface antigen vaccine in French haemodialysis units: I. Medical staff. Lancet, 1, 455-459

Crosnier, J., Jungers, P., Couroucé, A.M., Laplanche, A., Benhamou, E., Degos, F., Lacour, B., Prunet, P., Cerisier, Y. & Guesry, P. (1981b) Randomised placebo controlled trial of hepatitis B surface antigen vaccine in French haemodialysis units. II. Haemodialysis patients. Lancet, 1, 787-800

Desmyter, J., Colaert, J., De Groote, G., Reynders, M., Reerink-Brongers, E.E., Lelie, P.N., Dees, P.J., Reesink, H.W. & the Leuven Renal Transplantation Collaborative Group (1983) Efficacy of heat-inactivated hepatitis B vaccine in haemodialysis patients and staff. Double blind placebo controlled trial. Lancet, 2, 132301327

Francis, D.P., Hadler, S.C., Thompson, S.E., Maynard, J.E., Ostrow, D.G., Altman, N., Braff, E.H., O'Malley, P., Hawkins, D., Judson, F.N., Penley, K., Nylund, T., Christie, G., Meyers, F., Moore, J.N., Gardner, A., Doto, I.L., Miller, J.H., Reynolds, G.H., Murphy, B.L., Schable, C.A., Clark, B.T., Curran, J.W. & Redeker, A.G. (1982) The prevention of hepatitis B with vaccine. Report of the Centers for Disease Control multi-center efficacy trial among homosexual men. Ann. intern. Med., 97, 362-366

Heyward, W.L., Bender, J.R., Lanier, A.P., Francis, D.P., McMahon, B.J. & Maynard, J.E. (1982) Serological markers of hepatitis B virus and alpha-fetoprotein levels preceding primary hepatocellular carcinoma in Alaskan Eskimos. Lancet, 2, 889-891

Hollinger, F.B., Adam, E., Heiberg, D. & Melnick, J.L. (1982) Response to hepatitis B vaccine in a young adult population. In: Szmuness, W., Alter, H.J. & Maynard, J.E., eds, Viral Hepatitis, Philadelphia, The Franklin Institut Press, pp. 451-466

Maupas, P., Goudeau, A., Coursaget, P., Drucker, J. & Bagros, P. (1976) Immunization against hepatitis B in man. Lancet, 1, 1367-1370

Maupas, P., Chiron, J.P., Barin, F., Coursaget, P., Goudeau, A., Perrin, J., Denis, F. & Diop-Mar, I. (1981a) Efficacy of hepatitis B vaccine in prevention of early HBsAg carrier state in children. Controlled trial in an endemic area (Senegal). Lancet, 1, 289-292

Maupas, P., Chiron, J.P., Barin, F., Perrin, J., Denis, F., Coursaget, P., Goudeau, A. & Diop-Mar, I. (1981b) Vaccination against hepatitis B in an endemic area, prevention of the early HBsAg carrier state in children. In: Maupas, P. & Guesry, P., eds, Hepatitis B Vaccine (INSERM Symposium No. 18), Amsterdam, Elsevier-North-Holland, pp. 213-224

Maupas, P., Coursaget, P., Chiron, J.P., Goudeau, A., Barin, F., Perrin, J., Denis, F. & Diop-Mar, I. (1981c) Active immunization against hepatitis B in an area of high endemicity: Part I, Field design. Prog. med. Virol., 27, 168-184

Szmuness, W., Prince, A.M., Diebolt, G., Leblanc, L., Baylet, R., Masseyeff, R. & Linhard, J. (1973) The epidemiology of hepatitis B infections in Africa: Results of a pilot survey in the Republic of Senegal. Am. J. Epidemiol., 98, 104-110

Szmuness, W., Stevens, C.E., Harley, E.J., Zang, E.A., Oleszko, W.R., William, D.C., Sadovsky, R., Morrison, J.M. & Kellner, A. (1980) Hepatitis B vaccine: Demonstration of efficacy in a controlled clinical trial in a high risk population in the United States. New Engl. J. Med., 303, 833-841

Vulpillat, M. & Carbon, C. (1976) Tetanic antitoxin radio-immunoassay: a very highly sensitive method. Biomedicine, 25, 355-358

Yvonnet, B., Coursaget, P., Petat, E., Tortey, E., Diouf, C., Barin, F., Denis, F., Diop-Mar, I. & Chiron, J.P. (1984) Immunogenic effect of hepatitis B vaccine in children: comparison of two and three doses protocols. J. med. Virol. (in press)

USE OF HEPATITIS B VIRUS VACCINE IN AFRICA: RATIONALE AND PRACTICAL APPROACHES FOR EFFECTIVE UTILIZATION

A.M. Prince

The Laboratory of Virology,
The Lindsley F. Kimball Research Institute of
The New York Blood Center
New York, USA
and
Vilab II, The Liberian Institute for Biomedical Research
Robertsfield, Liberia

RESUME

Ce rapport considère les questions suivantes: (1) devra-t-on utiliser le vaccin contre le virus de l'hépatite B (HBV) en Afrique, s'il est un jour disponible en quantités suffisantes et à un prix abordable ? (2) Qui devra-t-on vacciner et quand ? (3) Quel type de vaccin HBV faudra-t-il utiliser ?

Les réponses à ces questions sont suggérées sur la base des connaissances actuelles de l'épidémiologie des infections HBV en Afrique, du rôle d'HBV dans l'étiologie du cancer primitif du foie et de la cirrhose, et de l'utilisation des différents vaccins expérimentaux actuellement disponibles.

SUMMARY

This report considers the following questions: (1) Should hepatitis B virus (HBV) vaccine be used in Africa, if and when adequate supplies become available at an affordable cost? (2) Who should receive the vaccine and when? (3) What type of HBV vaccine should be used?

Answers to these questions are suggested based on a review of available knowledge of the epidemiology of HBV infections in Africa, the role of HBV in the etiology of hepatocellular carcinoma and cirrhosis, and the utilization of various currently available and experimental HBV vaccines.

INTRODUCTION

Hepatitis B virus (HBV) vaccines are now available for use in many parts of the world. It is appropriate, therefore, to appraise the status of progress in this field, and especially to answer the following three questions:

1. Why should such a vaccine be used?
2. Who should receive it?
3. How should it be made and given?

The following discussion will focus on these questions in the context of medical priorities on a continent in which hepatitis B infection and its associated sequelae are highly prevalent, and where use of new vaccines must be considered in the light of other health-related needs which compete for severely limited available funds.

IS HEPATITIS B VIRUS VACCINE NEEDED IN AFRICA ?

To date, the major use of HBV vaccine has been to prevent acute HBV infections in high-risk groups in Western Europe and the United States. In these regions it is well established that the following groups are at high risk of developing such infections: haemodialysis patients and staff, multiply transfused patients, persons exposed to high-risk blood products, e.g., haemophiliacs, subjects accidentally or sexually exposed to HBV-infected blood or persons, infants of HBV-infected mothers, sexually promiscuous persons, e.g., male homosexuals, recreational parenteral drug users, and hospital and laboratory staff.

In the context of medicine in Africa most of the above 'high-risk' groups are of limited importance. Indeed, clinically evident acute hepatitis is relatively rare in Africa, as most acute infections occur early in childhood when subclinical infections predominate. Thus use of HBV vaccine for prevention of acute hepatitis would have low priority in Africa today.

However, it is now clear that in most of sub-Saharan Africa between 5 and 25% of the population develop the hepatitis B carrier state. That this type of infection can give rise to chronic hepatitis and cirrhosis first became apparent as a result of studies carried out in Korea in 1962 (Prince et al., 1964; Chung et al., 1964a,b) and in New York in 1968 and 1969 (Prince et al., 1969; Prince, 1971a,b) and has subsequently been confirmed by many reports. Of even greater importance is the fact that it is now becoming increasingly clear that the chronic HBV carrier state causes not only chronic active hepatitis and cirrhosis, but also hepatocellular carcinoma (HCC).

Although relatively rare in the United States, HCC is the most common malignancy occurring in males in many parts of the world, particularly in tropical regions of Africa and Asia.

Payet et al. (1956) and Steiner and Davis (1957) were the first to suggest that the extraordinarily high incidence of HCC in Africa might be related to the high prevalence there of viral hepatitis and post-hepatitic cirrhosis. Their speculations received serological support when it became possible to test for specific markers of HBV infection. When sensitive methods for detecting hepatitis B surface antigen (HBsAg) were employed, a striking association between the presence of HBsAg and HCC was observed in almost all studies. The closest association was found in Africa, where HBsAg was found in 63% of sera of HCC patients by radioimmunoassay (RIA), as compared with 11.7% in controls (Prince et al., 1975).

Recently, much more convincing data have become available which support the conclusion that HBV is the major cause of HCC in man.

Prospective studies

Beasley et al. (1981) and Beasley (1984) have reported on 22688 Taiwanese male civil servants over the age of 40 who have been followed prospectively with periodic alpha-fetoprotein determinations since 1978. A total of 3 435 of these subjects were HBV carriers, the remainder being free of detectable HBsAg. As shown in Table 1, 113 cases of HCC developed among the HBV carriers as compared to only 3 among the much larger control group. The relative risk of development of HCC was 217 times greater in HBV carriers than in the controls - the highest relative risk ever determined for any human carcinogenic factor.

The rarity of HCC in the non-carrier group indicates strongly that aflotoxins, which are likely to be relatively common in the hot and humid climate of Taipeh, are probably unable to initiate HCC carcinogenesis, at least in the absence of HBV. Furthermore, the observation that HBV carriers in New York, where aflatoxins are rare, have a much higher incidence of HCC than the population as a whole (Prince & Alcabes, 1982) suggests that aflatoxins are probably not essential co-factors in HBV-induced carcinogenesis.

Table 1. Results of Taiwan prospective study[a]

HBsAg	No. of subjects	No. of cases of HCC	Incidence (cases per 100 000)	Relative risk
+	3435	113	3272	
				217
–	19 253	3	16	

[a] Source: Beasley, 1984. Subjects were followed for 6 years (1978–1984)

A striking finding in this study was the observation that 54% of all deaths in HBV carriers were due to HCC (38%) or cirrhosis (16%) (Fig. 1).

The woodchuck hepatitis virus model

Additional support for the etiological role of HBV in HCC is provided by the discovery of a virus morphologically and bio-chemically similar to HBV which is prevalent in North American woodchucks (Summers et al., 1978). It is remarkable that HCC has been observed in 29% of woodchucks over the age of 4 (Snyder, 1968). All tumour-bearing animals are carriers of woodchuck hepatitis virus, and these animals usually also have chronic active hepatitis and/or cirrhosis.

FIG. 1. DEATHS IN MALE HBV CARRIERS IN TAIWAN

(From Beasley <u>et al.</u>, 1981)   HCC = hepatocellular carcinoma;
CIRRH = cirrhosis

```
40 -- HCC
17 -- CIRRH
48 -- OTHER
```

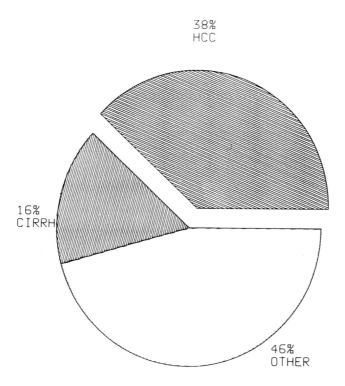

Evidence from molecular biological studies

The probable importance of HBV in HCC carcinogenesis has
been further underlined by molecular biological studies. Nucleic
acid hybridization (reviewed by Prince, 1981) has confirmed that
most HCC DNA contains HBV sequences, and has shown that the HBV
genome is usually integrated into host cellular DNA; such

integration occurs at a restricted number of sites. The molecular biological behaviour of the HBV genome thus resembles that
of known oncogenic DNA viruses, such as SV-40 and polyoma virus.
Additional cases of HBV integration into HCC DNA have been found
in anti-HBs-positive persons, suggesting that chronic HBV
carriers, in whom integration of DNA is also seen, may
'terminate' their (detectable) HBsAg carrier state yet continue
to carry the HBV genome, and that these persons remain at high
risk of development of HCC.

    All of the above lines of evidence point to an important
role for HBV in HCC carcinogenesis. It must, however, be
recognized that other actual or potential etiological factors
exist: other hepatitis viruses (e.g., non-A, non-B), alcoholism,
aflatoxins, vinyl chloride, certain steroids, etc.). The relative importance of such factors may differ in different geographical regions and occupational groups; however, none appears to
be as closely associated with HCC as is the HBV carrier state.

    The above considerations provide strong indications for
large-scale immunization with HBV vaccine in high- and interme-
diate-prevalence regions of the world. To the degree that
immunization is successful in eliminating the chronic carrier
state in future generations, the result is likely to be a reduction in the incidence of cirrhosis and of HCC, the most common
cancer of males in most of these regions.

            WHO SHOULD RECEIVE HEPATITIS B VACCINE IN AFRICA ?

    An age-specific incidence study was carried out in infants
living in rural villages in Liberia, a country with a 10-15%
prevalence rate for HBV chronic carriers, and thus probably fairly typical of much of sub-Saharan Africa (Prince et al., 1981).
This study revealed an annual incidence of HBV infection of
25-30% per year during the first 4 years of life. Clearly,
therefore, the vast majority of these infants are infected before
reaching school age. Interestingly, in contrast to findings in
Asia, only a minor proportion (about 12%) of infections were
associated with carrier mothers. Most infections were thus
probably due to spread from infant to infant.

Several important conclusions can be drawn from these findings. Firstly, it is clearly desirable to immunize African infants as early as possible - ideally at birth. This is especially important as the risk of developing the chronic carrier state is highest in those infected during the first year of life (when about 30% of infants will become infected). Secondly, immunization of children of school age or older, or of adults, is neither useful nor necessary; and lastly, passive-active immunization, as advocated for interruption of vertical transmission from e antigen (HBeAg)-positive HBV carrier mothers in Asia (Beasley et al., 1983), is not likely to have an important role in immunization practice in Africa, even if it were economically and logistically feasible.

It should be emphasized that, in Africa, the concept of 'high-risk groups', as usefully applied in selecting subjects requiring immunization in Europe and the United States, has no particular relevance. All infants in Africa constitute the high-risk group; all thus deserve and require immunization.

The quantities of vaccine required to attain these goals are not currently available, and will probably not become available during the next few years. For this reason, initial utilization should be limited to additional clinical trials - which are needed especially in high-prevalence regions - to determine optimal utilization strategies. Larger supplies of vaccine will, however, soon become available. This increase in supply will depend in part on the expansion of source plasma supply, e.g., if developing nations recognize that it is their responsibility to contribute to that supply, and in part on the development of alternative vaccines, such as recombinant DNA or synthetic products.

Dosage and frequency of administration

In clinical trials, HBV vaccines have proven efficacious when given in a variety of doses and frequencies of administration (Maupas et al., 1981; Guesry et al., 1981; Szmuness et al., 1980). However, some of the doses and schedules used may represent 'overkill'. Unfortunately, the actual doses used are difficult to compare since there has until recently been no international potency standard. Further work needs to be done to determine minimum doses and schedules required for adequate immunization.

To the extent that doses and schedules of administration can be minimized, vaccine cost will decrease, and supply increase; thus, the number of persons who can be protected will be increased.

HOW SHOULD HEPATITIS B VIRUS VACCINES BE MADE ?

The background to the development of HBV vaccine has been thoroughly reviewed (McAuliffe et al., 1980) and will not be repeated here. Table 2 summarizes some of the major properties of current licensed and candidate vaccines. Which vaccine is the best ? We simply do not know.

Table 2. Currently available HBV vaccines

Manufacturer	Source plasma	Purity	Inactivation steps	Dose (μg)	Efficacy	Approximate cost per dose
A. Licensed						
Merck, Sharp, & Dohme	HBeAg(+)	High	Purification pepsin-hydrochloride Urea Formalin	20	Good	$30
Institut Pasteur	Anti-HBe(+)	High	Purification Formalin	5	Good	$25
Korean Green Cross	HBeAg(+)	High	Purification Formalin	10	?	$10
B. Undergoing clinical trials						
Netherlands Red Cross	Anti-HBe(+)	Low	Purification 102°C for 90 s 65°C for 10 h	3	Very good	?
New York Blood Center	Anti-HBe(+)	High	Purification Tween 80 102°C for 90 s 65°C for 10 h	?	?	?

The most controversial point appears to be whether HBeAg-positive plasma, i.e., plasma that is Dane-particle-rich and highly infective, should be used as the starting material.

Is it safe to prepare a vaccine from HBeAg-positive plasma?

In the preparation of the first vaccines, e.g., the Netherlands Red Cross, Institut Pasteur, and Japanese Green Cross vaccines, those responsible were prevailed upon in the interests of 'safety' to avoid the use of HBeAg-positive plasma. This prohibition has apparently, as a consequence, found its way into the recommended requirements in the European Pharmacopoeia.

It soon became apparent, however, that HBeAg-negative plasma is a low HBsAg-titre source, making it difficult if not impossible to produce adequate amounts of vaccine.

In the United States, vaccine manufacturers (Gerin and Purcell at the National Institutes of Health; Merck, Sharpe and Dohme; The New York Blood Center) chose to use high HBsAg-titre source materials; these are almost all HBeAg-positive. It was reasoned that the purification and inactivation steps employed in manufacture were sufficient to guarantee a safe product, despite the higher initial infectivity of the source plasma.

This approach was endorsed and approved by the WHO Expert Committee on Standards for Hepatitis B Vaccine (1983), and is further approved by the US Food and Drug Administration, as evidenced by licensure of the Merck vaccine, which is made predominantly from HBeAg-positive plasma.

Production technique

Purification techniques have varied from the very elaborate (Adamowicz et al., 1981), presumably yielding a relatively pure product, to the comparatively simple, yielding a product composed predominantly of serum proteins with HBsAg as a minor constituent (Brummelhuis et al., 1981). The latter approach is somewhat more economical. However, it entails accepting theoretical, albeit so far unproven, dangers due to the inclusion of host antigenic components. The two types of product overlap, however, as even the purest preparations of HBsAg are found to harbour cryptic serum proteins when such proteins are sought for energetically (Neurath et al., 1974; Vnek et al., 1978).

It is too early to draw conclusions as to the relative immunogenicity or efficacy of these vaccines; all so far appear to be immunogenic. Careful comparative studies of immunogenicity and efficacy are needed. Meanwhile, any licensed vaccine will probably be reasonably immunogenic and efficacious. As HBV vaccine will be in short supply for a number of years, all available vaccines should be used to prevent hepatitis B infections.

The failure of the Merck, Sharpe, and Dohme vaccine to protect renal dialysis patients (Stevens et al., 1984), a group that is notoriously difficult to immunize, in contrast to the high efficacy shown by the Netherlands Red Cross vaccine in the same setting, suggests that one or more of the relatively harsh purification steps employed in preparing the Merck vaccine (i.e., pepsin-hydrochloride or urea treatment) may have impaired its immunogenicity.

Safety of plasma-derived vaccines

The vaccines produced so far appear to be entirely safe. More than 8 million doses have been administered without a single report of any serious adverse reaction, or inadvertent transmission of hepatitis or of the recently described AIDS syndrome.

The lack of infectivity of existing vaccines depends in part on the high process efficacy of the various purification steps in removing viable Dane particles. This can be estimated by following HBV DNA concentrations by means of sensitive and quantitative DNA hybridization techniques using ^{32}P-labelled cloned HBV DNA probes. The process efficacy of the various purification procedures used varies between 10^3 and 10^5 (i.e., 3-5 logs). Furthermore, each of the following frequently used procedures has been shown by studies in chimpanzees to inactivate 4-5 or more logs of HBV infectivity: pepsin-hydrochloride, 8 M urea, formalin 1:4000 for 3 days at 36°C, 102°C for 2 minutes, 10 h at 65°C (Tabor et al., 1982; Lelie, P.N., personal communication).

It is estimated that the aggregate process efficacy in HBV removal and inactivation in the purified HBV vaccines which have been produced to date is in the range 15-18 logs. This degree of process efficacy is sufficient to guarantee that less than 1 dose in 10^{12} will contain a single particle of viable HBV.

Safety is further confirmed by chimpanzee tests, which have been carried out with all lots of these vaccines so far. However, these tests are unsatisfactory in that they generally indicate only that there is no infectivity in 20-22 doses of vaccine, and therefore guard only against cross-contamination due to poor manufacturing practices. Thus, after a manufacturer has shown his ability to produce safe lots consistently, this test can probably be dispensed with if the manufacturing protocol includes steps giving an acceptable aggregate process efficacy.

Cost of plasma-derived HBV vaccines

The current cost of the licensed plasma-derived vaccines is clearly too high to permit their use in mass immunization campaigns in developing countries. This is due in part to the very considerable construction costs of complex plants and facilities, and the equally high cost of conducting large-scale efficacy trials. It is to be expected that, when these are amortized, costs will decline rapidly. Furthermore, newly developed vaccines (Netherlands Red Cross, and New York Blood Center) have been developed specifically with the aim of being simple and much more economical to produce. It is likely that these vaccines can be produced at a cost sufficiently low to permit mass utilization.

Should plasma-derived vaccines be produced in Africa?

Obvious economies could theoretically result if HBV vaccines could be produced in the developing world from locally available source plasma. The practicality of this approach must be considered in the light of the general absence of a stable and reliable infrastructure, e.g., electricity, water supply, equipment maintenance, as well as the shortage of trained personnel. The cost of introducing the required infrastructure and trained counterpart personnel can easily outweigh the hoped for economy of local production.

On the other hand, there is a natural and justifiable demand on the part of developing countries to attain self-sufficiency to the greatest possible extent.

It would appear desirable for leading developing countries to begin to collaborate with existing experienced manufacturers. Such collaboration should include training of personnel in all production and quality-control procedures. During the training period, appropriate personnel from the developing countries should carry out clinical trials, planned in collaboration with experienced epidemiologists, to determine appropriate immunization schedules and routes of administration that are effective and consonant with local realities and logistics.

Manufacturers will need to develop appropriate packaging for use under local conditions in different parts of the world, and may need to prepare the vaccines in a heat-stable form (Funakoshi et al., 1981) for use where adequate and reliable 'cold chains' do not exist.

Subsequently, importation of vaccine in bulk, followed by local filling and quality control, should be undertaken prior to eventual transfer of the entire production process.

Possible second- and third-generation vaccines

Newer candidate vaccines, summarized in Table 3, are also on the horizon, e.g., those based on recombinant DNA technology (Charnay et al., 1980; Dubois et al., 1980; Moriarty et al., 1981), and even some which are totally synthetic (Hopp & Woods, 1981; Hopp, 1981; Prince et al., 1982). It will be a number of years before the safety and efficacy of these newer candidate vaccines are established.

Vaccines based on antigens produced in cancer cells are of dubious acceptability. Those based on antigens produced in non-neoplastic cell cultures, or in yeast carrying recombinant plasmids, should prove acceptable if their cost and efficacy match or are superior to those of plasma-derived vaccines - neither of which has been demonstrated to date.

An exciting development is the demonstration that cells infected with vaccinia virus recombinants which carry the gene coding for HBsAg can yield immunogenic quantities of the antigen (Smith et al., 1983). Vaccines based on this principle could be

Table 3. Possible second- and third-generation vaccines

Type	Acceptability	Cost
Eukaryotic systems:		
HCC cells	Poor	?
Recombinant SV-40-transformed cells	?	?
Recombinant plasmid-transformed mammalian cells	$\pm$	?
Live vaccines:		
Recombinant vaccinia	?	Low
Synthetic peptide immunogens	?	?

produced at the low cost of recent smallpox vaccines. Such vaccines, however, entail acceptance of the well documented risk of generalized vaccinia, which can occur in 1-5 subjects per million immunized. From a risk-benefit public health point of view this would perhaps be acceptable, especially if other safer candidate vaccines cannot be produced at such low cost.

Synthetic peptide immunogens based on the synthesis of anti-genic epitopes may also provide an economical means of mass immunization. Peptide-carrier-adjuvant combinations would have to be developed that provide strong and long-lasting protective immune responses; these responses must be such that resistant organisms which are unaffected by the antibodies induced do not rapidly emerge by mutation, and it must be shown that the anti-bodies induced do not cross-react with host proteins to produce autoimmune complications.

It is unlikely that second- and third-generation vaccines will be acceptable for mass use in the near future. Safety and efficacy trials and production scale-up are likely to require a minimum of 3-5 years. By that time it is possible that the cost of plasma-derived vaccines may have become low enough for them to remain competitive, or even to be less expensive than the newer vaccines.

REFERENCES

Adamowicz, P.H., Gerfaux, G., Platel, A., Muller, L., Vacher, B., Mazert, M.C. & Prunet, P. (1981) Large scale production of an hepatitis B vaccine. In: Maupas, P. & Guesry, P., eds, Hepatitis B Vaccine (INSERM Symposium No. 18), Amsterdam, Elsevier-North Holland, pp. 37-50

Beasley, R.P., Hwang, L.-Y., Lin, C.-C. & Chien, C.S. (1981) Hepatocellular carcinoma and hepatitis B virus. A prospective study of 22 707 men in Taiwan. Lancet, 2, 1129-1133

Beasley, R.P., Huang, L.-Y., Lee, G., Lan, C.C., Roan, C.-H., Huang, F.Y. & Chen, C.L. (1983) Prevention of perinatally transmitted hepatitis B virus infections with hepatitis B immune globulin and hepatitis B vaccine. Lancet, 2, 1099-1102

Beasley, R.P. (1984) Epidemiology of hepatocellular carcinoma in viral hepatitis. In: International Symposium on Viral Hepatitis, San Francisco (in press)

Brummelhuis, H.G.J., Wilson-De-Sturler, L.A. & Raap, A.K. (1981) Preparation of hepatitis B vaccine by heat inactivation. In: Maupas, P. & Guesry, P., eds, Hepatitis B Vaccine (INSERM Symposium No. 18), Amsterdam, Elsevier-North Holland, pp. 51-56

Charnay, P., Gervais, M., Louise, A., Galibert, F. & Tiollais, P. (1980) Biosynthesis of hepatitis B surface antigen in Escherichia coli. Nature, 286, 893-895

Chung, W.K., Moon, S.K., Gershon, R.K., Prince, A.M., Park, Y.C. & Cho, Y.S. (1964a) Anicteric hepatitis in Korea. I. Clinical and laboratory studies. Arch. intern. Med., 113, 526-534

Chung, W.K., Moon, S.K., Gershon, R.K., Prince, A.M. & Popper, H. (1964b) Anicteric hepatitis in Korea. II. Serial histologic studies. Arch. intern. Med., 113, 535-542

Dubois, M., Pourcel, C., Rousset, S., Cheny, C. & Tiollais, P. (1980) Excretion of hepatitis B surface antigen particles from mouse cells transformed with cloned viral DNA. Proc. natl Acad. Sci. USA, 77, 4549-4553

Funakoshi, S., Ohmura, T., Fujiwara, T., Tajima, T., Kinoshita, K., Matsumoto, T. & Suyama, T. (1981) Hepatitis B vaccine - the production and testing. In: Maupas, P. & Guesry, P., eds, Hepatitis B Vaccine (INSERM Symposium No. 18), Amsterdam, Elsevier-North Holland, pp. 57-66

Guesry, P., Jungers, P., Courouce, A.M. et al. (1981) Double-blind randomized clinical trial of Pasteur hepatitis B vaccine in high-risk haemodialysis unit's staff. In: Maupas, P. & Guesry, P., eds, Hepatitis B Vaccine (INSERM Symposium No. 18), Amsterdam, Elsevier-North Holland, pp. 133-148

Hopp, T.P. & Woods, K.R. (1981) Prediction of protein antigenic determinants from amino acid sequences. Proc. natl Acad. Sci. USA, 78, 3824-3828

Hopp, T.P. (1981) A synthetic peptide with hepatitis B surface antigen reactivity. Mol. Immunol., 18, 869-872

McAuliffe, V.J., Purcell, R.H. & Gerin, J.L. (1980) Type B hepatitis: a review of current prospects for a safe and effective vaccine. Rev. infect. Dis., 2, 470-492

Maupas, P., Goudeau, A., Dubois, F. et al. (1981) Potency and efficacy of HB vaccine applied to a high risk population: a five year study. In: Maupas, P. & Guesry, P., eds, Hepatitis B Vaccine (INSERM Symposium No. 18), Amsterdam, Elsevier-North Holland, pp. 117-132

Moriarty, A.M., Hoyer, B.H., Shih, JW.-K., Gerin, J.L. & Hamer, D.H. (1981) Expression of the hepatitis B surface antigen gene in cell culture by using simian virus 40 vector. Proc. natl Acad. Sci. USA, 78, 2606-2610

Neurath, A.R., Prince, A.M. & Lippin, A. (1974) Hepatitis B antigen. Antigenic sites related to human serum proteins revealed by affinity chromatography. Proc. natl Acad. Sci. USA, 71, 2663-2667

Payet, M., Camain, R. & Pene, P. (1956) Le cancer primitif du foie; étude critique à propos de 240 cas. Rev. intern. Hépatol., 6, 1-86

Prince, A.M. (1971a) Role of viruses in chronic liver disease in man and animals. In: Liver Cancer (IARC Scientific Publications No. 1), Lyon, International Agency for Research on Cancer, pp. 51-57

Prince, A.M. (1971b) Role of serum hepatitis virus in chronic liver disease. Gastroenterology, 60, 913-921

Prince, A.M. (1981) Hepatitis B virus and hepatocellular carcinoma: molecular biology provides further evidence of an etiologic association. Hepatology, 1, 73-75

Prince, A.M. & Alcabes, P. (1982) The risk of development of hepatocellular carcinomas in hepatitis B virus carriers in New York. A preliminary estimate using death records matching. Hepatology, 2, (Suppl.), 15 S

Prince, A.M., Fuji, H. & Gershon, R.K. (1964) Immunohistochemical studies on the etiology of anicteric hepatitis in Korea. Am. J. Hyg., 79, 365-381

Prince, A.M., Hargrove, R.L. & Jeffries, G.H. (1969) The role of serum hepatitis virus in chronic liver disease. Trans. Assoc. Am. Physicians, 72, 265-277

Prince, A.M., Szmuness, W., Michon, J., Demaille, J., Diebolt, G., Linnard, J., Quenum, C. & Sankale, M. (1975) A case control study of the association between primary liver cancer and hepatitis B infection in Senegal. Int. J. Cancer, 16, 376-383

Prince, A.M., White, T., Pollock, N., Riddle, J., Brotman, B. & Richardson, L. (1981) The epidemiology of hepatitis B infection in Liberian infants. Infect. Immun., 32, 675-680

Prince, A.M., Ikram, H. & Hopp, T.P. (1982) Hepatitis B virus vaccine: identification of HbsAg/a,d but not HBsAg/y subtype antigenic determinants on a synthetic immunogenic peptide. Proc. natl Acad. Sci. USA, 79, 579-582

Reerink-Brongers, E.E., Lelie, P.N., Reesink, H.W., Dees, P.J., Brummelhuis, H.G.J., Van Aken, W.G. (1983) Immunogenicity and safety of heat inactivated hepatitis B vaccine (CLB) in low risk human volunteers and in patients treated with chronic haemodialysis in the Netherlands. Develop. Biol. Stand., 54, 197-203

Smith, G.L., Mackett, M. & Moss, B. (1983) Infectious vaccinia virus recombinants that express HBsAg. Nature, 302, 490-495

Snyder, R.L. (1968) Hepatomas of captive woodchucks. Am. J. Pathol., 52, 32

Steiner, P.E. & Davis, J.N.P. (1957) Cirrhosis and primary liver carcinomas in Uganda, Africa. Br. J. Cancer, 11, 523-534

Stevens, C.E., Alter, H.J., Taylor, P.E., Zang, E.P., Harley, E.J., Szmuness, W. & The Dialysis Vaccine Trial Study Group (1984) Hepatitis B vaccine in hemodialysis patients: immunogenicity and efficacy. New Engl. J. Med., 311, 496-501

Summers, J., Smolec, J.M. & Snyder, R. (1978) A virus similar to human hepatitis B virus associated with hepatitis and hepatoma in woodchucks. Proc. natl Acad. Sci. USA, 75, 4533-4537

Szmuness, W., Stevens, C.E., Harley, E.J., Zang, E., Oleszko, W., William, D., Sadovsky, R., Morrison, J. & Kellner, A. (1980) Hepatitis B vaccine. Demonstration of efficacy in a controlled clinical trial in a high risk population in the United States. New Engl. J. Med., 303, 833-841

Tabor, E., Buynak, E., Smallwood, L.A., Snoy, P., Hilleman, M. & Gerety, R.J. (1982) Inactivation of hepatitis B virus by three methods: treatment with pepsin, urea and formalin. J. med. Virol., 11, 1-9

Vnek, J., Prince, A.M., Hashimoto, N. & Ikram, H. (1978)
    Association of normal serum protein antigens with chimpanzee
    hepatitis B surface antigen particles. J. med Virol., 2,
    319–333

AN AFFORDABLE MULTIDETERMINANT PLASMA-DERIVED HEPATITIS B VIRUS VACCINE

A.M. Prince, J. Vnek & B. Brotman

The Laboratory of Virology,
The Lindsley F. Kimball Research Institute of
The New York Blood Center
New York, USA
and
Vilab II
The Liberian Institute of Biomedical Research
Robertsfield, Liberia

RESUME

On décrit ici un nouveau vaccin, qui contient l'antigène e du virus de l'hépatite B (AgHBe) et des déterminants pré-S, en plus de l'antigène de surface (AgHBs) hautement purifié. Cette approche est basée sur les données suivantes, qui montrent que les anticorps anti-HBe, les anticorps dirigés contre l'antigène central (anti-HBc) et les anticorps dirigés contre les déterminants pré-S peuvent jouer un rôle actif dans la prévention de l'infection HBV: (1) l'immunisation active de chimpanzés avec l'antigène HBe dénué d'AgHBs détectable les a protégés lors d'une confrontation ultérieure avec l'HBV; (2) l'immunisation passive de chimpanzés avec une immunoglobuline anti-HBe/anti-HBc dénuée d'anti-HBs et injectée par voie intraveineuse a retardé de façon significative et semble avoir atténué l'infection HBV à la suite d'une confrontation subséquente avec le virus; (3) l'anticorps dirigé contre les déterminants pré-S semble être capable de neutraliser l'HBV infectieux.

Le procédé de purification utilisé pour la production du vaccin du "New York Blood Center" a été élaboré de façon à obtenir une purification très poussée en utilisant le minimum d'équipements complexes. Cela peut faciliter l'utilisation éventuelle du vaccin à grande échelle pour la prévention de l'état de porteur d'HBV dans les régions du monde où la prévalence est élevée.

Le procédé utilise des précipitations par le polyéthylène
glycol et des étapes d'adsorption sur hydroxylapatite, suivies
d'une seule séparation isopycnique avec un rotor zonal, et permet
d'obtenir un vaccin débarassé des protéines sériques et de fragments détectables d'ADN d'HBV et contenant cependant l'Ag HBs,
l'Ag HBe et les déterminants pré-S.

Le vaccin original a été inactivé par le Tween 80 et le
formol. Quatre lots ont passé les tests de sécurité chez le
chimpanzé; deux de ces lots ont été testés dans des essais
cliniques.

Récemment, un vaccin amélioré a été développé, dans lequel
deux étapes d'inactivation par la chaleur sont utilisées à la
place de l'inactivation au formol. Cela a permis d'augmenter
encore l'antigénicité et l'immunogénicité, et d'obtenir une marge
supplémentaire de sécurité.

SUMMARY

A new vaccine is reported which contains hepatitis B virus
(HBV) e antigen (HBeAg) and pre-S determinants, in addition to
highly purified HBV surface antigen (HBsAg). The rationale for
this approach depends on the following data indicating that
anti-HBe and antibody to the core antigen (anti-HBc), and antibody to pre-S determinants may play an active role in preventing
HBV infection: (1) active immunization of chimpanzees with
HBeAg(s) devoid of detectable HBsAg protected against subsequent
challenge with HBV; (2) passive immunization of chimpanzees with
an anti-HBe/anti-HBc intravenous immunoglobulin devoid of anti-
HBs significantly delayed and appeared to attenuate HBV infection
following subsequent challenge with HBV; (3) antibody to pre-S
determinants appears to be able to neutralize infective HBV.

The purification procedure used for the production of the
New York Blood Center vaccine was designed to accomplish a high
degree of purification with minimal use of complex equipment.
This may facilitate eventual utilization of the vaccine on a mass
scale for prevention of the HBV carrier state in high-prevalence
regions of the world.

The procedure uses polyethylene glycol (PEG) precipitations
and hydroxylapatite adsorption steps, followed by only a single
isopycnic separation in a zonal rotor, to achieve a vaccine which

is substantially free of serum proteins and detectable HBV DNA yet contains HBsAg, HBeAg and pre-S determinants.

The original vaccine was inactivated by Tween 80 and formalin. Four lots passed chimpanzee safety tests; two of these have been tested in clinical trials.

Recently an improved vaccine has been developed in which two heat inactivation steps are used instead of formalin inactivation. This has resulted in further improvement in yields of antigenicity and immunogenicity, and provides an additional margin of safety.

INTRODUCTION

The development of a new hepatitis B virus (HBV) vaccine specifically designed to contain hepatitis e antigen (HBeAg) as well as hepatitis B surface antigen (HBsAg) was first reported in 1978 (Prince et al., 1978). This was based on the hypothesis that anti-HBe, in addition to anti-HBs, was a protective antibody in this infection. Inclusion of HBeAg was made possible by the fact that all forms of HBsAg-associated particles from HBeAg-positive plasma can be shown to contain HBeAg when treated with detergents (Vnek et al., 1979).

Recently, an update was presented on the procedures used in the preparation of this vaccine and on its properties, as well as additional data to support the hypothesis that anti-HBe is a protective antibody (Prince et al., 1983).

In the present report a brief account is given of the properties of this vaccine, and the procedures for its preparation, and improved inactivation procedures are described which provide better preservation of antigenicity and immunogenicity, as well as a greater margin of safety. Furthermore, it will be shown that pre-S determinants present in this vaccine may elicit antibodies which are protective.

METHODS

Purification of HBsAg

Pooled HBeAg-containing plasma obtained from chronic HBsAg carriers is adjusted to pH 4.6 and clarified at 10 000 rpm in a Westphalia continuous-flow centrifuge. The clarified supernatant is adjusted to 4% PEG 6000 at 4°C and stirred for 20 minutes. The precipitate is recovered by sedimentation for 2 hours without centrifugation and is solubilized with distilled water in one-fifth of the starting plasma volume by adjusting the pH to 7.5-8.0. The pH is then lowered to 5.0 and the resulting precipitate is recovered by centrifugation. The pH of the supernatant is then adjusted to 4.6 and PEG is added to a final concentration of 3%. After sedimentation over-night at 4°C, the precipitate is redissolved by neutralization and the suspension clarified after lowering the pH to 5.0 as before. The material is adjusted to pH 6.8 and, after addition of 0.005 M phosphate buffer, further purified by 2-3 consecutive adsorptions with equal volumes of packed hydroxylapatite. Subsequently the hydroxylapatite sediments are washed with 0.02 and 0.05 M phosphate buffer. Finally the original supernatants and the washes of the hydroxylapatite sediments are pooled, clarified by centrifugation and concentrated to about 0.3% of the starting plasma volume with an Amicon hollow fibre cartridge. The concentrated HBsAg is then adjusted to a density of 1.25 g/ml with solid potassium bromide and dynamically loaded under a linear 1.05-1.2 g/ml potassium bromide gradient over a 1.3 g/ml cushion into a Beckman T_1-14 rotor. The gradient is centrifuged for 18 h at 28 000 rpm and fractionated by pumping water into the centre of the rotor. Fractions corresponding to densities between 1.17 and 1.22 g/ml are pooled.

Determination of purity

The purity of the final preparation is determined as follows:: (1) the ultraviolet absorption spectrum is determined; it should show the characteristic shoulder at 290 nm (Adamowicz et al., 1981); (2) the purified antigen is tested at a concentration of $\geq$ 3 mg/ml by agar gel diffusion against polyvalent and monovalent anti-human-serum-protein antigen sera, which must not detect human serum proteins at a concentration of $\geq$ 2% of total protein; (3) sodium dodecyl sulfate/polyacrylamide gel electrophoresis (SDS-PAGE) must reveal no more than the characteristic HBsAg-associated polypeptides; (4) the ratio of total protein, as determined by OD_{280} $(E_{1cm}^{0.1\%} = 3.73)$, and of HBsAg antigenicity, as determined by quantitative radioimmunoassay (Prince et al., 1978), to the WHO international HBsAg standard (World Health Organization, 1982) should be 1:1 $\pm$ acceptable limits of test variability.

Inactivation procedure

In the initial lots, the purified antigen was adjusted to a concentration of 1 mg/ml (based on OD_{280}, $E_{1cm}^{0.1\%}$ = 3.73) and diluted with an equal volume of 2% Tween 80. After 1 hour at room temperature, the solution was filtered through a 0.22-μ Millipore filter and adjusted to 1:2000 formalin. The solution was incubated with slow magnetic stirring for 72 hours at $37^{o}C$, dialysed against normal saline containing 1:10 000 Thimerosol, and finally sterile filtered.

More recently the procedure has been modified as follows. After addition of Tween 80 and Millipore filtration, the antigen preparation is passed under pressure through a stainless steel (2 mm diameter) coil held at $102^{o}C$ in an oil bath at a rate such that the material will be held at that temperature for 2 minutes. The final alum-adsorbed vaccine is further treated for 10 hours at $65^{o}C$ as an additional inactivation step. Similar inactivation steps were introduced by Brummelhuis et al. (1981) for inactivation of an unpurified vaccine.

Quality controls

All quality controls recommended by the WHO Expert Committee on Biological Standardization (World Health Organization, 1980) were carried out. Specifically, tests for adventitious viruses were carried out on the plasma pools by inoculation of adult and suckling mice, chick embryos and Vero and WI-38 cell strains. The plasma pools were additionally tested for bacterial sterility and freedom from tubercle bacilli. The purified bulk antigen was tested for microbial sterility, blood-group substances, DNA polymerase, HBV DNA (by a blot hybridization assay capable of detecting about 1 pg HBV DNA), purity as described above and pyrogenicity; the chimpanzee safety test was also carried out. The final containers were subjected to the mouse and guinea-pig general safety test, and were also tested for microbial sterility, free formaldehyde (when used), Thimerosol (when used), alum, HBsAg-antigen content after removal of alum (see below), and mouse immunogenicity (by inoculation of 20 mice per dilution with serial dilutions of the alum-adsorbed vaccine). Mice were bled 1

month after injection and individual sera were assayed by a quantitative parallel-line radioimmunoassay (Ausab, Abbott Laboratories, North Chicago, IL, USA), and compared with the WHO International HBIg (anti-HBs) Standard (World Health Organization,
1982). The proportion of mice seroconverting and geometric mean
anti-HBs levels in mIU were plotted against vaccine dose.

Adjuvanting procedure

The initial lots were adjuvanted as follows. To the desired
concentration of antigen suspended in sterile saline, 1:10 000
Thimerosol, 1/10 volume of sterile filtered 0.2 M alum
$(AlK(SO_4)_2.12H_2O)$ was added. The pH was adjusted to 5.0 with
sterile 1 N sodium hydroxide and the suspension was stirred at
room temperature for 3 hours. The alum-precipitated antigen was
recovered by centrifugation for 10 minutes at 2000 rpm, resus-
pended in sterile normal saline containing 1:10 000 Thimerosol,
and filled under sterile conditions.

More recently, a presterilized aluminum phosphate adjuvant
has been employed, to which the inactivated diluted antigen is
added under sterile conditions to yield 0.6 mg aluminum phosphate
per ml.

Stability testing

To determine the stability of HBsAg adsorbed on to alum, the
antigen was recovered by resolubilizing the alum in 3% sodium
citrate followed by dialysis successively against 3% sodium
citrate and phosphate-buffered saline (0.1 M sodium chloride,
0.01 M phosphate buffer, pH 7.2) (PBS). HBsAg was then determined by parallel line radioimmunoassay against dilutions of a
purified HBsAg standard prepared by Dr John Gerin. The standard
was held frozen at -70^{0}C in the form of a 1:100 dilution made in
PBS/50% newborn calf serum.

EVIDENCE SUPPORTING THE RATIONALE
FOR A MULTIDETERMINANT VACCINE

Immunity to viral infection can theoretically result from
induction of antibody against a variety of virus-associated antigens. Evidence indicating that this applies also to hepatitis B
infection continues to accummulate, and is summarized below.

HBsAg as a protective antigen

The idea that anti-HBs could serve as a protective antibody first arose as a consequence of the observation that persons with preexisting anti-HBs are usually immune to hepatitis B infection when followed in high-risk settings, such as haemodialysis units (Snydman et al., 1976). This type of observation is, however, not as informative as it might seem since 'anti-HBs' includes a variety of antibodies reactive with various immunogenic regions (epitopes) on surface antigen particles. Which of these are of importance?

The so-called subtype antigens HBsAg/d and HBsAg/y do not appear to be important since vaccination with vaccines derived from HBsAg/ad effectively protects against infection with HBV/ay (Purcell & Gerin, 1978).

It has been demonstrated that immunization of chimpanzees with purified HBsAg polypeptide P25 can protect them against HBV infection (Hollinger et al., 1978). Thus protective epitopes must exist on this molecule. However, it is clear from studies with synthetic peptides (Lerner et al., 1981; Hopp, 1981; Dreesman et al., 1982; Bhatnagar et al., 1982) that there are numerous distinct immunogenic epitopes located along the length of this molecule. A similar concusion can be reached based on the variety of non-competing monoclonal antibodies which can react with the molecule. It is thus not at all clear which of the various epitopes can elicit protective antibody.

Hepatitis Be antigen (HBeAg) as a protective antigen

The generally low titres of HBV in anti-HBe-positive HBsAg carriers originally suggested the hypothesis that anti-HBe might modulate HBV replication (Prince et al., 1978). To test this hypothesis, two seronegative chimpanzees were immunized with 3 injections of HBeAg-containing plasma freed from detectable HBsAg and 32 weeks after the first immunization, both animals were challenged with $10^{3.5}$ chimpanzee infective dose CID_{50} of the NIH HBV/ayw challenge material. Neither of the HBeAg-immunized animals developed HBsAg (Prince et al., 1983).

Because of the difficulty of ruling out the possibility that the results reflected an effect of undetectable amounts of HBsAg in the antigen preparation used for immunization, this hypothesis was further evaluated by testing the effect of passive immunization with anti-HBe immunoglobulin (HBeIg), free of anti-HBs, on experimental HBV infection in the chimpanzee model.

Repeated administration of an intravenous immunoglobulin containing anti-HBe and antibody to the core antigen (anti-HBc), and free of anti-HBs, before and after the inoculation of $10^{4.9}$ CID_{50} HBV, markedly prolonged the incubation period of hepatitis B in experimentally infected chimpanzees (Prince et al., 1983). Similar administration of an immunoglobulin preparation containing anti-HBc but free of anti-HBe and anti-HBs, did not appear to modulate HBV infection. These observations suggested that anti-HBe, or an unidentified antibody associated with it, may have biological activity in the modulation of HBV replication.

HBeAg is a specificity present on the HBcAg polypeptide (Neurath & Strick, 1979; Takahashi et al., 1979). This polypeptide appears to be present on the membrane of HBV-infected liver cells, since HBcAg has been demonstrated by immunofluorescence on such cells after elution of bound anti-HBc (Trevisan et al., 1982) and sera containing anti-HBc and anti-HBe have been found to block the effect of cytotoxic T-cells on autologous infected liver cells in vitro (Eddleston et al., 1982). It is thus possible that anti-HBe combines with this polypeptide on the surface of infected liver cells resulting in a modulation of virus replication in a similar manner to that obseved in measles-virus-infected cells exposed to extracellular antibody to measles-virus proteins (Fujinami & Oldstone, 1981).

In a recent report, Tabor and Gerety (1984) provided evidence indicating that immunization of chimpanzees with purified hepatitis B core particles protected these animals against subsequent exposure to live HBV. These authors suggested that the protection observed may result from a combination of anti-HBc with the nucleoprotein core particle at some stage of replication. However, the high rate of HBV replication in HBeAg-positive chronic carriers, all of whom also have high titres of anti-HBc, suggests that this interpretation may not be correct. It appears more likely, especially in the light of the data cited above, that the HBeAg epitope on the core polypeptide may be responsible for the protective effect observed in these experiments.

Although the interpretation that anti-HBe is the biologically active antibody in the above studies has much to commend it,
the possibility that an unmeasured but associated antibody may be
responsible for the observed modulation of HBV replication cannot
be excluded. Rigorous proof that anti-HBe is involved could be
obtained only by active immunization with an HBeAg-specific peptide obtained by chemical synthesis or by the use of recombinant
DNA techniques, or by passive immunization with a monoclonal
chimpanzee or human anti-HBe.

The pre-S epitope as a protective antigen

It has been found that surface antigen particles from highly
infectious HBeAg-positive carriers contain elevated amounts of
polypeptides having a molecular weight of 33 000 and 36 000
daltons (Stibbe & Gerlich, 1983). These proteins contain 236
amino acids at their carboxy-terminal end in a sequence identical
to that of the 24 000 dalton HBsAg protein. However, the 55
amino acids at the N-terminal end are products of the pre-S
region of the HBV genome, which immediately precedes the surface
antigen gene.

It has been postulated that the pre-S region may contain the
ligand for the HBV acceptor on liver cells (Schaeffer & Sninsky,
1984).

Neurath et al. (1984) have synthesized a highly antigenic
region of the pre-S sequence. Antibody raised in rabbits to this
synthetic peptide has been found to neutralize the infectivity of
2×10^3 chimpanzee infectious doses of HBV (Prince et al., unpublished data). Thus, the pre-S region appears to contain a
third epitope potentially useful for immunization against HBV.

Desirability of a multideterminant vaccine

Based on the above considerations, it is considered to be
desirable to prepare HBV vaccine from HBeAg-positive plasma,
since HBsAg particles isolated from this source will contain
HBeAg (Vnek et al., 1979) which is immunogenic in experimental
animals (Vnek et al., 1983). Furthermore, these particles also
have a high content of pre-S determinants (Stibbe & Gerlich,
1983), which may provide additional protective immunogenicity.
Furthermore, it is necessary to avoid harsh chemical steps in
purification which may inactivate HBeAg and/or pre-S determinants.

It is hoped that the resulting vaccine will induce several protective antibodies, thus enhancing its effectiveness, as well as preventing the emergence of resistant strains of HBV.

INACTIVATION OF THE VACCINE

The procedure currently in use for the preparation of the New York Blood Center vaccine has already been described and is summarized in Figure 1. The preliminary PEG precipitation steps result in about 30-fold purification with quantitative recovery of HBsAg. After adsorption with hydroxylapatite, the recovery of HBsAg is about 60% and purification has risen to about 600-fold. The pooled main peak of antigen in the 1.17-1.22 g/cm density region of the potassium bromide gradient yields HBsAg at about 2000-fold purification.

Inactivation of infectivity is achieved by three approaches. Firstly, the major proportion ($\geq$ 99.99%) of the Dane particles are lost during the purification itself. The slight DNA polymerase activity still present after the hydroxylapatite steps bands at a position below that of the peak antigen pool used for vaccine production and is thus discarded. Secondly, the antigen is exposed to 1% Tween 80, a procedure which is known to strip the outer membranes from the core of purified Dane particles. Lastly, the purified antigen is exposed to 102°C for 2 minutes, a step which yields $\geq$ 5 logs of inactivation (Lelie, personal communication) with $\geq$ 70% recovery of antigenicity. After adsorption on to alum, the vaccine is further inactivated by exposure to 65°C for 10 hours, a procedure which is estimated to inactivate at least 4 logs of HBV (Shikata et al., 1978).

PROPERTIES OF THE VACCINE

Morphology

As shown in Figure 2, the bulk of the HBsAg after Tween 80 and heat treatment is in the form of ragged, hollowo-looking particles having a mean diameter of 16.2 nm. Dane particles have never been seen.

FIG. 1. OUTLINE OF THE PURIFICATION AND INACTIVATION TECHNIQUE
USED FOR PREPARATION OF THE PRESENT NEW YORK BLOOD CENTER
HEPATITIS B VACCINE

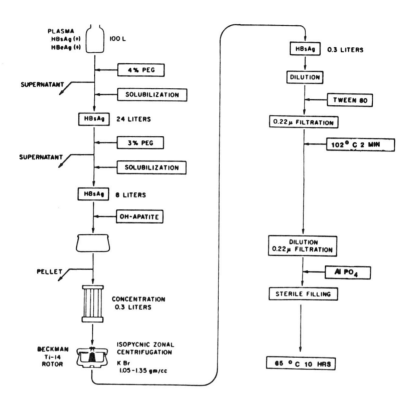

After exposure to 102°C for 2 minutes, many particles
aggregate into filament-like linear arrays (Fig. 3). These can
be disrupted to only a minor extent by sonication, indicating
that they have been produced by heat-induced membrane fusion.

FIG. 2. MORPHOLOGY OF HBsAg-ASSOCIATED PARTICLES
AFTER TWEEN 80 TREATMENT
PHOSPHOTUNGSTIC ACID NEGATIVE STAIN

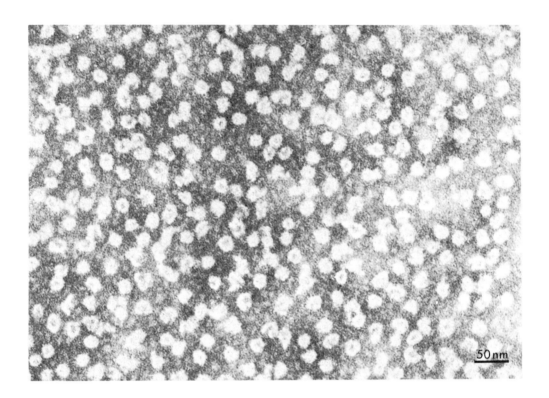

50 nm

Purity

To assess purity, immunoelectrophoresis of the final
purified HBsAg at a concentration of 4 mg/ml against polyvalent
anti-human-serum-protein antiserum, and gel diffusion against
monospecific antisera against albumin, C_3, $alpha_2$-macroglobulin,
beta-lipoprotein IgG transferrin, prealbumin, fibrinogen, and
IgM, are carried out. The sensitivity of these tests is
sufficient to detect any contaminating proteins present if these
amount to 0.1% of the total protein. In early lots, traces of
albumin, IgG and $alpha_2$-macroglobulin were detected at a total
concentration of 2-5% of total protein. The most recent lots did
not reveal any detectable serum proteins in these tests.

FIG. 3. APPEARANCE OF HBsAg PARTICLES AFTER EXPOSURE FOR
2 MINUTES TO 102°C SHOWING AGGREGATION TO FILAMENT-LIKE FORMS
PHOSPHOTUNGSTIC ACID NEGATIVE STAIN

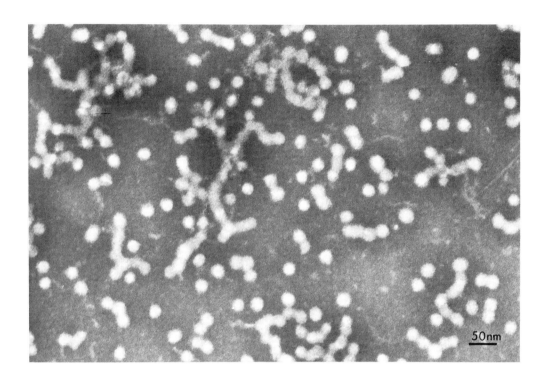

No HBV DNA has been detected using a Southern blot hybridization technique sensitive to about 1 pg of HBV DNA.

Stability

HBsAg in alum-adsorbed vaccine has been found to be stable
for at least 19 months (last sample tested) when stored at 4°C.
There was approximately a 50% loss of antigen during this period
when vaccine was stored at 20°C, and a 75% loss on storage at
37°C.

Safety tests in chimpanzees

Four lots of vaccine have been safety tested in chimpanzees. For each lot, 2 seronegative animals were injected intravenously with 40 μg HBsAg and 2 with 400 μg. Animals were followed with weekly blood specimens tested for HBV markers and transaminases, and biweekly liver biopsies, for 6 months. No evidence of infectivity has been observed.

Immunogenicity in mice

The results of titrations of immunogenicity in mice by injection of female 1CR strain Swiss mice, weighing 20-22 g, subcutaneously with 0.1 ml of alum-adjuvanted vaccine containing different concentrations of HBsAg have shown that 50% sero-conversion requires between 0.03 and 0.1 μg HBsAg (Prince et al., 1983).

Safety and immunogenicity in man

A group of 23 anti-HBs-seronegative volunteers received three intramuscular injections each of vaccine containing 40 μg HBsAg (Kaufmann et al., 1983). No rise in serum transminase activities occurred during the follow-up period, and none of the volunteers developed clinical signs related to viral hepatitis. Only minor side-reactions, such as burning or reddening at the site of injection, were reported by the volunteers, and 100% seroconversion occurred within 150 days after the first vaccina-tion. The subsequent two vaccinations caused a strong booster effect, with median anti-HBs levels of about 5000 mIU/ml developing 10 days after booster injections.

The minimal doses and the schedules required to yield satisfactory immunization, especially in infants, still remain to be determined.

DISCUSSION

The present vaccine was designed to be economical to pro-duce, while maintaining a high level of purity and immunogenici-ty. Furthermore, as the evidence summarized above suggests that HBeAg and pre-S epitopes may contribute to the development of a multivalent protective immunity, efforts were made to include these in the vaccine.

The high HBsAg titre of HBeAg-positive starting plasma, as well as the simple purification techniques employed, contribute to the economy of the production process. The lack of harsh inactivation steps, leading to improved immunogenicity, should further contribute to economic utilization by permitting smaller doses of HBsAg to be used. How small such doses can be is a critical question which must be answered, as this will be a major determinant of the final cost of immunization.

Careful comparisons need to be carried out between this and other available vaccines to provide further information on which optimal vaccine design can be based.

The safety of the present vaccine is guaranteed by the process efficacy of the purification and inactivation steps employed: purification about 4 logs; Tween 80 about 3 logs; $102^{o}C$ at 2 min $\geq$ 5 logs; 10 h at $65^{o}C$ $\geq$ 4 logs, i.e., a total process efficacy of $\geq$ 16 logs. Furthermore, since safety tests are carried out <u>prior to</u> alum adsorption, and thus prior to the final inactivation step, demonstration of lack of infectivity in about 20 doses by the chimpanzee safety test indicates that less than 1 dose in 20×10^{4} (the latter being the minimal process efficacy of the final $65^{o}C$, 10-h inactivation step) can contain residual infectivity. The extraordinary overall process efficacy, however, indicates that potential residual infectivity is many orders of magnitude less than this, i.e., less than 1 in 10^{12} doses. If good manufacturing practices are followed, this vaccine should be absolutely safe.

ACKNOWLEDGEMENTS

The studies described here were supported in part by NIH grant No. HE09011, and by grants in aid from the Institut Mérieux, The Biotest Serum Institute and Eugene Technical International, and by institutional funds from the New York Blood Center.

PRINCE ET AL.

REFERENCES

Adamowicz, P.H., Gerfaux, G., Platel, A., Muller, L., Vacher, B., Mazert, M.C. & Prunet, P. (1981) Large scale production of an hepatitis B vaccine. In: Maupas, P. & Guesry, P., eds, Hepatitis B Vaccine (INSERM Symposium No. 18), Amsterdam, Elsevier-North-Holland, pp. 37-50

Bhatnagar, P.K., Papas, E., Blum, H.E., Milich, D.R., Nitecki, D., Karels, M.J. & Vyas, G.N. (1982) A synthetic analogue of hepatitis B surface antigen sequence 139-147 produces immune response specific for the common a determinant. Proc. natl Acad. USA, 79, 4400-4404

Brummelhuis, H.G.J., Wilson-De-Sturler, L.A. & Raap, A.K. (1981) Preparation of Hepatitis B vaccine by heat inactivation. In: Maupas, P. & Guesry, P., eds, Hepatitis B Vaccine (INSERM Symposium No. 18), Amsterdam, Elsevier-North-Holland, pp. 51-56

Dreesman, G.R., Sanchez, Y., Ionescu-Matiu, I., Sparrow, J.T., Six, H.R., Peterson, D.L., Hollinger, F.B. & Melnick, J.L. (1982) Antibody to hepatitis B surface antigen after a single inoculation of uncoupled synthetic HBsAg peptides. Nature, 295, 158-160

Eddleston, A.L.W.F., Mondelli, M., Mieli-Vergani, G. & Williams, R. (1982) Lymphocyte cytotoxicity to autologous hepatocytes in chronic hepatitis B infection. Hepatology, 2, 122-127

Fujinami, R.S. & Oldstone, M.B.A. (1981) Alteration in expression of measles virus polypeptides by antibody: molecular events in antibody induced antigenic modulation. J. Immunol., 124, 78-85

Hollinger, F.B., Dreesman, G.R., Sanchez, Y., Cabral, G.A. & Melnick, J.L. (1978) Experimental hepatitis B polypeptide vaccine in chimpanzees. In: Vyas, G.N., Cohen, S.N. & Schmid, E., eds, Viral Hepatitis, Philadelphia, The Franklin Institute Press, pp. 557-567

Hopp, T.P. (1981) A synthetic peptide with hepatitis B surface antigen reactivity. Mol. Immunol., 18, 869-872

Kaufmann, R., Mondorf, A.W., Uthemann, H., Bauer, H. & Prince, A.M. (1983) Hepatitis B vaccine: safety study in anti-HBs seronegative human volunteers. Dev. biol. Standard., 54, 229-235

Lerner, R.A., Green, N., Alexander, H., Liu, F.T., Sutcliffe, J.G. & Shinnick, T.M. (1981) Chemically synthesized peptides predicted from the nucleotide sequence of the hepatitis B virus genome elicit antibodies reactive with the native envelope protein of Dane particles. Proc. natl Acad. Sci. USA, 78, 3403-3407

Neurath, A.R. & Strick, N. (1979) Association of hepatitis B e antigen (HBeAg) determinants with the core of Dane particles. J. gen. Virol., 42, 645-649

Neurath, A.R., Kent, S. & Strick, N. (1984) Location and chemical synthesis of a pre-S gene coded immunodominant epitope of hepatitis B virus. Science, 224, 392-395

Prince, A.M., Vnek, J., Brotman, B., Hashimoto, N. & Ende, M.C. (1978) Comparative evaluation of hepatitis B vaccines in chimpanzees and in man. In: Vyas, G.N., Cohen, S.N. & Schmid, E., eds, Viral Hepatitis, Philadelphia, The Franklin Institute Press, pp. 507-523

Prince, A.M., Vnek, J. & Stephan, W. (1983) A new hepatitis B vaccine containing HBeAg in addition to HBsAg. Dev. biol. Standard., 54, 13-22

Purcell, R.H. & Gerin, J.L. (1978) Hepatitis B vaccines: a status report. In: Vyas, G.N., Cohen, S.N. & Schmid, E., eds, Viral Hepatitis, Philadelphia, The Franklin Institute Press, pp. 491-505

Shikata, T., Karasawa, T., Abe, K., Takahasi, T., Mayumi, M. & Oda, T. (1978) Incomplete inactivation of hepatitis B virus after heat treatment at $60^{\circ}C$ for 10 hours. J. infect. Dis., 138, 242-244

Schaeffer, E. & Sninsky, J.J. (1984) Predicted secondary structure similarity in the absence of primary amino acid sequence homology: hepatitis B virus open reading frames. Proc. natl Acad. Sci. USA, 81, 2902-2906

Snydman, D.R., Bryan, J.A., Macon, E.J. & Gregg, M.B. (1976) Hemodialysis associated hepatitis: report of an epidemic with further evidence on mechanisms of transmission. Am. J. Epidemiol., 104, 563-570

Stibbe, W. & Gerlich, W.H. (1983) characterization of pre-S gene products in hepatitis B surface antigen. Dev. biol. Standard., 54, 33-43

Tabor, E. & Gerety, R.J. (1984) Possible role of immune responses to hepatitis B core antigen in protection against hepatitis B infections. Lancet, 1, 172

Takahashi, K., Akahane, Y., Gotanda, T., Mishoro, T., Imai, H., Miyakawa, Y. & Mayumi, M. (1979) Demonstration of hepatitis B e antigen in the core of Dane particles. J. Immunol., 122, 275-279

Trevisan, A., Realdi, G., Alberti, A., Ongaro, G., Pornaro, E. & Meliconi, R. (1982) Core antigen specific immunoglobulin G bound to the liver cell membrane in chronic hepatitis B. Gastroenterology, 82, 218-222

Vnek, J., Prince, A.M., Trepo, C., Williams, A.E., Mushahwar, I.K., Ling, C.M. & Overby, L.R. (1979) Cryptic association of e antigen with different morphological forms of hepatitis B surface antigen. J. med. Virol., 4, 187-199

Vnek, J., Hashimoto, N. & Prince, A.M. (1983) Immunogenicity of HBeAg in the New York Blood Center hepatitis B vaccine. Dev. biol. Standard., 54, 217-221

World Health Organization (1980) Biological substances: International standards, reference preparations and reference reagents, Geneva

World Health Organization (1982) Biological substances: International standards, reference preparations, and reference reagents, Geneva

NEW DEVELOPMENTS IN NUCLEIC ACID HYBRIDIZATION

H. Wolf, M. Haus, U. Leser, S. Modrow & M. Motz

Max von Pettenkofer Institute
University of Munich
Munich, Federal Republic of Germany

S.-Y. Gu

Institute of Virology
Beijing, People's Republic of China

N. Falser & I. Bandlow

ENT Clinic, University of Innsbruck
Innsbruck, Austria

W. Richter

ENT Clinic, University of Würzburg
Würzburg, Federal Republic of Germany

R. Pathmanathan

Institute of Pathology
University of Malaya
Kuala Lumpur, Malaysia

RESUME

L'hybridation des acides nucléiques est largement utilisée pour des applications scientifiques dans des laboratoires spécialisés. Ce papier décrit des sondes d'hybridation qui peuvent être préparées avec un équipement moins spécialisé. Un nouveau test indirect d'hybridation "en sandwich" est décrit; cette technique permet d'utiliser une seule sonde marquée universelle pour hybrider spécifiquement différentes séquences.

Les différentes techniques de marquage et d'hybridation sont
également discutées et comparées de façon critique. Pour
l'hybridation *in situ*, les possibilités d'utilisation de
matériaux fixés et inclus sont testées et évaluées.

SUMMARY

Nucleic acid hybridization is widely used for scientific
applications in specialized laboratories. This paper describes
hybridization probes that can be prepared with less specialized
equipment. A new indirect 'sandwich' hybridization test is
described which allows the use of only one universally usable
labelled probe for hybridization tests with specificities for
various sequences. The use of different labels and hybridization
techniques is also discussed and critically compared. For *in
situ* hybridization, the usability of fixed and embedded materials
is tested and evaluated.

INTRODUCTION

Nucleic acid hybridization is based on the tendency of
nucleic acids to form double-stranded hydrogen-bonded complexes
if strands of complementary sequences are incubated under appropriate salt and temperature conditions. The technique has been
widely applied to study mainly the following questions:

- Presence of genes;
- State of genes (free linear, circular, integrated);
- Localization of genes in specific tissues or
  cell types, or in subcellular structures;
- Transcriptional activity of genes.

EQUATIONS USED TO DESCRIBE HYBRIDIZATION CONDITIONS

The hydrogen bonds between two complementary strands of
nucleic acid can be reversibly broken. This can be achieved at
neutral pH and low ionic strength by the application of heat or,
in the case of DNA, by treatment with alkali. Neutralization and
rapid chilling as well as dilution reduce self-annealing. The
addition of single-stranded nucleic acids from other sources will
lead to the formation of hybrid molecules, the characteristic

which gives its name to this technique. The formation of double-stranded nucleic acid molecules occurs best about 18-32°C below the melting point of the product (T_m) (Gillis et al., 1970), which is identical to that of the parental species if these are completely homologous. Random sequence differences of the hybrid strands will lower the T_m of the product (see formula), which is also influenced by the base composition, the monovalent ion concentration and the dielectric constant of the solvent. The effect of the last of these is frequently used to lower T_m (by addition of formamide) and, as a consequence, the hybridization temperature (McConaughy et al., 1969). The same effect of lowered T_m can be observed if a significant fraction of the nucleotides is chemically modified. This can be observed, for example, with iodinated probes and may be compensated for by lowering the hybridization temperature.

For DNA-DNA hybridization, the value of T_m is given by (Howley et al., 1979):

$$T_m = 81.5 + 16.6 \log (Na^+) + 0.41 (\%GC) - 0.7 (\% \text{ formamide}) - 1.4 (\% \text{ mismatch})$$

The relative hybridization (to 0.18 M Na^+) rate is (Britten & Smith, 1970):

$$F = K^{0.42} (0.24/K)$$

where K = monovalent ion concentration, F = acceleration factor

It should be noted that the molar concentration of DNA molecules, not the concentration of nucleotides, influences the rate of renaturation. Consequently, DNA from smaller viruses hybridizes faster than DNA from larger viruses when similar concentrations of DNA as measured by optical density are used in the test. The relative hybridization rates are therefore directly correlated with the genetic complexity, if repetitive sequences are absent.

COMMONLY USED HYBRIDIZATION TECHNIQUES AND THEIR OBJECTIVES

Detection of certain genes in a mixture with unrelated nucleic acids

This technique is widely used to detect viral nucleic acid sequences in clinical specimens or specific plasmids in bacterial isolates. The particular advantage of nucleic acid hybridization is its independence of viral replication, which allows detection of viral genes in infected cells; this is important, especially in tumour virology, where virus production is not likely to occur. Hybridization was used to link Epstein-Barr virus (EBV) to neoplastic disease in man, and it thus became the first candidate human tumour virus (zur Hausen et al., 1979; Wolf et al., 1975).

The other important application of this technique is based on the possibility of detecting viral nucleic acids when biological activity may be too labile to be preserved or its detection too time-consuming, as is the case for cytomegalovirus (CMV) DNA in urine (Chou & Merigan, 1983). The presence of hepatitis B virus (HBV) DNA in surface antigen (HBsAg)-positive sera in the absence of detectable e/antigen, as in persons recovering from HBV infection, seems to be the best marker for infectivity and its detection is another important clinical application of nucleic acid hybridization (Scotto et al., 1983).

Some enteroviruses and viruses infecting the respiratory organs have been detected with nucleic acid hybridization, which may soon allow rapid characterization of the isolates (Flores et al., 1983). Another application which may be of considerable value is the type-specific detection of human papilloma viruses in laryngeal and cervical materials[1].

The detection of EBV DNA in aspirated cells from a group defined by serological pretesting as at high risk of developing nasopharyngeal carcinoma is under investigation for its diagnostic and prognostic value (Gu et al., 1984) and may be one of the first mass screening tests for neoplastic and preneoplastic conditions in man based on nucleic acid hybridization.

---

[1] See Gissman, this volume

Filter hybridization techniques

The most frequently used technique is based on the immo-
bilization of one hybridization partner on DNA-binding membranes
(Gillespie & Spiegelman, 1965; Alwine et al., 1977). Extracted
nucleic acid is denatured and fixed to membranes, so as to avoid
self-annealing. Labelled single-stranded nucleic acid is then
added and its binding is monitored. The labelled probe can be
removed by heat treatment under low salt conditions and the
filters, which retain the sample nucleic acid, can be rehy-
bridized with probes of different specificity (Thomas, 1980).

Colony hybridization test

A very helpful modification of this technique was introduced
by Grunstein and Hogness (1975), who circumvented the need for
extracting the nucleic acids by directly lysing cells on the
membrane. This technique has been adapted to eukaryotic cells
with good success (Brandsma & Miller, 1980; Wolf, 1981).

Spot hybridization

The large number of specimens that have to be tested for
clinical purposes call for an economic method of hybridization.
Multichannel microfiltration units are now widely used for
application of series of samples on membranes (Schleicher &
Schuell, Keene, NH, USA). These can then be hybridized by
standard procedures. Bresser succeeded in using suspensions of
biological materials without phenol extraction and was able to
selectively bind DNA or RNA with concentrated sodium iodide
(Bresser et al., 1983). The applicability of this technique is
determined by the binding capacity of the membrane for nucleic
acid per unit area, which limits the power to detect very rare
sequences in a vast excess of unrelated ones. Digestion of DNA
with restriction enzymes, separation of the fragments and transfer to membranes has been used with excellent success to overcome
these problems (Southern blot technique) (Southern, 1975;
Desgranges et al., 1982). The same technique has been used in a
most elegant way to describe areas of higher and lower homology
between related viruses by adding varying amounts of formamide at
a constant hybridization temperature to replica blots to control
the melting point and thereby the stringency of the hybridization
conditions (Howley et al., 1979).

Reassociation kinetics

This technique has been widely used to detect sequences of low abundance and partial homologies, and to determine the relative concentrations of certain sequences. The principle of this technique is that both hybrid-forming components are kept in solution. The labelled sequence must be present at a very low concentration so as to minimize self-annealing. The rate of conversion of the labelled sequence into double-stranded nucleic acid is measured and compared to that of self-annealing in a control experiment. This technique requires the amount of label converted into double-stranded nucleic acid to be determined by chromatographic procedures (Kohne & Britten, 1971) or by digestion of the single-stranded fraction with the specific nuclease S_1 followed by determination of the activities found in the fractions. Large amounts of DNA (up to 5 mg) are necessary for the detection of 1-0.1 single-copy genes (for application and limitations of the method and further references, see Frenkel et al., 1986). For this reason, and because of the time-consuming protocol, this procedure is now frequently replaced by other methods.

Detection of the state of genes

The use of appropriate restriction enzymes in connection with blot hybridization allows the determination of the status of the genes under investigation (free linear, circular or integrated). When DNA from tissues is digested with restriction enzymes and the fragments are separated, blotted on membranes and hybridized with nucleic acid sequences from the ends of the gene under investigation, fragments of expected molecular weight deriveable from the free linear form signal free sequences. If the bands appear at different molecular-weight regions, this is likely to be due to circularization or integration (Botchan et al., 1976).

Localization of sequences in specific cells

Certain genes or genomes have frequently to be localized in certain cell types or even subcellular structures, such as chromosomes. Although tissue fractionation has been used successfully to locate viral sequences in specific cell types (Desgranges et al., 1975), in situ hybridization is the method of choice for this purpose (Gall & Pardue, 1969).

The first application of this technique in human medical virology was the successful detection of EBV DNA in the epithelial tumour cell fraction of nasopharyngeal carcinoma (Wolf et al., 1973). Since then, it has found widespread application in cytological and virological problems. Recently, it has been used to identify cells in the lumen of parotid glands as sites of life-long production of EBV following primary infection (Wolf et al., 1984). This powerful technique has also been used for localizing viral genes on specific chromosomes (Wolf et al., 1975; Gerhard et al., 1981; Henderson et al., 1983). In the presence of proteins, this technique can produce signals unrelated to specific hybridization. Carefully controlled experiments, experience in evaluation and, ideally, confirmation by independent techniques are therefore necessary.

Detection of transcription

Separation of mRNA by molecular weight and hybridization of the fractions with fragments of specific genomic areas have been widely used to study transcription (Thomas, 1980). The availability of single-stranded hybridization probes in the direction of transcription and in the reverse orientation, after comparison of the hybridization results, allows the detection of transcribed genes directly by in situ hybridization. This approach has been used with clones from HBV in m13 phage DNA. These clones span the HBsAg- and HBV core antigen (HBcAg)-encoding regions, respectively (Fig. 1). Transcription of viral genes (encoding for HBs) has been detected in a human hepatocellular carcinoma cell line. Hybridization with the complementary strand of viral DNA was negative at the resolution obtained in this test (Modrow et al., unpublished data).

WOLF ET AL.

FIG. 1. DETECTION OF TRANSCRIPTION

Upper part: Diagram of the genome of HBV and the directions in which the genes are transcribed (inner circles). The outer lines show the length and position of the individual ml3 phage DNA clones of HBV.

Lower part: Characterization of the individual ml3 phage DNA HBV clones by digestion with the appropriate restriction endonucleases (indicated below) and electrophoresis in 0.7% agarose gels to define the direction in which the HBV fragments were inserted. M13 HB1, 3, 4 and 5 were cloned into the BamHl site, ml3 HB2 into the BamHl-EcoRl sites of ml3 mp8

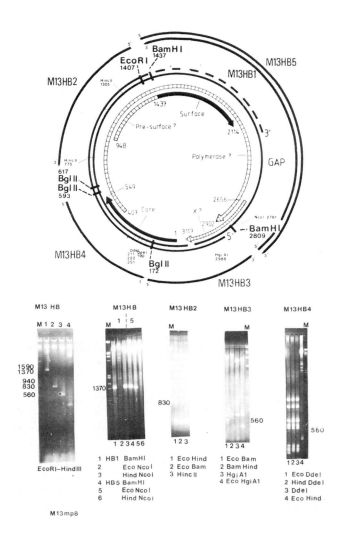

PREPARATION OF LABELLED HYBRIDIZATION PROBES

In vivo labelled probes

The most important application of nucleic acid hybridization ocncerns the preparation of hybridization probes. In vivo labelling of nucleic acids by metabolic pathways has been used to obtain such probes. The main difficulties are the usually limiting low specific activity (Frenkel et al., 1976), the difficulty in obtaining enough labelled material, and the problem of unspecific or cross-reacting sequences. These sequences may appear to be due to incomplete purification of the desired gene, for example, from cell lysates, or can be due to sequences within the genome used as probe. CMV DNA is a typical example, as several areas of the viral genome cross-hybridize with DNA from uninfected human cells (Peden et al., 1982).

In vitro labelled probes

Various procedures have been used to introduce labels into nucleic acids. DNA can be transcribed in vitro into cRNA in the presence of radioactive ribonucleoside triphosphates, using RNA polymerases. By analogy, RNA can be reverse-transcribed into cDNA. The original template can be destroyed with appropriate nucleases. Although of great importance in earlier studies, these techniques have been largely replaced by others.

The most frequently used protocol is based on the use of E. coli DNA polymerase I. This enzyme acts on DNase-introduced nicks in double-stranded DNA as a 5'-3'-exonuclease and a 5'-3'-synthetase which allows the efficient and random introduction of label. With ^{32}P-labelled nucleotides, specific activities of 10^8-10^9 cpm/μg DNA can be obtained.

Single-stranded nucleic acids and, with reduced efficiency, also double-stranded nucleic acids can be labelled by chemical introduction of ^{125}I into the cytosines of DNA or RNA (Commerford, 1971; Gu et al., 1983; Han & Harding, 1983; Prensky, 1976). The specific advantage of chemical modification is easy scaling up for the mass production of labelled probes.

Problems with the specificity of probes are effectively controlled by means of recombinant DNA techniques. Sequences without the cross-reacting portions can be cloned in plasmids and prepared with good yields. Wherever the plasmid part introduces a danger of unwanted signals, it can be replaced by another vector or removed by restriction-enzyme digestion and electrophoretic separation. The desired sequence can be eluted from the gel by means of special procedures (Langridge et al., 1980; Vogelstein & Gillespie, 1979), which abolish otherwise observed inhibitory effects of remaining contaminants from the gel matrix. Recently, the single-stranded DNA phage ml3 has been used as a cloning vehicle for probes (Messing, 1983). This approach is very helpful as ml3 sequences rarely occur in natural specimens and thus do not have to be removed, and the recombinant phage DNA can be purified in large amounts without the use of ultracentrifuges or other special equipment. Single-stranded DNA can be labelled either by primer-directed synthesis of a second strand which spans all or part of the ml3 sequences or by chemical reactions (Hu & Messing, 1982; Gu et al., 1983).

Selection of label

Tritium has been widely used for most labelling procedures. Because of its weak radiation, the resolution obtainable in the commonly used autoradiographic systems is rather low. However, for in situ hybridization this label gives readily locatable signals and good resolution, if the samples are exposed after dipping in photoemulsion. ^{32}P-labelled nucleotides give the highest specific activity, and ^{32}P is still the label of choice, if the highest resolution is required, in all variations of filter hybridization. It is not suitable for in situ hybridization, as the signals are relatively weak and diffuse. The main disadvantage of ^{32}P is its short half-life of 2 weeks.

^{35}S-nucleoside triphosphates may be used to replace ^{32}P where longer shelf-life is required (half-life 87 days) and where a slightly reduced sensitivity is acceptable. Probes labelled with this isotope should be acceptable for in situ hybridization (Vincent et al., 1982). ^{125}I labelling can be efficiently achieved with simple chemical procedures, especially if single-stranded probes are used. The sensitivity of labelled samples is comparable to that of ^{32}P-labelled samples when used in filter assays. ^{125}I-labelled probes can also be used for in situ hybridization with slightly less satisfying results than those obtained with tritium because of the higher background (Commerford, 1971; Prensky, 1976; Gu et al., 1983).

Thanks to the simple labelling procedure, the acceptable half-life of 60 days and their suitability for <u>in situ</u> and filter hybridization tests, ^{125}I-labelled probes seem very attractive for routine use. The modification in the cytosine may lower the melting point by a few degrees centigrade.

Non-radioactive labels have been used to detect hybridization (Langer <u>et al.</u>, 1981). At present, biotin covalently linked with nucleic acids via a molecular spacer is the most popular non-radioactive label. It is currently introduced into DNA by using appropriately altered nucleoside triphosphates in the nick-translation reaction. The biotin is detected in further steps by standard procedures, using either avidin or antibiotin antibodies covalently linked to fluorochromes or enzymes used in ELISA tests (beta-galactosidase or horse radish peroxidase).

These labels offer the greatest advantages for routine laboratories, as they would avoid the handling of radioactive materials with all its decontamination problems and because the keeping of usable stocks of probes would be facilitated. This advantage becomes even greater if only one labelled probe for the sandwich-hybridization technique is kept.

The sensitivity of the reaction has been found in direct comparisons not to be quite as high as with radiolabelled probes, especially in the filter-hybridization test. It will be interesting to see whether sandwich hybridization can increase the sensitivity to fully acceptable levels.

Chemical introduction of the label would further facilitate the mass production of probes which will become possible if only one labelled sequence is used in the sandwich technique. This procedure should significantly reduce the cost per test.

Indirect 'sandwich' hybridization

Recently (Wolf, unpublished data) a new approach has been developed which overcomes the need to introduce label into each specific hybridization probe by taking advantage of the recombinant DNA technique and linking the specific sequence 1 to another sequence 2, which can conveniently be m13 DNA. Figure 1 shows the establishment of such clones for HBV DNA. These readily available probes are used in a first hybridization step unlabelled and in high concentrations, which favours fast and complete hybridization. After removal of excess probe, a second probe is added which is homologous to sequence 2 and ideally contains both orientations of the DNA strands. This second probe can be universally applied and can, under appropriate conditions, form a network on top of sequence 2. An example is shown in Figure 2 where, with appropriate exposure time, as little as 200 fg of the specific sequences represented in the probe were found in the test DNA. This procedure gives an amplification of the hybridization signal of up to 100-fold when non-radioactive 'second probes' were utilized. This technique has been used to detect a fragment of EBV DNA in Southern blots, using a ^{32}P-labelled double-stranded replicative form of ml3 for second-step hybridization, and was able to detect 0.5 pg of the fragment.

PREPARATION OF TEST MATERIALS

In many instances, the collection of samples is theoretically easy because the lesions which yield the test materials are accessible without operation. However, the lack of specialized equipment for sample collection enforces compromises in relation to sample quality or quantity. By means of newly designed equipment (for diagram, see Figure 3), it was possible to use a new type of probe (Richter et al., 1983) (also available from Haselmeier, Stuttgart, Federal Republic of Germany). This has a slim head and a cylinder connected via parallel tubing to a buffer reservoir and a vacuum source. Pressing the head on to a suspected area creates a vacuum which leads to aspiration of buffer and a continuous swirl of liquid over the mucosal area, moving liquid providing only the force used in cell collection. This procedure is painless in most cases. The stream of isotonic buffer exfoliates cells from the mucosa and transports them to a membrane filter composed of nitrocellulose ester, where they are concentrated.

FIG. 2. INDIRECT 'SANDWICH' HYBRIDIZATION

Variable amounts of Raji cell (50 EBV genomes per cell) DNA were
digested with <u>Bam</u>Hl restriction enzyme, separated on an agarose
gel, blotted on to a nitrocellulose membrane and used for
sandwich hybridization. For the first hybridization step, 0.13
μg/ml (total 1 μg/blot) of ml3 phage containing a fragment of the
<u>Bam</u>W piece of EBV was hybridized at 68°C in 0.99 M Na^{+}; for the
second step 10^{7} cpm of ^{32}P-labelled heat-denatured probes
prepared by nick translation of the replicative form of wild-type
ml3 phage (1.25 cpm/μg) was hybridized at 63°C in Na^{+}.

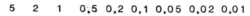

5   2   1   0.5 0.2 0.1 0.05 0.02 0.01

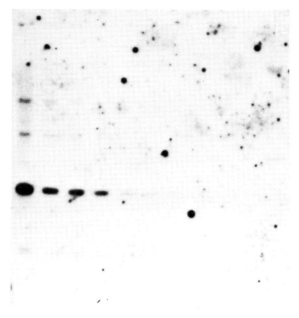

FIG. 3.   COLLECTION OF SAMPLES

The diagram shows a modified method of using the instrument for
collecting cells (Richter _et al._, 1983) for nucleic acid hybridization.   This modification speeds up work with the patient and
gives greater flexibility in using cells for different modifications of the hybridization test.

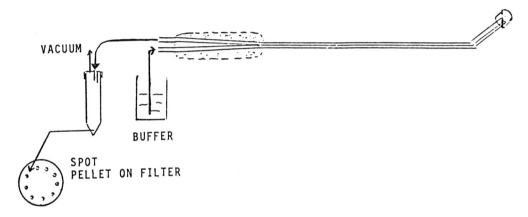

Alternatively, the cells can be collected with the buffer in
a trap and pelleted.   The maintainance of isotonic conditions
minimizes cell damage and allows the specimen to be used for
cytological examination as well as for nucleic acid hybridization.   Both techniques may be carried out directly on the filter
membranes (Richter _et al._, 1983; Wolf, 1981).

Where histological conditions are important, sections of the
material under investigation must be used.   Frozen sectioning has
been successfully used to locate viral genomes in tumour cells
(Wolf _et al._, 1973) or to identify 'virus factories' in biopsy
material (Wolf _et al._, 1984).   Frequently, fresh samples are not
available or fixation is important in obtaining better results in
the cytological and histological examination by light or electron
microscopy.

Glutaraldehyde-fixed,   paraffin-embedded   materials   were
successfully used to detect HBV DNA (Brigati _et al._, 1983; Gowans
_et al._, 1981) in liver tissue and pseudorabies virus DNA in brain
tissue (Falser _et al._, unpublished data) after removal of
paraffin and _in situ_ hybridization.

Especially when tissue with cartilage is used, paraffin blocks are not suitable for sectioning. Several alternative embedding media have been tested and it was found that sections from materials embedded in the acrylate-based K4M (Balzers, Frankfurt, Federal Republic of Germany) gave acceptable hybridization signals. K4M has the advantage that it still polymerizes at temperatures as low as $-20^{\circ}C$. The use of osmium tetroxide treatment following glutaraldehyde fixation did not further reduce the hybridization signal. Formalin fixation for 20 minutes drastically reduced hybridization efficiency.

DISCUSSION

Nucleic acid hybridization has long been considered a technique usable only in highly specialized laboratories. More efficient labelling procedures for nucleic acids have increased the sensitivity of detection to about 10^{-19} M of a specific sequence under optimal conditions, and the signal can be associated with cellular structures. This powerful technique has still not found widespread use, however, in clinical testing. This may have been due in part to a lack of information, but the main problem seems to be the apparent need for specialized and expensive equipment and for highly qualified personnel to perform the complex experimental procedures. This review gives some approaches to solving these problems.

REFERENCES

Alwine, J., Kemp, D. & Stark, G. (1977) Method for detection of specific RNAs in agarose gels by transfer to diazobenzyl-oxymethyl-paper and hybridization with DNA probes. Proc. natl Acad. Sci. USA, 12, 5350-5354

Botchan, M., Topp, W. & Sambrook, J. (1976) The arrangement of simian virus 40 sequences in the DNA of transformed cells. Cell, 9, 269-287

Brandsma, J. & Miller, G. (1980) Nucleic acid spot hybridization: rapid quantitative screening of lymphoid cell lines for Epstein-Barr viral DNA. Proc. natl Acad. Sci. USA, 6851-6855

Bresser, J., Doering, J. & Gillespie, D. (1983)   Quick-blot:
    Selective mRNA or DNA immobilization from whole cells. DNA,
    2, 243-254

Brigati, D., Myerson, D., Leary, J., Spalholz, B., Travis, S.,
    Fong, C., Hsiung, G. & Ward, D. (1983)   Detection of viral
    genomes in cultured cells and paraffin-embedded tissue
    sections using   biotin-labeled   hybridization   probes.
    Virology, 126, 32-50

Britten, R. & Smith, J. (1970) A bovine genome. Carnegie Inst.
    Washington Yearb., 68, 378-386

Chou, S. & Merigan, T. (1983)   Rapid detection and quantitation
    of human cytomegalovirus in urine through DNA hybridization.
    New Engl. J. Med., 308, 921-925

Commerford, S. (1971)   Iodination of nucleic acids in vitro.
    Biochemistry, 10, 1993-1999

Desgranges, C., Wolf, H., de-Thé, G., Shanmugaratnam, K.,
    Cammoun, N., Ellouz, R., Klein, G., Lennert, K., Munoz, N. &
    zur Hausen, H. (1975) Nasopharyngeal carcinoma. X. Presen-
    ce of Epstein-Barr genomes in separated epithelial cells of
    tumors in patients from Singapore, Tunisia and Kenya.   Int.
    J. Cancer, 16, 7-15

Desgranges, C., Bornkamm, G., Zeng, Y., Wang, P., Zhu, J., Shang,
    M. & de-Thé, G. (1982) Detection of Epstein-Barr viral DNA
    internal repeats in the nasopharyngeal mucosa of Chinese
    with IgA/EBV-specific antibodies. Int. J. Cancer, 29, 87-91

Flores, J., Purcell, R., Perez, I., Wyatt, R., Boeggeman, E.,
    Sereno, M., White, L., Chanock, R. & Kapikian, A. (1983) A
    dot hybridization assay for detection of rotavirus. Lancet,
    1, 555-558

Frenkel, N., Locker, H., Cox, B., Roizman, B. & Rapp, F. (1976)
    Herpes simplex virus DNA in transformed cells: Sequence
    complexity in five hamster cell lines and one derived
    hamster tumor. J. Virol., 18, 885-893

Gall, J. & Pardue, J. (1969) Formation and detection of RNA-DNA hybrid molecules in cytological preparations. Proc. natl Acad. Sci. USA, 63, 378-383

Gerhard, D., Kawasaki, E., Bancroft, F. & Szabo, P. (1981) Localization of a unique gene by direct hybridization in situ. Proc. natl Acad. Sci. USA, 78, 3755-3759

Gillespie, D. & Spiegelman, S. (1965) A quantitative assay for DNA/RNA hybrids with DNA immobilized on a membrane. J. mol. Biol., 12, 829-842

Gillis, M., De Ley, J. & De Cleene, M. (1970) The determination of molecular weight of bacterial genome DNA from renaturation rates. Eur. J. Biochem., 12, 143-153

Gowens, E., Burrell, C., Jilbert, A. & Marmion, B. (1981) Detection of hepatitis B virus DNA sequences in infected hepatocytes by in situ cytohybridisation. J. med. Virol., 8, 67-78

Grunstein, M. & Hogness, D. (1975) Colony hybridization: A method for the isolation of cloned DNAs that contain a specific gene. Proc. natl Acad. Sci. USA, 72, 3961-3965

Gu, S., Wolf, H. & Yi, Z. (1983) Cloning fragments of EBV-DNA in single-stranded phage M13 mp8. I. Preparation and identification of cloned DNA. Cancer (China), 129-135

Han, J. & Harding, J. (1983) Using iodinated single-stranded M13 probes to facilitate rapid DNA sequence analysis - nucleotide sequence of a mouse lysine tRNA gene. Nucleic Acids Res., 11, 2053-2064

Henderson, A., Ripley, S., Heller, M. & Kieff, E. (1983) Chromosome site for Epstein-Barr virus DNA in a Burkitt tumor cell line and in lymphocytes growth-transformed in vitro. Proc. natl Acad. Sci. USA, 80, 1987-1991

Howley, P., Israel, M., Law, M. & Martin, M. (1979) Rapid methods for detecting and mapping homology between heterologous DNAs. J. biol. Chem., 254, 4876-4883

Hu, N. & Messing, J. (1982) The making of strand-specific M13 probes. Gene, 17, 271-277

Kohne, D. & Britten, R. (1971)   Hydroxyapatit techniques for nucleic acid reassociations. Proced. Nucleic Acid Res., 2, 500-512

Langer, P., Waldrop, A. & Ward, D. (1981) Enzymatic synthesis of biotin-labeled polynucleotides: Novel nucleic acid affinity probes. Proc. natl. Acad. Sci. USA, 78, 6633-6637

Langridge, J., Langridge, P. & Bergquist, P. (1980) Extraction of nucleic acids from agarose gels. Anal. Biochem., 103, 264-271

McConaughy, L., Laird, C. & McCarthy, B. (1969) Nucleic acid reassociation in formamide. Biochemistry, 8, 3289-3295

Messing, J. (1983) New M13 vectors for cloning. Methods Enzymol., 101, 20-78

Peden, K., Mounts, P. & Hayward, G. (1982) Homology between mammalian cell DNA sequences and human herpesvirus genomes detected by a hybridization procedure with high-complexity probes. Cell, 31, 71-80

Prensky, W. (1976) The radioiodination of RNA and DNA to high specific activities. Methods cell Biol., 13, 121-152

Richter, W., Gu, S., Seibl, R. & Wolf, H. (1983) A new method for examination of carcinomas of the nasopharynx. In: Prasad, U., Ablashi, D.V., Levine, P.H. & Pearson, G.R., eds, Nasopharyngeal Carcinoma: Current Concepts, University of Malaya Press, pp. 25-32

Scotto, J., Hadchouel, M., Hery, C., Yvart, J., Tiollais, P. & Bréchot, C. (1983) Detection of hepatitis B virus DNA in serum by a simple spot hybridization technique: comparison with results for other viral markers. Hepatology, 3, 279-284

Southern, E. (1975) Detection of specific sequences among DNA fragments separated by gel electrophoresis. J. mol. Biol., 98, 503-517

Thomas, P. (1980) Hybridization of denatured RNA and small DNA fragments transferred to nitrocellulose. Proc. natl Acad. Sci. USA, 77, 5201-5205

Vincent, M., Beltz, W. & Ashton, S. (1982) Preparation of DNA labelled with high specific activity S^{35}-deoxy- adenosine 5'- (a-thio) triphosphate; the use of ^{35}S-labeled nucleic acids as molecular hybridization probes. In: Ahmed, F., ed., Miami Winter Symposium, Vol. 19

Vogelstein, B. & Gillespie, D. (1979) Preparative and analytical purification of DNA from agarose. Proc. natl Acad. Sci. USA, 76, 615-619

Wolf, H. (1981) Die Verwendung verschiedener Nuklein-säure-Hybridisierungstechniken am Beispiel von Epstein-Barr-Virus korrelierter Erkrankungen. Verh. dtsch Ges. Pathol., 65, 47-57

Wolf, H., zur Hausen, H. & Becker, V. (1973) EB viral genomes in epithelial nasopharyngeal carcinoma cells. Nature New Biology, 138, 245-247

Wolf, H., zur Hausen, H., Klein, G., Becker, V., Henle, G. & Henle, W. (1975) Attempts to detect virus-specific DNA sequences in human tumors. III. Epstein-Barr viral DNA in non-lymphoid nasopharyngeal carcinoma cells. Med. Micro-biol. Immunol., 161, 15-21

Wolf, H., Haus, M. & Wilmes, E. (1984) Persistence of Epstein-Barr virus in the parotid gland. J. Virol., 51, 795-798

zur Hausen, H., Diehl, V., Wolf, H. & Schulte-Holthausen, H. (1973) EB virus associated macromolecules in cells derived from human tumors. In: Molecular Studies in Viral Neopla-sia, 25th MD Anderson Annual Symposium on Fundamental Cancer Research, Houston, 1972, pp. 517-530

zur Hausen, H., Schulte-Holthausen, H., Klein, G., Henle, W., Henle, G., Clifford, P. & Santesson, L. (1979) EBV DNA in biopsies of Burkitt tumours and anaplastic carcinomas of the nasopharynx. Nature, 228, 1056-1058

REPORT OF THE OAU/STRC AD HOC COMMITTEE ON HEPATITIS B VACCINATION IN AFRICA[1]

TERMS OF REFERENCE

To review the present status of hepatitis B vaccines.

To make recommendations concerning vaccination against hepatitis in Africa and consequent prevention of liver cancer.

1. PREAMBLE

1.1 Hepatocellular carcinoma (HCC) is one of the commonest malignant tumours in the world. Its prevalence is particularly high in tropical Africa, where it affects young adults and middle-aged Africans. It is rapidly fatal, with or without attempts at treatment.

1.2 There is abundant and convincing evidence that hepatitis B virus (HBV) infection is causally related to the development of HCC in Africa and other parts of the developing world.

---

[1] Members of the Committee

E.A. Ayoola (Chairman), Nigeria
C. Chuwa, WHO (Observer)
P. Coursaget, Senegal
B. Fritzell, IPP, France
A.O.K. Johnson, Nigeria
C.L.M. Olweny, Zambia/Uganda
J. Perrin, Burundi
O. Sobeslavsky, WHO (Observer)
P. Touré, Senegal
F. Tron, IPP, France

1.3 HBV infections are very common in tropical Africa, where the majority of the estimated 200 million chronic HBV surface antigen (HBsAg) carriers of the world live. This infection is acquired during infancy and early childhood in most tropical populations. Such infections lead to chronic liver diseases, such as liver cirrhosis, with high morbidity and mortality.

1.4 More data concerning the epidemiology of HBV infections are continually being acquired. They indicate that the rates of chronic carriers, acute hepatitis and chronic liver diseases are increasing. This requires immediate intervention.

1.5 In the causation of HCC, additional factors such as mycotoxins may play a role. The control of contamination of food grains by mycotoxins must depend on agriculture workers and planners.

1.6 It is clear that, if HBV infection is prevented early by active immunization, the incidence of HCC will be markedly reduced.

2. HEPATITIS B VACCINES: PRESENT STATUS

2.1 Availability

Two commercially available vaccines have now been introduced in Africa and effectively used on a limited basis:

(a) Institut Pasteur (Hevac B) vaccine, which contains 5 μg/ml of bivalent (ad + ay) antigen, and is applied subcutaneously.

(b) MSD (Heptavax) vaccine, which contains 20 μg/ml of monovalent (ad) antigen and is given intramuscularly.

2.2 Safety

Available data indicate that the vaccines already tested are safe. No significant untoward effects have so far been reported.

2.3 Cost

It is estimated that US$ 40-80 per vaccination schedule would be needed for each vaccine. Institut Pasteur vaccines cost US$ 40-50 per schedule per person (i.e., 2- or 3-dose schedule).

2.4 Efficacy/Potency

(a) Available vaccines are highly immunogenic in the populations already tested.

(b) Neonates are capable of an adequate immunogenic response to the vaccines.

(c) Passively transferred maternal antibodies do not interfere with the response to the vaccine.

(d) Those who respond to vaccination are protected against HBV infection, with particular reference to acute hepatitis and HbsAg carriage.

2.5 Application: routes of vaccination

(a) Intramuscular injections (MSD) and subcutaneous (Pasteur) injections require:

(i)   trained manpower;
(ii)   disposable sterile materials;
(iii) privacy during vaccination (if adults are vaccinated).

(b) Available data suggest that the intradermal route is effective, but more studies are desirable. If this is confirmed, it may be the fastest and most economical route.

2.6 Stability of vaccines

(a) Freezing is undesirable and detrimental to vaccines.

(b) It is recommended that vaccines be kept at 2-8°C.

(c) Information is lacking on the potency of vaccines kept at ambient temperature.

3. RECOMMENDATIONS

The need for a vaccination programme against HBV infection is imperative.

3.1   It is **mandatory** that neonates and infants should be vaccinated.

3.2   It is **desirable** that older children should be vaccinated.

3.3   In view of the cost, the manpower required and the epidemiological data, the routine vaccination of adults is not recommended.   Susceptible adults in some populations may, however, be vaccinated under defined circumstances.

3.4   Multicentre programmes, using standard protocols, should be carried out to assess the efficacy of all vaccines in tropical populations.

3.5   Training of personnel and research on field trials and laboratory diagnosis in the area of hepatitis should be incorporated in the vaccination programmes of African countries.

3.6   Additional data should continuously be acquired in areas such as the best route of vaccination, the stability of vaccines not kept in a cold chain, the optimal minimum dose, and most importantly the cumulative influence of vaccination on the prevalence and incidence of chronic liver diseases and HCC.

3.7   The urgent and ultimate goal should be to encourage a marked reduction in the cost of these vaccines.   Establishment of production centres in Africa should ensure production of cheaper vaccines.

3.8   It is highly desirable to provide an international standard for HBV vaccines, as has already been done for immunoglobulins and some vaccines (e.g., tetanus).

3.9   A follow-up symposium should be held in 2-4 years time to review the progress made in vaccination against hepatitis and the control of liver cancer in Africa, with particular reference to the progress and additional information accruing from the use of second-generation vaccines.

RAPPORT DU COMITÉ AD HOC OUA/CSTR SUR LA VACCINATION CONTRE L'HÉPATITE B EN AFRIQUE[1]

TERMES DE REFERENCE

Buts

Evaluer la situation présente en ce qui concerne les vaccins contre l'hépatite B.

Fournir des recommandations quant à la vaccination contre l'hépatite en Afrique, et la prévention conséquente du cancer du foie.

1. PREAMBULE

1.1 Le cancer primitif du foie (CPF) est une des tumeurs malignes les plus communes dans le monde. Sa prévalence est particulièrement élevée en Afrique tropicale, où il affecte les jeunes adultes et les sujets d'âge moyen. Il est rapidement fatal, avec ou sans tentatives de traitement.

1.2 Des preuves nombreuses et convaincantes indiquent que l'infection par le virus de l'hépatite B (HBV) est liée de façon causale au développement du CPF en Afrique et dans d'autres parties du monde en voie de développement.

---

[1] Membres du Comité

E.A. Ayoola, Président, Nigéria
C. Chuwa (OMS), Observateur
P. Coursaget, Sénégal
B. Fritzell, IPP, France
A.O.K. Johnson, Nigéria
C.L.M. Olweny, Zambie/Ouganda
J. Perrin, Burundi
O. Sobeslavsky, OMS (Observateur)
P. Touré, Sénégal
F. Tron, IPP, France

1.3 Les infections HBV sont très communes en Afrique tropicale, où vit la majorité des porteurs chroniques de l'antigène de surface du virus HB (Ag HBs), estimés à 200 millions.

1.4 On acquiert continuellement des données supplémentaires sur l'épidémiologie des infections HBV. Ces données indiquent que les taux de porteurs chroniques, d'hépatites aiguës et de maladies chroniques du foie sont en augmentation. Ceci nécessite une intervention immédiate.

1.5 Dans l'étiologie du CPF, des facteurs additionnels tels que les mycotoxines peuvent jouer un rôle. Le contrôle de la contamination des graines alimentaires par les mycotoxines doit reposer sur ceux qui travaillent dans l'agriculture et ceux qui la planifient.

1.6 Il est clair que, si l'infection HBV est prévenue de façon précoce par une immunisation active, l'incidence de CPF sera réduite de façon notable.

2. VACCINS CONTRE L'HEPATITE B: SITUATION ACTUELLE

2.1 Disponibilité

Deux vaccins commercialement disponibles ont maintenant été introduits en Afrique et utilisés de façon effective sur une base limitée:

(a) Le vaccin de l'Institut Pasteur (Hevac B), qui contient 5 g/ml d'antigène bivalent (ad + ay), et qui s'administre par voie sous-cutanée;

(b) Le vaccin MSD (Heptavax), qui contient 20 g/ml d'antigène monovalent (ad) et qui s'administre par voie intramusculaire.

2.2 Sécurité

Les données disponibles indiquent que les vaccins déjà testés sont sûrs. Aucun effet néfaste significatif n'a été rapporté jusqu'ici.

2.3 Coût

On estime qu'il faut compter 40-80 US$ par vaccination pour chacun des vaccins. Les vaccins de l'Institut Pasteur coûtent 40 à 50 US$ par vaccination et par personne (une vaccination correspond à 2 à 3 doses).

2.4 Efficacité/Activité

(a) Les vaccins disponibles se sont révélés hautement immunogènes dans les populations déjà testées.

(b) Les nouveau-nés présentent une réponse immunologique correcte à ces vaccins.

(c) Les anticorps maternels transmis passivement n'interfèrent pas avec la réponse au vaccin.

(d) Ceux qui répondent à la vaccination sont protégés contre l'infection HBV, et en particulier contre l'hépatite aiguë et le portage chronique de l'AgHBs.

2.5 Application: voies d'administration des vaccins

(a) Les injections intramusculaires (MSD) et sous-cutanées (Pasteur) nécessitent:

(i) une main-d'oeuvre entraînée
(ii) du matériel stérile
(iii) un certain isolement pendant la vaccination (pour les adultes qui sont vaccinés)

(b) Les données disponibles suggèrent que la voie intradermique est efficace, mais des études complémentaires sont souhaitables. Si son efficacité se confirme, cette voie d'administration peut être la plus rapide et la plus économique.

2.6 Stabilité des vaccins

(a) La congélation n'est pas souhaitable; elle est préjudiciable aux vaccins.

(b) Il est recommandé de conserver les vaccins entre 2 et 8°C.

(c) On manque d'information sur l'activité des vaccins conservés à la température ambiante.

3. RECOMMANDATIONS

La nécessité d'un programme de vaccination contre l'infection HBV est impérative.

3.1 Il faut imposer que les nouveau-nés et les nourrissons soient vaccinés.

3.2 Il est souhaitable que les autres enfants soient vaccinés.

3.3 Du fait de son coût, de la main d'oeuvre qu'elle implique et des données épidémiologiques, on ne peut recommander la vaccination systématique des adultes. Cependant, dans certaines populations les adultes sensibles pourraient être vaccinés dans des circonstances définies.

3.4 Des programmes multicentriques utilisant des protocoles standardisés devraient être réalisés afin d'évaluer l'efficacité de tous les vaccins dans les populations tropicales.

3.5 La formation du personnel et la recherche sur le terrain comme sur le diagnostic de laboratoire, dans le domaine de l'hépatite devraient être incorporées dans les programmes de vaccination des pays africains.

3.6 Des données complémentaires devraient être acquises de façon continue dans des domaines tels que la meilleure voie d'administration des vaccins, leur stabilité en dehors de la chaîne du froid, la dose optimale minimale, et, plus important encore, l'influence cumulative de la vaccination sur la prévalence et l'incidence des maladies chroniques du foie et du CPF.

3.7 L'objectif urgent et le but final à atteindre devraient être d'encourager une réduction notable du prix de ces vaccins. L'installation de centres de production en Afrique devrait assurer la production de vaccins meilleur marché.

3.8 Il est hautement souhaitable de fournir un standard international pour les vaccins HBV, comme cela a déjà été fait
pour les immunoglobulines et certains vaccins (tels que le
tétanos).

3.9 Un autre Symposium devrait se tenir dans 2 à 3 ans, pour
évaluer les progrès réalisés dans la vaccination contre
l'hépatite et la prévention du cancer du foie en Afrique.
Il permettrait en particulier d'évaluer les progrès et les
informations nouvelles recueillies dans l'utilisation des
vaccins de la deuxième génération.

GENITAL CANCERS

HUMAN PAPILLOMAVIRUS DNA IN GENITAL TUMOURS

L. Gissmann

Institute for Virus Research of the
German Cancer Research Centre
Heidelberg, Federal Republic of Germany

RESUME

On a identifié les papillomavirus humains (HPV) de type 16 et 18 dans deux différents épithéliomas du col utérin. Les ADN viraux ont été clonés et utilisés comme sondes pour tester un grand nombre de tumeurs génitales par la technique de transfert de Southern. On a retrouvé des séquences de HPV-16 ou de HPV-18 dans un pourcentage élevé d'épithéliomas du col, mais seulement dans un petit nombre de condylomes acuminés ou de condylomes plats. Cependant, la majorité de ces dernières lésions conte- naient respectivement des séquences de HPV-6 ou de HPV-11, qui n'étaient par contre que rarement détectées dans les épithéliomas in situ ou invasifs. On a observé une distribution similaire des différents papillomavirus quand on a testé les frottis du col par hybridation in situ.

SUMMARY

Human papillomaviruses (HPV) types 16 and 18 have been identified in two different human cervical carcinomas. The viral DNAs were molecularly cloned and used as probes to screen a large number of genital tumours by Southern blot analysis. HPV 16 or HPV 18 sequences were found in a high percentage of cervical carcinomas but only in a small number of condylomata acuminata or flat condylomas. The majority of the latter lesions, however, contained HPV 6 or HPV 11 sequences, respectively, which, in contrast, were detected only rarely in carcinoma in situ or invasive carcinomas. A similar distribution of the different papillomaviruses was observed when cell scrapings taken from the cervix were tested by in situ hybridization.

INTRODUCTION

The involvement of an infectious event in the development of human cancer of the uterine cervix has been suspected for many years, based mainly on epidemiological studies which showed that the time of first intercourse and the number of sexual partners were the most important factors associated with cervical neoplasia (reviewed by Thomas, 1973). Women whose husbands have had multiple sexual partners are also at relatively higher risk (Martin, 1967). The possibility that herpes simplex virus (HSV), among other agents, might be associated with cervical carcinoma has been extensively investigated. Serological data, in fact, support the hypothesis that this virus may play a role in tumour development, but nearly all attempts to detect viral DNA in biopsies have failed (for review, see zur Hausen, 1983). On the other hand, human papillomaviruses have been under consideration in recent years as possible candidates (zur Hausen, 1977) for the following reasons:

(i)   The oncogenic potential of some papillomaviruses, e.g., of the Shope papillomaviruses and bovine papillomavirus, is well documented (reviewed by Pfister, 1984; Gissmann, 1984).

(ii)   The possible malignant conversion of certain virus-induced human papillomas (e.g., laryngeal papillomas, genital warts, lesions in epidermodysplasia verruciformis patients) has been reported (for review, see zur Hausen, 1977; Gissmann, 1984).

(iii)   Venereally transmitted papillomavirus infections of the genital tract are very common. Approximately 2% of randomly selected women were shown to be affected by genital papillomas (Meisels et al., 1982).

(iv)   It has become clear, thanks mainly to the investigations by Meisels and co-workers (1982), that cervical lesions which have been diagnosed as mild dysplasia are in fact papillomavirus-associated condylomas (Meisels & Fortin, 1976; Purola & Savia, 1977). It is also known that such dysplasias progress in some cases to cervical intra-epithelial neoplasia grades II and III and to invasive cancer.

HUMAN PAPILLOMAVIRUSES IN GENITAL WARTS

Human papillomaviruses represent a very heterogeneous group. At least 24 different virus types have been identified thus far (reviewed by Gissmann and Schwarz, 1984);   they are found in various lesions and their genomes show only limited sequence homology with each other, if any. It is not surprising, therefore, that the first attempts to detect papillomavirus DNA in genital tumours were unsuccessful, since DNA prepared from skin wart viruses was used as the probe in these hybridization experiments (zur Hausen et al., 1974; Gissmann et al., 1977).

The concentration of papillomavirus particles in genital warts is extremely low. Since no permissive cell system for virus replication has so far been established (for review, see Pfister, 1984), molecular cloning of the DNA was a prerequisite to investigating its presence in different tumours. It has been shown by Southern blot analysis that the majority of genital warts (96 of 106 tested) contained sequences of HPV 6 or HPV 11 (Gissmann et al., 1982a, 1983; Ikenberg et al., unpublished data). The DNA of the latter was first isolated and cloned from a laryngeal papillomatosis (Gissmann et al., 1982b). The two viruses are closely related (Gissmann et al., 1982b) and no type-specific differences in clinical appearance or in the histological picture could be observed between the individual papillomas containing either virus (Gross et al., unpublished data). In what follows, therefore, the respective lesions will be classified as HPV-6 or HPV-11 positive. Of flat condylomas associated with dysplasias of different severity, 42% contained HPV 6 or HPV 11 which, in contrast, have been found only once in 29 cases of cervical carcinoma biopsies tested thus far (Gissmann et al., 1983; Ikenberg et al., unpublished data).

HUMAN PAPILLOMAVIRUSES IN CERVICAL CARCINOMA

As stated above, many of the different human papillomavirus DNAs do not cross-react with each other under hybridization conditions of high stringency (20°C below the denaturation temperature (T_m)). If the temperature of hybridization is lowered to 40°C below T_m, papillomavirus sequences of even more distantly related types can be detected (Howley et al., 1980; Gissmann, unpublished data). Under these conditions, two hitherto unknown human papillomaviruses, HPV 16 and HPV 18 were identified in two different cervical carcinomas (Dürst et al., 1983; Boshart et al., unpublished data). After cloning, the DNAs of these viruses could be used as probes to screen additional tumours by Southern blot analysis under stringent conditions of hybridization. It turned out that either HPV 16 or HPV 18 was present in only 6.1% of condylomata acuminata and 16.7% of flat condylomas but in 43.9% of carcinomata in situ and in 57.4% of cervical cancers (Dürst et al., 1983; Boshart et al., unpublished data; Ikenberg et al., unpublished data). This clearly shows a preferential association of these two viruses with malignant tumours and may indicate an elevated risk for patients infected with HPV 16 or HPV 18.

A similar correlation was found when epithelial cells of the cervix, as regularly taken for routine Papanicolaou smears, were hybridized in situ with HPV 11 and with a mixture of HPV 16 and HPV 18 (Gissmann et al., unpublished data). No positive reaction with HPV 16 or HPV 18 was seen in 36 different patients with normal Pap smears, in 6 out of 13 cases cytologically diagnosed as mild or moderate dysplasia, and in 15 out of 22 carcinomata in situ. HPV 6 or HPV 11 sequences were found in these materials at frequencies of 4/36, 6/13 or 4/22, respectively. It will be of interest to follow up those patients where a clear diagnosis could not be made from the Pap smear but which were positive for HPV 11 or for HPV 16 and HPV 18. It would be expected that only in the HPV-16/18 positive cases will definite dysplastic changes be observed within the next few months.

The fact that HPV 16 and HPV 18 DNA occurs only rarely in condylomata acuminata or flat condylomas excludes the possibility that the DNA derived from carcinomas which contain those sequences might have been contaminated by adjacent genital warts. On the other hand, it raises the question as to which primary lesions are induced by HPV 16 or HPV 18, especially in the male population. It is tempting to speculate that the very often inconspicuous but quite common Bowenoid papules on the glans penis or the vulva (Gross, personal communication) may represent the reservoir for virus spread, at least in the case of HPV 16, since viral sequences of this type could be found in the majority of such Bowenoid papulosis lesions (Ikenberg et al., 1983).

CONCLUSIONS

The high frequency of occurrence of certain papillomaviruses within human genital carcinomas does not, of course, per se prove that they have a causative role in tumour development. Epidemiological data clearly indicate that other factors are involved, e.g., herpes simplex virus infection, which may act synergistically with these viruses in cell transformation (zur Hausen, 1982). Present knowledge of the specific virus-cell interactions concerned, however, is still inadequate and additional studies on the biological features of the papillomaviruses in vivo and in vitro are required to improve our understanding of their role in human genital cancer.

REFERENCES

Dürst, M., Gissmann, L., Ikenberg, H. & zur Hausen, H. (1983) A papillomavirus DNA from a cervical carcinoma and its prevalence in cancer biopsies from different geographic regions. Proc. natl Acad. Sci. USA, 60, 3812-3825

Gissmann, L. (1984) Papillomaviruses and their association with cancer in animals and in man. Cancer Surv. (in press)

Gissmann, L. & Schwarz, E. (1984) Cloning papillomavirus DNA. Dev. mol. Virol., 5 (in press)

Gissmann, L., Pfister, H. & zur Hausen, H. (1977) Human papillomaviruses (HPV): Characterization of four different isolates. Virology, 76, 569-580

Gissmann, L., de Villiers, E.M. & zur Hausen, H. (1982a) Analysis of human genital warts (condylomata acuminata) and other genital tumors for human papillomaviruses type 6 DNA. Int. J. Cancer, 29, 140-143

Gissmann, L., Diehl, V., Schultz-Coulon, H.J. & zur Hausen, H. (1982b) Molecular cloning and characterization of human papillomavirus DNA derived from a laryngeal papilloma. J. Virol., 44, 393-400

Gissmann, L., Wolnik, L., Ikenberg, H., Koldovsky, U., Schnürch, H.G. & zur Hausen, H. (1983) Human papillomavirus type 6 and 11 DNA sequences in genital and laryngeal papillomas and in some cervical cancers. Proc. natl Acad. Sci. USA, 80, 560-563

Howley, P.M., Law, M.F., Heilman, C., Engel, L., Alonso, M.C., Israel, M.A. & Lowy, D.R. (1980) Molecular characterization of papillomavirus genomes. In: Essex, M., Todaro, G. & zur Hausen, H., eds, Viruses in Naturally Occurring Cancers (Cold Spring Harbor Conferences on Cell Proliferation, Vol. 7), Cold Spring Harbor, NY, Cold Spring Harbor Laboratory, pp. 233-247

Ikenberg, H., Gissmann, L., Gross, G., Gruszendorf-Conen, E.I. & zur Hausen, H. (1983) Human papillomavirus type 16 related DNA in genital Bowen's disease and in Bowenoid papulosis. Int. J. Cancer, 32, 563-565

Martin, C.E. (1967) Epidemiology of cancer of the cervix. II. Marital and coital factors in cervical cancer. Am. J. Public Health, 57, 803-814

Meisels, A. & Fortin, R. (1976) Condylomatous lesions of the cervix and vagina. I. Cytological patterns. Acta Cytol., 20, 505-509

Meisels, A., Morin, C. & Casas-Cordero, M. (1982) Human papillomavirus infection of the uterine cervix. Int. J. Gynecol. Pathol., 1, 75-94

Pfister, H. (1984) Biology and biochemistry of papillomaviruses. Rev. physiol. biochem. Pharmacol. (in press)

Purola, E. & Savia, E. (1977) Cytology of gynecologic condyloma acuminatum. Acta Cytol., 21, 26-31

Thomas, D.B. (1973) An epidemiologic study of carcinoma in situ and squamous dysplasia of the uterine cervix. Am. J. Epidemiol., 98, 10-28

zur Hausen, H. (1977) Human papillomaviruses and their possible role in squamous cell carcinomas. Curr. Top. Microbiol. Immunol., 78, 1-30

zur Hausen, H. (1982) Human genital cancer - synergism between
    two virus infections or synergism between a virus infection
    and initiating events. Lancet, 2, 1370-1372

zur Hausen, H. (1983)   Herpes simplex virus in human genital
    cancer. Int. Rev. exp. Path., 25, 307-325

zur Hausen, H., Meinhof, W., Schreiber, W. & Bornkamm, G.W.
    (1974) Attempts to detect virus-specific DNA sequences in
    human tumors: I. Nucleic acid hybridizations with
    complementary RNA of human wart virus. Int. J. Cancer, 13,
    650-656

EPIDEMIOLOGICAL ASPECTS OF CERVICAL CANCER
IN TROPICAL AFRICA

R. Schmauz & R. Owor

Institute of Pathology,
Medizinische Hochschule Lübeck
Lübeck, Federal Republic of Germany
and
Department of Pathology
Makerere University
Kampala, Uganda

RESUME

Le cancer du col utérin est une des tumeurs malignes les
plus communes en Afrique tropicale, et représente près d'un quart
des cas de cancers féminins en Ouganda. Il est vraisemblable que
tous les cas ne soient pas rapportés et les taux d'incidence disponibles sont probablement des sous-estimations grossières. La
transmission se fait par les contacts sexuels. La promiscuité
aussi bien féminine que masculine et une hygiène sexuelle insuf-
fisante entraînent une incidence élevée dans une communauté
donnée. Un certain nombre d'investigations montrent que le risque de cancer du col varie peu, que le partenaire masculin ait
été circoncis ou non, et ces résultats semblent indiquer seulement qu'une extrême propreté est plus efficace que la circoncision seule. Les populations de l'Ouganda qui pratiquent la circoncision ont une incidence plus faible que celles qui ne la
pratiquent pas, ce qui est en faveur de l'hypothèse selon
laquelle cette coutume confère une protection partielle. Le
virus Herpes simplex de type 2 (HSV-2) reste un agent cancérogène
possible, mais les résultats d'études séroépidémiologiques
comparant les titres d'anticorps dirigés contre ce virus de
malades et de témoins sont variables, non seulement en Ouganda,
mais aussi dans d'autres régions du monde. Les papillomavirus
humains jouent un rôle nettement plus important. Les analyses de
la répartition du cancer en Ouganda, selon la situation géographique et selon l'âge, basées sur les résultats d'un service de
biopsie couvrant tout le pays, montrent que les cáncers du col,

de la vulve, du vagin et du pénis partagent des étiologies
communes et sont liés aux verrues génitales. Récemment, un
certain nombre de papillomavirus différents ont été trouvés dans
différentes formes de néoplasmes spino-cellulaires de l'appareil
génital, et il serait intéressant de réaliser des études similaires en Afrique tropicale.

SUMMARY

Cervical cancer is one of the most common malignant tumours
in tropical Africa accounting, for example, for nearly one-
quarter of female cancer cases overall in Uganda. The disease is
likely to be under-reported and available incidence rates are
probably gross underestimates. Spread is through sexual
contacts. Both female and male promiscuity and a low standard of
sexual hygiene lead to a high incidence within a given community.
A number of investigations show that the risk of cervical cancer
varies little, whether or not the male partner has been circumcised, but these findings seem to indicate only that extreme
cleanliness is more effective than circumcision alone. Populations of Uganda who practise male circumcision have a lower
incidence than those who do not, favouring the view that partial
protection is provided by this custom. Herpes simplex virus type
2 remains a candidate oncogenic agent, but the results of comparative seroepidemiological surveys of titres among cases and
controls are inconsistent, not only in Uganda, but also in other
areas of the world. Human papillomaviruses are clearly more
important. Analyses of the geographical and age distribution of
cancer in Uganda, based on the results of a country-wide biopsy
service, show that cervical cancer and cancer of the vulva,
vagina, and penis share common causes and are related to genital
warts. Recently, a number of different papillomaviruses have
been found in various forms of squamous-cell neoplasia of the
genital tract, and similar studies would be worthwile in tropical
Africa.

***

It has been repeatedly suggested that a viral agent might be
the cause of cervical cancer (Rotkin, 1973, 1981). This is in
agreement with observations closely linking the risk of developing the disease with the sexual behavioural pattern of the
female. Recent investigations have added a considerable amount

of new information and show that this cancer can be viewed as a communicable disease which is transmitted sexually. This review attempts to discuss the more complete picture of this disease now available with special emphasis on tropical Africa.

RISK FACTORS

In the past, too much blame was placed on the female partner. Young age (under 18 years) at the time of first sexual contact and the number of sexual partners were considered to be the key variables which explain why multiple marriages, divorce, and prostitution carry an excess risk for the disease (Rotkin, 1973). Recent findings, however, show that the sexual behaviour of the male is just as important (Buckley et al., 1981; Singer et al., 1976). Even if she has no other sexual partners, the wife may contract the disease from a promiscuous husband who has had pre- or extra-marital relationships. In particular, the very high incidence of cervical cancer observed at the beginning of this century in Europe may be attributable to the former wide-spread habit of casual contacts with prostitutes (Skegg et al., 1982). Similarly, the advent of more liberal attitudes which have reduced the need to use prostitutes has contributed consi-derably to the present decrease in cervical cancer in Western countries. Other factors responsible for the decline are the increasing number of hysterectomies and cytology screening pro-grammes (Doll & Peto, 1981). The usefulness of the latter is beyond doubt (Clark & Anderson, 1979), but often overestimated; a marked change in incidence was observed before the Second World War, long before such preventive measures were instituted. The general standard of cleanliness has also improved considerably, and this should also be taken into consideration. Indirect evidence is adduced in one investigation which shows that the dental hygiene of patients with cervical cancer is much poorer than among patients with other female genital cancers (Keller et al., 1979).

Religion can have a major impact on the way of life. The classic finding of an extremely low incidence of cervical cancer among nuns was the first clue to the nature of the disease (Scotto & Bailar, 1969; Fraumeni et al., 1969). The low frequencies observed in North America among the Mormons and the Amish (Gardner & Lyon, 1977; Cross et al., 1968) seem to be attributable to stable marital relationships and the rarity of contacts with individuals from other social groups. These examples demonstrate that endemicity of transmissible agents is an important determinant of cervical cancer in any population. A closed society and a relationship with one partner only throughout life characterize the Orang Asli aborigines who live in the jungle of Malaysia. Sexual activity starts early, but under such conditions spread of infectious agents is minimal, as is the incidence of cervical cancer (Sumithran, 1976).

The low incidence of cervical cancer in Jewish women has still to be explained. The disease is still rare in Israel (Katz & Steinitz, 1977) (Table 1), even in the younger generation, where an increase has been observed recently in Western societies (MacGregor & Teper, 1978). Because of this low incidence among Jews, circumcision of the male newborn was once believed to offer full protection (Garvin & Persky, 1966). However, there are communities in Lebanon and in Fiji where circumcised Moslems live together with uncircumcised Christians or immigrant Hindus, and no differences could be detected between such groups in the overall low and moderately high incidence of cervical cancer, respectively (Abou-Daoud, 1967; Boyd et al., 1973). However, an earlier report had found a higher incidence in the Indians of Fiji than in the natives who practise circumcision (Lyster, 1967). In Western countries, case-control studies show that the circumcision status of the husband does not appreciably alter the risk of cervical cancer in the female partner (Dunn & Buell, 1959; Rotkin, 1973), and there are areas in Africa where cervical cancer is common in spite of male circumcision (Huber, 1960). Can these inconsistent findings be reconciled by the confounding effect of personal hygiene? The Lugbara of Uganda, who are uncircumcised but have a high standard of cleanliness and a low incidence of both cervical and penile cancer (Cook-Mozzafari, 1981; Schmaux & Jain, 1971), can be taken as an example to show that extreme cleanliness is more effective than circumcision. That this practice may be of some value is shown by the fact that the highest incidence rates of cervical cancer are recorded from parts of the world where all men are uncircumcised, namely Latin America, the Caribbean, and the Hindu societies of India (Parkin et al., 1984; Wahi et al., 1969). Similarly, the proportional incidence of cervical cancer was markedly lower in the tribes of Uganda that practise circumcision as compared to those that do not (Dodge et al., 1973).

Features of cervical cancer in Africa that are frequently quoted include the extremely high incidence, the early onset among young persons, and an early peak in age distribution (Ojwang & Mati, 1978). Reports from a number of cancer registries, however, do not confirm these impressions, which were derived from patients seen in hospital (Table 1). Throughout Africa, the incidence appears to be only moderately high and similar to rates recorded from Europe. Nothing corresponding to the epidemic in Colombia has been found. As would be expected from the increase among young people in Europe (MacGregor & Teper, 1978), a very early onset of cervical cancer is observed in Birmingham, England, and in the German Democratic Republic. In Africa, considerable differences are found between the areas surveyed, and the late onset seen in Bulawayo, Zimbabwe, and in Ibadan, Nigeria, is remarkable. While a peak incidence in middle age is found both in European and African countries, peak incidences rates among the old, as observed in Asia and South America, were not recorded by the African registries. Apart from geographical variations in incidence patterns, shortcomings in reporting may account for the discrepancy between clinical observations and the findings of the cancer registries. Under-reporting of cancer in a deep site such as the uterine cervix is probably very marked in tropical Africa. This is in part due to lack of trained medical personnel, so that many cases remain undiagnosed, but also to the reluctance of people to attend hospital, particularly among the elderly. When an allowance is made for such distortions, the incidence in some regions of Uganda seems to be as high as 30 or 40 per 100 000 per year (Cook-Mozzafari, 1982). When rates from cytology laboratories are compared, cervical cancer is about 10 times more prevalent in Kampala than in Quebec (Table 2). The incidence would therefore amount to 108 per 100 000 per year. Admittedly, this incredibly high rate may be inflated since the comparison is only approximate and not standardized. However, the possibility remains that in some parts of tropical Africa cervical cancer is a very common disease and probably nearly as frequent as liver cancer, the most common type of cancer in the Third World (Parkin et al., 1984).

Table 1. Epidemiological features of cervical cancer in tropical
Africa and world-widea

Age at onset and cancer registry[b]	Peak incidence[c]	Age-group	Overall incidence[d]
10-14 years			
German Democratic Republic (1975)	79.4	55-59	30.1
Birmingham, UK (1975)	37.4	55-59	12.0
15-19 years			
Poona, India (1975)	93.4	55-59	30.4
Senegal (1972)	67.4	50-59	17.2
Quebec (1975)	38.0	65-69	10.8
20-24 years			
Cali, Colombia (1974)	205.0	75+	52.9
Maputo, Mozambique (1956)	94.3	55-59	22.5
Kyadondo, Uganda (1957)	71.4	55-59	18.1
Miyagi, Japan (1975)	71.6	75+	12.1
25-29 years			
Bulawayo, Zimbabwe (1970)	222.2	60-64	28.4
Shanghai, China (1975)	111.4	75+	22.1
Ibadan, Nigeria (1965)	98.1	60-64	21.9
Israel: Jews born in Europe and America (1974)	21.8	75+	3.8
30-34 years			
Varese, Italy (1976)	52.0	55-59	11.7

[a] Source: Doll et al., 1966, 1970; Waterhouse et al., 1976, 1982

[b] Midpoint of the time-period of the survey in parentheses

[c] Age-specific rate per 100 000 per year

[d] Age-adjusted rate (world standard population) per 100 000 per year

Table 2. Prevalence of precancerous and cancerous lesions of the uterine cervix recorded in cytology laboratoriesa

Type of lesion	Quebec (1976)	Munich (1976)	Kampala (1964-1971)
CIN I + II	5.1	4.2	13.0
CIN III	0.8	1.6	7.0
Invasive cancer	0.7	0.3	6.0

a Source: Meisels et al., 1977; Soost et al., 1982; Leighton et al., 1975. Figures are crude rates per 1000 vaginal smears. CIN = cervical intraepithelial neoplasia

ROLE OF VIRUSES AND BACTERIA

Ever since its isolation from the smegma of males (Rawls 1968) herpes simplex virus type 2 (HSV-2) has been a candidate virus for cervical cancer.   Several observations indicate that HSV-2 might be able to initiate cervical neoplasia (zur Hausen, 1982).   However, the main objection to such an association is that, in contrast to human papillomaviruses (HPV) viral DNA has been found within the cancer cells in only one case (Frenkel et al., 1972). Furthermore, many studies have shown a steady increase in the proportional frequency of HSV-2 antibody titres among cases of intraepithelial neoplasia and invasive cancer as compared to controls, but an early study in Uganda (Adam et al., 1972) and recent investigations in several different countries (Mendis et al., 1981) and in Czechoslovakia (Vonka et al., 1984) have failed to confirm this relationship. Chlamydia trachomatis has been implicated in a small proportion of cases.   Titres against this bacterial organism have been found in 8 and 18% of cases with intraepithelial and invasive squamous-cell neoplasia, respectively, but only in 1% of controls (Hare et al., 1982). Whether administration of tetracycline will lead both to a reduction in infection and to the regression of neoplastic changes, is under investigation. At present, the evidence is undoubtedly strongest in favour of HPV as a promoter of cervical cancer (zur Hausen, 1982). Several types of viral DNA have been identified in the various forms of squamous-cell neoplasia of the uterine cervix, vulva and vagina, and the penis, while HPV-6, -10 and -11 were found mainly in genital warts and dysplasias, and HPV-16 and -18 in various cancers (Dürst et al., 1983; Gissmann, this volume).

CHEMICAL CARCINOGENS

An important finding is that women who have had cancer of the uterine cervix have a 4-5-fold excess risk for cancer of the lung, the larynx and the oral cavity (Newell et al., 1975), which points to a common cause of these cancers. It is not surprising, therefore, that several case-control studies have now shown an association between cigarette smoking and cervical cancer (Helberg et al., 1983). This habit may produce tumours either by immunosuppression (Burton, 1983) and/or by direct action of the carcinogen, which may perhaps be excreted and concentrated in the cervical mucus. Constituents of sperm and smegma have repeatedly been implicated. An altered protamin ratio in the head of the spermatozoa might also be a factor (Reid et al., 1978). In mice, painting of the skin and the uterine cervix with smegma produced squamous-cell carcinomas, although a chemical carcinogen could not be isolated (Wynder, 1972). In a promiscuous male, smegma probably contains both herpesviruses (Rawls et al., 1968) and papillomaviruses, in addition to remnants of the ejaculate. Chemical agents cannot account for the transmissibility of cervical cancer, but may still be the sole cause in occasional patients. At present, the majority, but not all cases can be related to a viral infection (zur Hausen, 1982; Gissmann, this volume).

GEOGRAPHICAL ASSOCIATION WITH OTHER TUMOURS

An association has been reported between cervical and penile cancer both world-wide and in China (Sorahan & Crombie, 1981; Li 1982). In Africa, the quality of the medical services available varies markedly and reporting of cervical cancer is much more likely to be distorted than that of penile cancer, a readily accessible disease. A hospital survey carried out in East

Africa, Zambia and Malawi, perhaps for this reason, found only a slight association between the two diseases (Cook-Mozzafari, 1982). In Uganda, a small country with marked variations in climate and ethnic composition and, at the time of the survey, well developed hospital services, much more accurate regional patterns of cancer incidence were determined for many sites including the penis, thanks to a country-wide biopsy service (Hutt & Burkitt, 1965; Schmauz & Jain, 1971). When the geographical distributions were compared for the 18 districts of the country, the correlation was very marked, not only between penile and cervical, but also between vulvar and vaginal cancer (Schmauz et al., 1984). This shows clearly that cancer of the lower female genital tract and the penis is an entity with common causes applicable to both sexes. It should be noted, however, that differences do also exist. By far the highest incidence is found for the uterine cervix, where nearly twice as many cases were recorded as for the penis (Table 1). Vulvar and vaginal cancer are seen only rarely; the frequency of these two tumours is less than 10% of that of cervical cancer. A possible explanation is that the transformation zone found in the uterine cervix but not in the external genitalia, has a much higher turnover of epithelial cells, and this may render the cervical squamous-cell layer much more vulnerable (Coppleson, 1970).

In addition to malignant tumours, the biopsy service, which was used extensively by the many hospitals throughout Uganda, collected any lesion requiring excision, including cases of genital warts (condylomata acuminata). Again, very markedly similar geographical distributions were noted for these warts and for cases of cancer of the vulva, vagina, cervix uteri, and penis (Schmauz & Owor, 1980a; Schmauz et al., 1983). As cervical condylomata acuminata are recorded only rarely in biopsy services, vulvar and vaginal condylomata were used instead for the comparison with cervical cancer. This seems justifiable, since vulvovaginal lesions often extend to the cervix uteri. To exclude the possibility that these associations merely reflect differences in practices in taking biopsies, genital warts were also compared with other malignant tumours seen frequently in Uganda. Except for Kaposi's sarcoma among men, these correlations always had lower coefficients, and were not statistically significant in the case of Burkitt's lymphoma and cancer of skin of leg. These findings are in line with the suggestion made a long time ago that genital warts can undergo malignant degeneration (Buschke & Löwenstein, 1931), and indicate that the viral agent(s) underlying these lesions may produce squamous-cell

genital cancer. Further epidemiological support for this conclusion is obtained from investigations which found a higher frequency of both warts and cervical cancer among immunosuppressed
renal transplant recipients (Schneider et al., 1983).

When these associations were explored in Israel by again
using the biopsy records of a pathology department, it was found
that genital warts are not more common on the glans of the circumcised penis than the extremely rare cases of cancer, whereas
on the vulva both warts and cases of cancer were recorded much
more frequently (Schmauz & Schachter, 1982). In males, the
penile urethra was the most frequent site of genital warts, but
cases of cancer were encountered as rarely as on the glans of the
penis. In genital sites, therefore, the risk of malignant degeneration appears to be higher than in the urethra, where wart
virus infection alone only rarely leads to cancer. For such a
progression, additional factors seem to be required, and since
the urethra is always kept clean by the urinary flow, the low
incidence of cancer in that site favours the long held view that
lack of hygiene is important. The other conclusion is that the
male urethra might harbour and transmit oncogenic agents, and
this might explain why in many populations there is a high
incidence of cervical cancer in spite of the widespread practice
of circumcision among males (Huber, 1960).

AGE DISTRIBUTION OF GENITAL WARTS AND CANCER

Age distribution is another classical tool for assessing
relationships. Genital warts are a heterogeneous group of
lesions showing a bimodal age distribution. Analyses of biopsy
reports from pathology departments in three different countries,
namely in Kampala, Uganda, Jerusalem, Israel, and Lübeck, Federal
Republic of Germany, showed that genital warts of the external
genitalia occur not only in young age-groups, but also in a
smaller proportion of the middle-aged (Schmauz & Schachtner,
1982). The warts preceded the development of cancer by decades
and years, respectively, which suggests a low risk of malignant
change in young people and a higher risk among the elderly. A
recent report from the north-west of the United States (Chuang et
al., 1984) confirmed the observation of the bimodal age distribution of condylomata acuminata first described for cases in Uganda
(Fig. 1; Schmauz & Owor, 1976). Subsequent histological review
of the African cases revealed 7 types of warts varying to some
extent in age distribution and thus reflecting the diversity of

FIG. 1. AGE-DISTRIBUTION OF CONDYLOMATA ACUMINATA
AND CANCER OF THE VULVA, VAGINA, AND PENIS IN UGANDA
OVER THE PERIOD 1964-1968

The cases were taken from the files of the country-wide biopsy
service (Schmauz & Owor, 1976). The lack of a second group of
cases for vulva and vagina can be explained by deficiencies in
ascertainment.

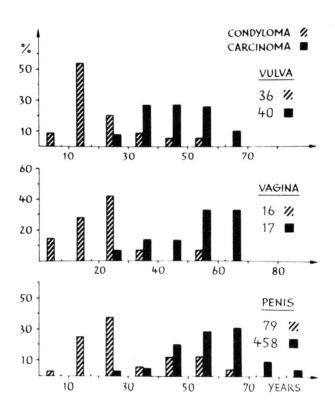

these tumours and the differences in the risk of developing
cancer (Schmauz & Owor, 1980b). In young persons, changes
resembling those of a cytocidal viral infection were most frequent, namely, isolated cell necroses and cytoplasmic vacuolation, whereas atypias and proliferative changes predominated
among the elderly. Concerted efforts would seem worthwhile to
relate the many types of HPV to particular condylomatous lesions
in the genital area.

For the cervix uteri, the age distribution of warts showed only one peak around the age of 20 (Meisels et al., 1977). Further groups of lesions occurring in middle age, as seen on the external genitalia, have not been demonstrated. This difference, however, only reflects differences in categorization. Cervical warts, mainly flat and composed of cells showing cytoplasmic vacuolation (Meisels et al., 1977; Purola & Savia, 1977), do not encompass precancerous lesions, as on the external genitalia, where warts are seen mainly as condylomata acuminata and defined by the macroscopic appearance of a papillary tumour alone. Many cases of dysplasia and carcinoma in situ of the uterine cervix have been shown to contain HPV DNA (zur Hausen, 1982; Gissmann, this volume), and are therefore warty lesions. If included, the age distribution of warty precursor lesions would be similar throughout the genital tract, and could be used to distinguish between a number of groups varying in risk of subsequent cancer.

CONCLUSIONS

Since cervical cancer is very common in at least some areas of tropical Africa, it is important that the patterns of frequency should be determined more accurately and comparisons made between areas of low and high incidence so as to gain an insight into the nature of the disease. This could be done conveniently through cytology laboratories; the establishment of such laboratories should therefore be encouraged. It is likely that cervical cancer and its precursor lesions are to some extent different diseases in tropical Africa; thus cigarette smoking is not so widespread as to contribute substantially to the high incidence rates. Among cases collected in the Federal Republic of Germany, traces of papillomaviruses were found in nearly 70%; in tumour tissue from Kenyan patients, however, this frequency amounted only to 30% (Dürst et al., 1983). Since the different papillomaviruses appear to give rise to distinct types of tumours, histological comparisons between African and European cases may provide further etiological clues. Sexual life-styles need to be explored in order to identify both the individuals and the communities at high risk. The decrease in the overall incidence noted in Western countries shows that, with the inevitable advent of social change, the overall risk of cervical cancer may diminish, while increasing in particular groups, as in young people in those same countries.

ACKNOWLEDGEMENTS

This work was supported by the Deutsche Forschungsgemeinschaft (Schm 392/6-1).

REFERENCES

Abou-Daoud, K.T. (1967) Epidemiology of carcinoma of the cervix uteri in Lebanese Christians and Moslems. Cancer, 20, 1706-1714

Adam, E., Sharma, S.D., Zeigler, O., Iwamoto, K., Melnick, J.L., Levy, A.H. & Rawls, W.E. (1972) Seroepidemiologic studies of herpesvirus type 2 and carcinoma of the cervix. II. Uganda. J. natl Cancer Inst., 48, 65-72

Boyd, J.T., Doll, R. & Gurd, C.H. (1973) Cancer incidence in Fiji. Int. J. Epidemiol., 2, 177-187

Buckley, J.D., Harris, R.W.C., Doll, R., Vessey, M.P. & Williams, P.T. (1981) Case-control study of the husbands of women with dysplasia or carcinoma of the cervix uteri. Lancet, 2, 1010-1015

Burton, R.C. (1983) Smoking, immunity and cancer. Med. J. Aust., 2, 411-412

Buschke, A. & Löwenstein, L. (1931) Beziehungen der spitzen Kondylome zu den Karzinomen des Penis. Dermat. Syph., 163, 31-46

Chuang, T.-Y., Perry, H.O., Kurland, L.T. & Ilstrup, D.M. (1984) Condyloma acuminatum in Rochester, Minn. 1950-1978. I. Epidemiology and clinical features. Arch. Dermatol., 120, 469-475

Clark, E.A. & Anderson, T.W. (1979) Does screening by "Pap" smears help prevent cervical cancer? A case-control study. Lancet, 2, 1-6

Cook-Mozzafari, P. (1982) Symposium on tumours in the tropics. Carcinomas of the oesophagus, bladder, cervix uteri and penis. Trans. Roy. Soc. trop. Med. Hyg., 76, 157-163

Coppleson, M. (1970) The origin and nature of premalignant lesions of the cervix uteri. Int. J. Gynecol. Obstet., 8, 539-550

Cross, H.E., Kennel, E.E. & Lilienfeld, A. (1968) Cancer of the cervix in an Amish population. Cancer, 21, 102-108

Dodge, O.G., Owor, R. & Templeton, A.C. (1973) Tumours of the male genitalia. Recent Results Cancer Res., 41, 132-144

Doll, R., Payne, & Waterhouse, J., eds (1966) Cancer Incidence in Five Continents, Berlin, Heidelberg, New York, Springer-Verlag

Doll, R., Muir, C. & Waterhouse, J., eds (1970) Cancer Incidence in Five Continents, Vol. II, Berlin, Heidelberg, New York, Springer-Verlag

Doll, R. & Peto, R. (1981) The Causes of Cancer, Oxford, Oxford Medical Publications, p. 1290

Dunn, J.E., Jr & Buell, P. (1959) Association of cervical cancer with circumcision of sexual partner. J. natl Cancer Inst., 22, 749-764

Dürst, M., Gissmann, L., Ikenberg, H. & zur Hausen, H. (1983) A papillomavirus DNA from a cervical carcinoma and its prevalence in cancer biopsy samples from different geographic regions. Proc. natl Acad. Sci. USA, 80, 3812-3815

Fraumeni, J.F., Lloyd, J.W., Smith, E.M. & Wagoner, J.K. (1969) Cancer mortality among nuns: role of marital status in etiology of neoplastic disease in women. J. natl Cancer Inst., 42, 455-468

Frenkel, N., Roizman, B., Casai, E. & Nahmias, A. (1972) A DNA fragment and its transcription in human cervical cancer tissue. Proc. natl Acad. Sci. USA, 69, 3734-3789

Gardner, J.W. & Lyon, J.L. (1977) Low incidence of cervical cancer in Utah. Gynecol. Oncol., 5, 68-80

Garvin, C.H. & Persky, L. (1966) Circumcision: Is it justified in infancy? J. natl Med. Assoc., 58, 233-238

Hare, M.J., Taylor-Robinson, D. & Cooper, P. (1982) Evidence for an association between Chlamydia trachomatis and cervical intraepithelial neoplasia. Br. J. Obstet. Gynaecol., 89, 489-492

zur Hausen, H. (1982) Human genital cancer: synergism between two virus infections or synergism between a virus infection and initiating events? Lancet, 2, 1370-1372

Helberg, D., Valentin, J. & Nilsson, S. (1983) Smoking as a risk factor in cervical neoplasia. Lancet, 2, 1497

Huber, A. (1960) Uteruskarzinom und Zirkumzision. Wien med. Wschr., 110, 571-574

Hutt, M.S.R. & Burkitt, D.P. (1965) Geographical distribution of cancer in East Africa: A new clinico-pathological approach. Br. med. J., 2, 719-722

Katz, L. & Steinitz, R. (1977) Cancer in Israel. Facts and Figures, 1967-1971, Jerusalem, Ministry of Health

Keller, E., Schmelzle, R., Meier, W. & Schindler, A.E. (1979) Mundhygiene bei Frauen mit Genitalkarzinom. Arch. Gynecol., 228, 441-442

Leighton, P.C., Zeigler, O., Trussel, R.R. & Sharma, S.D. (1975) Cervical cytology in a developing country. Trop. Doctor, 5, 79-83

Li, J.-Y., Li, F.P., Blot, W.J., Miller, R.W. & Fraumeni, J.F. (1982) Correlation between cancers of the uterine cervix and penis in China. J. natl Cancer Inst., 69, 1063-1065

Lyster, W. (1967) Uterine cancer in the circumcised and uncircumcised populations of Fiji. Med. J. Aust., 2, 993

MacGregor, J.E. & Teper, S. (1978) Mortality from carcinoma of cervix uteri in Britain. Lancet, 1, 774-776

Meisels, A., Fortin, R. & Roy, M. (1977) Condylomatous lesions of the cervix. II. Cytologic, colposcopic and histopathologic study. Acta Cytol., 21, 379-390

Mendis, L.N., Best, J.M., Senarath, L., Chiphangwi, J., Vestergaard, B.F. & Banatvala, J.E. (1981) A geographical study of antibodies to membrane antigens of HSV-2 infected cells and HSV-2-specific antibodies in patients with cervical cancer. Int. J. Cancer, 28, 535-542

Newell, G.R., Krementz, E.T. & Roberts, J.D. (1975) Excess occurrence of cancer of the oral cavity, lung, and bladder following cancer of the cervix. Cancer, 36, 2155-2158

Ojwang, S.B.O. & Mati, J.K. (1978) Carcinoma of the cervix in Kenya. East Afr. med. J., 55, 194-198

Parkin, P.M., Muir, C.S. & Stjernswärd, J. (1984) Estimates of the world-wide frequencies of 12 major cancers. Bull. World Health Org., 62, 163-182

Purola, E. & Savia, E. (1977) Cytology of gynecologic condyloma acuminatum. Acta Cytol., 21, 26-31

Rawls, W.E., Laurel, D., Melnick, J.L., Glicksman, J.M. & Kaufman, R.H. (1968) A search for viruses in smegma, premalignant and early malignant cervical tissues. The isolation of herpesviruses with distinct antigenic properties. Am. J. Epidemiol., 87, 647-655

Reid, B.L., Singer, A. & Hagan, B.E. (1978) Sperm basic proteins in cervical carcinogenesis: Correlation with socioeconomic class. Lancet, 2, 60-62

Rotkin, I.D. (1973) A comparison review of key epidemiological studies in cervical cancer related to current searches for transmissible agents. Cancer Res., 33, 1353-1367

Rotkin, I.D. (1981) Etiology and epidemiology of cervical cancer. Curr. Top Pathol., 70, 82-110

Schmauz, R. & Jain, D.K. (1971) Geographical variation of carcinoma of the penis in Uganda. Br. J. Cancer, 25, 25-32

Schmauz, R. & Owor, R. (1976) Altersverteilung der spitzen Condylome und der Carcinome der Vulva, Vagina und des Penis. Verh. Dtsch. Ges. Pathol., 60, 458

Schmauz, R. & Owor, R. (1980a) Epidemiology of malignant degeneration of condylomata acuminata in Uganda. Pathol. Res. Pract., 170, 91-103

Schmauz, R. & Owor, R. (1980b) Condylomatous tumours of vulva, vagina, and penis. Relation between histological appearance and age. J. clin. Pathol., 33, 1039-1046

Schmauz, R. & Schachter, A. (1982) Geographical clues from Israel for a relationship between condylomata acuminata and cancer. In: Gundmann, E., Clemmesen, J. & Muir, C.S., eds, Geographical Pathology in Cancer Epidemiology, Stuttgart, New York, Gustav Fischer Verlag, pp. 249-253

Schmauz, R., Claussen, C.P., Cordes, B. & Owor, R. (1983) Genital warts and their possible relationship to cancer of the uterine cervix. Case report and geographical observations. Acta Cytol., 27, 533-539

Schmauz, R., Owor, R. & Schachter, A. (1984) Condylomata acuminata and squamous cell genital cancer. The patho-anatomical and epidemiological basis. J. Cancer Res. clin. Oncol. (in press)

Schneider, V., Kay, S. & Lee, H.M. (1983) Immunosuppression: High risk factor for the development of condyloma acuminatum and squamous neoplasia of the cervix. Acta Cytol., 27, 220-224

Scotto, J. & Bailar, J.C. (1969) Rigoni-Stern and medical statistics. A ninteenth century approach to cancer research. J. Hist. Med., 24, 65-75

Singer, A., Reid, B.L. & Coppleson, M. (1976) A hypothesis: the role of a high risk male in the etiology of cervical carcinoma. Am. J. Obstet. Gynecol., 126, 110-115

Skegg, D.C.G., Corvin, P.A., Paul, C. & Doll, R. (1982) Impor-
    tance of the male factor in cancer of the cervix. Lancet,
    2, 581-583

Soost, H.-J., Bockmühl, B. & Zock, H. (1982) Results of cyto-
    logical mass screening in the Federal Republic of Germany.
    Acta Cytol., 26, 445-451

Sorahan, T. & Crombie, I.K. (1981) Cancer of the cervix and
    cancer of penis. Lancet, 2, 1419-1420

Steinitz, R. (1976) Israel. In: Waterhouse, J., Muir, C.S.,
    Correa, P. & Powell, J., eds, Cancer Incidence in Five
    Continents. III, Lyon, International Agency for Research on
    Cancer, pp. 248-267

Sumithran, E. (1976) Rarity of cancer of the cervix in Malaysian
    Orang Asli despite the presence of known risk factors.
    Cancer, 39, 1570-1572

Vonka, V., Kanka, J., Hirsch, J., Zadova, H., Krcmar, M.,
    Suchankova, A., Rezacova, D., Broucek, J., Press, M.,
    Domorazkova, E., Svoboda, B., Havrankova, A. & Jelinek, J.
    (1984) Prospective study on the relationship between
    cervical neoplasia and herpes simplex type 2 virus. II.
    Herpes simplex type 2 antibody presence taken at enrolment.
    Int. J. Cancer, 33, 61-66

Wahi, P.N., Saraswati, M. & Luthra, V.K. (1969) Factors influ-
    encing cancer of the uterine cervix in North India. Cancer,
    23, 1221-1226

Waterhouse, J., Muir, C., Correa, P. & Powell, J., eds (1976)
    Cancer Incidence in Five Continents, Vol. III (IARC Scien-
    tific Publications No. 15), Lyon, International Agency for
    Research on Cancer

Waterhouse, J., Muir, C., Shanmugaratnam, K. & Powell, J., eds
    (1982) Cancer Incidence in Five Continents, Vol. IV (IARC
    Scientific Publications No. 42), Lyon, International Agency
    for Research on Cancer

Wynder, E.L. (1972) <u>Die Epidemiologie des Korpus- (Endometrium-)</u> <u>und Zervixkarzinoms</u>. In: Käser, O., Friedberg, F., Ober, K.G., Thomsen, K. & Zander, J., eds, <u>Gynäkologie und</u> <u>Geburtshilfe</u>, Vol. III, Stuttgart, Georg Thieme Verlag

CARCINOMA OF THE CERVIX:
CAN A VIRAL ETIOLOGY BE CONFIRMED?

B. Adelusi

Department of Obstetrics and Gynaecology
College of Medicine
University College Hospital
Ibadan, Nigeria

RESUME

Le rôle étiologique des virus dans les cancers des animaux est maintenant bien établi. Un rôle similaire dans les cancers humains reste encore à confirmer. En effet, jusqu'à une période toute récente, les infections virales n'étaient considérées comme responsables que d'une faible proportion de la pathologie humaine; et rien n'indiquait que les virus puissent être des agents étiologiques des tumeurs malignes chez les humains. L'introduction des techniques d'immunovirologie les plus avancées a permis de mieux comprendre et de mieux définir le rôle des virus dans des syndromes dont l'étiologie était jusque-là obscure.

En 1964, l'Emory University Group a émis pour la première fois l'hypothèse d'une association entre l'infection par les virus Herpès simplex (HSV) et le cancer du col, à la suite d'une étude effectuée sur un enfant présentant une infection néonatale par le HSV et sur sa mère présentant une infection du col de l'utérus par le HSV. Cette hypothèse reposait sur l'observation selon laquelle les femmes porteuses du HSV génital (HSV de type-2 ou HSV-2) ont une fréquence du cancer du col plus élevée que les autres femmes. Des enquêtes démographiques sur le cancer du col ont suggéré que la maladie pouvait se transmettre par voie sexuelle.

De même, on a montré que l'infection par le HSV-2 est sexuellement transmissible. On a alors postulé que ce virus pouvait être un agent cancérigène, initiateur ou promoteur, transmis à la femme pendant l'acte sexuel.

Par des approches multicentriques effectuées à différents
niveaux, allant des études épidémiologiques aux études molécu-
laires on a tenté de confirmer cette association. Bien qu'on ait
accumulé des preuves indirectes à la suite de recherches
intensives, on n'a pu établir aucune relation définitive de cause
à effet entre le virus et le cancer du col. La question se pose
cependant de savoir s'il est possible de confirmer une
association étiologique entre le virus et la maladie.

Des études complémentaires sont nécessaires. L'isolement,
la purification et la caractérisation des antigènes associés à la
tumeur du col, leur comparaison aux antigènes du HSV-2 pourraient
aider à démontrer cette association.

SUMMARY

The etiological role of viruses in various animal cancers is
no longer in doubt; a similar role in human cancers is, however,
yet to be confirmed. Indeed, until recently, virus infections
were considered to be responsible for only a small proportion of
the clinical states encountered in humans and the view that
viruses may be etiological agents for human malignant tumours was
not seriously entertained. With the introduction of more
advanced techniques in immunovirology, the role of viruses in
clinical syndromes the etiology of which had been obscure became
clearer.

The Emory University Group first postulated in 1964 an association between herpes simplex virus (HSV) infection and cervical
neoplasia, following studies of an infant with neonatal HSV
infection and his mother's cervical HSV infection. This postulate was based on the observation that women with genital HSV
(herpes simplex virus type-2 (HSV-2)) infection have a greater
frequency of cervical neoplasia than women in the general
population. Demographic surveys of cancer of the cervix have
established patterns of high risk that strongly suggest that the
disease may be transmitted venereally. Similarly, evidence has
accumulated to show that HSV-2 is a sexually transmitted disease.
It has thus been postulated that this virus may be an initiating
or promoting carcinogenic factor transmitted to the female during
sexual intercourse.

Various multicentric approaches, from epidemiological studies to molecular studies, have been employed to substantiate this association. Even though the weight of circumstantial evidence supporting the role of HSV-2 in human carcinoma of the cervix has increased, no definitive 'cause-and-effect' association has been established between the virus and carcinoma of the cervix. The question arises, therefore, whether or not an etiological association between the virus and the disease can be confirmed. To prove a definitive cause-and-effect relationship, further studies will be required, such as the recent demonstration of the involvement of papillomavirus.

INTRODUCTION

The role of herpesviruses in the etiology of certain animal cancers is no longer in doubt. It is now known, for example, that Marek's disease, a contagious lymphoproliferative and neuropathic disease of the domestic fowl, is caused by Group-B cell-associated herpesviruses (Churchill & Biggs, 1967; Solomon et al., 1968; Nazerian et al., 1968). Apart from the development of antigen-antibody reactions in affected fowls (Chubb & Churchill, 1968), experimental laboratory studies have shown that attenuated strains of Marek's disease virus have been able to offer a considerable degree of protection against later infection with a virulent strain of the virus (Churchill et al., 1969; Edison & Anderson, 1971; von Bulow, 1971). In like manner, the etiological role of another group of herpesviruses in the pathology of the renal adenocarcinoma of the North American leopard frog has been demonstrated by Fawcett (1956). Other confirmatory evidence has been presented associating this virus with the Lucké renal tumour (Granoff et al., 1965, 1969; McKinnell & Tweedell, 1970).

Even though the first indication that herpesviruses might be oncogenic dates back to 1956 (Fawcett, 1956), it is only in recent years that such viruses have been recognized as candidate oncogenic agents of man. Indeed, Cowdry (1964), as late as 1964, believed that, while it would be foolish to deny the possibility that man, like the lower animals, might occasionally be afflicted with 'cancer viruses', there was little reason to seriously entertain the view that viruses might be etiological agents in human malignant tumours.

However, studies by the group at Emory University School of Medicine, Atlanta, Georgia, USA, of an infant with neonatal herpes simplex virus (HSV) infection, together with the mother's cervical HSV infection, provided the first clue of an association between the virus and cervical carcinoma (CaCx). This was based on the premise that women with cytologically detected genital herpes had a greater frequency of cervical neoplasia as compared with women in the general population (Naib et al., 1966). A later finding (Nahmias & Dowdle, 1968) showed that about 95% of cases of genital herpes simplex virus infection are caused by a different viral type, namely herpes simplex virus Type-2 (HSV-2), as distinct from that isolated from non-genital herpetic infections (HSV-1). This provided the means whereby the frequency of HSV-2 antibodies could be compared in women with and without cervical neoplasia (Nahmias et al., 1970a).

Demographic surveys of cancer of the cervix have established patterns of high risk that strongly suggest that it may be a sexually transmitted disease (Nahmias & Dowdle, 1968; Nahmias et al., 1980). There is also a good deal of evidence to show that HSV-2 infection is equally a sexually transmitted disease (Hutfield, 1968; Rawls et al., 1971; Josey et al., 1972; Duenas et al., 1972; Adelusi et al., 1976a; Kessler, 1977; Doll, 1977). It has thus been postulated that the virus might be the sexually transmitted initiating or promoting carcinogenic agent responsible for the development of carcinoma of the cervix (Naib et al., 1966; Nahmias et al., 1970; Rawls et al., 1973; Adelusi et al., 1977).

POSSIBLE CAUSE-AND-EFFECT RELATIONSHIP OF HSV-2 AND CaCx

Consequent on the postulate of an association between HSV-2 and CaCx, various approaches have been employed to substantiate a possible cause-and-effect relationship between them. These have varied from serological and epidemiological studies (Rawls et al., 1969; Nahmias et al., 1970a; Aurelian et al., 1970; Royston & Aurelian, 1970; Rotkin, 1973; Adelusi et al., 1976b, 1980), in vitro and animal experimental studies (Nahmias et al., 1970b; Duff & Rapp, 1971; Munoz, 1973; Kimura et al., 1975; Copple & McDougall, 1976; Skinner, 1976; Minhu et al., 1980) to molecular studies (Feorino & Palmer, 1973; Anzai et al., 1975; Aurelian et al., 1976; Camacho & spear, 1978; Heise et al., 1979; Shortland et al., 1979). These studies have all raised the question of the possible cause-and-effect relationship between the virus and the malignancy but none has so far confirmed it.

Apart from serological tests, for example, the oncogenic potential of HSV-2 has been demonstrated by the fact that intra-peritoneal and intrathoracic inoculation of newborn hamsters with the virus has been shown to be associated with the development of sarcomas at the site of inoculation (Nahmias et al., 1970b). Such tumour-bearing hamsters have been shown to possess HSV-2 antibodies in their sera and HSV-2 antigens can be demonstrated in a varying number of tumour cells (Rapp & Duff, 1973; Kimura et al., 1975). Direct genital infection with the virus has also been shown to produce lesions identical to atypia and carcinoma in situ (Nahmias et al., 1971; Munoz, 1973).

Further convincing evidence of the oncogenic potential of HSV-2 has been provided by the transformation of hamster cells in vitro by the virus (Duff & Rapp, 1971). Similarly, the virus has been shown to transform rat (McNab, 1974) and mouse (Kimura et al., 1975) cell cultures, and the cell lines derived from these transformations, when inoculated into other animals, have been shown to produce tumours consistently (Duff et al., 1974; Copple & McDougall, 1976; Skinner, 1976). Such interaction in vitro between HSV-2 and most, if not all cells, results in lysis. Experimental transformation was achieved by eliminating viral infectivity, e.g., by ultraviolet inactivation (Duff & Rapp, 1971), or by using subgenomic sequences of viral DNA (Camacho & Spear, 1978). Of possible relevance also was the in vitro demonstration that the DNA of some of the virus strains was defective (Roizman & Furlong, 1974).

Various attempts have been made to detect HSV-2 antigens in cervical cells or biopsy tissues by the immunofluorescence, immunoperoxidase and radioimmunoassay techniques. For example, the indirect immunofluorescence technique was applied to ex-foliated cells (Royston & Aurelian, 1970; Aurelian, 1973; Adelusi et al., 1976), and the anti-complement immunofluorescence techni-que to biopsy materials (Nahmias et al., 1975). In contrast, exfoliated cervical cells from patients without carcinoma of the cervix did not show evidence of viral antigens, except in those women diagnosed clinically as having herpetic cervicitis.

HSV-2 is a DNA virus and therefore unlikely to be demonstrated in transformed cells. However, significant portions of the
viral genome and readily identifiable virally induced RNA have
been found in cancer cells by molecular biological studies using
hybridization techniques (Frenkel et al., 1972; Collard et al.,
1973; Copple & McDougall, 1976; Minson et al., 1976). Unfortunately the detection of viral DNA or RNA in cancer cells by such
techniques has been limited by the sensitivity of the assays; if
only a small fraction of the viral genome is present, the assay
is not sensitive enough to detect it. Furthermore, in the cancer
tissue being tested, the proportion of cancer cells and normal
cells must be determined, since it is crucial for the assay that
cancer cells should comprise the large majority of the cells in
the tissue. In the case of in situ hybridization techniques performed on tissue sections (McDougall et al., 1980), problems of
non-specific positive reactions are also limiting factors.

Increasing evidence for the presence of HSV-associated antigens in carcinoma of the uterine cervix has accumulated
(Hollinshead et al., 1972, 1973, 1976; Gall & Haines, 1974;
Ibrahim et al., 1975; Notter & Docherty, 1976; Notter et al.,
1978). Among these antigens, the membrane-associated HSV
tumour-associated antigen (HSV-TAA) (Hollinshead et al., 1972,
1973, 1976) has been demonstrated in cancer of the cervix, and in
human cultured cells infected with herpesvirus, but not in
control tissues or uninfected control cultures (Hollinshead et
al., 1972, 1973).

Antibodies to HSV-TAA have been found at much higher frequencies in sera of patients with squamous-cell carcinomas of the
cervix than in control sera or sera from patients with other
types of malignancies (Hollinshead et al., 1976; Notter &
Docherty, 1976). The recent identification, separation and
characterization of the two polypeptide chains which comprise
HSV-TAA, has enabled highly specific hyperimmune antisera to
these antigens to be produced (Hollinshead et al., 1976;
Hollinshead & Stewart, 1979) and such antisera have been used to
ascertain whether HSV-TAA can be demonstrated in cell lines of
human carcinomas of the cervix (Auersperg et al., 1980).

Following the demonstration of tumour-associated antigens in
several animal and human cancers by a variety of in vitro and in
vivo techniques (Hellström & Hellström, 1969; Notter & Docherty,
1976; Notter et al., 1978), another twist was introduced into the
search for a possible cause-and-effect relationship between HSV-2

and CaCx when attempts were made to show TAA in sarcomas produced after inoculation of newborn hamsters with herpes simplex virus Type-2 (Nahmias et al., 1970b) by the immuno-adsorption-in-gel method (Ibrahim et al., 1975).   Cross-reactivity between anti-HSV-2 sera and the HSV-2 associated hamster tumours (OT-I and OT-II) was demonstrated (Ibrahim et al., 1976).   Anti-HSV-2 serum also reacted by passive haemagglutination with the purified TAA of OT-II, whereas anti-HSV-I serum did not react with any of the tumours.   Absorption of the anti-HSV-2 serum with HSV-2 removed homologous as well as heterologous reactivity with OT-I and OT-II.   This clearly indicates the presence of common antigens between HSV-2, OT-I and OT-II.

With the same technique, antisera prepared against partially purified preparations of cancer of the cervix, absorbed with pooled normal human plasma and normal cervix preparations, reacted reproducibly with CaCx tissue antigen preparations and HSV-2 antigen preparations, thus indicating that the two have common antigens.   Rabbit antisera to normal cervix, similarly absorbed, did not react with either the homologous or the hetero-logous antigens.   Similarly, antisera prepared against HSV-2 reacted with both HSV-2 and CaCx, whereas the antisera prepared against HSV-1 did not react with the CaCx antigen.   Absorption of the anti-HSV-2 serum with HSV-2 eliminated reaction with CaCx, suggesting that the common antigen may be specific to HSV-2.

The results of these studies have demonstrated a possible etiological role of HSV-2 in human carcinoma of the cervix.   The weight of the circumstantial evidence supporting such a role has been shown to be heavy.   On the other hand, evidence supporting a similar role for many other DNA viruses as etiological agents of human cancer is lacking (Rangan et al., 1968).   Nevertheless, a definitive proof of a causal relationship still requires further confirmatory studies.

CAN A VIRAL ETIOLOGY BE CONFIRMED ?

In order to place the current status of the genital herpes-carcinoma of the cervix problem in perspective it may be appro-priate to adopt again the criteria originally proposed by Nahmias et al. (1972) for determining whether a causal relation exists between virus and neoplasm, namely: (1) coherence;   (2) consis-tency;   (3) strength;   (4) specificity;   and (5) temporal relation-ship.

Coherence

This criterion requires coherence with known facts in the natural history and biology of the disease. It is essential, for example, that the herpesvirus infecting the female genital tract should differ from that infecting other sites. Evidence now abounds to confirm that there are numerous differences, both antigenic and biological, between the genital and non-genital herpesviruses (Nahmias & Dowdle, 1968; Nahmias et al., 1971). Crucial to the coherence of the association is the need to establish that genital herpes affects the cervix, since it had generally been thought that the virus affected only the external genitalia. Not only has the cervix been shown to be a common site of HSV infection, it has also been found to be the one most commonly affected, although the majority of the cervical infections are asymptomatic (Josey et al., 1968; Nahmias et al., 1971).

It has always been considered that the epidemiological characteristics of genital herpes and carcinoma of the cervix should be similar for the coherence criterion to be satisfied. Here again, evidence has been provided to show that the prevalence of both entities is the same in various groups of women, and that both the virus and the neoplasm have the epidemiological characteristics of sexually transmitted diseases (Josey et al., 1968; Nahmias et al., 1969; Beral, 1974). Of course, other studies have shown evidence of coherence of the association, e.g., where sarcomas developed after inoculation of newborn hamsters (Nahmias et al., 1970b) or cervical neoplasms were observed after genital inoculation of mice with HSV-2 (Nahmias et al., 1971; Munoz, 1973). Furthermore, common antigens to both HSV-2 and CaCx have been found (Royston & Aurelian, 1970; Adelusi et al., 1976, 1983; Ibrahim et al., 1976).

Consistency

The results of numerous studies (Rawls et al., 1969; Aurelian et al., 1970; Nahmias et al., 1970a; Adelusi et al., 1977, 1980) have demonstrated a consistent association between HSV-2 and CaCx. These studies have used a variety of serological tests to detect HSV Type-2 antibodies in women with carcinoma of the cervix and healthy control groups. This does not mean, of course, that minor variations have not been noticed (Rawls et al., 1972).

Strength

The strength of the association between HSV-2 and CaCx in the various studies has been shown to be related to the dose effect. For example, it was shown that the strength of the association may depend on whether HSV-2 infection is primary or recurrent (Nahmias et al., 1972), since a higher frequency of cervical neoplasia was noted in the recurrent infections than in the primary cases, thus suggesting that transformation may occur during a recurrence as well, and that it may take longer for neoplasia to develop after a primary than a recurrent infection.

Specificity

The question of the specificity of the various serological tests for HSV-2 antibodies in women with and without CaCx has generated a great deal of argument. Of the various serological tests used in the studies, it has been suggested that the reproducibility of any one, when carried out in the same laboratory, is no better than 80%, and as little as 50% when comparative serum samples are submitted to different laboratories (Nahmias et al., 1972).

Various studies have shown that there is cross-reactivity between HSV-1 and HSV-2, thereby presenting problems with regard to the specificity of the various serological tests for HSV-2. The need for improved serological tests to detect type-2 antibodies has never been in doubt. Since it is believed that the cross-reactivity between HSV-1 and HSV-2 and their homologous sera is more likely to be a one-way cross, the immunodiffusion technique has been introduced to demonstrate distinct precipitin lines for Type-1 and Type-2 HSV, as well as common lines (Schneweis & Nahmias, 1971).

Temporal relationship

In the search for the viral etiology of cervical neoplasia, it would be significant if the observed time interval between maximum viral growth and tumour response noted in some animals was also seen in women. Thus, the search should be carried out prior to the appearance of clinically obvious cervical neoplasms in patients with such lesions as dysplasia and carcinoma in situ, which are apparently present for months or even years before the development of an invasive lesion. Furthermore, the median age

for genital herpes, detected by cytological or virological techniques, has been put at about 10 years earlier than that for
cervical dysplasia, which in itself is about 10 years earlier
than carcinoma in situ and invasive cancer (Nahmias et al.,
1969). This has provided further support for the theory of a
causative association rather than both the infection and the
disease being co-variables of promiscuity.

CONCLUSIONS

The various difficulties that have been encountered in the
search for a possible cause-and-effect role of HSV-2 in carcinoma
of the cervix notwithstanding, the weight of circumstantial
evidence supporting that role in human carcinoma of the cervix is
considerable. Evidence supporting a similar role for many other
DNA viruses as etiological agents of human cancer, on the other
hand, is lacking. However, the final proof of a causal relationship between viruses and carcinoma of the cervix requirs further
studies, such as the recent demonstration of the involvement of
papillomavirus (see Gissman, this volume).

REFERENCES

Adelusi, B. (1983) Common antigens of herpes simplex virus
    type-2 (HSV-2) and carcinoma of the cervix uteri. West Afr.
    J. Med. (submitted for publication)

Adelusi, B., Ayeni, O., Fabiyi, A. & Osunkoya, B.O. (1976a)
    Serological evidence for the venereal mode of transmission
    of herpes virus type-2 infection in Ibadan. Niger. med. J.,
    6, 386-391

Adelusi, B., Osunkoya, B.O. & Fabiyi, A. (1976b) Herpes type-2
    virus antigens in human cervical carcinoma. Obstet.
    Gynecol., 47, 544-548

Adelusi, B., Osunkoya, B.O. & Fabiyi, A. (1977) Herpes type-2
    virus antibody status in groups of patients with neoplasia
    in Nigeria. Afr. J. med. Sci., 5, 297-301

Adelusi, B., Naib, Z.M., Muther, J. & Nahmias, A.J. (1980) Epidemiological studies relating genital herpes simplex virus (HSV-2) to cervical neoplasis - An update. In: Nahmias, A., Dowdle, W. & Shinazi, R., eds, The Human Herpes viruses - An Interdisciplinary Perspective, New York, Elsevier-North Holland, p. 627

Anzai, T., Dreasman, G.R., Courtney, R.V., Adam, E., Rawls, W.E. & Benyesh-Melnick, M. (1975) Antibody to herpes simplex virus type-2 induced nonstructural proteins in women with cervical cancer and in control groups. J. natl Cancer Inst., 54, 1051-1059

Auersperg, N., Hollinshead, A.C., Lee, O.B. & Wong, K.S. (1984) Detection of herpes simplex virus tumour associated antigens in human cell-lines after long term cultivation (submitted for publication)

Aurelian, L. (1973) Virus and antigens of herpes virus type-2 in cervical carcinoma. Cancer Res., 33, 1539-1547

Aurelian, L., Royston, I. & Davis, H.J. (1970) Antibody to genital herpes simplex virus: Association with cervical atypia and carcinoma in situ. J. natl Cancer Inst., 45, 455-464

Aurelian, L., Smith, F. & Garnish, J.D. (1976) IgM antibody to a tumour associated antigen (AG-4) induced by herpes simplex virus type-2. Its use in location of the antigen in infected cells. J. natl Cancer Inst., 56, 471-477

Beral, V. (1974) Cancer of the cervix - a sexually transmitted infection? Lancet, 1, 1037-1040

von Bulow, V. (1971) Studies on the diagnosis and biology of Marek's disease virus. Am. J. vet. Res., 32, 1275-1288

Camacho, A. & Spear, P.G. (1978) Transformation of hamster embryo fibroblasts by a specific fragment of the herpes simplex virus genome. Cell, 15, 993-1002

Chubb, R.C. & Churchill, A.E. (1968) Precipitating antibodies associated with Marek's disease. Vet. Rec., 83, 4-7

Churchill, A.E. & Biggs, P.M. (1967) Agent of Marek's disease in tissue culture. Nature, 215, 528-530

Churchill, A.E., Payne, L.N. & Chubb, R.C. (1969) Immunization against Marek's disease using a live attenuated vaccine. Nature, 221, 744-747

Collard, W., Thomton, H. & Green, M. (1973) Cells transformed by HSV-2 transcribe virus specific RNA sequences shared by herpes virus Types 1 and 2. Nature New Biol., 243, 264-266

Copple, C.J. & McDougall, J.K. (1976) Clonal derivatives of a herpes type-2 transformed cell line (333-8-9) - cytogenetic analysis, tumorigenicity and virus sequence detection. Int. J. Cancer, 17, 501-510

Cowdry, E.V. (1964) Factors in cancer production. Surg. Clin. North Am., 34, 985-993

Doll, R. (1977) Introduction. In: Hiatt, H.H., Watson, J.D. & Winsten, J.A., eds, Origins of Human Cancer, Cold Spring Harbor, NY, Cold Spring Harbor Laboratory, pp. 1-12

Duenas, A., Adam, E., Melnick, J.L. & Rawls, W.E. (1972) Herpes virus type-2 in a prostitute population. Am. J. Epidemiol., 95, 483-489

Duff, R. & Rapp, F. (1971) Oncogenic transformation of hamster cells after exposure to herpes simplex virus type-2. Nature New Biol., 233, 48-50

Duff, R., Kreider, J.W., Levy, B.M., Katz, M. & Rapp, F. (1974) Comparative pathology of cells transformed by herpes simplex virus type 1 or type 2. J. natl Cancer Inst., 53, 1159-1164

Edison, C.S. & Anderson, D.P. (1971) Immunization against Marek's disease. Avian Dis., 15, 49-55

Fawcett, D.W. (1956) Electron microscope observations of intra-cellular virus-type particles associated with the cells of the Lucké renal adenocarcinoma. J. biophys. biochem. Cytol., 2, 725-742

Feorino, P.M. & Palmer, E.L. (1973) Incidence of antibody to envelope antigen of herpes simplex virus type-2 among patients with cervical carcinoma. J. infect. Dis., 127, 732-735

Frenkel, N., Roizman, D., Cassai, E. & Nahmias, A. (1972) A DNA fragment of herpes simplex-2 and its transcription in human cervical cancer tissue. Proc. natl Acad. Sci. USA, 69, 3784-3789

Gall, J.A. & Haines, P. (1974) Cervical carcinoma antigens and the relationship to HSV-2. Gynecol. Oncol., 2, 451-459

Granoff, A., Cane, P.E. & Rafferty, K.A. (1965) The isolation and properties of viruses from Rana pipiens. Their possible relationship to the renal adenocarcinoma of the leopard frog. Ann. N.Y. Acad. Sci., 126, 237-255

Granoff, A. & Darlington, R.W. (1969) Viruses and renal carcinoma of Rana pipiens. 8. Electron microscopic evidence for the presence of herpesvirus in the urine of a Lucké tumor bearing frog. Virology, 38, 197-200

Heise, E.R., Kucera, L.S., Raben, M. & Homesley, H. (1979) Serological response patterns to herpes virus type-2 early and late antigens in cervical carcinoma patients. Cancer Res., 39, 4022-4026

Hellström, K.E. & Hellström, I. (1969) Cellular immunity against tumor antigens. Adv. Cancer Res., 12, 167-223

Hollinshead, A.C., Stewart, T.M. & Takita, H. (1979) Tumor-associated antigens: their usefulness as biological drugs. Prog. Cancer Res. Ther., 11, 501-520

Hollinshead, A.C., Lee, O.B., McKelway, W., Melnick, J.L. & Rawls, W.E. (1972) Reactivity between herpes virus type-2 related soluble cervical tumour cell membrane antigens and matched cancer and control sera. Proc. Soc. exp. Biol. Med., 145, 688-693

Hollinshead, A.C., Lee, O.B., Chretien, P.B., Tarplay, J.L.,
    Rawls, W.E. & Adam, E. (1973) Antibodies to herpes virus
    "non virion" antigens in squamous carcinoma. Science, 182,
    713-715

Hollinshead, A.C., Chretien, P.B., Lee, O.B., Tarplay, J.L.,
    Kerney, J.E., Silverman, N.A. & Alexander, V.C. (1976) In
    vivo and in vitro measurements of the relationship of human
    squamous carcinomas to herpes simplex virus tumour associa-
    ted antigens. Cancer Res., 36, 821-828

Hutfield, D.C. (1968) Herpes genitalis. Br. J. vener. Dis., 44,
    241-250

Ibrahim, A.N., Ray, M. & Nahmias, A.J. (1975) Tumor antigens in
    hamsters with sarcomas associated with herpes virus type-2.
    Proc. Soc. exp. Biol. Med., 148, 1025-1028

Ibrahim, A.N., Ray, M., Megaw, J., Brown, R. & Nahmias, A.J.
    (1976) Common antigens of herpes simplex virus type-2
    associated hamster tumors and human cervical cancer. Proc.
    Soc. exp. Biol. Med., 152, 343-347

Josey, W.E., Nahmias, A.J. & Naib, Z.M. (1968) Genital herpes
    simplex infection. Present knowledge and possible relation-
    ship to cervical cancer. Am. J. Obstet. Gynecol., 101,
    718-729

Josey, W.E., Nahmias, A.J. & Naib, Z.M. (1972) The epidemiology
    of type-2 (genital) herpes simplex virus infection. Obstet.
    gynecol. Surv., 27, 296-302

Kessler, I.I. (1977) Venereal factors in human cervical cancer.
    Cancer, 39, 1912-1919

Kimura, S., Flannery, V.L., Levy, B. & Schaffer, P.A. (1975)
    Oncogenic transformation of primary hamster cells by herpes
    simplex virus type-2 (HSV-2), and HSV-2 temperature sensi-
    tive mutant. Int. J. Cancer, 15, 786-789

McDougall, J.K., Galloray, D.A. & Fenoglio, C.M. (1980) Cervical
    carcinoma - detection of herpes simplex virus DNA in cells
    undergoing neoplastic change. Int. J. Cancer, 25, 1-8

McKinnell, R.G. & Tweedell, K.S. (1970)   Induction of renal tumors in triploid frogs. J. natl Cancer Inst., 44, 1161-1166

McNab, J.C.M. (1974)   Transformation of rat embryo cells by temperature-sensitive mutants of herpes simplex virus. J. gen. Virol., 24, 143-153

Minhui, C., Yu, S., Qida, Z. & Yousing, C. (1980) Experimental studies on induction of cervical carcinoma in mice by genital herpes simplex virus. In: Nahmias, A.J., Dowdle, W. & Schinazi, R., eds, The Human Herpes Viruses - An Interdisciplinary Perspective, New York, Elsevier-North Holland, p. 633

Minson, A.C., Thouless, M.E., Eglin, R.P. & Darby, C. (1976) the detection of virus DNA sequences in a herpes type-2 transformed hamster cell line (333-8-9). Int. J. Cancer, 17, 493-500

Munoz, N. (1973)   Effect of herpes virus type-2 and hormonal imbalance on the uterine cervix of the mouse. Cancer Res., 33, 1504-1508

Nahmias, A.J. & Dowdle, W. (1968)   Antigenic and biologic differences in herpes virus hominis. Prog. med. Virol., 10, 110-159

Nahmias, A.J., Dowdle, W.E., Naib, Z.M., Josey, W.E., McClone, D. & Domescik, G. (1969) Genital infection with type-2 (HSV-2) herpesvirus hominis - a commonly occurring venereal disease. Br. J. vener. Dis., 45, 294-298

Nahmias, A.J., Josey, W.E., Naib, Z.M., Luce, C.F. & Guest, B.A. (1970a) Antibodies to herpesvirus hominis types 1 and 2 in humans. II. Women with cervical cancer. Am. J. Epidemiol., 91, 547-552

Nahmias, A.J., Naib, Z.M., Josey, W.E., Murphy, F.A. & Luce, C.F. (1970b) Sarcomas after inoculation of newborn hamsters with herpes virus hominis type-2 strains. Proc. Soc. exp. Biol. Med., 134, 1065-1069

Nahmias, A.J., Naib, Z.M. & Josey, W.E. (1971) Herpes virus hominis type-2 infection. Association with cervical cancer and perinatal disease. Perspect. Virol., 7, 73-88

Nahmias, A.J., Naib, Z.M. & Josey, W.E. (1972) Genital herpes and cervical cancer - can a causal relation be proven? - a review. In: Biggs, P.M., de-Thé, G. & Payne, L.N., eds, Oncogenesis and Herpesviruses (IARC Scientific Publications No. 2), Lyon, International Agency for Research on Cancer, pp, 403-408

Nahmias, A.J., Del Buono, I. & Ibrahim, I. (1975) Antigenic relation between herpes simplex viruses, human cervical cancer and HSV-associated hamster tumours. In: de-Thé, G., Epstein, M.A. & zur Hausen, H., eds, Oncogenesis and Herpesviruses II (IARC Scientific Publications No. 11), Lyon, International Agency for Research on Cancer, pp. 309-313

Nahmias, A.J., Josey, W.E. & Oleske, J.M. (1976) Epidemiology of cervical cancer. In: Evans, A.S., ed., Viral Infections of Humans, New York, John Wiley & Sons, pp. 501-518

Naib, Z.M., Nahmias, A.J. & Josey, W.E. (1966) Cytology and histopathology of cervical herpes simplex virus infection. Cancer, 19, 1026-1031

Nazerian, K., Solomon, J.J., Witter, R.L. & Burmester, B.R. (1968) Studies on the etiology of Marek's disease. II. Finding of a herpes virus in cell culture. Proc. Soc. exp. Biol. Med., 127, 177-182

Notter, F.M.D. & Docherty, J.J. (1976) Comparative diagnostic aspects of herpes simplex virus tumour associated antigens. J. natl Cancer Inst., 57, 483-488

Notter, F.M.D., Docherty, J.J., Mortel, R. & Hollinshead, A.C. (1978) Detection of herpes simplex virus tumour associated antigen in uterine cervical cancer tissue: Five case studies. Gynecol. Oncol., 6, 574-581

Rangan, S.R.S., Mukherjee, A.L. & Bang, F.B. (1968) Search for adenovirus etiology of human oral and pharyngeal tumours. Int. J. Cancer, 3, 819-828

Rapp, F. & Duff, R. (1973)   Transformation of hamster embryo fibroblasts by herpes simplex virus types 1 and 2. Cancer Res., 33, 1527-1534

Rawls, W.E., Tompkins, W.A.F. & Melnick, J.L. (1969) The association of herpesvirus type-2 and carcinoma of the uterine cervix. Am. J. Epidemiol., 89, 547-554

Rawls, W.E., Gardner, H.L., Flanders, R.W., Lowry, S.P., Kaufman, R.H. & Melnick, J.L. (1971) Genital herpes in two social groups. Am. J. Obstet. Gynecol., 110, 682-689

Rawls, W.E., Adam, E. & Melnick, J.L. (1972) Geographical variation in the association of antibodies to herpesvirus type-2 and carcinoma of the cervix. In: Biggs, P.M., de-Thé, G. & Payne, L.N., eds, Oncogenesis and Herpesviruses (IARC Scientific Publications No. 2), Lyon, International Agency for Research on Cancer, pp, 424-427

Rawls, W.E., Adam, E. & Melnick, J.L. (1973) An analysis of seropeidemiologic studies of herpesvirus type-2 and carcinoma of the cervix. Cancer Res., 33, 1477-1483

Roizman, B. & Furlong, D. (1974) The replication of herpesviruses. In: Frenkel-Conrat, H. & Wagner, R.R., eds, Comprehensive Virology, Vol. 3, New York, Plenum, pp. 229-382

Rotkin, I.D. (1973) A comparative review of key epidemiologic studies in cervical cancer related to current searches and transmissible agents. Cancer Res., 33, 1353-1367

Royston, I. & Aurelian, L. (1970) Immunofluorescent detection of herpes virus antigens in exfoliated cells of human cervical carcinoma. Proc. natl Acad. Sci. USA, 67, 204-221

Schneweis, K.E. & Nahmias, A.J. (1971) Antigens of herpes simplex virus types 1 and 2 - immunodiffusion and inhibition passive haemagglutination studies. Z. ImmunForsch. exp. Ther., 141, 479-487

Shortland, N.R., Monsansy, K., Fees, R.C. & Potter, C.W. (1979) Tumorigenicity of herpesvirus hominis type-2 transformed cells (line 333-8-9) in adult hamsters. J. Pathol., 129, 169-178

Skinner, G.R.B. (1976) Transformation of primary hamster embryo fibroblasts by type-2 herpes simplex virus - evidence of a "hit and run" mechanism. Br. J. exp. Pathol., 57, 361-376

Solomon, J.J., Witter, R.L., Nazerian, K. & Burmester, B.R. (1968) Studies on the etiology of Marek's disease. Propagation of the agent in cell culture. Proc. Soc. exp. Biol. Med., 127, 177-182

CONTROL OF CANCER OF THE CERVIX: FEASIBILITY OF SCREENING FOR PREMALIGNANT LESIONS IN AN AFRICAN ENVIRONMENT

J.K.G. Mati, S. Mbugua & M. Ndavi

Department of Obstetrics and Gynaecology
University of Nairobi
Nairobi, Kenya

RESUME

Le cancer du col utérin est une maladie commune en Afrique sub-Saharienne, et qui tend à être diagnostiquée plus tardivement que dans les pays développés. La maladie est de ce fait associée à une mortalité importante. De plus, elle survient à un âge beaucoup plus précoce en Afrique qu'en Europe et en Amérique du Nord.

On ne connaît pas son étiologie, mais on a montré que les malades atteintes de cancer avaient eu des relations sexuelles précoces plus souvent que les témoins. Le mariage des enfants, qui existe dans beaucoup de pays d'Afrique, peut donc contribuer à la maladie. Par contre, les études réalisées dans différents groupes ethniques du Kenya n'ont pas confirmé l'hypothèse selon laquelle la circoncision des hommes réduirait l'incidence des cancers du col.

Puisque le cancer du col peut se développer chez les femmes Africaines avant l'âge de 20 ans, le dépistage doit commencer dès que les femmes deviennent sexuellement actives, dans le but premier de diagnostiquer de façon précoce une éventuelle maladie invasive. Comme le nombre de gynécologues disponibles est faible, les infirmiers et les sages-femmes doivent apprendre à pratiquer l'examen du col. Au Kenya, un laboratoire de recherche cytologique créé en 1981 a réalisé trois campagnes de dépistage chez des femmes asymptomatiques. Les résultats de ces campagnes montrent que les taux de cytologies anormales sont beaucoup plus élevés que ceux décrits dans les pays développés.

SUMMARY

Cancer of the cervix is a common disease in sub-Saharan Africa and tends to be diagnosed later than in the developed countries. The disease is therefore associated with a high mortality under African conditions. In addition, it occurs at a much earlier age in Africa than in Europe and North America.

The etiology is unknown, but early adolescent sexual exposure has been shown to occur more frequently in cancer patients than in controls. Child marriage, found in many African countries, may therefore be a contributing factor. In contrast, the suggestion that male circumcision reduces the incidence of cancer of the cervix has not been confirmed by studies of different ethnic groups in Kenya.

Since cervical intraepithelial neoplasm may develop in African women before the age of 20, screening must be started as soon as women become sexually active, and early diagnosis of invasive disease must be the first aim. As the number of gynaecologists available is small, nurses and midwives must be instructed in examination of the cervix. In Kenya, a cytology research department was established in 1981 and has carried out three surveys of asymptomatic women. The survey data suggest much higher prevalence rates of abnormal cytology than those reported in the developed countries.

***

In sub-Saharan Africa, cancer of the cervix is a very common disease, accounting for 25-30% of all cancers of the female genital tract, as shown in Table 1 (Ojwang et al., 1980; Asuen & Ahnaimugan, 1980; Megafu & Uche, 1980; Adelusi & Babatunda, 1980). In contrast, cancer of the corpus uteri is a rare disease and the ratio of cancer of the cervix to that of the corpus has been shown to be as high as 29-30:1 in Nairobi and Enugu (Ojwang et al., 1980; Megafu & Uche, 1980). In the developed countries, this ratio is approaching unity, mainly because of the marked reduction in the incidence of invasive cervical carcinoma, and some possible increase in the incidence of carcinoma of the corpus in recent decades.

Table 1. Cancer of the cervix and of the corpus uteri in some African hospitals

Hospital	Cancer of the cervix as a percentage of all cancers of the genital tract[a]	Ratio cervix:corpus
Kenyatta National Hospital, Nairobi, Kenya	80.2 (501)	29:1
University of Benin Teaching Hospital, Benin City, Nigeria	74.4 (90)	8:1
Enugu Hospital, Nigeria	73.2 (82)	30:1
Khartoum Hospital, Sudan	51.7 (327)	4:1

[a] Figures in parentheses are numbers of patients

   Another feature of cancer of the cervix as seen in Africa is the late diagnosis. Table 2 shows the distribution of the various stages as seen in the Kenyatta National Hospital (KNH) in Nairobi compared to that in some selected hospitals in developed countries. It will be seen that only 10.2% of the cases diagnosed are in stage I and 61.7% present at stages III and IV. This situation is completely the opposite of what happens in developed countries. As a consequence, cancer of the cervix is associated with a high mortality in Africa, particularly as the facilities for treatment are inadequate. An example of the effect of early diagnosis on mortality rates is provided by data from the USA, where in 1930, when only less than 20% of cases presented in stage I, the death rate was 27.5 per 100 000. This had dropped to 8 per 100 000 by 1976 at a time when 50% of cancer of the cervix was diagnosed at stages 0 and 1.

Table 2. Staging of cancer of the cervix in Kenya and in some
developed countries

Stage	Kenyatta National Hospital, Nairobi, Kenya[a] (%)	Chelsea Hospital for Women, London London, UK[b] (%)	Umeå, Sweden[a] (%)	Houston Texas, USA[c] (%)
I	10.2	28	45.6	40.3
II	28.1	42	36.3	43.9
III	56.0	22	11.2	13.0
IV	5.7	8	6.9	2.8

[a] Source: Ojwang et al., 1980
[b] Source: Blaikley et al., 1969
[c] Source: Wall et al., 1966

Cancer of the cervix in Africa occurs at a much younger age
than is the case in Europe and North America, where its peak
incidence is in the 50-60-year age-group. Table 3 shows that 42%
of cases at KNH were under 40 years old and 72.6% were under 50
years. The appreciation of this difference is important when
considering the institution of measures for early detection.

Table 3. Age distribution of cancer of the cervix at Kenyatta
National Hospital, Nairobi, Kenya

Age (years)	No.	%
20-29	39	9.7
30-39	139	32.3
40-49	123	30.6
50-59	76	18.8
60-69	20	5.0
70-79	8	2.0
Unknown	6	1.5

ETIOLOGY

Although the actual cause of cervical cancer remains unknown, certain factors are known to influence the prevalence of
the disease. Of central importance is sexual exposure, and this
has led to the hypothesis that the carcinogenic stimulus is
either irritation or an agent (or agents) introduced to the
cervical epithelium during coitus. Among the sexual factors that
have been identified are: early start of coitus, frequency of
intercourse, and multiplicity of sexual partners.

Table 4 is derived from the work of Adelusi (Adelusi &
Babatunda, 1980) in Ibadan, and demonstrates that, in a case-
control study, early adolescent sexual exposure occurred more
frequently in cancer patients than in controls. The practice of
child marriage found in many African countries may therefore
contribute to the high incidence of cervical cancer.

Table 4. Age at first coitus among cases of cancer of the cervix
and controls[a]

Age at first coitus (years)	Cancer of the cervix		Controls	
	No.	%	No.	%
11–15	36	31.6	11	10.4
16–20	55	48.2	72	67.9
21–25	22	19.3	18	17.0
> 25	1	0.9	5	4.7
TOTAL	114	100.0	106	100.0

[a] Based on the data of Adelusi and Babatunda,
1980

A male factor in the etiology of cervical cancer has been suggested because of the observation that the disease is rare among nuns and virgins, but has a higher incidence among prostitutes and women attending sexually transmitted disease clinics. The observation of a low incidence of cervical cancer among Jewish women has led to the suggestion that male circumcision reduces the risk of cancer of the cervix. This association, however, has not been observed in Kenya, where no difference in the incidence of the disease has been found between those ethnic groups that practise male circumcision and those that do not.

In 1976, Singer and Reid proposed that arginine-rich histone in the sperm may be capable of bringing about the malignant transformation of DNA, and introduced the concept of the 'high-risk' male, depending on the amount of arginine-rich histone in the sperm. Further studies are needed along these lines.

Finally, a viral etiology has been proposed because of the finding of herpes simplex virus Type-2 (HSV-2) antibodies in the serum of cervical cancer patients as well as HSV-2 antigen in exfoliated cervical cells from cervical cancer patients (Adelusi & Babatunda, 1980). However, a cause-and-effect relationship remains to be established.

NATURALLY HISTORY OF CANCER OF THE CERVIX

Figure 1 is a schematic representation of what is thought to be the natural history of cervical cancer. Starting with a normal cervical epithelium, histological changes pass through mild to moderate, through severe (or marked) dysplasia to carcinoma in situ or cervical intraepithelial neoplasm (CIN). The changes up to this stage are considered to be reversible. Further change to invasive carcinoma is, however, irreversible.

Epidemiological data, mostly from Europe and North America, has suggested that these progressive changes are slow, and that it may take 10-15 years for CIN to change into invasive carcinoma. The peak age for invasive carcinoma is in the fifth and sixth decades of life while for CIN it is in the early and late 30s. This makes it possible, therefore, to institute screening procedures before invasive disease develops. However, the age distribution of cancer patients previously discussed shows that, in Africa, the disease affects much younger women, and that the peak age of invasive disease is in the 30s and 40s.

FIG. 1. NATURAL HISTORY OF CANCER OF THE CERVIX

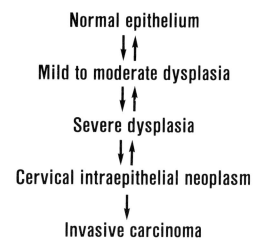

Normal epithelium

↓↑

Mild to moderate dysplasia

↓↑

Severe dysplasia

↓↑

Cervical intraepithelial neoplasm

↓

Invasive carcinoma

Based on the observed length of time that elapses between the invasive and the in situ stages in Europe and North America, CIN could thus be observed before the age of 20 in Africa. This means, therefore, that for screening to be effective, it must be started as early as a woman becomes sexually active, irrespective of the age.

The finding of advanced disease at an early age also raises the question as to whether the disease necessarily has the same natural history in all women, or whether in some cases the invasive cancer stage may be reached without the intermediate stages of dysplasia and CIN. Could this be a biologically different disease or a reflection of etiological differences ? Further work in this area is needed.

APPROACHES TO THE CONTROL OF CERVICAL CANCER IN AFRICA

The first aim in the control of cervical cancer in Africa should be the early diagnosis of invasive disease because this offers better chances of long-term survival. The responsibility of making such early diagnosis should not be left to gynaecologists alone because they are too few. It is essential that

emphasis should be placed on the importance of speculum visuali-
zation of the cervix in all examinations of women and by all
doctors. Medical students are taught the importance of taking
blood pressure at any available opportunity; they need to be
taught the same as far as examination of the breast and the
cervix are concerned.

Nurses and midwives also need to be instructed in examination of the cervix and its importance. In many parts of Africa,
nurses and midwives see the majority of antenatal, postnatal and
family planning patients. They can therefore be taught to
recognize an abnormal cervix and to refer the patient to a
doctor.

The second aim should be institution of measures to detect
preinvasive disease through exfoliative cervical cytology.
Population screening in British Columbia and New Zealand has been
followed by a decrease in the incidence of invasive disease and,
in the Canadian experience, a reduction in mortality from cancer
of the cervix (Boyes et al., 1977; Green, 1978). The most
important constraint on planning such population screening is the
inadequacy of financial resources. However, in a continent where
cancer of the cervix is an important public health problem, the
costs of screening should be considered in the same way as those
of communicable disease control. Another fear that has been
expressed is that treatment facilities may not be able to cope
with the large number of cases diagnosed. It is true that, in
the initial stages, many cases of advanced disease will be un-
earthed which will overtax the limited radiotherapy facilities.
Gradually, however, these will largely be replaced by earlier
cases which will be amenable to surgical treatment as well as
radiotherapy.

CYTOLOGY SERVICES IN KENYA

Cytology services became available at the Kenyatta National
Hospital in 1969. At first, only patients attending the gynaecology clinics had smears taken, and the facility was not available for research purposes or for screening of asymptomatic
women. In 1981, through the support of WHO, a cytology research
laboratory was established in the Department of Obstetrics and
Gynaecology and this has made it possible to screen asymptomatic
women. Table 5 shows the results of three surveys that have been

Table 5. Results of screening of asymptomatic women in Kenya

Group	Stage						Total
	I	II	III		IV		
	No.	No.	No.	Preva-lence[a]	No.	Preva-lence[a]	
Women attending gynaecology clinics	2330	2479	81	16.5	19	3.9	4909
Women using depo-provera	368	932	35	28.5	1	0.8	1236
Women attending family planning clinic	484	978	33	22.0	2	1.3	1497
Total	3182	4389	149	19.5	22	2.9	7642

[a] Per 1000

carried out. The first covered 4909 women seen at the gynaeco-logy clinics (Kirima, 1981), and the second 1236 women who had an initial smear taken before starting on depot medroxyprogesterone acetate (depo-provera) for contraception purposes. The last group consisted of 1497 women who attended a rural family plan-ning clinic, the smears having been taken before a contraceptive method was adopted. In the three groups of women, the prevalence of abnormal cytology varied from 20.4 per 1000 in the gynaecology clinic patients to 29.3 per 1000 in women who adopted depo-provera. Dabancens et al. (1974) also observed a higher preva-lence of abnormal cytology in women who chose depo-provera for contraception. However, follow-up of depo-provera users over a

5-year period has not shown higher incidence of cervical cancer.
In the third year, the incidence in 1061 users was 16/1000, and
5-year follow-up of 497 cases showed an incidence of 10/1000.

On the whole, these data suggest much higher prevalence
rates of abnormal cytology in Kenya than those reported in
Europe, North America and New Zealand, and this by itself is an
important reason why cytology screening should be made available
for all women visiting organized clinics.

The rural population to which the 1497 women screened belong
occupies a well defined area where the age structure is known.
It has therefore been possible to calculate the age-specific prevalence rates of abnormal cytology, and these are shown in Table
6.   It can be seen that the prevalence in the 15-19-years age-
group was 7.5 per 1000, and that it more than doubled in women
aged 20-24 years;   there was then a further rise to a plateau
(except for the age-group 30-34 years) between 25 and 49 years.
It is obvious, therefore, that in this environment an arbitrary
age when screening should start cannot be fixed;   rather, it
should be offered to all sexually active women irrespective of
age.

Table 6. Age distribution of abnormal smears in a rural population in Kenya

Age (years)	Stages I and II	Stages III and IV	Total	Prevalence of stages III and IV (per 1000)
15-19	133	1	134	7.5
20-24	407	7	414	16.9
25-29	265	9	274	32.8
30-34	304	7	311	22.5
35-39	200	7	207	33.8
40-44	123	4	127	31.5
45+	30	0	30	0
Total	1462	35	1497	23.4

ESTABLISHMENT OF A NATIONAL SCREENING PROGRAMME

Apart from financial restrictions, the major constraint on any large-scale screening programme is the lack of trained personnel to obtain the smears from patients and to process them in the laboratory. In Africa, where most maternal/child health and family planning services are provided by nurse-midwives, this offers the opportunity of using this category of personnel to collect the cervical smears. No difficulty has been found in training nurses to use the vaginal speculum, obtain the smear and fix it. This type of training needs to be introduced into the nursing and midwifery curricula, and certainly into any family planning course.

Technicians who have handled microscopes previously can be trained over a period of 3 months in the technique of staining the smears, as well as in identifying doubtful smears which require greater expertise. Since every district hospital is expected to have a microscope for other diagnostic work, what is needed most is the training of the technicians. It is also possible to arrange for slides to be examined at the central or provincial hospitals, where trained technicians can be located.

The next step is for the screening of all women attending antenatal, postnatal, family planning and sexually transmitted disease clinics to be made a routine practice, since such women comprise a large proportion of the 'at-risk' women presenting themselves at health facilities. Such groups need to be covered before whole-population screening is embarked upon.

Finally, it is important to ensure that, before the programme begins, arrangements have been made for good record keeping. This will permit, not only the referral and follow-up of cases, but also allow prevalence studies in different areas or communities. By repeat screening of the same individuals over a period of time, incidence data can also be obtained. Such studies are urgently needed since the epidemiology of cervical cancer in Africa remains unexplored.

REFERENCES

Adelusi, B. & Babatunda, C. (1980) Cancer of the cervix. Factors associated with causation. In: Ojo, O.A., Aimakhu, V.E., Akinla, O. et al., eds, Obstetrics and Gynaecology in Developing Countries. The Nigeria conference, Lund, Broderna Ekstrands Tryckeri, pp. 446-458

Asuen, M.I. & Ahnaimugan, S. (1980) A review of cervical cancer at the University of Benin Teaching Hospital, Benin City, Nigeria from 1st April 1973 - 31st March 1977 - a four year period. In: Ojo, O.A., Aimakhu, V.E., Akinla, O. et al., eds, Obstetrics and Gynaecology in Developing Countries. The Nigeria Conference, Lund, Broderna Ekstrands Tryckeri, pp. 427-433

Blaikley, J.B., Lederman, P. & Pollard, N. (1969) Carcinoma of the cervix in Chelsea Hospital for Women. J. Obstet. Gynaecol. Br. Commonw., 76, 729-740

Boyes, D.A., Nichols, T.M., Millner, A.M. & Worth, A.J. (1977) Recent results from the British Columbia screening program for cervical cancer. Am. J. Obstet. Gynecol., 128, 692-693

Dabancens, A., Prado, R., Larraguibel, R. & Zanartu, J. (1974) Intraepithelial cervical neoplasia in women using intrauterine devices and long acting injectable progesterones as contraceptives. Am. J. Obstet. Gynecol., 119, 1052-1056

Green, G.H. (1978) Cervical cancer and cytology screening in New Zealand. Br. J. Obstet. Gynaecol., 85, 881-886

Kirima, J. (1981) Retrospective Study on Cervical Smears. Diagnostic Value and Influencing Factors, Thesis, University of Nairobi

Megafu, U. & Uche, G.O. (1980) Cancer of the female genital tract among the Igbo women. In: Ojo, O.A., Aimakhu, V.E., Akinla, O. et al., eds, Obstetrics and Gynaecology in Developing Countries. The Nigeria Conference, Lund, Broderna Ekstrands Tryckeri, pp. 437-442

Ojwang, S.B.O., Mati, J.K.G. & Makokha, A.E. (1980) The problem of gynaecological cancer in Kenya with reference to some practical problems in radiotherapy management of carcinoma of the uterine cervix in developing countries. In: Ojo, O.A., Aimakhu, V.E., Akinla, O. et al., eds, Obstetrics and Gynaecology in Developing Countries. The Nigeria Conference, Lund, Broderna Ekstrands Tryckeri, pp. 344-352

Singer, A. & Reid, B.L. (1976) Causes of cervical carcinoma: new ideas. Comp. Ther., 2, 29-37

Wall, A.J., Vincent, P.C., Philip, T.H. et al. (1966) Carcinoma of the cervix. Am. J. Obstet. Gynecol., 96, 57

ANTIBODIES TO MEMBRANE ANTIGENS OF HERPES SIMPLEX VIRUS TYPE-2 INFECTED CELLS AND HSV-2 SPECIFIC ANTIBODIES IN PATIENTS WITH CERVICAL CANCER IN MALAWI

J.D. Chiphangwi

P.O. Box 95
Blantyre, Malawi

RESUME

Dans le cadre d'une étude géographique englobant le Royaume-Uni, le Soudan, Sri Lanka et le Malawi, on a prélevé des sérums chez 27 patientes du Malawi atteintes de cancer du col utérin et chez 18 témoins appariés pour l'âge, l'origine ethnique et le statut socio-économique. Les anticorps IgG et IgA dirigés contre les antigènes de membrane du virus Herpes simplex de type 2 (HSV-2) ont été dosés par immunofluorescence indirecte. Les résultats ont montré qu'il n'y avait pas de différence significative aux titres de 1:4 entre les patientes et les témoins du Malawi, mais aux titres du 1:16 la différence était significative. On a trouvé que 73% des patientes avaient des anticorps spécifiques anti-HSV-2 (mesurés par la technique ELISA) alors que seulement 30,7% des témoins en possédaient.

SUMMARY

In a geographical study involving the United Kingdom, Sudan, Sri Lanka and Malawi, sera were taken from 27 Malawian patients with cervical cancer and 18 controls matched for age, ethnic origin and socioeconomic status. The sera were tested by indirect immunofluorescence for IgG and IgA antibodies to membrane antigens of herpes simplex virus type-2 (HSV-2). The results showed that there was no significant difference at titres 1:4 between Malawian patients and controls, but at titres 1:16 the difference was significant. It was found that 73% of patients had HSV-2 specific antibodies (measured by ELISA) as compared with 30.7% of controls.

INTRODUCTION

Carcinoma of the cervix uteri is the commonest type of cancer among women in Malawi, accounting for 36.8% of all histologically proven cancers in women (Lowe et al., 1981). The majority of the diagnoses (60%) are made when the cancer has already progressed to stages III and IV (Table 1). The age distribution (with a peak in the fifth decade) is similar to that found in series from other parts of Africa (Fig. 1).

Table 1. Age at diagnosis and staging of patients with carcinoma of the cervix in Malawi

Stage	Total	Age at diagnosis					
		20-29	30-39	40-49	50-59	60-69	70-79
I	41	2	11	17	7	3	1
II	95	6	18	36	22	13	0
III	70	3	18	24	13	11	1
IV	93	4	12	31	18	20	8
Total	299	15	59	108	60	47	10

Many seroepidemiological studies all over the world have tended to implicate herpes simplex virus type-2 (HSV-2) either partially or totally in the development of cervical cancer. Most of these studies tend to measure both latent and past infections with HSV-2. Mendis et al. (1981a) have suggested that IgA against membrane antigens (MA) may reflect latent infection while the ELISA method measures antibodies resulting from previous infections. This study of Malawian patients and controls was part of a geographical study that involved the United Kingdom, Sri Lanka, Sudan and Malawi (Mendis et al., 1981b).

FIG. 1. AGE AT DIAGNOSIS OF PATIENTS
WITH CARCINOMA OF THE CERVIX IN MALAWI

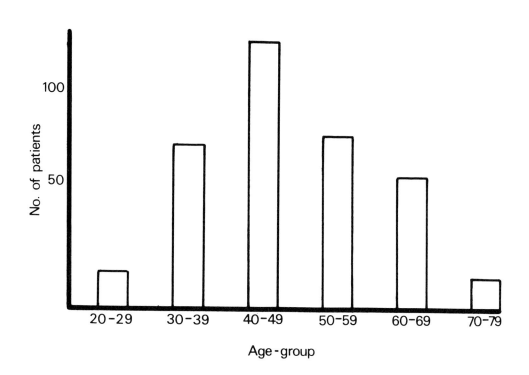

MATERIALS AND METHODS

The Malawian study group consisted of 27 patients with histologically proven cervical cancer (treated at Queen Elizabeth Central Hospital (QECH) Blantyre) and 18 controls who were matched for age, parity, ethnic group and socioeconomic status, and were also attending QECH for conditions other than malignancy. Sera from patients and controls were sent to the Virology Department, St. Thomas's Hospital Medical School, London, for testing.

IgG anti-MA and IgA anti-MA antibodies were measured by indirect immunofluorescence as described by Mendis et al. (1981), live HSV-2 infected RK 13 cells being used as antigen.

HSV-2 specific antibodies were assayed by the ELISA method as described by Vestergaard & Grauballe (1979a,b).

RESULTS

All patients and controls had IgG anti-MA at titres ≫ 1:8 (Table 2). There was no significant difference in the prevalence of IgA anti-MA at titres ≫ 1:4, but at titres ≫ 1:16 the difference was significant in that 18 out of 27 patients (66%) had IgA anti-MA, while only 7 out of 18 controls (38%) possessed this antibody.

Table 2. Prevalence and reciprocal geometric mean titre (GMT) of IgG anti-MA and IgA anti-MA and prevalence of HSV-2 specific antibodies in patients and controls in Malawi

Item	No. Positive	No. Tested	%	GMT
IgG anti-MA:				
patients	27	27	100	692
controls	18	18	100	362
IgA anti-MA:				
patients	25	27	93	21.2
controls	15	18	83	7.7
HSV-2 antibodies:				
patients	19	26	73	
controls	4	13	30.7	

It was found by the ELISA method that 19 out of 26 patients (73%) had HSV-2 specific antibodies, whereas only 4 out of 13 controls (30.7%) did so (Table 2). There was also a greater prevalence of these antibodies in patients under 60 years of age

as opposed to those over 60, but the difference was not statistically significant (Table 3).

Table 3.   Prevalence of HSV-2 specific antibodies (by ELISA)
among patients according to age at diagnosis.

Country	Age						p
	Less than 60			Over 60			
	Total	+ve	%	Total	+ve	%	
Malawi	23	18	78	5	3	60	NS[a]
Sri Lanka	23	15	65	6	5	83	NS[a]
United Kingdom	46	29	63	20	7	35	0.05

[a] Not significant

DISCUSSION

The results of this study show a greater prevalence of HSV-2
specific antibodies in patients than in controls, and in this
respect, they agree with those of the majority of studies on this
subject.   However 27% of patients did not have these antibodies.
It has been suggested that some of these may be false negatives.

Of Malawian controls, 83% possessed IgA anti-MA, as demonstrated by using HSV-2 infected cells.   It is suggested that this
may be due to a high background level of herpes simplex type-1
(HSV-1) infection or to an alteration in the immune response
induced by some parasitic infections.   Sogbetun et al. (1979) and
Montefiore et al. (1980) have also suggested that, in Nigeria,
under conditions of poor hygiene and in a hot humid climate,
HSV-2 infections can occur non-venereally.

REFERENCES

Lowe, D., Jorizo, J., Chiphangwi, J. & Hutt, M.S.R. (1981)
    Cervical carcinoma in Malawi. A histopathologic study of
    460 cases. Cancer, 47, 2493-2495

Mendis, L.N., Best, J.M. & Banatvala, J.E. (1981a) Class-specific
    antibodies (IgG and IgA) to membrane antigens of herpes
    simplex type 2 infected cells in patients with cervical dys-
    plasia and neoplasia. Int. J. Cancer, 27, 669-677

Mendis, L., Best, J., Senarath, L., Chiphangwi, J., Vestergaard,
    B. & Banatvala, J. (1981b) A geographical study of anti-
    bodies to membrane antigens of HSV-2-infected cells and
    HSV-2-specific antibodies in patients with cervical cancer.
    Int. J. Cancer, 28, 535-542

Montefiore, D., Sogbetun, A.O. & Anong, C.N. (1980) Herpes virus
    hominis type 2 infection in Ibadan. Problem of non-venereal
    transmission. Br. J. Venereol., 56, 49-53

Sogbetun, A.O., Montefiore, D. & Anong, C.N. (1979) Herpesvirus
    hominis antibodies among children and young adults in
    Ibadan. Br. J. Vener. Dis., 1, 44-47

Vestergaard, B.F. & Grauballe, P.C. (1979a) Isolation of the
    major herpes simplex virus type 1 (HSV-1) specific glyco-
    protein by hydroxylapatite chromatography and its use in
    enzyme-linked immunosorbent assay for titration of human
    HSV-1 specific antibodies. J. clin. Microbiol., 10, 772-777

Vestergaard, B.F. & Grauballe, P.C. (1979b) ELISA for herpes
    simplex type-specific antibodies in human sera using HSV
    type-1 and type-2 polyspecific antigens blocked with type
    heterologous rabbit antibodies. Acta path. microbiol.
    scand., 87, 261-263

DÉPISTAGE CYTOLOGIQUE DES LÉSIONS DU COL UTERIN: RÉSULTATS D'UNE CAMPAGNE MENÉE AU SÉNÉGAL

P. Touré, J.M. Afontou, A. Diab-D.N'Dao

Dakar, Senegal

SUMMARY

The authors have analysed the results of 5131 Papanicolaou tests carried out in Senegal between November 1980 and July 1983. They emphasize the importance of classes II and III, which correspond to lesions that can be treated so as to ensure prevention of cervical cancer.

The classical etiopathogenic factors of this type of cancer are studied, and results obtained from a group tested systematically are compared with those of a group that were tested only at the time of a gynaecological examination for another purpose. This comparison demonstrated the usefulness of systematic screening.

The authors propose a scheme for organizing the prevention and screening of this type of cancer at the subregional level in Africa.

RESUME

Les auteurs ont analysé les résultats de 5 131 tests de Papanicolaou effectués au Sénégal de novembre 1980 à juillet 1983. Ils insistent sur l'importance des classes II et III, qui correspondent à des lésions dont le traitement assure la prévention du cancer du col utérin.

Les facteurs étiologiques classiques de ce type de cancer sont étudiés, et les résultats de tests réalisés de façon systématique sont comparés à ceux de tests orientés par un examen gynécologique préalable, ce qui permet de noter la supériorité du dépistage systématique.

Les auteurs proposent enfin un schéma d'organisation de la prévention et du dépistage de ce type de cancer à l'échelle sous-régionale africaine.

INTRODUCTION

Toutes les études consacrées au cancer en Afrique soulignent la grande fréquence du cancer du col utérin.

Au Sénégal, le cancer du col vient au troisième rang de tous les cancers après le cancer primitif du foie et les cancers cutanés. Chez la femme, c'est le cancer le plus fréquent: il représente 21% des cancers et son incidence est estimée à 12,4 pour 100 000 (8,4 pour le cancer du sein).

Une étude préliminaire effectuée à l'Institut du Cancer de Dakar et portant sur 600 cas de cancers du col confirmés histologiquement, a montré le pronostic défavorable de cette affection, diagnostiquée le plus souvent à un stade très avancé (77% aux stades III et IV).

Cette étude a montré également:

- qu'il existe un pic de fréquence entre 46 et 54 ans;

- que ce cancer prédomine chez les multipares; en particulier chez les femmes ayant eu des grossesses précoces (16 ans en moyenne au Sénégal à l'âge de la première grossesse).

- que la majorité des malades ont un niveau socio-économique faible et sont exposées à un grand nombre de facteurs de risque (infections génitales répétées et non traitées, rapports sexuels précoces, traumatismes répétés du col utérin).

Certains mesures, telles que l'éducation des jeunes filles, l'information du corps médical et du public, devraient permettre de réduire la fréquence de cette affection. Parallèlement, l'organisation de centres de dépistage devrait permettre d'en améliorer considérablement le pronostic.

Cette dernière mesure nous paraissant de première importance; nous avons, dans le cadre d'une collaboration pluridisciplinaire, procédé à une campagne de dépistage cytologique des lésions du col utérin chez les femmes de l'agglomération dakaroise. L'objectif d'une telle campagne était de démontrer l'intérêt du diagnostic cytologique.

MATERIEL ET METHODS

L'étude a été menée dans plusieurs centres sanitaires du Cap-Vert. Cette région regroupe près d'un million et demi d'habitants, répartis entre Dakar et sa banlieue. Cette population est représentative des différentes classes socio-économiques rencontrées au Sénégal. De novembre 1980 à juillet 1983, 5 131 tests colpocytologiques ont été pratiqués chez des femmes qui peuvent être réparties en deux groupes:

- un premier groupe de 3 804 femmes chez qui le frottis a été pratiqué de façon systématique;

- un second groupe de 1 327 patientes chez qui l'indication de frottis a été orientée par un examen préalable du col au spéculum.

Chaque test a comporté 3 prélèvements selon les recommandations d'Ayre: un du cul de sac vaginal postérieur, un grattage de l'exocol et frottis endocervical à la ponction cylindropavimenteux.

RESULTATS

Les résultats de l'examen cytologique peuvent être ainsi résumés (Tableau 1):

- 394 frottis (7,7%) n'ont pu être interprétés, soit pour des raisons techniques (frottis trop épais ou panci-cellulaires), soit en raison de la cytolyse ou de l'inflammation trop marquées, imposant le renouvellement de l'examen;

- 412 frottis (8,0%) ont été jugés normaux (classe I)

- 4 059 frottis (60%) ont été attribués à la classe II, qui regroupe l'ensemble des frottis inflammatoires, (de sévérité légère à modérée).

Tableau 1. Résultats globaux.

Résultats	Nombre de cas	Pourcentage
Frottis ininterprétables	394	7,7 %
Frottis normaux (classe I)	412	8,0 %
Frottis inflammatoires (classe II)	4 059	79,1 %
- Après biopsie		
cancers préinvasifs	27	
cancers invasifs	22	
- Non biopsiés	4	
Dysplasies (classe III)	213	4,2 %
Frottis à caractère malin (classe IV et V)	53	1,0 %
TOTAL	5 131	100 %

- 436 frottis (8,5%) ont tout d'abord été considérés comme douteux, et attribués à la classe III. Un traitement local a été administré à ces patientes, et la cytologie de contrôle a permis alors de ramener à 213 (4,2%) le nombre de frottis de classe III. Ce fait met en relief les difficultés rencontrées par les cytologistes et la nécessité d'un entraînement suffisamment long et de l'application d'une technique rigoureuse.

- 53 frottis (1%) ont présenté un caractère franchement malin (classes IV et V).   Un contrôle biopsique a été effectué dans 49 cas.   Le caractèere pré-invasif a été confirmé dans un peu plus de la moitié d'entre eux (55%).

Ces résultats nous permettent d'estimer à 15 pour 1000 le nombre de lésions malignes du col qui pourraient être diagnostiquées par la pratique des frottis, la moitié de ces lésions pouvant être détectées au stade pré-invasif.

Nous avons tenté de dégager quelques facteurs épidémiologiques caractéristiques de la population étudiée.

Age

L'âge des patientes chez qui la cytologie a été pratiquée varie de 13 à 71 ans. La répartition de la population étudiée par tranches de 10 années montre que plus de 80% des femmes examinés ont entre 21 et 50 ans (Tableau 2).

Tableau 2. Répartition selon l'âge.

Tranches d'âge	Nombre de frottis pratiqués	Pourcentage de frottis pratiqués
10 à 20 ans	318	6,2
21 à 30 ans	2 192	42,7
31 à 40 ans	1 023	19,9
41 à 50 ans	983	19,2
51 à 60 ans	316	6,2
61 à 71 ans	299	5,8
TOTAL	5 131	100 %

Il est à noter une plus grande facilité de l'examen chez les femmes en période d'activité génitale que chez les femmes plus âgées; en effet, les femmes en période d'activité génitale se prêtent volontiers aux examens gynécologiques, surtout lorsqu'il existe des centres de formation sanitaire.

Parité

En ce qui concerne la parité, la répartition des différents frottis est présentée dans le Tableau 3.

Tableau 3. Répartition selon la parité

Parité	Nombre de frottis pratiqués	Poucentage de frottis pratiqués
Nullipares	531	10,4 %
Primipares	612	11,9 %
Multipares	2 892	56,4 %
Grandes multipares	1 096	21,4 %
TOTAL	5 131	100 %

Il aurait été intéressant d'étudier les résultats des frottis en fonction de l'âge et de la parité. Cela n'a malheureusement pas été possible.

Dépistage systématique et dépistage orienté

La comparison entre les résultats du dépistage systématique et du dépistage orienté à partir d'une lésion d'appel constatée cliniquement fait apparaître certaines différences:

- le dépistage orienté chez 1 327 femmes a permis de découvrir des frottis très infectés avec un grand nombre de frottis ininterprétables. Dans ce cas, le nombre de frottis classés 'normaux' est faible. Par ailleurs, les lésions carcinomateuses diagnostiquées à partir du dépistage orienté sont déjà invasives;

- le dépistage systématique chez 3 804 femmes s'est révélé nettement supérieur en ce qui concerne le diagnostic des dysplasies. Ce fait est important étant donné que la dysplasie est l'étape qui précède le cancer in situ lequel peut ensuite devenir invasif.

La rentabilité des examens systématiques est donc supérieure.

DISCUSSION

Les résultats obtenus dans la lutte contre le cancer du col utérin dans les pays dévelopés démontrent qu'il est également possible en Afrique de réduire la fréquence de ce type de cancer. Cette réduction passe par la modification progressive de certaines habitudes sociales (nuptialité et maternité précoces, grande multiparité), l'amélioration du niveau économique et l'éducation sanitaire.

La prévention par le dépistage et le traitement des lésions du col doit permettre à court terme de faire baisser la fréquence des lésions invasives.

Un système de dépistage peut s'articuler sur les structures habituelles et ne nécessite donc pas de création de nouvelles structures. Il peut se structurer selon une pyramide à 3 niveaux:

- A la base, un système de prévention sera instauré au niveau des cases de santé, des maternités rurales et communales. Ce système s'articulera autour des sages-femmes et des infirmiers, qui devront recevoir une formation en gynécologie carcinologique. Ils devront être capables de réaliser les prélèvements pour les cytologies cervicales, d'effectuer des examens du sein et du col utérin, et d'orienter si besoin les malades vers le niveau suivant.

- Le niveau intermédiaire sera constitué par une antenne départementale et régionale de dépistage, tenue par un cyto-technicien capable de pratiquer des prélèvements, et d'éffectuer leur coloration et leur lecture sous l'autorité du médecin-chef de la circonscription médicale. Ceci conduira à la sélection des classes II, à traiter sur place, et des classes III et IV à orienter au niveau supérieur de la pyramide de dépistage.

- Ce niveau supérieur de la pyramide sera constitué par le Centre National de dépistage. Celui-ci sera intégré à l'Institut du Cancer ou, à défaut, au Laboratoire d'Anatomie Pathologique.

Au Sénégal, la supervision et la coordination de toutes ces activités reviendraient à un Centre National de Dépistage du Cancer, rattaché à l'Institut du Cancer de Dakar, où doivent aboutir toutes les malades présentant des lésions précancéreuses ou cancéreuses. L'équipement de ce Centre de traitement des tumeurs constitute, bien sûr, l'objectif prioritaire car il ne servirait à rien de dépister des cancéreux sans leur apporter l'assistance nécessaire.

Contrairement à ce qui se disait il y a encore une dizaine d'années, le cancéreux n'est pas voué à une mort certaine. Le pronostic vital est fonction du stade auquel est dépistée la maladie.

ÉTUDE RÉTROSPECTIVE DES CANCERS DU COL DE L'UTERUS OBSERVÉS À CASABLANCA 1971–1972

B. El Gueddari, A. El Hafed, A. Kahlain, F. Kettani
A. Bouih, M. El Morchid & A. Allami

Institut National de Lutte contre le Cancer
Rabat

SUMMARY

The authors present a retrospective study of 383 cases of cervical cancer seen at the Bergonié Centre in Casablanca in 1971 and 1972. An epidemiological analysis of this cancer is given, as well as the results of a clinical and therapeutic study. The long-term results for this series are very satisfactory, since survival at five years for carcinomas, which are the most frequent, was 30%, despite the variety of therapeutic regimens used at the time of treatment.

RESUME

Les auteurs présentent l'étude rétrospective de 383 cancers du col utérin vus au Centre Bergonié de Casablanca en 1971 et 1972. Ils dressent le profil épidémiologique de ce cancer, et présentent les résultats de l'étude clinique et thérapeutique. Les résultats à long terme de cette série sont très satisfaisants, puisqu'on obtient une survie à 5 ans de l'ordre de 30% pour les épithéliomas qui sont les plus fréquents, et ce malgré la diversité et la disparité des attitudes thérapeutiques adoptées à l'époque.

INTRODUCTION

Au cours des consultations de surveillance que nous donnons actuellement, nous avons rencontré un certain nombre de femmes guéries d'un cancer du col utérin qui avaient été traitées pendant les années 1971 et 1972. Aussi nous a-t-il paru intéressant de reprendre les dossiers des malades traitées pendant cette période.

MATERIEL ET METHODES

Les dossiers des malades ayant été traitées pour un cancer du col utérin au Centre Bergonié de Casablanca, entre le 2 janvier 1971 et le 31 décembre 1972 ont été revus rétrospectivement.

Ces dossiers comportent de nombreuses lacunes, en particulier quant au bilan d'extension de la tumeur: l'urographie intraveineuse, la lymphographie, la radiographie pulmonaire, la cytoscopie et la rectoscopie n'ont pas été pratiquées de façon systématique.

D'autre part, la surveillance des malades n'a pas été régulière: 20% d'entre elles ont été perdues de vue dès la première année.

Aussi, le nombre de cas analysés varie selon le paramètre étudié.

RESULTATS

Fréquence

Nous avons colligé 383 cas de cancer du col utérin parmi les 3 171 nouveaux cas de cancer diagnostiqués au Centre Bergonié durant la même période. Le cancer du col représente 12% des cancers de la femme; c'est le 2ème par ordre de fréquence, après les tumeurs cutanées.

Age

L'âge des malades varie de 25 à 80 ans, avec un âge moyen de 47 ans. La répartition par classes d'âge (Fig. 1) fait apparaître un pic de fréquence entre 30 et 50 ans: 66,3% des cancers du col sont diagnostiqués durant cette période.

FIG. 1. REPARTITION DES CANCERS DU COL UTERIN SELON L'AGE

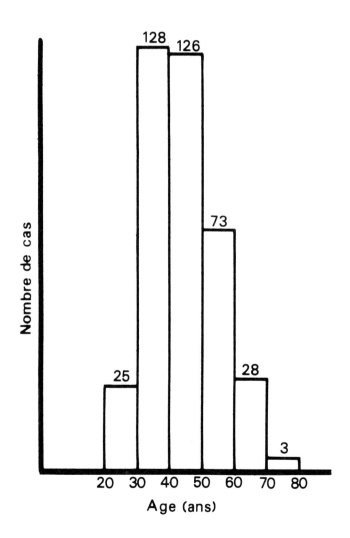

Parité

Le nombre d'enfants a pu être connu pour 195 malades: 80% d'entre elles avaient plus de 3 enfants (Tableau 1).

Tableau 1. Parité des patientes atteintes de cancer du col utérin

Parité	Nombre de malades	%
Nullipare	8	4,1
< 3 enfants	31	15,9
> 3 enfants	156	80,0
Total	195	100

Stade clinique au moment du diagnostic

Les données cliniques ont permis de classer 342 malades selon le stade de leur cancer, d'après la classification de la FIGO (Tableau 2). Les subdivisions des stades I et II n'ont pas pu être effectuées.

Tableau 2. Répartition des cancers du col utérin selon le stade (classification de la FIGO)

Stades	I	II	III	IV	Total
Nombre de cas	38	116	162	26	342
%	11,1	33,9	47,4	7,6	100

Les chiffres rapportés montrent que 55% des patientes consultent à un stade avancé: stade III (47,4%) et stade IV (7,6%).

Classification anatomo-pathologique

L'étude anatomo-pathologique, réalisée chez 348 malades,
montre une nette prépondérance des épithéliomas (94%) (Tableau
3).

Tableau 3.   Répartition des cancers du col utérin selon l'histologie

Histologie	Nombre de cas		%
Epithéliomas	327	)	94,0
Adenoépithéliomas	16	)	4,6
Epithéliomas mixtes	3	) 348	0,9
Sarcomes	2	)	0,6
Non pratiquée	35		9,13

Les figures 2 et 3 montrent les caractéristiques histopa-
thologiques.

Résultats thérapeutiques - Survie

Seize malades (4,2%) n'ont reçu aucun traitement. Les 367
autres patientes ont reçu différents traitements, du fait de leur
provenance assez disparate et en fonction des modalités thérapeutiques appliquées en dehors du Centre Bergonié.

Ainsi, 65% des malades ont été traitées exclusivement par
radiothérapie (Tableau 4);   55% d'entre elles présentaient des
tumeurs aux stades III et IV. Les patientes de stade I et II ont
surtout été traitées par des associations chirurgie/radiothérapie
(Tableau 5).

FIG. 2. EXOCOL: CONDYLOME PLAT

Présence d'hyperacanthose avec bourgeonnement dans le chorion.
Présence de nombreux koïlocytes au niveau du corps muqueux.
Haematoxyline et éosine

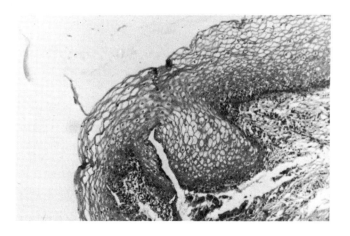

FIG. 3. JONCTION ENDO-EXOCOL: CONDYLOME DYSPLASIANT

Présence d'atypies cellulaires mêlées à quelques koïlocytes rési-
duels. Le chorion est inflammatoire. Haematoxyline et éosine

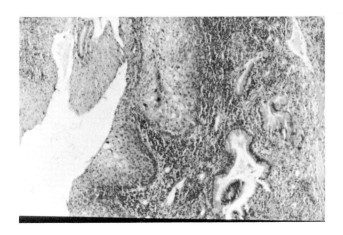

Tableau 4. Distribution des malades selon le type de traitement
(curie = curiethérapie; RTE = radiothérapie; chir. = chirurgie;
chimio = chimiothérapie)

Type de traitement		Nombre de cas	%
Radiothérapie	curie seule	16	4,4
exclusive	RTE + curie	78	21,3
242 (65,9%)	RTE seule	148	40,3
Associations	curie + chirurgie	8	2,2
radio-	chir + curie	5	1,4
chirurgicales	curie + chir + RTE	6	1,6
116 (31,6%)	chir + curie + RTE	18	4,9
	RTE + curie + chir	8	2,2
	RTE + curie + chir + RTE	6	1,6
	chir + RTE	62	16,9
	chir + RTE + curie + RTE	3	0,8
Association	RTE + chimio	6	1,6
radioth. +	chimio + RTE + curie	3	0,8
chimio 9 (2,4%)			
Total		367	100

La survie des malades est difficile à évaluer, car 60%
d'entre elles ont été perdues de vue durant les deux années qui
ont suivi le début du traitement. Ce taux élevé est probablement
dû au fait que la majorité des malades appartenaient à des classes défavorisées, pour qui il est difficile de se déplacer pour
des consultations de surveillance.

C'est pourquoi nous avons étudié le taux de survie pour
chacune des année à partir du début du traitement.

EL GUEDDARI ET AL.

Tableau 5. Répartition des différents types de traitement selon le stade des cancers

Traitement	Stades				
	I	II	III	IV	NP
Radiothérapie exclusive					
Curie seule	10	5	1	–	–
RTE + curie	5	47	26	–	–
RTE seule	3	27	102	13	3
Associations radiochirurgicales					
Curie + chir.	6	2	–	–	–
Chir + Curie	2		2		1
Cur + chir + RTE	2	4	–		–
Chir + Cur + RTE	3	5	1		9
RTE + cur + chir	3	3	2		–
RTE + cur + chir + RTE	1	3	2		–
Chir + RTE	2	15	10	7	27
Chir + RTE + Cur + RTE	2	1	–	–	–

NP, non précisé

La survie globale brute est de 24,8% à 5 ans, et de 8,1% à 10 ans. Si on élimine de cette étude 53 malades non traitées (16 malades n'ont reçu aucun traitement et 37 ont abandonné la radio-thérapie à moins de 30 Gy), et si l'on ne considère que les épi-théliomas traités (285 patientes), la survie à 5 ans passe à 33,3%, et la survie à 10 ans à 10,2% (Tableau 6).

Tableau 6. Survie des malades atteintes de cancer du col utérin

Nombre d'années écoulées depuis le début du traitement	0	1	2	3	4	5	6	7	8	9	10
Cancers du col diagnostiqués											
Nombre de survivantes	383	256	155	125	114	95	81	64	52	40	31
%		66,8	40,5	32,6	29,8	24,8	21,1	16,7	13,6	10,4	8,1
Epithéliomas traités											
Nombre de survivantes	285	251	155	125	113	95	79	64	51	39	29
%		88,1	54,4	43,9	39,6	33,3	27,7	22,5	17,9	13,7	10,17

L'analyse des résultats thérapeutiques en fonction du stade des épithéliomas au moment du diagnostic (Tableau 7) montre que le traitement des stades I et II a un effet assez médiocre. Par contre, les résultats du traitement des stades III sont comparables à ceux de la littérature (Kottmeier, 1962; Chaplain, 1978; Fenton & Decroix, 1979; Duran et coll., 1980; Gerbaulet et coll., 1981). Ils sont bien meilleurs quand le traitement a consisté exclusivement en une radiothérapie. Pour les stades I et II, les résultats les meilleurs sont obtenus par l'association de la chirurgie et de la radiothérapie.

Enfin, en raison du nombre important des malades perdues de vue, il nous a semblé intéressant d'étudier le contrôle local à un an (Tableau 8). Ces résultats sont très satisfaisants, notamment pour les stades III et IV.

Tableau 7. Survie des patientes atteintes d'un épithélioma du col utérin selon le stade et le type du traitement

Stade	Traitement	Nombre de patientes	Survie à 5 ans		Survie à 10 ans	
			No. de survivantes	%	No. de survivantes	%
I	Tous types	35	17	48,6	9	25,7
	Radiothérapie exclusive	17	5	29,4	2	11,8
	Association radiothérapie-chirurgie	18	12	66,7	7	38,9
II	Tous types	99	36	36,4	10	10,1
	Radiothérapie exclusive	70	26	37,1	6	8,6
	Association radiothérapie-chirurgie	29	10	34,5	6	20,7
III	Tous types	109	28	25,7	6	5,5
	Radiothérapie exclusive	95	26	27,4	5	5,3
	Association radiothérapie-chirurgie	14	2	14,3	2	14,3
IV	Tous types	13	1	7,7	0	0
	Radiothérapie exclusive	10	1	10,0	0	0
	Association radiothérapie-chirurgie	3	0	0	0	0
NP	Tous types	29	5	17,2	3	10,3
	Radiothérapie exclusive	3	0	0	0	0
	Association radiothérapie-chirurgie	26	5	19,2	3	11,5

NP, non précisé

Tableau 8. Contrôle local (à 1 an) selon le type de traitement

Stade	Radiothérapie exclusive (%)	Radiothérapie + chirurgie (%)
I	88,2	90,0
II	78,7	75,8
III	60,7	60,7
IV	40,2	14,3
NP	66,7	85,3

NP, non précisé

En ce qui concerne les récidives, 30 cas seulement ont été relevés dans les dossiers des malades qui ont pu être suivies (Tableau 9).

Tableau 9. Récidives

Stade	Récidives (30 cas)	%
I	2	6,6
II	9	30,0
III	12	40,0
NP	7	23,3

NP, non précisé

DISCUSSION

L'étude rétrospective des cancers du col utérin traités il y a 12 ans, dans des conditions difficiles, montre l'importance de ce cancer au Maroc. Sa fréquence est en progression, puisque ce cancer représente actuellement 23% des cancers au Centre Bergonié.

La majorité des cancers du col qui frappent une population relativement jeune (moyenne d'âge, 47 ans), sont des épithéliomas.

La parité semble jouer un rôle important dans l'apparition de ces cancers, ainsi que l'ont confirmé des études réalisées au Maroc (Ben Amor, 1981; Ben Kirane, 1982). Cependant, le rôle de la parité est actuellement contesté en Europe. Ce paramètre pourrait en fait être lié à un autre facteur de risque, l'âge précoce au mariage.

Une étiologie virale est actuellement de plus en plus évoquée. L'agent en cause serait un virus du groupe Papova (HPV16). Celui-ci détermine des lésions cytologiques et histologiques typiques (koilocytose, hyperacanthose, caryolyse...). L'association de ces atypies avec des états dysplasiques est fréquente (Meisels et coll., 1976). Des études dans ce sens sont actuellement en cours, notamment au Maroc.

Malgré la diversité des attitudes thérapeutiques adoptées, le contrôle local de la tumeur a été obtenu dans bon nombre de cas, et la survie reste appréciable, compte-tenu du nombre de patientes perdues de vue. On peut alors estimer que les faibles moyens qui ont pu être mis en oeuvre ont tout de même permis de guérir un nombre assez important de malades.

L'ouverture prochaine de l'Institut National de Lutte contre le Cancer à Rabat, l'application d'un protocole de traitement bien défini, un meilleur suivi des malades, devraient permettre d'obtenir des résultats plus satisfaisants.

A l'heure actuelle, le dépistage et le diagnostic précoce du cancer du col utérin représentent encore un des principaux problèmes vis-à-vis de ce cancer au Maroc.

REFERENCES

Ben Amor, Z. (1981) Aspects du cancer du col utérin au Maroc à propos de 1131 cas relevés au Centre anti-cancéreux de Casablanca. Thèse Méd. Rabat, No. 316

Ben Kirane, M.J. (1982) Approche épidémiologique des cancers génitaux à propos de 225 cas. Thèse Méd. Rabat, No. 102

Chaplain, G. (1978) Radiothérapie exclusive des cancers du col utérin. Résultats préliminaires d'une étude inter-centres à propos de 777 cas. Thèse Méd. Nancy I

Duran, J.C., Pilleron, J.P., Cleophax, J.P., Hamelin, J.P., Carcia, J.C. & Lefrance, J.P. (1980) Cancers du col utérin au début. Traitement par association radiochirurgicale. Bull. Cancer, 67, 48-57

Fenton, J. & Decroix, Y. (1979) Radiothérapie exclusive des épithéliomas du col utérin de stade II distal et III. Résultats et complications thérapeutiques de 393 cas traités à l'Institut Curie. Bull. Cancer, 66, 542-548

Gerbaulet, A., Chassagne, D. & Castaigne, D. (1981) Traitement des épithéliomas du col utérin, T_2 distal et T_3. Rev. Prat., 31, 1927-1932

Kottmeier, H.L. (1962) Ten years results of radiological treatment of carcinoma of the cervix. Act. Obstet. Gynecol., 41, 195-203

Meisels, A., Forlin, R. & Roy, M. (1976) Condylomatous lesions of the cervix (I) cytologic patterns. Acta Cytol., 20, 505-509

CARCINOMA OF THE PENIS IN UGANDA

R. Owor

Makerere University Medical School
Kampala, Uganda

RESUME

En Ouganda, l'épithélioma du pénis est le cancer le plus fréquent chez les sujets de sexe masculin, en particulier dans les groupes ethniques qui ne pratiquent pas la circoncision. Les grandes variations de fréquence de ce cancer observées néanmoins entre ces différents groupes suggèrent que d'autres facteurs peuvent jouer un rôle important. Les infections peuvent constituer un de ces facteurs, et la circoncision pourrait, de ce fait, intervenir uniquement en permettant une meilleure hygiène du pénis. Les condylomes acuminés sont également fréquents en Ouganda, et peuvent ressembler à des épithéliomas tant sur le plan clinique que sur le plan histologique.

SUMMARY

Carcinoma of the penis is the commonest cancer of males in Uganda, particularly among the different uncircumcised ethnic groups. The great variations in frequency among those groups, however, suggest that other factors may play an important role. These factors may be infections, so that circumcision may act only by permitting better penile hygiene. Condylomata acuminata are also common in Uganda and can resemble carcinoma both clinically and histologically.

***

Carcinoma of the penis is the commonest cancer of males in Uganda. The clinical records of Mengo Hospital, Kampala, show that Dr Albert Cook diagnosed carcinoma of the penis as early as the beginning of this century (Davies et al., 1964). The proportional rate in males for carcinoma of the penis during the years 1897-1956 was 14.9%; most were diagnosed clinically. The

Kampala Cancer Registry shows that during the period 1952-1960, the proportional rate was 12.2%, while from 1964 to 1968, it was 12.0% (Dodge et al., 1973). This suggests that the frequency of this tumour in Uganda, and presumably the incidence, has not changed since the beginning of this century.

More detailed epidemiological studies of carcinoma of the penis in Uganda started with the establishment of the Kampala Cancer Registry in 1952. A review of carcinoma of the penis in Uganda and Kenya shows that the tumour is much commoner in the uncircumcised ethnic groups (Dodge & Linsell, 1963). In Uganda, only a small proportion of the male population is circumcised, e.g., the Bakonjo in the west, the Bagisu in the east, and Moslems, who constitute about 5% of the population.

The Department of Pathology, Makerere University, Kampala, provides a histopathology service for the whole country and is also responsible for the Cancer Registry, which records all cancers seen in the country. The present report gives an analysis of the cases of carcinoma of the penis recorded in the Cancer Registry over the period 1964-1978.

During this period there were 1290 cases of carcinoma of the penis aged between 25 years and over 100 years. Table 1 shows the age distribution. Most of the tumours were seen in patients over 50 years; the majority were well differentiated squamous-cell carcinomas. It can be difficult occasionally to differentiate such carcinomas from condylomata acuminata, particularly when only a small biopsy is available.

The geographical distribution of the tumour was as shown in Table 2. The Southern Region has the highest number of cases, but this is the area where Kampala, the capital, is situated and where the medical services are relatively more readily available than in the rest of the country. Availability of medical services alone may not, however, explain the marked variation between the different regions.

Table 1. Age distribution of carcinoma of the penis in Uganda, 1964-1978

Age (years)	No. of cases
0 - 19	0
20 - 29	22
30 - 39	105
40 - 49	202
50 - 59	324
60 - 69	382
70 +	220
'Adult'	35
Total	1290

Table 2. Regional distribution of carcinoma of the penis in Uganda, 1964-1978

Region	No. of cases
East	274
West	390
North	88
South	500

Analysis by ethnic group yields a different picture (Table 3). The Banyoro and Batoro, who come from the Western region, have the highest proportional rates. The general pattern is that the rates are high in non-circumising ethnic groups, but there is considerable variation even within these groups. It is possible that there are differences in social habits between the different

ethnic groups and that these may lead to differences in penile
hygiene and hence to differences in the incidence of penile
cancer. All the ethnic groups concerned are of low socioeconomic
status.

Table 3. Proportional rates of carcinoma of the penis in
different ethnic groups in Uganda

Ethnic group	Proportional rate (%)
Banyoro	40.0
Batoro	32.0
Teso	24.0
Banyankole	15.0
Baganda	12.0
Rwanda/Rundi	10.0
Acholi	10.0
Basoga	8.0
Bakiga	3.0
Lango	3.0
Lugbara	2.9
Circumcising ethnic groups	2.0

In a different paper at this Symposium Dr Schmauz and myself
have discussed the possible relationship between condylomas and
carcinoma of the penis. Our studies strongly suggest that a
virus may play a part in the causation of some of these penile
tumours.

REFERENCES

Davies, J.N.P., Elmes, S., Hutt, M.S.R., Mtimavalye, L.A.R., Owor, R. & Shaper, L. (1964) Cancer in an African community 1897-1956. An analysis of the records of Mengo Hospital, Kampala, Uganda. Br. med. J., 1, 259-264

Dodge, O.G., Owor, R. & Templeton, A.C. (1973) Tumours of the male genitalia. In: Templeton, A.C., ed., Tumours in a Tropical Country, Berlin, Springer-Verlag

Dodge, O.G. & Linsell, M.D. (1963) Carcinoma of the penis in Uganda and Kenya Africans. Cancer, 16, 1255-1263

NASOPHARYNGEAL CARCINOMA

NASOPHARYNGEAL CANCER IN NIGERIA

F.D. Martinson

Department of Otorhinolaryngology
College of Medicine
University College Hospital
Ibadan, Nigeria

P.U. Aghadiuno

Department of Pathology, College of Medicine
University College Hospital
Ibadan, Nigeria

RESUME

On admet maintenant que le cancer du nasopharynx, jadis considéré comme inexistant ou rare en Afrique, est relativement commun. Cette maladie a été étudiée au Nigéria sur une période de 15 années. Comme ailleurs, la maladie est plus fréquente chez les hommes que chez les femmes. Le pic d'incidence selon l'âge est inférieur à celui que l'on observe dans le monde occidental. Les cancers d'origine épithéliale sont les plus fréquents. Le signe précurseur le plus courant est une adénopathie cervicale supérieure profonde, qui n'est pas toujours accompagnée de symptômes nasaux et/ou auditifs. L'implication du nerf crânien a été décelée au stade précoce dans environ 30% des cas; dans certains cas, elle peut constituer l'unique symptôme ou signe à la première consultation et l'origine de ce trouble ne peut être identifiée que si l'on pense à suspecter la maladie.

Les différentes étiologies virales, liée à l'environnement, sont examinées. Les patients se présentent en général tardivement à l'hôpital et le stade de la maladie est souvent tellement avancé qu'on ne peut leur proposer recevoir qu'un traitement palliatif. Il n'est pas surprenant alors que les taux de guérison et de survie soient faibles. Une meilleure connaissance de

la prévalence de la maladie aux différents âges et une grande
vigilance dans la détection des divers signes d'appel devraient
permettre d'effectuer un diagnostic précoce, et d'améliorer ainsi
les résultats du traitement. Il faut éliminer les facteurs
étiologiques   environnementaux   suspects   et   fournir   une
immunisation contre les virus en cause pour réduire l'incidence
de la maladie.

SUMMARY

Nasopharyngeal cancer, once considered to be non-existent or
rare in the African, is now accepted as being far from uncommon.
Experience of this disease in Nigeria over a 15-year period is
presented.   As elsewhere there is a preponderance of males over
females, but the peak age of incidence is lower than that
observed in the Western world.   Cancers of epithelial origin
predominate.   The commonest early sign of the disease is upper
deep cervical adenopathy usually, but not always, with nasal
and/or aural symptoms. Cranial nerve involvement has been
observed early in about 30% of cases and occasionally this may be
the only symptom or sign at first presentation and so may require
a high index of suspicion to discover its origin.

Viral, environmental and other possible etiological factors
are considered. Delay in seeking or being referred for hospital
treatment is common, and patients often present at such an
advanced stage that only palliation can be offered. The cure and
survival rates, not surprisingly, are low. Increasing awareness
of the prevalence of the disease at all ages and alertness in
recognizing its various presenting features are essential, as are
early diagnosis and improved facilities for treatment. Elimination of suspected environmental and other controllable etiologies, and efforts to provide immunization against the viruses
concerned are needed to help in reducing the incidence of the
disease.

INTRODUCTION

Nasopharyngeal cancer (NPC) was once considered to be non-
existent or at worst rare in the African, a view based on records
and observations in East and West Africa, Rhodesia and South
Africa (Elmes & Baldwin, 1946; Gelfand, 1949; Shapiro et al.,
1955; Edington, 1956; Davies, 1961).   In retrospect, it is

possible that some of the factors which may have contributed to these findings among some communities were the scarcity of doctors in the countries concerned, transport and economic problems, which made journeys to hospitals difficult, perhaps the unshakeable faith in traditional medicine which attracted many patients away from the few available hospitals, and opposition, in some communities, to post mortem examinations. In 1961, however, Clifford reported a high incidence of the disease in parts of Kenya, and various published records and communications from other parts of Africa since then (Clifford, 1965) have confirmed that the disease not only does occur in the African but also is far from uncommon.

In a review of NPC seen in University College Hospital (UCH), Ibadan, from 1960 to 1965 (Martinson, 1968), 55 patients, an average of 9 per annum, were recorded and these constituted about 9% of all head and neck cancers and about 0,6% of all cancers in the hospital register. At that time, UCH was one of three teaching hospitals to which most of such cases in the country were referred. During the following 15 years, 1966-1980, with which this review deals, when three additional teaching hospitals with otorhinolaryngology units took on a share of the load, 180 new cases (Table 1), an average of 12 per annum, were seen in Ibadan, only 25% of these having been referred from outside the state in which the hospital is situated.

Table 1. NPC: incidence by age and sex in 180 new cases (1966-1980)

Sex	Age (years)														
	0-5	6-10	11-15	16-20	21-25	26-30	31-35	36-40	41-45	46-50	51-55	56-60	61-65	66-70	Total
M	-	1	1	3	2	2	1	2	3	2	1	-	1		19
F	-		2	1	-	1	-	1	1	2	1	-	-	1	10
M	-	2	4	5	9	9	5	4	11	4	4	5	1	4	67
F	-	1	3	5	2	4	3	2	3	5	2	3	1	2	36
M	-	4	2	1	3	3	2	5	3	2	4	5	2	-	36
F	-	2	-	-	-	2	0	2	2	1	1	1	1	-	12
Total		10	12	15	16	21	11	16	23	16	13	14	6	7	180

In this series, the ratio of males to females is just over
2:1. Their ages range from 6 to over 65 years, with a peak age
incidence between 35 and 45 years; this is lower than in the
Western world and 20% of the cases are under the age of 20 years.
Our figures are similar in pattern but not in numbers to those of
Clifford in East Africa in 1964 (Clifford, 1965).

SYMPTOMS

The stated duration of symptoms ranges from 3 months to 3
years and a half, the very short durations often being open to
doubt or belied by the apparent advanced stage of the lesion.
Among the earliest symptoms complained of (Table 2) are a
swelling in the neck due to metastatic lymphadenopathy, usually
unilateral at first, nasal obstruction, epistaxis or blood-
stained discharge, and aural complications due to eustachian
obstruction. Cranial nerve palsies are common (Table 3), but the
extent and gravity of the features due to the main disease may so
overshadow the relatively minor inconvenience caused by some
neuropathies that the presence of the latter may be revealed only
when they are specially sought for. The 3rd, 4th, 5th, 6th, 9th,
and 10th nerves are most often affected, but all of the cranial
nerves have been involved singly or in different combinations,
early or late in the disease, and their paralysis may occasionally be the first and sole presenting features. This may be mis-
leading unless a high index of suspicion exists or the discovery
of a tell-tale hard cervical gland prompts the examiner to seek
the cause in the nasopharynx. Other symptoms and signs depend on
the rate of growth, direction of spread, invasiveness of the
tumour, and production of regional or distant metastases.

Table 2. NPC: main presenting symptoms

Symptom	No. of patients
Swelling in neck	100
Nasal obstruction	85
Blood-stained discharge or epistaxis	80
Aural symptoms	60
Nerve lesions (diplopia, facial weakness, dysphagia, weakness in legs)	30

Table 3. NPC: presenting signs

Sign	No. of patients
Enlarged cervical glands	100
Nasal or pharyngeal mass, palatal bulge	50
Proptosis	30
Ptosis	10
Aural signs:	
otorrhoea, deafness, serous otitis	45
acute suppurative otitis media	4
Meningitis	4
Cranial nerve palsies	80
Trismus	12
Parotid swelling	8
Pulmonary metastases	6
Paralysis of lower limbs	2

GROSS PATHOLOGY

Four gross pathological types of tumours have been encountered, namely the ulcerative, the nodular or polypoidal, whose names are descriptive of their appearance, the obstructing dome-like exophytic lesion and, least common, the sinister infiltrating lesion which, like the snake in the grass, advances for a long time hidden beneath apparently normal mucosa. This may therefore be easily missed on inspection or when random or 'blind biopsies' of the suspected area are taken. It has also been known to be associated with widespread metastases out of all proportion to the apparent size or superficial appearance of the primary lesion.

HISTOPATHOLOGY

As most observers have found elsewhere, tumours of epidermoid origin predominate (Table 4). The well-differentiated carcinomas form only a small proportion, in this case 5.3% of all tumours in this group of carcinomas, including those diagnosed from gland biopsies only. They have also been seen in patients

of 50 years and above and are more slowly growing than the less
differentiated types.

Table 4. NPC: histological types in 170 cases

Histological type	No. of patients
Squamous-cell carcinomas:	
well differentiated	8
lymphoepithelioma	15
variously differentiated and anaplastic[a]	101
Other carcinomas	30
Sarcomas:	
lymphosarcomas	12
plasmacytoma	4

[a] Biopsy from nasopharynx: 87; biopsy from
cervical gland: 14

DIAGNOSIS

Although biopsies of glandular metastases from carcinomas
may, as noted by Owor (1982), sometimes be difficult to differentiate from Hodgkin's disease or malignant lymphomas, a number of
our cases have been diagnosed from such material, each diagnosis
being corroborated by clinical examination in order to exclude
the chance of the primary being outside the head and neck.
Before biopsies were taken, other possible diagnoses have been
considered, particularly in the light of local patterns of
disease. When cervical lymphadenopathy is the only presenting
feature, tuberculosis and lymphomas have had to be excluded, and
this sometimes causes delay before referral to the otolaryngolo-
gist or head and neck surgeon. The early stages of NPC presenting as nasal obstruction with an occasional streak of blood
in the discharge forcibly expressed from the nose, may excusably
be diagnosed at first as chronic rhinosinusitis or even vasomotor
rhinitis because of the very high local prevalence of these

diseases, but this optimistic diagnosis must always be followed by investigation to justify maintaining it. Diseases encountered which have simulated NPC are angiofibroma, Wegener's granulomatosis, antrochoanal polyp in an adult of 42 (which incidentally resurfaced 5 years postoperatively as a sarcoma), a tuberculoma, a gummatous lesion associated with aural complications, craniopharyngioma, persistently enlarged adenoids in a man of 40, aspergilloma and rhinoentomophthoromycosis, all presenting as nasopharyngeal masses. Some parotid swellings with facial paralysis have proved to be metastatic lymphadenopathy.

ETIOLOGY

The viral theory has gained strength since Old et al. (1966), in studies on the sera of patients with NPC, found precipitating antibodies to an antigen prepared from Burkitt's lymphoma cells. This led to the suggestion that the Epstein-Barr virus (EBV) or a similar one might be involved. Henle et al. (1973) demonstrated changes in the serum titre of antibodies to EBV in patients that correlated with periods of remission or advance of the disease.

The idea that ethnic predisposition and genetic factors are involved has been prompted by the incidence of the disease in certain ethnic groups, notably those of south-east Chinese origin, whether resident in their own country or abroad (Digby et al., 1941; Pang, 1959), and the low incidence in India (Das et al., 1954). Among some Chinese communities, however, a dietary factor has been incriminated, namely a type of salted fish which from early childhood has been a regular item in the daily diet of members of the community affected (Ho, 1971).

Environmental factors have been suggested, such as prolonged exposure to smoke and soot as seen in the poorly ventilated homes of some tribes in Kenya (Clifford, 1965). The soot has been analysed and found to contain benzo(a)pyrene, benzanthracene, benzofluanthene and other carcinogenic agents (Clifford, 1965). We have so far not observed any relationship between similar living conditions among the poor in Nigeria and the incidence or distribution of the disease. Admittedly the concentrations of soot and smoke in huts may not be as high as those described in some areas of Kenya; the idea that the type of vegetation used in the fires may be the important factor has been discounted.

Certain Bantu tribes among whom the incidence of NPC is high are reputed to indulge in the use of snuff mixed with the ash of certain plants (Keen, 1964); some others use a liquid snuff (Linsell, 1963), but the evidence in favour of an association between these habits and NPC, in contrast to their association with cancer of the anterior nasal passages, is, according to these authors, slender.

Another theory which has not yet been tested clinically is the hormonal one (Allbrook, 1956; Politzer & Tucker, 1958), which associates a low level of male hormone and high oestrinization with increased susceptibility to the disease. Hypovitaminosis and poor nutritional states, which have also been said to play a role in the etiology (Wynder & Hoffman, 1965), may be found in the large majority of patients in Ibadan with and without the disease. However, this deficiency, it is claimed, might predispose to the disease because of its possible oestrinizing effect.

A theory which has much to recommend it is that of the possible role of vasomotor rhinitis and rhinosinusitis, diseases which are extremely common in West Africa. Ho (1978) believes that three factors are together responsible, namely EBV, genetically determined susceptibility and environmental factors.

TREATMENT

Cytotoxic drugs have been used, either alone or in combination with irradiation therapy, depending on the availability of facilities. This irregularity in therapy combined with the late stage of presentation often makes prognosis poor and the therapist's only possible aim one of palliation. Nevertheless, a few cures have been achieved and followed up for 2-5 years before the patients have decided optimistically to default. Among these have been extramedullary plasmocytomas, reticulum-cell sarcomas, some lymphomas and lymphoepithelioma.

DISCUSSION

A large proportion of patients in Ibadan (about 70%) come from the lower socio-economic strata (usually associated with the adverse environmental and nutritional conditions considered by some authors to be contributory etiological factors). These and other suggested etiologies may in fact be predisposing or precipitating factors needed to 'soften up' host resistance to invasion by the ubiquitous and opportunistic EBV.

The increase in incidence of the disease in this series, as compared with the previous one, may be more apparent than real and could be due to the progressive elimination of those factors suggested earlier as being contributory to previous low hospital records. On the other hand, one cannot rule out the possibility that the increase may in fact be real and might be due to changing patterns of disease, environmental conditions, modes of living and even therapeutic regimes, Western or traditional, for unrelated conditions. Until a national cancer register can be organized and can produce really representative figures, estimates of the incidence of the disease will remain inaccurate. Early detection of the disease and increased availability of treatment facilities should improve the results and give better survival rates than those so far achieved. Attempts at prevention by efforts to eliminate the suspected environmental, nutritional and other controllable contributing agents will also be necessary, if not imperative. Since a viral agent may be the most important member of the complex group of suspected etiological factors, preparation of some form of vaccine against EBV or other related viruses so far under suspicion may prove to be the only hope of reducing the incidence of what Lambert (1960) referred to as the most lethal and distressing condition of the speciality.

REFERENCES

Allbrook, D. (1956) Size of adrenal cortex in East African males. Lancet, 2, 606-607

Clifford, P. (1961) Contribution to the treatment of cancer of the head and neck. East Afr. med. J., 38, 491

Clifford, P. (1965) Carcinoma of the nasopharynx in Kenya. East Afr. med. J., 42, 373-396

Davies, J.N. (1961) The pattern of African cancer in Uganda. East Afr. med. J., 38, 486-491

Digby, K.H., Fook, W.L. & Che, Y.T. (1941) Nasopharyngeal
    cancer. Br. J. Surg., 28, 517-537

Edington, G.M. (1956) Malignant disease in the Gold Coast. Br.
    J. Cancer, 10, 595-608

Elmes, B.G.T. & Baldwin, R.B.T. (1947) Malignant disease in
    Nigeria. An analysis of a thousand tumours. Ann. trop.
    Med. Parasit., 41, 321-328

Gelfand, M. (1949) Malignancy in African. South Afr. med. J.,
    23, 1010-1016

Henle, W., Ho, H.C., Henle, G. & Kwan, H.C. (1973) Antibodies to
    Epstein-Barr-virus-related antigens in nasopharyngeal carci-
    noma. Comparison of active cases with long term survivors.
    J. natl Cancer Inst., 51, 361-369

Ho, J.H.C. (1978) An epidemiologic and clinical study of naso-
    pharyngeal carcinoma. Int. J. Radiol. Oncol. Biol. Phys.,
    4, 183-198

Keen, P. (1964) In U.I.C.C. Symposium on Cancer of the Naso-
    pharynx and Accessory Nasal Sinuses

Linsell, C.A. (1964) Nasopharyngeal cancer in Kenya. Br. J.
    Cancer, 18, 49-57

Old, I.J., Boyse, E.A., Oettgen, H.F., DeHarven, E., Geering, G.,
    Williamson, B. & Clifford, P. (1966) Precipitating antibody
    in human serum to an antigen present in cultured Burkitt's
    lymphoma cells. Proc. natl Acad. Sci. USA, 56, 1699-1704

Owor, R. (1982) Nasopharyngeal cancer. In: Cancer in Africa,
    pp. 33-49

Pang, L.Q. (1959) Carcinoma of the nasopharynx. An analysis of
    34 cases and a preliminary report on palatal fenestration in
    its management. Ann. Otol. (St Louis), 68, 356-371

Politzer, W.M. & Tucker, B. (1958) Urinary 17-ketosteroid and
    17-ketogenic steroid execretion in South African Bantu.
    Lancet, 2, 778-779

Shapiro, M.P., Keen, P., Cohen, L. & de Moor, N.G. (1955) Malignant disease in the Transvaal. _South Afr. med. J._, _29_, 95-101

LE CANCER DU NASOPHARYNX AU MAROC:
APPROCHE ÉPIDÉMIOLOGIQUE

B. El Gueddari, A. El Hafed, A. Bouih, M. El Morchid & A. Kahlain

Institut National de Lutte contre le Cancer
B.P. 6213 RI
Rabat

SUMMARY

Between 1 April 1980 and 30 Septembre 1983, 412 cases of nasopharyngeal carcinoma were seen at the Bergonié Cancer Centre in Casablanca (the sole centre in the country), representing 4.76% of all malignant tumours diagnosed in that period. This percentage is low, since the majority of these tumours are not diagnosed outside the big towns but indicates that Morocco is an area of moderate incidence for this cancer.

We have studied the epidemiological aspects of our series; there is a predominance of males (sex ratio, 2.25: M:F); the average age is 43 years with a large proportion of young people (24.6% are less than 30 years old). A high incidence is observed in the north of the country, where, however, more medical facilities are available.

Advanced tumours are common: 15% cannot be treated; 32.5% are in stage T4, and 70% have metastatic cervical nodes. Pathologically, 90% are undifferentiated carcinomas of the nasopharyngeal type.

The results of the immunological study do not exclude a viral (Epstein-Barr virus) contribution.

Prospective epidemiological studies are needed to elucidate the exact profile of this cancer in our country.

RESUME

Du ler avril 1980 au 30 septembre 1983, 412 cas de cancer du nasopharynx ont été observés au Centre Bergonié de Casablanca (seul centre de radiothérapie au Maroc), ce qui représente 4,76% des tumeurs diagnostiquées durant cette période. Cette fréquence est sûrement une sous-estimation, car un grand nombre de cas, survenant en dehors des grandes villes, échappent au diagnostic.

Un certain nombre de données épidémiologiques ont pu être dégagées de cette étude. Il existe, pour ce cancer, une nette prédominance masculine (sex-ratio H:F, 2,25). L'âge moyen est de 43 ans, avec une large proportion de sujets jeunes (24,6% des malades ont moins de 30 ans).

Une incidence élevée est observée dans le Nord du pays, plus médicalisé. La plupart des malades consultent à un stade avancé: 15% sont au-delà de toute ressource thérapeutique, 32,5% au moins sont au stade T4, et 70% présentent des adénopathies métastatiques.

Sur le plan anatomopathologique, il existe une nette prépondérance des épithéliomas de type nasopharyngé (90%).

La recherche des marqueurs de l'infection par le virus d'Epstein-Barr est en cours.

Des études prospectives et l'établissement d'un registre du cancer sont indispensables pour mieux cerner les problèmes de ce néoplasme.

INTRODUCTION

Il est actuellement classique de considérer le Maroc et les pays du Maghreb comme des pays à incidence du cancer du nasopharynx modérément élevée. Cette incidence se situe entre celle des pays de l'Asie du Sud-Est, où elle est la plus élevée, et celle des pays occidentaux, où elle est la plus faible (Ellouz et coll., 1975; Muir, 1975; Ho, 1978; Lefebvre et coll., 1983).

Les études marocaines concernant ce type de cancer sont restées jusqu'à présent assez disparates. Nous pouvons néanmoins citer les études les plus significatives, telles que celle de Alj et coll. (1980) et de Guerbaoui et coll. (1981).

Nous nous proposons de fournir ici de nouvelles données, basées sur le recrutement du Centre de Radiothérapie de Casablanca.

MATERIEL ET METHODES

L'étude a été menée du 1er avril 1980 au 30 septembre 1983, au Centre Bergonié du C.H.U. Ibn Rochd de Casablanca, seul centre de radiothérapie du Maroc. Avril 1980 correspond à la restructuration de ce service, qui fonctionne depuis 1923.

Durant cette période, 8 648 nouveaux cas de cancer ont été enregistrés, dont 412 cancers du nasopharynx (NPC) chez des Marocains. Ce chiffre a été utilisé pour calculer les taux d'incidence de la maladie, et a été rapporté aux données démographiques du dernier recensement général de la population (Bulletin Officiel du Maroc, 1981).

L'examen des dossiers a fait apparaître que le compte-rendu anatomopathologique faisait défaut pour 34 observations. L'analyse a donc porté sur 378 cas de cancer du nasopharynx confirmés histologiquement.

Les anticorps dirigés contre le virus d'Epstein-Barr (EBV) ont été recherchés dans le sérum et la salive de certains malades, essentiellement les malades qui ont été adressés au Centre par les services d'O.R.L. des C.H.U. de Rabat et de Casablanca. Les analyses ont été effectuées dans le service de Biologie de l'Hôpital Militaire d'Instruction de Rabat (Professor Nejmi) avec la collaboration du CIRC.

RESULTATS

Incidence et répartition géographique

Nous avons colligé 412 cas de cancer du nasopharynx parmi les 8 648 nouveaux cas de cancer enregistrés pendant la période d'étude. Le NPC représente donc 4,8% des cancers. Ce taux est inférieur à celui obtenu en Tunisie, qui est de 8,3% (Ellouz et coll., 1975). Il correspond très certainement à une sous-estimation, due à des insuffisances tant humaines que matérielles. En effet, le Centre Bergonié, qui est le seul service de radiothérapie du royaume, ne dispose que de deux radiothérapeutes, d'une

bombe au cobalt, d'un télécésium, et de 40 lits d'hospitalisation.   Il ne peut assurer le traitement de tous les cancers du
pays.

L'incidence minimale du cancer du nasopharynx au Maroc est de
1,84 cas pour 100 000 habitants, pour la période considérée, mais
elle varie selon les régions.

L'incidence du NPC a été calculée pour chaque région et
reportée sur une carte du Maroc.   Le découpage par région est
très significatif:

Région	Pourcentage de la population marocaine étudiée	Incidence (pour 100 000)
Centre et Nord	35,7	2,36
Nord-Ouest	13,2	2,04
Centre-Nord	17,8	2,67
Nord-Est	6,7	2,11
Province d'Alhoceima		0,32
Région de Casablanca-Rabat	17,8	2,94
Zone de la Chaouia	9,3	1,53
Su-Ouest	22,9	0,96
Sud-Est (région semi-désertique)	7,0	0,90

Un seul cas a été répertorié dans le Grand Sud à Eddakhla.

L'incidence est élevée (2,65 pour 100 000) dans la moitié
nord du pays (région de Casablanca-Rabat comprise), plus médica-
lisée où le climat est méditerranéen.   Dans la région sud, où le
climat est plutôt continental, elle n'est environ que de 1 pour
100 000, et ceci malgré l'existence d'une forte concentration de
population dans la région de Marrakech.

Dans le nord, la faible incidence observée dans la province d'Alhoceima est probablement due à la difficulté des communications entre la chaîne du Rif et Casablanca; seule une faible proportion des malades peut venir se faire soigner au Centre.

Age et sexe

Des 378 patients dont le diagnostic de cancer du cavum a été confirmé histologiquement, 262 (70%) étaient de sexe masculin, et 116 (30%) de sexe féminin, ce qui donne un sex-ratio de 2,25 hommes pour une femme.

L'âge n'a pas pu être précisé pour quatre hommes et une femme, ce qui ramène à 371 le nombre de malades retenus pour l'étude de ce paramètre.

Les âges extrêmes sont de 7 et 80 ans, l'âge moyen de 42 ans. Il est de 43,4 ans chez l'homme, et de 38,8 ans chez la femme. Ces résultats sont comparables à ceux de Guerbaoui et coll. (1981).

L'étude de la répartition des NPC par tranches d'âge (Fig. 1) fait apparaître un premier pic de fréquence entre 20 et 30 ans: 15% des NPC se situent dans cette tranche d'âge; 24,6% des malades enregistrés au Maroc ont moins de 30 ans.

Un deuxième pic de fréquence, plus important, apparaît entre 40 et 60 ans.

La répartition par âge et par sexe confirme l'existence des deux pics, aussi bien chez l'homme que chez la femme (Fig. 2).

FIG. 1.   REPARTITION DES CANCERS DU NASOPHARYNX SELON L'AGE

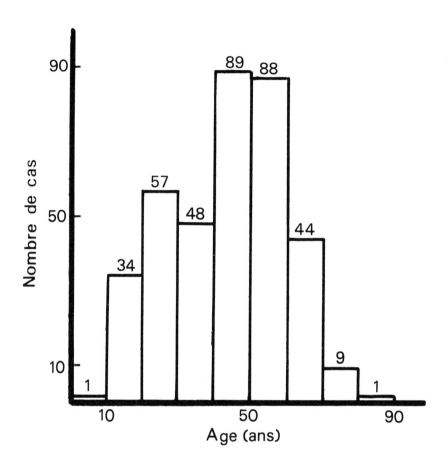

FIG. 2. REPARTITION DES CANCERS DU NASOPHARYNX
SELON L'AGE ET LE SEXE
▲, FEMMES; ●, HOMMES

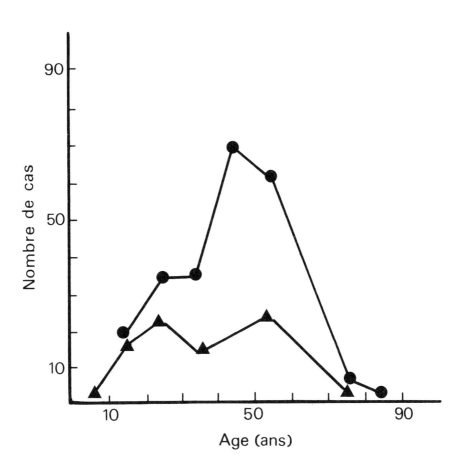

Données cliniques

Elles sont malheureusement peu fournies. Quarante-deux dossiers restent inexploitables, du fait de la pauvreté des renseignements cliniques. Les patients arrivent souvent au Centre sans le moindre bilan d'extension tant sur le plan clinique que sur le plan radiologique.

Les éléments cliniques présentés ici proviennent donc de
l'examen réalisé par les deux radiothérapeutes du Centre chez 336
patients.

Signes cliniques	Nombre de cas (336)	Pourcentage
Signes rhinologiques:		
Epistaxis	175	52,0
Obstruction nasale	106	31,5
Signes otologiques	141	42,0
Signes neurologiques (avec atteinte prépondérante du VI)	48	14,3
Exophtalmie	8	2,4
Trismus	46	13,7

Ces signes sont le plus souvent associés.

Le stade de la maladie a pu être évalué selon la classification TNM chez seulement 124 malades:

         T1   5 cas
         T2   7 cas
         T3   3 cas
         T4 cliniquement évident   109 cas

La présence d'adénopathies a été notée chez 230 des 336
patients examinés (69%):

         N0   6 cas
         N1   1 cas
         N2   36 cas
         N3   21 cas
         NX sans précision du   172 cas
            nombre, du siège,
            ni du caractère

Des métastases (M1) ont été signalées dans 8 cas.

Aspect anatomopathologique

Parmi les 378 cancers du nasopharynx confirmés histologiquement, 373 étaient des épithéliomas, qui ont pu être classés en deux catégories, selon la classification de Micheau (1975):

- Les épithéliomas de type nasopharyngé (UCNT), chez 339 malades et regroupant:

  -- les épithéliomas épidermoïdes peu différenciés
  -- les épithéliomas indifférenciés et ce que l'on appelait jadis, les lymphépithéliomas

- Les épithéliomas épidermoïdes bien différenciés kératinisants, retrouvés chez 34 patients (9%).

Les cinq patients restants étaient porteurs de formes rares de NPC avec:

- 2 lymphomes malins non Hodgkiniens: un chez un homme de 66 ans et un chez une femme de 70 ans;
- 1 localisation de maladie de Hodgkin chez une femme de 25 ans;
- 1 rhabdomyosarcome embryonnaire chez une fillette de 7 ans;
- 1 plasmocytome solitaire chez une femme de 55 ans.

Données thérapeutiques

Parmi les 378 malades dont le diagnostic de NPC a été confirmé histologiquement:

- 57 (15,0%) ont été jugés au-dessus de toute ressource thérapeutique;

- 321 (84,9%) ont été traités par radiothérapie, dont:

  -- 166 (43,9%) ont reçu une dose curatrice de 65 à 70 Gy
  -- 155 (41,0%) ont reçu une dose non tumoricide, inférieure à 45 Gy.

Etiologie

Les résultats préliminaires de la recherche d'anticorps
anti-EBV ont déjà été publiés (Alj et coll., 1980), et montrent:

- dans le sérum: la présence d'anticorps dirigés contre
  l'antigène précoce du virus d'Epstein-Barr (anti-EA) et
  d'anticorps dirigés contre la capside virale (anti-VCA)
  dans 80% des cas

- dans la salive: la présence d'anticorps anti-VCA dans 36,8%
  des cas.

Chez les jeunes, la positivité du sérum est faible: seulement 6% des malades de moins de 21 ans possèdent des anticorps.

DISCUSSION

Au Maroc, la fréquence du cancer du nasopharynx (évaluée à
4,8% des cancers d'après cette étude) est sûrement sous-estimée,
du fait de l'infrastructure médicale peu développée en dehors de
Casablanca-Rabat et des moyens de diagnostic très limités en
province.

La distribution des cancers du cavum selon le sexe et l'âge
se rapproche de celle des autres séries, en particulier des
séries tunisiennes (Ellouz et coll., 1975). La proportion de cas
survenant chez des sujets jeunes est élevée: 24,6% des malades
de notre série ont moins de 30 ans. Toutefois, les études tunisiennes montrent que 15,8% des cancers du cavum surviennent chez
des sujets de moins de 19 ans, alors que dans notre étude, 15%
des cancers sont observés entre 20 et 30 ans. Le sex-ratio
(2,25) est voisin de celui obtenu dans les autres études (Ellouz
et coll., 1975; Muir, 1975; Ho, 1978; Guerbaoui, 1981).

La répartition géographique montre une incidence élevée (2,65
pour 100 000) dans la moitié nord du pays, de climat méditerranéen, contrastant avec celle observée dans le sud du pays.

Les renseignements cliniques quoiqu'insuffisants permettent
de noter que la plupart des malades consultent à un stade avancé
de la maladie: 15% sont au-delà de toute ressource thérapeutique, près de 70% présentent des adénopathies (Brugère et coll.,
1975).

L'histologie montre une prépondérance des épithéliomas de type nasopharyngé (90% des UCNT).

Les études préliminaires sont en faveur d'une participation virale, mais ne permettent pas de conclure de façon définitive sur une relation de cause à effet (Alj et coll., 1980; Micheau et coll., 1980).

Cette contribution à l'étude du cancer du nasopharynx est encore modeste, du fait de nos moyens limités. Cependant, nous pouvons espérer qu'avec l'ouverture prochaîne de l'Institut National de Lutte contre le Cancer, une étroite collaboration avec les différents services des autres installations hospitalières verra le jour, qui permettra d'établir un registre national du cancer. Ce registre devrait permettre de définir de façon plus précise le profil épidémiologique du cancer du nasopharynx et d'en évaluer l'importance.

REFERENCES

Alj, S.A., Ouazzani, H., Tahiri Kzadri, M., Nejmi, S., Lenoir, G. & Desgrange, C. (1980) Les cancers du cavum (N.P.C.) au Maroc. Epidémiologie et circonstances de découverte. Ebauche d'une étude immunologique. Revue de Laryngologie, 101, 487-493

Brugère, J., Eschwege, F., Schwaab, G., Micheau, C. & Cachin, Y. (1975) Les carcinomes du nasopharynx (cavum): Aspects cliniques et évolutifs. Bull. Cancer, 62, 319-330

Bulletin Officiel du Royaume du Maroc (1983) Recencement de la population du Maroc. B.O. No. 3679, du 4 Mai 1983

Ellouz, R., Cammoun, M., Zaouche, A., Benattia, R. (1975) Les cancers du nasopharynx en Tunisie: Aspects épidémiologiques et anatomo-cliniques. Bull. Cancer, 62, 295-306

Guerbaoui, M., Iraqi, A., El Gueddari, B., El Jai, J. & Ouazzani, H. (1981) Le carcinome du nasopharynx au Maroc. Travail présenté aux assises Ana-path, Bruxelles, 26-27 mars 1981

Ho, J.H.C. (1978) An epidemiologic and clinical study of naso-
    pharyngeal carcinoma. Radiat. Oncol. Biol. Phys., 4, 183-198

Lefebvre, J.L., Madelain, M., Adenis, L., Demaille, M.C.,
    Delobelle, A. & Demaille, A. (1983) Les épithéliomas naso-
    pharyngés: Expérience du centre régional de lutte contre le
    cancer de Lille (79 cas de 1970 à 1982). Bull. Cancer, 70,
    294-299

Micheau, C. (1975) Anatomie pathologique et essai de classifica-
    tion des EOA du nasopharynx. Bull. Cancer, 62, 277-286

Micheau, C., de-Thé, G., Orofiamma, B., Schwaab, G., Brugère, J.,
    Sancho-Garnier, H. & Cachin, Y. (1980) carcinome du nasopha-
    rynx: Relation entre types histologiques et sérologie anti-
    virus Epstein-Barr. Nouv. Presse méd., 9, 21-24

Muir, C.S. (1975) L'épidémiologie du cancer du cavum. Bull.
    Cancer, 62, 261-264

STRATEGIES FOR THE ECONOMIC PREPARATION OF EPSTEIN-BARR VIRUS PROTEINS OF DIAGNOSTIC AND PROTECTIVE VALUE BY GENETIC ENGINEERING: A NEW APPROACH BASED ON SEGMENTS OF VIRUS-ENCODED GENE PRODUCTS

H. Wolf, M. Motz, R. Kühbeck, R. Seibl, W. Jilg & G.J. Bayliss

Max von Pettenkofer Institute
Munich, Federal Republic of Germany

B. Barrell

Medical Research Council
Cambridge, United Kingdom

E. Golub

Oral Health Center
Philadelphia, USA

Y. Zeng & S.-Y. Gu

Institute of Virology
Beijing, People's Republic of China

RESUME

L'immunoprécipitation des protéines du virus d'Epstein-Barr (EBV) par différents sérums provenant d'adultes normaux, de patients ayant une mononucléose infectieuse récente ou un épithélioma du nasopharynx a été utilisée pour identifier les antigènes permettant de déterminer l'état immunitaire d'un individu vis-à-vis du virus et caractéristique de chacune de ces maladies. On a localisé les gènes codant pour certains de ces antigènes sur le génome du virus d'Epstein-Barr par traduction de fragments d'ARN

sélectionnés par hybridation. A partir des données sur la
séquence, ces gènes ont pu ensuite être subclonés à partir de
l'ADN du virus EB et exprimés dans des cellules eucaryotes et
procaryotes. Les données sur l'expression de ces gènes sont
présentées, et l'application de ces méthodes à la production de
réactifs de diagnostic et de vaccins est discutée.

SUMMARY

Immunoprecipitation of Epstein-Barr viral proteins with
various sera from normal adults, patients with fresh infectious
mononucleosis or nasopharyngeal carcinoma was used to identify
antigens which are of importance in the determination of immune
status and characteristic of a particular disease. Some genes
coding for of these antigens have been localized on the Epstein-
Barr virus (EBV) genome by hybrid-selected translation. With the
use of sequence data, these genes could then be subcloned from
EBV DNA and expressed in eukaryotic and prokaryotic cells. Data
on the expression are presented and the application of the
methods described for the production of diagnostic reagents and
vaccines is discussed.

INTRODUCTION

The first suggestive evidence that Epstein-Barr virus (EBV)
might be causally related to nasopharyngeal carcinoma (NPC) and
African Burkitt's lymphoma was derived from serological data (for
review, see Epstein & Achong 1979). Using mainly indirect
immunofluorescence on cells producing virus or at least early
viral genes, significantly higher antibody titres to these antigens were found in patients' sera. Although helpful in establish-
ing a relationship between EBV and these diseases, these first
tests which detected unspecified immunoglobulin classes against a
group of proteins called early antigen (EA) and another group of
proteins called virus capsid antigens (VCA) were of limited value
for definite diagnosis of the malignancies from a single serum,
and could not be used for the control of therapy. Furthermore,
antigen preparation and test evaluation were not easy and
restricted use of the diagnostic procedure to a limited number of
laboratories.

The introduction of antigen and antibody class-specific tests, specifically the determination of peripheral IgA anti-bodies for the two antigen families EA and VCA, and also the first attempts to subdivide at least the EA family (into EA diffuse (D) or restricted (R); Henle et al. 1971), led to remarkable improvements in the diagnostic and prognostic value of the tests. However, the test systems did not allow automatic reading and thus did not favour mass testing. The preparation of single polypeptides from antigen classes promised a better corre-lation with disease status (Modrow et al., 1981). Attempts were made to develop ELISA tests from the lysates of antigen-producing cells, but these tests suffer from variable degrees of unspeci-ficity due to contaminating cellular materials that cannot be eliminated by inexpensive procedures. The use of highly purified antigens should overcome the problems of unspecificity and increase the diagnostic resolution. Because EBV does not effect-ively replicate in tissue culture, it is not feasible to purify viral antigens from infected cells, and genetic engineering seems to offer a way out of this dilemma.

MATERIALS AND METHODS

Cells

The EBV-producing, membrane antigen (MA)-positive cell line P3HR1, the EBV-positive, non-producing Raji cell line and the EBV-negative line BJAB were used. When the cells reached a density of about 10^6/ml, they were diluted with an equal volume of fresh medium. For induction of EBV antigens, P3HR1 cultures were treated with 40 μg/ml phorbol-12-mystrate-13-acetate (modified from zur Hausen et al., 1978) and 3 mM butyric acid immediately after subculture. Cells were harvested for labelling 1-2 days later.

Labelling of cells with ^{35}S-methionine

Cells were collected by low-speed centrifugation and resus-pended at a density of 2 x 10^6 cells/ml in methionine-free Eagle's minimum essential medium (MEM) containing between 50 and 100 μCi/ml ^{35}S-methionine. The cells were incubated at 37°C in 5% carbon dioxide for 4 h. The labelled cells were washed with cold Hanks' phosphate-buffered saline (PBS) and resuspended in cold IP buffer (1% Triton-x-100, 0.1% sodium dodecylsulfate (SDS); 0.137 M sodium chloride; 1 mM calcium chloride; 1 mM

magnesium chloride;   10% glycerol;   20 mM Tris-hydrochloride, pH
9.0;   0.01% NaN$_3$;   1 μg/ml phenylmethylsulfonyl fluoride; (Merck,
Darmstadt, Federal Republic of Germany) at a concentration of 5 x
10^6 cells/ml.   The cells were disrupted by sonication and incubated on ice for 60 min.   The extracts were clarified by centrifugation at 100 000 g for 30 min at 4°C.

Labelling of cell-surface proteins with ^{125}iodine

Lactoperoxidase-catalysed   iodination   of   cell-surface
proteins was performed according to Hubbard and Cohn (1975) with
some modifications.   Iodinated cells were suspended in PBS at a
concentration of 2 x 10^7 per ml and mixed with an equal volume of
1% Nonidet P-40 (NP-40) in PBS supplemented with Trasylol (Bayer,
Leverkusen, Federal Republic of Germany;   final concentration 200
KIU/ml) and phenylmethylsulfonyl fluoride (final concentration 2
mmol).   After incubation for 30 min on ice, the cells were
centrifuged at 2000 g for 30 min and the supernatant filtered
through Sephadex G-25.   The first radioactive peak containing the
labelled membrane protein was used for immunoprecipitation.

Immunoprecipitation

^{35}S-Methionine labelled extracts were immunoprecipitated
exactly as described by Bayliss and Wolf (1981).   Immunoprecipitation of ^{125}I-labelled membrane proteins was carried out as
previously described by Jilg and Hanning (1981).   Briefly, the
^{125}iodine-labelled cell extracts were first precleared with a
rabbit   antiserum   directed   against   human   peripheral   blood
lymphocytes (PBL) in order to remove most of the lymphocyte-
specific proteins and also to remove proteins which bind non-
specifically to immobilized Staphylococcus aureus protein A.   The
precleared extract was mixed with 10 μl of the serum to be tested
and incubated overnight in the cold.   Immune complexes were
isolated.   The beads were thoroughly washed, suspended in electrophoresis sample buffer (50 mM Tris-hydrochloride, pH 7.0, 2%
SDS;   5% 2-mercaptoethanol, 3% sucrose) and heated to 100°C for 5
min.

Preparation of RNA and hybrid-selected translation

RNA was prepared by lysing the cells with 4M guanidine iso-
thiocyanate and 0.5 M 2-mercaptoethanol 2 days after induction
(Chirgwin et al., 1979).   The lysate was centrifuged for 1 hour
at 20 000 rpm and the supernatant layered on top of 2 ml caesium

chloride, density 1.8 g/cm^3. After centrifugation for 17 hours at 150 000 g, the RNA pellet was precipitated with ethanol, and 100 g total cellular RNA was hybridized for 2.5 hours at 52°C in 65% formamide and 0.4 M sodium chloride to 16 g cloned EBV DNA, which was sonicated and denatured and spotted on small nitro-cellulose filters. Bound mRNA was eluted by boiling the filters in water. The RNA was translated in vitro with a mRNA-dependent rabbit reticulocyte lysate. The translation products were immunoprecipitated using 5 l of a pool of human sera for one assay after preincubation with a protein extract from unlabelled EBV-negative BJA-B cells, as previously described (Bayliss et al., 1983). The immune complexes were bound on protein A-sepha-rose, washed, eluted by boiling the beads in electrophoresis sample buffer and loaded on to SDS-polyacrylamid gels.

Cloning of viral DNA for expression

DNA of a plasmid containing the desired reading frame plus additional viral sequences in pBR 322 (Skare & Strominger, 1980) were digested with restriction enzymes and separated on agarose gels. The desired bands were electroeluted, purified through Elutip columns (Schleicher & Schuell, Keene, New Hampshire) and cloned by standard procedures into the selected vectors: pUC8 and pUC9 (Messing & Vieira, 1982) and pUR228 (Ruether & Müller-Hill, 1983). Strains JM83 and MBH 71-18 of E. coli were transfected by standard procedures and the clones with inserts were tested in rapid lysis assays, using appropriate restriction enzymes to determine the orientation of the insert relative to the plasmid. Clones with correct orientation and reading frame were grown, induced with isopropyl-13-0-thiogalactopyranoside (IPTG) (1 mM) and incubated for another 1 1/2 hours. The bacterial proteins were separated on reducing SDS-polyacrylamide gels.

RESULTS

Finding antigens important for the diagnosis of NPC

By the use of immunoprecipitation, it has been shown that EA and VCA are not single antigens, but that both consist of several polypeptides (Bayliss & Wolf, 1981). This technique has been used to test sera for the presence of antibodies to specific proteins. The results are shown in Figure 1. Whereas IgG anti-bodies very early after infection are not very dominant, it was

possible to show that antibodies to p150 and p143 are invariably
present in healthy individuals, even long after primary contact
with EBV, and in NPC patients. Antibodies to p138 were regularly
present in sera from NPC patients but only occasionally present
in some other sera. For this reason, this antigen was considered
to be of value in the diagnosis of NPC.

In a similar manner, patients' sera were tested for antibodies against the EBV-specific membrane antigen gp 250.   These
antibodies, which have neutralizing capacity, were present in
individuals with a history of past EBV infection and in high
concentrations in NPC patients; they were not found in patients
with acute and chronic persistent infection (Fig. 1b)

FIG. 1a. TESTING SERA FOR THE PRESENCE OF ANTIBODIES
TO SPECIFIC PROTEINS

Raji cells were superinfected with P3HR1 virus. Cells were
labelled with ^{35}S-methionine from 12-16 hours post infection and
immunoprecipitated with sera from different patients.   The
proteins were analysed on polyacrylamide gels.   Antibodies
against p 150 and p 143 could be used as indicators of the immune
status of the patients. Antibodies against p 138 were regularly
found in sera from NPC patients and are therefore suitable for
the initial serological screening of sera.

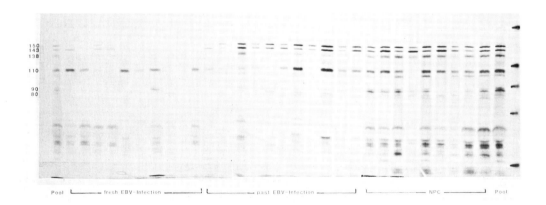

FIG. 1b. EXAMINATION OF PATIENTS' SERA FOR ANTIBODIES
AGAINST THE EBV-SPECIFIC MEMBRANE ANTIGEN gp 250

P3HR1 cells were surface-labelled with ^{125}iodine and membrane
proteins extracted as described under Materials and Methods.
Patients' sera were used to immunoprecipitate the labelled
extracts.   Sera were taken from patients with fresh EBV
infection, past EBV infection, and NPC.   A pool of high-titre
sera was used as a positive control, and sera from EBV-negative
persons as a negative control.

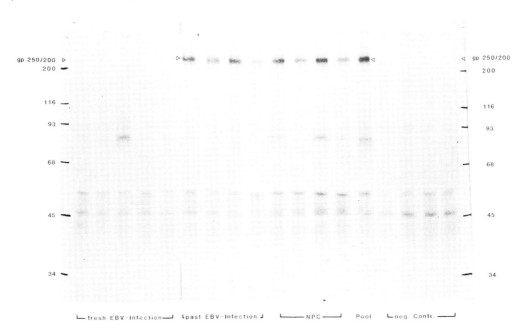

Localizing antigens on the EBV genome

By the use of cloned viral DNA immobilized on nitrocellulose
filters, mRNA originally transcribed from a particular segment of
the genome can be selected.   This mRNA can be eluted, translated
in vitro and the translation products analysed on a polyacrylamide gel.   This procedure has allowed the physical mapping of a
number of viral proteins on the viral genome (Fig. 2).   Protein
138 was localized on the BamH1 fragment of the EBV genome.   From
sequence data, it was possible to identify an appropriate open
reading frame in the l direction.

FIG. 2. MAP OF <u>IN VITRO</u> TRANSLATED PROTEINS WITH HYBRID-SELECTED RNA FROM INDUCED P3HR1 CELLS AND INDUCED RAJI CELLS

The <u>Bam</u>Hl fragments were cloned from B95-8-derived EBV DNA. By hybridizing to sheared fragments of EBV DNA cloned in Charon 4A a finer map of the coding regions of some proteins could be achieved. The narrow coding regions for the 18-kd, 90-kd, 47-kd, 73-kd and 69-kd proteins in the induced Raji cells are based on the assumption that these proteins correspond to proteins with the same molecular weights in P3HR1 cells (Seibl & Wolf, unpublished data).

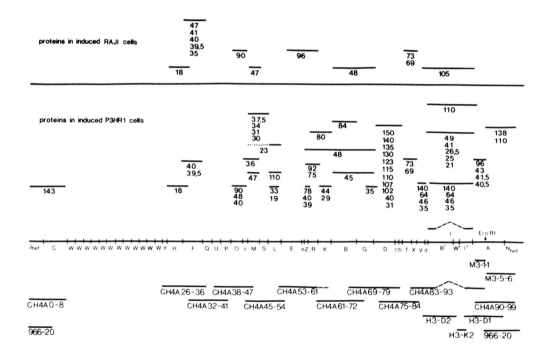

Expression of viral information in prokaryotes

Initially, an attempt was made to express a large segment of the gene coding for p138 in several bacterial expression vectors. This attempt was partially successful, but the yield of p138 was small due to its large size and to its degradation by bacterial proteases (data not shown). It was therefore decided to dissect the gene coding for this antigen. It was assumed that there might be a few antigenic epitopes and that these could be identified in the products of the recombinant hosts. Figure 3 shows computer graphics which give a suggested structure of the protein on the basis of the algorithms derived by Chou and Fasman (1974). Superimposed on the suggested structure are the hydrophilic (open) and hydrophobic (filled circles) values of the respective area (average of 5 neighbouring amino acids). Based on these graphics, amino-acid sequences near position 520 and at the n-terminus of p 138 should be antigenic and therefore recognizable by NPC sera. To test this hypothesis, the viral p 138 coding region was dissected into small segments (200-750 base-pairs (bp)) which were cloned into the expression vector pUR288 behind the beta-galactosidase reading frame. The resulting products are fusion proteins of the large beta-galactosidase (116 kD) fragment and the respective region of p 138 (Fig. 3). These proteins are stable due to the large bacterial protein fused to them. Electrophoretic transfer of proteins from bacterial lysates separated on SDS-polyacrylamide gels on to nitrocellulose membranes (western blot) allowed the detection of the antigenic fragments of p 138 (Fig. 4b), of which only two, p 600 and p 540, are antigenic. This is in good agreement with the prediction based on considerations of the structural and hydrophobic properties of the primary amino-acid sequence. The P600 but not the P540 region could be expressed after cloning in plasmid pUC 8; the resulting protein has a small portion of the bacterial beta-galactosidase (Fig. 4c). It is probable that the large beta-galactosidase fragment in the pUR 288 product protects the eukaryotic peptide from bacterial protease degradation. For successful expression of a eukaryotic antigenic determinant without a large bacterial protein fused to it, the following two conditions must be fulfilled: (1) the antigenic site must be determined; and (2) this site and its surrounding amino acids must form a structure which is resistant to attack by bacterial proteases.

WOLF ET AL.

FIG. 3. COMPUTER PLOT OF A CHOU-FASMAN (1974) CALCULATION
OF THE p 138 SECONDARY STRUCTURE

The hydrophobic (closed circles) and hydrophilic (open circles)
regions are also indicated.   Antigenic sites can be expected in
hydrophilic regions with a beta-turn.   This situation exists in
the p 600 region and at the c-terminus of the protein.

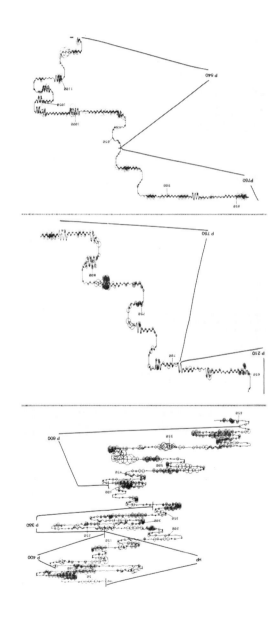

FIG. 4a. COOMASIE BRILLIANT BLUE STAINED SDS-POLYACRYLAMIDE
SLAB-GEL ANALYSIS OF LYSATES OF IPTG-INDUCED BACTERIA
CARRYING THE VARIOUS PLASMIDS

Fusion proteins with molecular weights between 120 and 150 kd are
indicated by closed circles. Track M: molecular-weight markers
tracks pUR400-pUR540 lysates of bacteria carrying plasmids
containing the regions of p138, as shown in Figure 3.

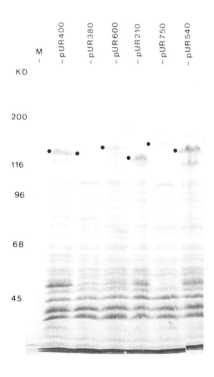

FIG. 4b.   AN ENZYME-LINKED IMMUNOABSORBENT ASSAY
OF PROTEINS TRANSFERRED FROM A GEL
(SIMILAR TO THAT SHOWN IN PANEL a)
ON TO NITROCELLULOSE PAPER

After electrophoretic transfer of the proteins (western blot) and
saturation of the blot with bovine serum albumin (BSA), a pool of
high titre antiserum was applied and, after washing, the bound
immunoglobulins were visualized by sequential reaction with peroxidase coupled to antibodies against human IgG and diaminobenzi-
dine.   Only fusion proteins from bacteria containing pUR600 and
pUR540 show specific reactions.   Plasmid pUC 635 contains almost
the whole of the p138 coding region, but the protein is unstable
and is rapidly degraded.   Puc8 is the negative control containing
the vector plasmid free from EBV-derived sequences.

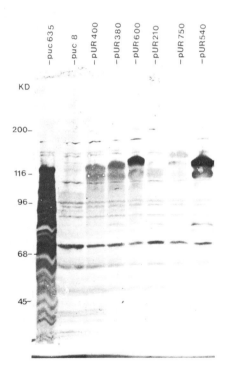

FIG. 4c. A WESTERN BLOT SIMILAR TO THAT SHOWN IN b
BUT ANALYSING pUC PLASMIDS CONTAINING THE VARIOUS REGIONS
SHOWN IN FIGURE 3

Clone pUC HG covers the same region as pUC HP, but contains an additional 100 base pairs. Only bacteria containing clone pUC600 produce stable antigenic products.

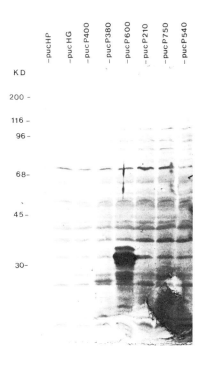

DISCUSSION

A powerful strategy has been developed for producing viral antigens that may be almost as fast as, and is certainly more reliable than the synthesis of oligopeptides. The advantage of this procedure is that the products are less vulnerable to rapid changes in antigenicity with minor variations in the length of the product. The same approaches and computer programs used to predict antigenic determinants for peptide synthesis make it possible to select those clones which will probably yield anti-genic products. Although the construction of the clones is restricted to specialized laboratories, the preparation of anti-

gens from established recombinant bacteria should be very
inexpensive and it should be possible to do this in developing
countries. It can be expected that highly specific products will
allow cheaper, more widely usable and standardizeable diagnostic
tests, which will also have an increased diagnostic value,
especially in conjunction with antibody class-specific test
protocols. A similar approach to the development of clones
expressing antigens suitable for use in vaccines should also be
of value. This would involve the identification of regions of
proteins with the known potential to induce neutralizing antibodies and their subsequent cloning in the vectors described
above. Polypeptides containing not only oligopeptides as antigenic sites but including flanking sequences may have advantages
over in vitro synthesized shorter oligopeptides, which frequently
elicit weak immune responses even when used in combination with
strong adjuvants.

REFERENCES

Bayliss, G.J. & Wolf, H. (1981) The regulated expression of
    Epstein-Barr virus. III. Proteins specified by EBV during
    the lytic cycle. J. gen. Virol., 56, 105-118

Bayliss, G.J., Deby, G. & Wolf, H. (1983) An immunoprecipitation
    blocking assay for the analysis of EBV induced antigens. J.
    virol. Methods, 7, 229-239

Chirgwin, J.M., Przybyla, A.E., MacDonald, R.J. & Rutter, W.J.
    (1979) Isolation of biologically active ribonucleic acid
    from sources enriched in ribonuclease. Biochemistry, 18,
    5294-5299

Chou, P. & Fasman, G. (1974) Conformational parameters for amino
    acids in helical, beta-sheet and random coil regions
    calculated from proteins. Biochemistry, 13, 211-245

Epstein, M.A. & Achong, B.G., eds (1979) The Epstein-Barr Virus,
    Berlin, Heidelberg, New York, Springer Verlag

Henle, G., Henle, W. & Klein, G. (1971) Demonstration of 2 distinct components in the early antigen complex of Epstein-Barr virus infected cells. Int. J. Cancer, 8, 272-282

Hubbard, A.L. & Cohn, Z.A. (1975) Externally disposed plasma membrane proteins. I. Enzymatic iodination of mouse cells. J. cell Biol., 64, 438-460

Jilg, W. & Hanning, K. (1981) Lymphocyte surface proteins recognized by an antithymocyte globulin. Hoppe-Seyler's Z. physiol. Chem., 362, 1475-1485

Messing, J. & Vieira, J. (1982) A new pair of M13 vectors for selecting either DNA strand of double-digest restriction fragments. Gene, 19, 269-276

Modrow, S., Schmidt, H. & Wolf, H. (1983) Immunoprecipitation as a tool for studying humoral immunity of natural and experimental hosts of Herpesvirus saimiri. Cancer Res., 43, 3398-3402

Rüther, U. & Müller-Hill, B. (1983) Easy identification of cDNA clones. EMBO J., 2, 1791-1794

Skare, J. & Strominger, J. (1980) Cloning and mapping of BamH1 endonuclease fragments of DNA from the transforming B95-8 strain of Epstein-Barr virus. Proc. natl Acad. Sci. USA, 77, 3860-3864

zur Hausen, H., O'Neill, F.J., Freese, U.K. & Hecker, E. (1978) Persisting oncogenic herpesvirus induced by the tumour promoter TPA. Nature, 272, 373-375

KAPOSI'S SARCOMA

ETIOLOGY OF ENDEMIC KAPOSI'S SARCOMA

C.L.M. Olweny

Harare, Zimbabwe

RESUME

L'étiologie exacte du sarcome de Kaposi (SK) demeure encore inconnue. Certaines observations suggèrent une étiologie virale; ce sont: (a) la régression spontanée de certaines formes cliniques; (b) l'apparition fréquente de tumeurs primitives secondaires; (c) le développement multifocal du SK.

Des études au microscope électronique ont révélé la présence de particules de virus de type herpès qui, du point de vue morphologique, ressemblent au cytomégalovirus (CMV). Les sérums provenant de malades atteints du SK en Europe et en Amérique renferment plus d'anticorps anti-CMV que ceux des témoins, contrairement à ceux des malades africains dont le titre d'anticorps anti-CMV n'est pas significativement différent de celui des témoins. Cette disparité peut être liée au fait que l'ensemble de la population africaine possède des taux d'anticorps anti-CMV relativement élevés.

Des études utilisant la technique d'hybridation moléculaire ont révélé la présence d'ADN du CMV dans le tissu de certains SK africains.

Le rôle possible du virus des leucémies/lymphomes T humains (HTLV) dans l'étiologie du SK est discuté à la lumière de la démonstration récente de son association avec le syndrome d'immuno déficience acquise (SIDA). De même, un éventuel rôle prédisposant du type HLA-DR5 chez ces malades atteints de SIDA ou de SK est examiné.

SUMMARY

The exact etiology of Kaposi's sarcoma (KS) remains unknown. Certain observed features suggest a possible viral etiology, including: (a) the spontaneous regression of indolent forms; (b) the frequent occurrence of second primary malignancies; (c) the multifocal nature of KS.

Electron microscopic studies have revealed herpesvirus-type particles which morphologically resemble cytomegalovirus (CMV). Sera from KS patients in Europe and America have higher anti-CMV antibodies than controls, in contrast to African patients, whose CMV antibody titres are not significantly different from those of controls. This difference may be related to the high background of CMV antibody in the general African population.

Nucleic acid hybridization studies have revealed CMV DNA in some African KS tissue.

The possible role of human T-cell leukaemia/lymphoma virus (HTLV) in the causation of KS is discussed in the light of recent evidence of its association with acquired immunodeficiency syndrome (AIDS). Similarly, the possible predisposing role of HLA-DR5 in patients with AIDS and KS is considered.

INTRODUCTION

Kaposi's sarcoma (KS) has recently attracted world-wide attention mainly because of its close association with acquired immunodeficiency syndrome (AIDS). Epidemiologically, KS occurs in sporadic, endemic or epidemic forms, each of which correlates with definite clinical varieties (Table 1).

The sporadic form is the classical disease described by Kaposi in 1872 and this is the type previously seen in Europe and North America. The disease runs a protracted course and is indolent in behaviour.

Table 1. Classification of Kaposi's sarcoma

Epidemiological	Clinical forms	Clinical behaviour
Sporadic	Cutaneous-nodular	Indolent
Endemic	1. Cutaneous-nodular or cutaneous-plaque	Indolent
	2. Locally aggressive	Aggressive
	3. Generalized aggressive	Aggressive
Epidemic	Generalized aggressive	Aggressive

Endemic KS exists in three varieties, as follows:

(a) The cutaneous nodular or plaque forms, which are similar in behaviour to the classic disease.

(b) The locally aggressive, which includes florid (vegetative or cauliflower) or infiltrative varieties.

(c) The generalized aggressive, which is usually lymphadenopathic, visceral or osseous and clinically resembles epidemic KS.

Epidemic KS is associated with AIDS and is aggressively malignant and often lymphadenopathic.

The spectrum of KS is thus similar to what is observed in leprosy, with tuberculoid disease at one end of the scale, passing through borderline cases and ending with lepromatous disease at the other. Like leprosy, the host's immune state appears to determine the clinical pattern of KS. Those with good immune mechanisms will develop indolent disease, occasionally remitting spontaneously, while those with a poor immune state will develop the aggressive generalized form of KS.

ROLE OF GENETIC FACTORS

Despite the increasing knowledge of the epidemiology, clinical features and therapy of KS, the etiology of the disease remains speculative. There are reports of familial occurrence (Templeton & Dhru, 1975; Finlay & Marks, 1979), but this may merely point to common agent exposure. Evidence is now available which suggests that certain HLA phenotypes (HLA-DR5) may be commonly associated with epidemic KS but whether this is true in the endemic form is yet to be determined. Although several HLA loci have been examined, so far only the DR locus is associated with KS. The mechanisms underlying the association are not clearly understood but several suggestions have been put forward, including: (a) population stratification; (b) HLA itself may be a cause of susceptibility, the antigen perhaps acting as a receptor for, say, a virus, or there may be antigen cross-reactivity; (c) linkage disequilibrium with a susceptibility locus.

GEOGRAPHICAL FACTORS

Although most available evidence would tend to point to an environmental factor or factors as responsible for the development of KS, the distribution of endemic KS does not seem to fit or coincide with that of any known geographical factors (temperature, humidity, rainfall, altitude). There have been suggestions that KS is associated with high-rainfall regions, such as the Delta region of Nigeria, but other rainfall belts of Africa or South America do not seem to show a similar distribution of this tumour.

VIRUSES

Certain clinical observations have been taken to suggest a possible viral etiology, including inter alia:

(a) the occurrence of spontaneous regression in certain clinical varieties (cutaneous nodular); this would tend to suggest an immune host response similar to that in virus-induced animal tumours;

(<u>b</u>)   the frequent occurrence of second primary neoplasms; this may indicate a persistent tumour inducer. In Uganda, second primaries have been observed either presenting concurrently or following treatment of KS and these have in the main been lymphoreticular malignancies;

(<u>c</u>)   the multifocal nature of KS; this is thought to be compatible with a virus infection.

Serological studies of European and American patients with sporadic classical KS revealed higher antibodies to cytomegalo-virus (CMV) than corresponding controls. However, African endemic KS sera did not have significantly higher anti-CMV titres, probably because of the high background of CMV antibody in the African population (Giraldo <u>et al.</u>, 1981). However, CMV DNA has been found by nucleic acid hybridization in endemic KS tissues from Uganda (Giraldo <u>et al.</u>, 1981). Thus, endemic KS may be initiated by a common virus, possibly CMV, which causes trans-formation of the target cell. The infection probably occurs early in life, and remains silent, but can be reactivated. The transformed cell would need a co-factor, probably malaria or some other immunosuppressive condition, to cause proliferation.

In the case of epidemic KS occurring in association with AIDS, the epidemiological evidence leads to the virtually inescapable conclusion that it is due to a transmissible agent, probably a virus. Recent evidence would tend to suggest the possible involvement of human T-cell leukaemia virus (HTLV) a T-cell-tropic virus, and AIDS is characterized by marked depletion of helper T-cells. Initial studies have demonstrated an increased prevalence of antibodies against HTLV cell-membrane antigens among patients with AIDS (Essex <u>et al.</u>, 1983). More recently Gallo at the National Cancer Institute, Bethesda, MD, USA, has convincingly demonstrated integrated HTLV-like proviral sequences in DNA from fresh as well as cultured lymphocytes from two AIDS patients (Gallo <u>et al.</u>, 1983). However, transformation <u>in vitro</u> with HTLV has largely been accomplished using co-culti-vation techniques, implying that HTLV may require cell-to-cell contact. It is possible that HTLV would have to interact with some other virus, such as CMV or Epstein-Barr virus (EBV), to produce AIDS. In a recent study of endemic KS in Zambia, all 16 patients had antibodies to CMV, 15 had antibodies to EBV, and 13 had antibodies to HTLV (Downing <u>et al.</u>, 1984).

It is possible that HTLV and other viral infections observed in both epidemic and endemic KS may merely represent an epiphenomenon related to profound immune deficiency and increased susceptibility to infection.

REFERENCES

Downing, R.G., Eglin, R.P. & Bayley, A.C. (1984)   African Kaposi's sarcoma and AIDS. Lancet, 1, 478-480

Essex, M., McLane, M.F., Lee, T.H., Falk, L., Howe, C.W.S., Mullins, J.I., Cabradilla, C. & Francis, D.P. (1983) Antibodies to cell membrane antigens associated with human T-cell leukemia virus in patients with AIDS. Science, 220, 859-862

Finlay, A.Y. & Marks, R. (1979) Familial Kaposi's sarcoma. Br. J. Dermatol., 100, 323-326

Gallo, R.C., Sarin, P.S., Gelmann, E.P., Robert-Guroff, M., Richardson, E., Kalyanaraman, V.S., Mann, D., Sidhu, G.D., Stahl, R.E., Zolla-Pazner, S., Leibowitch, J. & Popovic, M. (1983) Isolation of human T-cell leukemia virus in acquired immune deficiency syndrome (AIDS). Science, 220, 865-867

Giraldo, G., Beth, E. & Kyalwazi, S.K. (1981) Aetiological implications of Kaposi's sarcoma. Antibiot. Chemother., 29, 12-29

Kaposi, M. (1872) Idiopathisches multiples Pigment Sarkom der Haut. Arch. Dermatol. Syph., 4, 265-273

Templeton, A.C. & Dhru, D. (1975) Kaposi's sarcoma in half brothers. Trop. geogr. Med., 27, 324-327

KAPOSI'S SARCOMA IN ZAIRE

P.L. Gigase & A. de Muynck

Prince Leopold Institute of Tropical Medicine
Antwerp, Belgium

M. de Feyter

Fondation Médicale de l'Université de Louvain en Afrique Centrale
Katana, Bukavu (Kivu), Zaire

RESUME

Le sarcome de Kaposi (SK) a été reconnu en 1948 au Zaïre, où il a probablement toujours existé à l'état endémique. En 1957, on a trouvé que le SK représentait 9% de tous les cancers pour lesquels une biopsie avait été effectuée. L'incidence présente des fluctuations à l'intérieur du pays, avec une incidence plus élevée dans l'Est, où elle a été estimée en 1960 à environ 5 à 10 cas par 100 000 et par an chez les sujets de sexe masculin, avec un ratio Homme:Femme (H:F) supérieur à 1:10. Plus récemment, au nord-est du Zaïre, le SK représentait respectivement chez les hommes et chez les femmes 17% et 2% environ des tumeurs malignes ayant fait l'objet d'une biopsie (1969-1983). En deux années (1982-1983), on a confirmé histologiquement 26 cas de SK chez des hommes et 5 chez des femmes, dans une région du Zaïre oriental dont la population est d'approximativement 300 000 personnes.

On a suggéré, sur les bases de cette incidence élevée de SK et de l'identification récente de cas africains de SIDA, que l'agent transmissible supposé du SIDA pourrait avoir son origine en Afrique Centrale. La fréquence du SK dans les cas de SIDA africains est basse (16%) comparée à celle observée aux Etats-Unis. Le ratio H:F du SIDA est de 6:4, et celui du SK associé au SIDA de 1:1. Les cas associés au SIDA ont été observés chez de jeunes adultes; ils étaient généralisés et fulminants. Le SK survient chez les Africains à un âge modal plus précoce que chez les Caucasiens. Cela résulte de la conjonction de deux facteurs:

l'augmentation de l'incidence avec l'âge, et le fait que la proportion de jeunes est élevée dans la population africaine;   et
cela ne signifie pas que le risque soit plus élevé chez les
hommes jeunes, comme c'est le cas pour le SIDA. La plupart des
cas africains de SK ont une évolution plutôt indolente, comparable à celle du SK classique. Le ratio H:F élevé des SK africains
ne s'observe pas dans les cas de SIDA africains. La distribution
du SK au Zaïre diffère de celle du lymphome de Burkitt.

Il faudrait donner la priorité à l'investigation de l'immunité à médiation cellulaire, ainsi qu'au développement d'une
méthode de traitement efficace, sans danger et peu coûteuse.

SUMMARY

Kaposi's sarcoma (KS) was recognized in 1948 in Zaire, where
it has probably always been endemic. In 1957 a relative frequency of KS of 9% of all biopsied cancers was found.   There are
fluctuations in incidence within the country, with a higher
incidence in the east, where it was estimated in 1960 at about
5-10 cases per 100 000 per year in males, with a relative frequency of 14% of all malignant male tumours and a M/F ratio
higher than 10/1. More recently KS accounted for roughly 17% in
males and 2% in females of all malignant biopsied tumours in
north-east Zaire (1969-1983). In 2 years (1982-1983), 26 male
and 5 female KS cases were histologically confirmed in an area of
eastern Zaire with a population of roughly 300 000 people.

It has been suggested, on the basis of this high incidence
of KS and of the recent identification of African AIDS cases,
that the hypothetical transmissible agent in AIDS might originate
from Central Africa. The frequency of KS in African AIDS cases
was low (16%) as compared to that in the USA. The M/F ratio of
AIDS was 6/4 and that of AIDS-associated KS 1/1. AIDS-associated
cases occurred in young adults and were generalized and fulminating. African KS occurs at a younger modal age than in Caucasians, which is the combined result of increasing incidence with
age and of the high proportion of young people in the population
in Africa but not of a higher risk for younger male adults, as in
AIDS. Most African KS cases have a rather indolent evolution,
comparable to that of classical KS. The high M/F ratio of
African KS is not observed in African AIDS cases. The distribution of KS in Zaire differs from that of Burkitt's lymphoma.

Investigation of cell-mediated immunity in African KS should be given priority, together with the development of an efficient, harmless and inexpensive method of treatment.

INTRODUCTION

In 1935 a typical case of Kaposi's sarcoma (KS) from Zaire, then the Belgian Congo, was described and illustrated by Mattlet and Portois, but was not identified as such. The first correctly diagnosed case from Zaire was published by Dupont et al. in 1945 (Dupont et al., 1948). A series of 230 histologically confirmed cases of KS from the medical laboratory of Kisangani (Stanleyville) was the first large series to be reported from the country (Thijs, 1957). De Clippele in 1957 described the clinical and some epidemiological features of 42 cases reported from hospitals around Bukavu at the southern tip of Lake Kivu in eastern Zaire, from a well-defined population at risk. In 1959, a cancer survey was started by Clemmesen, Maisin and Gigase (unpublished data) in the area centred on the rural hospital of Katana, 45 km north of Bukavu along the western shore of Lake Kivu. The survey was cut short early in 1961. It confirmed the high prevalence of KS, but the number of cases observed in that short period was too small to provide reliable incidence figures. After 1960 little information on KS in Zaire was available, but sporadic observations confirmed the high frequency of KS in most parts of the country. This paper is based on data from the Laboratory of Pathology of the Institute of Tropical Medicine in Antwerp and on information collected in Katana (eastern Kivu) in 1959-1961 and 22 years later at the same place in 1983-1984.

KAPOSI'S SARCOMA CASES IN THE BIOPSY MATERIAL
OF THE DEPARTMENT OF HISTOPATHOLOGY
AT THE INSTITUTE OF TROPICAL MEDICINE, ANTWERP, BELGIUM

Over a period of 18 years, 168 cases of KS from Zaire were diagnosed more than half of them in the last 3 years. The series does not include cases from other African countries. More than 100 of these KS cases came from Kivu (eastern Zaire). There were 138 male patients (82.2%) and 22 female patients (13%). The sex of 8 patients was not stated (4.8%). The M/F ratio was 6.3/1.

Age was given in 96 cases. The mean age was 42.5 years for male patients (77 cases) and 39.4 years for females (19 cases). There were, in addition, 3 'young' male patients, 55 male and 2 female 'adult' patients and 3 male and 1 female 'elderly' patients. No indication of age was given in 9 cases. The distribution by age of the 96 cases is presented in Table 1.

Table 1. Age and sex distribution of 96 KS cases (1971-1984) from Zaire

Sex	Age (years)							
	< 5	5-14	15-24	25-34	35-44	45-54	55-64	> 65
M	1	3	7	9	20	19	14	4
F	-	-	4	4	2	6	2	1

The distribution of the lesions by site is based on the available information, which is usually scanty. Mention is often made of multiplicity of lesions and of oedema or lymphoedema of the affected extremity. Enlarged inguinal lymph-nodes are sometimes described or biopsied. Histological involvement of lymphnodes by KS appears, however, to be unforeseeable clinically. The reported localizations of the lesions are given in Table 2. The two children, 4 and 8 years old, presented with cervical lymphadenopathies, but there is no mention of skin lesions. Four biopsies came from patients with an acquired immune deficiency syndrome: an atypical skin lesion from a fulminating case from Kinshasa, two Zairian male patients, 29 and 39 years old, with initial cervical lymphadenopathies followed by generalized visceral involvement confirmed at necropsy, and an isolated KS lesion of the palate in a patient from eastern Zaire, clinically conforming to the definition of AIDS and dying in less than one year.

Table 2. Distribution of lesions by site

Site	No. of cases
Cutaneous involvement (156 cases)	
Lower limbs	102
Upper limbs	31
Male genitals	7
Generalized	4[a]
No localization mentioned	31
Extracutaneous involvement (12 cases)	
Inguinal lymph-nodes (with or without mention of skin lesions on lower limbs)	4
Cervical lymph-nodes	4
Palate (without other localizations)	1[b]
Stomach (without other localizations)	1
Generalized visceral involvement (autopsy cases)	2[b]

[a] One case associated with AIDS-like disease

[b] Associated with AIDS-like disease

The majority of biopsies displayed a mixed cellular pattern histologically. Few cases were of monocellular or anaplastic type. The diagnosis of KS has undoubtedly been missed in some of these cases, in the absence of clinical information. Nevertheless, the total number of spindle-cell sarcomas or anaplastic tumours of the extremities in the collection is small.

KAPOSI'S SARCOMA IN KATANA (KIVU, EASTERN ZAIRE)

In 1960, a retrospective study of cancer cases was performed at the Katana hospital. From 1953 to 1960, 388 cases of cancer had been seen, 204 in males and 184 in females, including 29 male KS and 2 female KS cases. The relative ratios in all, and in male and female patients, were respectively 8%, 14% and 1.1%. Of these cancer cases, 284 originated in a well defined area around Katana, for which precise and recent demographic information was available. In this population 16 male KS cases out of a total of 99 male cancers were identified in a 5-year period. The population consisted of 47 400 males and 50 300 females. A tentative crude incidence, based on these figures, of 3.3 per 100 000 per year for the total population and of 6.7 per 100 000 per year for the male population was proposed.

If cases confirmed by biopsy are alone taken into account, the relative frequency of KS in this area reaches 17% in males (19/108) and 1.5% (2/134) in females.

Early in 1984, a collaborative study of KS was initiated by the Fondation Médicale de l'Université de Louvain en Afrique Centrale (FOMULAC) at Katana and the Institute of Tropical Medicine of Antwerp. The high prevalence of KS was confirmed. In the locality of Katana, next to the hospital, with a population of 40 000 people, at least 14 patients with histologically confirmed and advanced KS are known to be living (10 males and 4 females), which gives a prevalence of roughly 50 per 100 000 in males and 20 per 100 000 in females. No confirmed cases of AIDS have so far been reported from this rural area. In all the patients, the disease is the classical African form, essentially localized to the lower and upper limbs and usually slowly progressive.

DISCUSSION

The view that KS occurs with high frequency in Africa was based initially on relative frequency figures in cancer series, but it is well known that a number of factors can affect the reliability of the results. The prolonged course of the disease means that KS cases are repeatedly admitted to hospital and biopsied (Table 3). Since identification of patients by name is often difficult, this can lead to overestimation through repeated registration of the same patient.

Table 3. Frequency of admissions for malignant diseases (Katana, 1953-1960)

Disease	Number	Admissions	Frequency
KS	21	38	1.81
All other cancers	265	341	1.29

On the other hand, not all cases are necessarily reported. In a systematic examination of the population in 1959-1960, we detected four 'new' cases of KS who had never been admitted. One of these patients was said to have been suffering from KS for 13 years. The cases in eastern Zaire are nearly always advanced to very advanced. It is possible that incipient or attenuated forms of KS are overlooked.

In a passive and probably incomplete survey of admitted and reported KS cases from eastern Kivu, De Clippele found, in 1957, 20 male and 2 female KS cases originating from a population of 215 659 males and 228 576 females, corresponding to a prevalence of 9.3 per 100 000 for males and of 0.9 per 100 000 for females. These figures are consistent with our own prevalence and incidence figures for the same area.

The ratio and age distribution of the cases reported here conform to the usual African pattern.

That KS is an ancient disease among the Shi tribes of Kivu is suggested by the fact that the disease is known to the population under its own name of lubambo and is attributed to a spell. A clear distinction is made between KS and endemic elephantiasis, known as bikimbo. The frequency of KS is not considered to be on the increase, in contrast to elephantiasis, which is said to have become more frequent in recent years.

The survival of KS cases is currently being investigated in the area. Eight KS patients from Katana are known to have survived more than 3 years after diagnosis, namely for periods of 7-24 years. Thus, one case was diagnosed in 1960 at the age of 30 years as a light nodular form and was retrieved 24 years later

in 1984 spontaneously cured. Four patients are known to have
died 3, 4, 8 and 11 years after diagnosis. The cause of death
is, however, not known. Some patients are cured after amputation, but recurrences are unforeseeable.

There are few records of familial KS. Templeton and Dhru
(1975) reported the first familial African case in two half-
brothers in Uganda. Three familial cases are currently being
investigated in Kivu. One of them concerns two brothers, 13 and
15 years old, both with histologically confirmed nodular lesions
of the left leg. Their father is said to have died from the same
disease.

The recent occurrence in Zaire of a syndrome of acquired
immuno deficiency similar to AIDS, though occurring in different
risk groups, complicates the epidemiology of KS in Africa.
Kaposi's sarcoma is one of the clinical presentations but its
frequency in Zairian AIDS is low (16%) and the sex ratio of KS in
these cases is 1/1 (Piot et al., unpublished data). The current
investigation in Katana is aimed at defining the status of cell-
mediated immunity of patients with African KS, the incidence in
the population, familial cases and clustering, and obtaining
material for electron microscopy and for immunohistochemistry,
and serum and tumour tissues for virological identification. In
this way we hope to contribute to the 'leap forward in our knowledge of this fascinating tumour' (Hutt, 1981).

ACKNOWLEDGEMENTS

The collaboration of Dr M. Paluku and Citoyen Infirmier
Chizungu from FOMULAC, Katana, in the 1984 study is gratefully
acknowledged. The present investigation of Kaposi's sarcoma in
Kivu is supported by the Oeuvre Belge du Cancer. Investigations
in 1959-1960 have been supported by grant C-4309 from the
National Cancer Institute of the USA.

REFERENCES

De Clippele, M. (1957) Le Sarcome de Kaposi, Thesis, Institute of Tropical Medicine, Antwerp

Dupont, A., Chabeuf & Van Breuseghem, R. (1948) Angiomatose de Kaposi chez des noirs. Arch. belges Dermatol. Syph., 4, 132-136

Hutt, M. (1981) The epidemiology of Kaposi's sarcoma. Antibiot. Chemother., 29, 3-8

Mattlet, G. & Portois, J. (1935) Tumeur d'origine nerveuse chez un Noir. Ann. Soc. belge Méd. trop., 15, 527-528

Templeton, A.C. & Dhru, D. (1975) Kaposi's sarcoma in half-brothers. Trop. geogr. Med., 27, 324-327

Thijs, A. (1957) L'angiosarcomatose de Kaposi au Congo belge et au Ruanda-Urundi. Ann. Soc. belge Méd. trop., 37, 295-307

CLINICOPATHOLOGICAL FEATURES
OF KAPOSI'S SARCOMA IN ZAIRE

M.M.R. Kalengayi & L. Kashala

Department of Pathology
Medical Faculty, and Kinshasa University Hospital
University of Kinshasa
Kinshasa, Zaire

RESUME

Les 299 cas de sarcome de Kaposi (SK) diagnostiqués au Zaïre sur une période de 21 ans ont été revus au Département d'Anatomie Pathologique de l'Hôpital Universitaire de Kinshasa.

Cette étude a révélé la prédominance de l'atteinte cutanée (268 cas, soit 89,6%) avec, dans 51,8% des cas, une localisation aux membres inférieurs; 31 cas (10,4%) avaient une localisation extra-cutanée, touchant en majorité (71,0%) les ganglions lympha-tiques. La maladie de Kaposi affecte plus sévèrement les adultes (67,6%) que les enfants (6,7%), les hommes (79,6%) que les femmes (12,8%) avec un ratio H:F de 4,8:1. La plus grande fréquence de la maladie a été observée dans la Province de l'Equateur (24,7%). Dans un cas (0,3%) un autre cancer était associé au SK. Histolo-giquement, 4 types de SK ont été rencontrés: angiomateux, granu-lomateux, sarcomateux et mixte, les deux derniers· représentant respectivement 42,5% et 49,2% des cas. La fréquence relative du sarcome de Kaposi a été évaluée à 5,3% des tumeurs malignes dia-gnostiquées dans le Département sur une période de 5 ans.

Cette étude rétrospective fournit des données anatomopatho-logiques et épidémiologiques essentielles pour une étude ulté-rieure du syndrome d'immunodéficience acquise (SIDA) au Zaïre.

SUMMARY

A total of 299 cases of Kaposi's sarcoma (KS) occurring in
Zaire over a 21-year period have been reviewed in the Department
of Pathology, Kinshasa University Hospital.

Of these, 268 were localized in the skin (89,6%) with the
majority (51.8%) in the lower limbs; 31 (10.4%) were located
elsewhere, chiefly in the lymph nodes (71.0%). Adults were more
severely affected (67.6%) than children (6.7%). The proportion
of females (12.8%) was much less than that of males (79.6%) and
the adjusted M:F ratio was 4.81:1. The highest frequency (24.7%)
of KS was found in Equator Province. Only 1 KS-associated cancer
was observed (0.3%). Histopathologically, angiomatous, granulomatous, sarcomatous and mixed types were encountered, with the
last two predominating and accounting for 42.5% and 49.2%, respectively. KS accounted for 5.3% of all cancers registered in
the Department over a 5-year period.

This retrospective study of KS describes some major pathological and epidemiological features of the disease that may be
of great importance in relation to further studies of acquired
immunodeficiency syndrome (AIDS) in Zaire.

INTRODUCTION

Since Kaposi's sarcoma (KS) was first reported in Vienna
(Kaposi, 1872), this disease has been recognized and extensively
documented in several countries (Dörffel, 1932; Symmers, 1948;
Bluefarb, 1957; Tedeschi, 1958; Cox & Helwig, 1959; Dutz & Stout,
1960; Rothman, 1962a), and in Africa (Quenum & Camain, 1958;
Basset & Payet, 1962; Davies & Lothe, 1962; Lothe, 1963; MacLean,
1963; Oluwasanmi et al., 1969; Slavin et al., 1969; Taylor et
al., 1971b; D'Oliveira & Torres, 1972; Templeton, 1972), where it
was first described by Hallenberger (1914).

In Zaire, KS was first reported by Mathieu (1948) and by
Dupont et al. (1948); Thijs (1957) gave a full account of the
disease, dealing mainly with cases encountered in eastern Zaire.

KS was subsequently observed in patients undergoing chemo-
and radiotherapy (Moe, 1966; Siegal et al., 1969; Klepp et al.,
1978; Hoshaw & Schwartz, 1980; Guillet et al., 1980; Leung et
al., 1981; Meynadier et al., 1981) for different conditions and
in recipients of renal transplants (Rudolf, 1977; Penn, 1979;
Zisbrod et al., 1980).

KS has recently been increasingly reported to occur in the
course of acquired immunodeficiency syndrome (AIDS) in patients
from different countries (Thomsen et al., 1981; Centers for
Disease Control, 1982; Fauci, 1982; Friedman-Kien et al., 1982),
including Zaire (Clumeck et al., 1983; Offenstadt et al., 1983;
Sonnet & De Bruyère, 1983; Taelman et al., 1983). Several
reports have mentioned the occurrence of this syndrome in Zaire
(Clumeck et al., 1983; Sonnet & De Bruyère, 1983; Taelman et al.,
1983). There is therefore clearly a need for further retrospective as well as prospective studies in order to clarify the
possible relationship between these two conditions.

This paper is a part of a series in progress in our Department devoted to the study of the profile of cancer in Zaire. It
deals mainly with a retrospective analysis of the pathology of KS
in Zaire based on biopsy material from the Department of Pathology, Kinshasa University Hospital, which serves at least four-
fifths of the entire country. Such a study should provide some
interesting data for further epidemiological investigations of
AIDS in Zaire and on the possible relationship between AIDS and
KS.

MATERIALS AND METHODS

Biopsy material

The study covers the period from 1963 to 1983 and deals with
the pathological specimens sent to the Department of Pathology,
Kinshasa University Hospital, from different provinces of Zaire,
including Kinshasa City.

All the biopsies with a diagnosis of KS were reviewed and
the conclusion confirmed or corrected. Moreover, all biopsies of
the skin, lymph-nodes, viscera and soft tissues where differen-
tion from KS was necessary were also revised; in this way,
further cases of KS were found and a total of 299 cases of histologically proven KS were retained.

The biopsy material was usually fixed in 10% formalin solution or in Bouin's fluid. It was paraffin embedded and the slides were routinely prepared and stained with haematoxylin and eosin. If necessary, special stains were used, e.g., Masson's trichrome, Gomori's reticulin, PAS and Perl's technique for iron staining.

Analysis of cases

The 299 cases were analysed for the following parameters: anatomical site, age and sex distribution, clinical presentation, histopathological features, geographical distribution and relative frequency of KS in all cancers diagnosed in the Department compared to that of malignant melanoma over a 5-year period (study still in progress).

From our experience and the proposals for the histological typing of KS by other authors (Dörffel, 1932; Montgomery, 1967; Lever, 1969; Taylor et al., 1971b), we tentatively divided KS lesions into 4 basic histological types:

- the granulomatous type: this is characterized by a clearly inflammatory background associated with a proliferation of small spindle cells, culminating in the formation of multiple, small thin-walled blood vessels containing small erythrocytes and with areas of haemorrhage; this histological type has been referred to as 'early lesion' (Montgomery, 1967; Lever, 1969) or as 'granulomatous, inflammatory stage' (Dörffel, 1932);

- the angiomatous type: this shows predominantly and characteristically a proliferation of very numerous and more highly developed blood vessels, sometimes with perivascular clear hyalinized areas; this form corresponds to the predominantly angiomatous pattern of the 'monomorphic type' of Templeton (1973) and of Taylor et al. (1971b), to the angiomatous stage of Dörffel (1932) and to the predominantly angiomatous late lesion of Lever (1969);

- the sarcomatous type: in this type, the proliferation of larger spindle cells with typical intermingled fascicular patterns predominates with the appearance of vascular slits throughout; this form is referred to as the 'tumoral stage'

(Dörffel, 1932; Montgomery, 1967; Ten Seldam et al., 1975), the 'monomorphic type with spindle cell predominance' (Taylor et al., 1971b; Templeton, 1973), the 'fibroblastic type' (Lever, 1969) and the 'sarcomatous stage' (Dörffel, 1932);

- the mixed type: this is characterized by the combination of at least 2 of the patterns described above; it corresponds to the 'mixed cellular pattern' of Templeton (1973) and of Taylor et al. (1971b) and to the mixed form of late lesion of Lever (1969).

In all these forms, a variable degree of cytonuclear atypism can be observed, but is clearly more pronounced in the sarcomatous type, which is then referred to as the 'anaplastic variant' (Taylor et al., 1971b; Templeton, 1973).

RESULTS

As far as the anatomical localization is concerned, 268 out of 299 cases were found in the skin (89,6%) and were distributed over the body, as shown by Table 1. Localizations other than skin were seen in 10.4% of cases, mainly in the lymph-nodes (7.4%), as also shown in Table 1.

Most KS patients (67.6%) were adults aged from 15 to 64 years. Only 4.0% were aged 65 years or more and 6.7% were less than 15 years (Table 2). Furthermore, when age and anatomical sites were considered together, it was observed that, up to 14 years, the disease was found exclusively in lymph-nodes in 25% of cases, while that localization was found in only 7.9% of adults (Table 2).

The disease was found predominantly in males with a global M:F ratio of 6.26:1. However, the sex ratio was very low in the younger age-groups, increasing significantly in the older ones (Table 3). Furthermore, the adjusted M:F ratio in patients for whom both age and sex were recorded (233 cases) is 4.8:1 (Table 3).

Table 1. Anatomical localization of KS lesions

Site	No. of cases (% of all sites)
Cutaneous (268; 89.6%)	
Lower limb	155[a] (51.8)
Upper limb	52 (17.4)
Penis	4 (1.3)
Head	4 (1.3)
Vulva	2 (0.7)
Back	1 (0.3)
Abdomen	1 (0.3)
Unrecorded or multiple	49 (16.4)
Extracutaneous (32; 10.4%)	
Lymph-nodes	22 (7.4)
Ear, nose and throat[b]	5 (1.7)
Gastrointestinal tract[c]	4 (1.3)
Total	299

[a] Including 2 Belgians

[b] Nose: 3 cases (including 1 Italian); ear: 1 case;
tonsils: 1 case

[c] Rectum: 2 cases; anus: 1 case; ileum: 1 case

Table 2. Distribution of KS by age and by age and site

A. Distribution of KS by age

Age	No. of cases	Frequency (%)
< 15 years	20	6.7
15-64 years	202	67.6
≥ 65 years	12	4.0
Age not given	65	21.7

B. Distribution of KS by age and site

Age	No. with nodal involvement/Total No.	Frequency (%)
< 15 years	5/20	25
Adults	17/214	7.9

The clinical presentation of the 268 cutaneous cases of KS was recorded in 190 patients (63.54%). In 97.89% of these cases, the lesion presented as typical (sometimes ulcerated) nodules, reddish or violet in colour, while it presented as a 'fungating mass' in only 2.11% of cases. However, it has been shown by dermatologists that a 'fungating mass' represents very old and altered nodule(s). The cases of KS localized to the lymph-nodes were clinically described as peripheral or subcutaneous lymphadenomegalies simulating tuberculosis, leukaemia or lymphomas.

Histologically, different patterns were encountered: 127 sarcomatous forms (42.47%), 16 granulomatous (5.35%), and 9 angiomatous (3.01%), while the mixed forms accounted for 147 cases (49.16%), as shown in Table 4. No predilection for any particular anatomical site, age or sex was found in connection with the different histopathological types.

Table 3. Distribution and M:F ratio of KS in 233 patients (both age and sex determined)

Age group	No. of cases	Sex			
		M	F	M:F	Unrecorded
0 - 4	8	6	2	3:1	0
5 - 9	9	6	3	2:1	0
10 - 14	3	3	0	3:1	0
15 - 19	10	9	1	9:1	0
20 - 24	13	7[a]	5	1.4:1	1
25 - 29	24	21	2	10.5:1	1
30 - 34	31	26	4	6.5:1	1
35 - 39	22	20	2	10:1	0
40 - 44	26	21[a]	5	4.2:1	0
45 - 49	24	20	3	6.66:1	1
50 - 54	31	25[b]	5	5:1	1
55 - 59	9	7	2	3.5:1	0
60 - 64	11	9	1	9:1	1
65 - 69	6	4	1	4:1	1
70 - 74	4	2	1	2:1	1
75 - 79	1	1	0	1:1	0
80 -	1	1	0	1:1	1
Total	233	187	37	4.81:1[c]	9

[a] Including 2 Belgians

[b] Including 1 Italian

[c] Mean M:F of 6.21:1 when sex alone recorded

Table 4. Histopathological patterns of KS

Microscopic type	No. of cases	Other names used	Authors
Granulomatous (G)	16	Early (granulomatous) lesion	Lever, 1969
		Granulomatous + inflammatory stage	Dörffel, 1932
Angiomatous (A)	9	Late lesion (angiomatous form)	Lever, 1969
		Angiomatous stage	Dörffel, 1932
		Monomorphic (angiomatous predominance)	Taylor et al., 1971b
Sarcomatous (S)	127[a]	Late lesion (fibroblastic form	Lever, 1969
		Sarcomatous stage	Dörffel, 1932
		Monomorphic (spindle-cell predominance) and anaplastic variant	Taylor et al., 1971b
Mixed[b]	147	Late lesion (mixed forms)	Lever, 1969
		Mixed cellular, mixed pattern	Taylor et al., 1971b; Templeton, 1973

[a] Of these, 9 were frankly anaplastic

[b] Made up as follows: S and G: 5; A and G: 12; A, G and S: 27; S and A: 103

With regard to the geographical distribution, KS was found in people from all the provinces and ethnic groups of Zaire, with a clear predominance in Equator Province in terms both of absolute number of cases diagnosed and of numbers of biopsy samples originating from this part of the country and sent to our Department (Table 5).

Table 5. Geographical distribution of KS in Zaire

Province	No. of cases	Frequency (%)
Equator	74	24.74
Kivu	46	15.38
Lower Zaire	42	14.04
Kinshasa City	34	11.37
Bandundu	30	10.03
Upper Zaire	23	7.69
Eastern Kasai	15	5.01
Western Kasai	10	3.34
Shaba	4	1.33
Not specified	18	6.02
Whites	3	1.00

The relative frequency of KS among all malignancies in Zaire was found to be 5.31% for the period considered, while it was of 3.58% for malignant melanoma, as shown in Table 6.

DISCUSSION

This study, which was on a larger scale than previous ones on KS in Zaire (Thijs, 1957), provided information on some important pathological and epidemiological features of the disease that were hitherto lacking from its profile in Zaire, and particularly in the lower, central and north-western areas of the country, which account for at least four-fiths of the total population, i.e., about 24 million people.

As pointed out in other studies by Bluefarb (1957), Gigase (1965), D'Oliveira and Torres (1972) and Templeton (1973), most KS in Zairians is seen in the skin (89.63%), mainly in the upper and lower limbs, as shown in Table 1. However, it is worthwhile mentioning that, in children under 15 years of age, the disease was exclusively found in lymph-nodes in 25% of cases, while nodal involvement was found in only 7.9% of adult patients. The frequency of exclusive nodal involvement in children in the

Table 6. Relative frequencies of KS and malignant melanoma (MM) in Zaire[a]

Year	No. of malignant tumours	KS		MM	
		No.	%	No.	%
1977	260	13	5.0	10	3.84
1978	229	12	5.24	4	1.74
1979	208	7	3.36	7	3.36
1980	196	11	5.61	12	6.12
1981	176	13	7.38	5	2.84
Total	1096	56	5.31[b]	38	3.58[b]

[a] Recorded between 1 January 1977 and 31 December 1981

[b] Mean relative frequency

present study proved to be very low, as compared with that found by Slavin et al. (1970) in children aged from 0 to 16 years. However, it should be pointed out that all the children with KS in the lymph-nodes in our series were less than 5 years old, so that our findings are similar to those of Dutz and Stout (1960). This nodal involvement in very young African children has been stressed by previous workers (Thijs, 1957; Quenum & Camain, 1958; Bhana et al., 1970; Slavin et al., 1970; Templeton, 1973). A visceral location was observed only in 4 out of 299 cases (1.37%), which is a very low frequency as compared with that reported by other investigators: 10% by Tedeschi (1958) and Ecklund and Valaitis (1962), 6-10% by Bluefarb (1957) and 91.17% by Templeton (1972) in a series of 102 autopsies. These discrepancies can be explained by the fact that our study is essentially based only on biopsy material. This is also a quite frequent situation in other parts of Africa, where autopsies are uncommon. The lack of autopsies must certainly mask a number of isolated or skin-associated visceral KS lesions.

The general features of the sex distribution (Table 3) in our material (M:F = 6.26:1 when sex only is recorded; mean M:F = 4.81:1 when both sex and age are recorded) show a clear male predominance, as reported in other countries (Bluefarb, 1957; D'Oliveira & Torres, 1972; Templeton, 1973). In our study, females accounted for 12.70% of all cases. This frequency is comparable with that previously found in Zaire by Thijs (1957), but very high as compared with that reported in other African countries (Maclean, 1963; Slavin et al., 1970; D'Oliveira & Torres, 1972; Templeton, 1972). Table 7 shows the frequency of female cases in some African and non-African countries. The reason why KS is predominantly a male disease is still unknown (Templeton, 1972, 1973) and the question remains a debatable one (Hurlbut & Lincoln, 1949; Tedeschi, 1958; Oettlé, 1962; Taylor et al., 1971b; Templeton, 1972).

Table 7. Frequency of female cases of KS in different countries

Authors	No. of cases	% Female	Country
Lothe (1963)	211	2.9	Uganda
Templeton (1972)	624	5.4	Uganda
Slavin et al. (1969)	117	7.5	Tanzania
D'Oliveira and Torres (1972)	98	2.14	Mozambique
Bluefarb (1957)	144	12.5	World
Choissier and Ramsey (1939)	434	5.9	World
O'Brien and Brasfield (1966)[a]	63	18.0	USA
Reynolds et al. (1965)	70	8.5	USA
Thijs (1957)	230	10.4	Zaire
Present study	299	12.7	Zaire

[a] Quoted by Templeton (1972)

The clinical presentation of KS skin lesions in our cases is similar to the characteristic dark nodules profusely described and illustrated by a number of authors (Bluefarb, 1957; Thijs, 1957; Quenum & Camain, 1958; Lothe, 1963; Taylor et al., 1971b; Templeton, 1972).

The histopathology of KS has been the subject of several tentative classification schemes (see above, under Materials and Methods). Our proposed classification is based only on the histological appearance and includes all the microscopic aspects which can be encountered in KS lesions at any stage of evolution of the disease. Our cases of KS showed a great majority of sarcomatous as well as mixed types (91.63%). According to some authors, the sarcomatous forms, particularly those with marked anaplasia, had a poorer prognosis (Cox & Helwig, 1960; Templeton & Bhana, 1975). In our retrospective study of biopsies originating from different areas of the interior of the country, correlation of prognosis with histopathology was not feasible. Furthermore, we found no relationship between age, anatomical site and histopathological form of KS; Gigase (1965) also failed to find any such relationship. These aspects will be investigated in an interdisciplinary study of KS by the Department of Dermatology, Kinshasa University Hospital (study in progress).

With regard to the frequency of KS in different provinces of Zaire, the present study found the highest frequency in Equator Province, with 74 of 299 registered cases of KS, i.e., 24.74%. This high frequency in Equator Province was found both in terms of the absolute number of cases in relation to the population of this Province, and of the number of pathological specimens sent from this part of Zaire to our Department. The figures for the geographical distribution of KS in Zaire are in conflict with previous data by Thijs (1957), who found that KS was most frequent in the eastern Province of Kivu (40 out of 207 Zairian cases, i.e., 19.32%), which is close to Rwanda, Burundi and Uganda, but his study partially covered the central and eastern and north-eastern parts of the country. In our study, Kivu Province comes second in terms of frequency (15.54%). Further population-based studies are needed in order to explain the highly variable frequencies from one area to another. The geographical distribution of KS is said to be reminiscent of that of Burkitt's lymphoma (BL) in Central Africa (Burkitt, 1970). In our material, no such parallel between KS and BL was observed. Of 115 cases of BL registered in Zaire, 47 (40.80%) were found in Kinshasa City, while only 10.4% originated from Equator

Province. Table 8 shows the geographical distribution of KS and BL in Zaire.

Table 8. Geographical distribution of KS and BL in Zairians

Province	KS		BL	
	No. of cases	%	No. of cases	%
Equator	74	24.74	12	10.43
Kivu	46	15.38	6	1.79
Lower Zaire	42	14.04	23	20.00
Kinshasa	34	11.37	47	40.86
Bandundu	30	10.03	6	1.79
Higher Zaire	23	7.69	6	4.34
Eastern Kasai	15	5.0	11	9.56
Western Kasai	10	3.34	5	4.34
Shaba	4	1.33	0 (10)[a]	0 (8.69)[a]
Total	278		115	

[a] 10 cases observed in our Department

Association of KS with other primary malignancies is commonly reported (Bluefarb & Webster, 1953; Moertel, 1966; Berg, 1967; Safai et al., 1980), in particular with malignant lymphomas (Safai et al., 1980). In Africa, such an association is uncommon (Gigase, 1965; Templeton, 1972; D'Oliveira & Torres, 1972). We found only 1 epidermoid carcinoma of the skin in a KS patient in the present series.

The relative frequency of KS was found to be 5.31%. This figure is lower than that previously obtained by Thijs (1957) in Zaire 27 years ago, i.e., 9.06%, but higher than that reported in Mozambique (2.11%) by D'Oliveira and Torres (1972), and in Kenya (2.4%) and in Uganda (4.7%) by Oettlé (1962). However, more recent studies have found a higher relative frequency (10%) in Kenya (Kungu & Gatei, 1981) and in Uganda (Templeton, 1981). The cause of this variability in the endemicity of KS in different African countries remains to be determined.

The etiopathogenesis of KS is still unknown (Degos, 1981; Fauci et al., 1984) and is the subject of many fascinating although speculative hypotheses (Becker & Tatcher, 1938; Rothman, 1962b; Oettlé, 1962). The occurrence of KS in association with several immunodeficiency conditions has been widely reported (Master et al., 1970; Taylor, 1973; Taylor & Ziegler, 1974; Templeton, 1981), including the organ recipient state (Dobosy et al., 1973; Stribling et al., 1978), immunosuppressive therapy (Myers et al., 1974; Gange & Jones, 1978; Harwood et al., 1979; Klepp et al., 1978; Penn, 1979), autoimmune disease (Klein et al., 1974), malignant lymphomas and other cancers (Weschler et al., 1979; Safai et al., 1980) and immunodepressive states of unknown origin (Templeton, 1981). More significant and intriguing is the recent finding of the occurrence of KS in individuals suffering from AIDS (Durack, 1981; Centers for Disease Control, 1982; Fauci, 1982; Friedman-Kien et al., 1982; Pitchenic et al., 1983; Sonnet & De Bruyère, 1983).

Alternatively, an infectious agent, most probably cytomegalovirus (CMV) is increasingly incriminated (Giraldo et al., 1972, 1975, 1978, 1980a,b). Furthermore, the possible etiological role of human T-cell leukemia viruses (HTLV) in the development of AIDS has been investigated (Barre-Sinoussi et al., 1983; Essex et al., 1983; Gallo et al., 1983; Gelmann et al., 1983 quoted by Kreiss et al., 1984; Gottlieb et al., 1983). However, a predisposing genetic factor (HLA-DR5) may have favoured the action of viral factors (Friedman-Kien et al., 1982).

Several reports have mentioned the occurrence of AIDS in Zairians and described the development of KS in the course of this disease (Sonnet & De Bruyère, 1983; Taelman et al., 1983, unpublished data). Because this new syndrome is being reported increasingly in Zairians and because of the well known high frequency of KS in Zaire, it is clearly necessary to undertake further retrospective as well as prospective investigations in order to clarify the relationship, if any, between AIDS and KS, in conjunction with CMV and HTLV surveys in Zaire. In particular, it would be of great interest to assess the predictive value of the carrier state of CMV and/or HTLV markers with regard to the eventual future development of AIDS or of KS in the course of

AIDS. Such a study will soon be undertaken on a collaborative
basis in this country.

ACKNOWLEDGEMENTS

The authors wish to thank Mrs Mamba Diyoyo for her
secretarial help.

REFERENCES

Barré-Sinoussi, F., Chermann, J.C., Rey, F., Nugeyre, M.T.,
Chamaret, S., Gruest, J., Dauguet, C., Axler-Blin, C.,
Vezinet-Brun, F., Rouzioux, C., Rozenbaum, W. & Montagnier,
L. (1983) Isolation of a T-lymphotropic retrovirus from a
patient at risk for acquired immune deficiency syndrome
(AIDS). Science, 220, 868-887

Basset, A. & Payet, M. (1962) Caractères cliniques de la maladie
de Kaposi dans l'Ouest Africain. Différences avec le Kaposi
Européen. Un. Int. Cancr. Acta, 18, 376-379

Becker, S.W. & Tatcher, H.W. (1938) Multiple idiopathic hemorrhagic sarcoma of Kaposi. Historical review. Nomenclature
and theories relative to the nature of the disease and
experimental studies in two cases. J. invest. Dermatol., 1,
379-398

Berg, J.W. (1967) The incidence of primary multiple cancers. I.
Development of further cancers in patients with lymphomas,
leukemias and myeloma. J. natl Cancer Inst., 38, 141-152

Bhana, D., Templeton, A.C., Master, S.P. & Kyalwazi, S.K. (1970)
Kaposi's sarcoma of lymph nodes. Br. J. Cancer, 24, 464-470

Bluefarb, S.M. & Webster, J.R. (1953) Kaposi's sarcoma associated with lymphosarcoma. Arch. intern. Med., 91, 97-105

Bluefarb, S.M. (1957) Kaposi's Sarcoma. Multiple Idiopathic
Hemorrhagic Sarcoma, Springfield, IL, C.C. Thomas

Burkitt, D. (1970) <u>Geographical distribution</u>. In: Burkitt, D.P. & Wright, D.H., eds, <u>Burkitt's Lymphoma</u>, Edinburgh, Livingstone, pp. 186-187

Centers for Disease Control (1982) Task force on Kaposi's sarcoma and opportunistic infections: epidemiological aspects of the current outbreak of Kaposi's sarcoma and opportunistic infections. <u>New Engl. J. Med.</u>, <u>306</u>, 248-252

Choissier, R.M. & Ramsey, E.M. (1939) Angioreticuloendothelioma (Kaposi's disease) of the heart. <u>Am. J. Pathol.</u>, <u>15</u>, 155-177

Clumeck, N., Mascart-Lemone, F., De Maubeuge, J., Brenez, D. & Marcelis, L. (1983) Acquired immune deficiency syndrome in black Africans. <u>Lancet</u>, <u>1</u>, 642

Cox, F.H. & Helwig, E.B. (1959) Kaposi's sarcoma. <u>Cancer</u>, <u>12</u>, 283-298

Davies, J.N.P. & Lothe, F. (1962) Kaposi's sarcoma in African children. <u>Un. Int. Cancr. Acta</u>, <u>18</u>, 394-399

Degos, R. (1981) <u>Maladie de Kaposi</u>. In: Degos, R., ed., <u>Dermatologie</u>, Tome II, Paris, Flammarion, pp. 924-928

Dobosy, A., Husz, S., Hunyadi, J., Berko, G. & Simon, N. (1973) Immune deficiencies and Kaposi's sarcoma. <u>Lancet</u>, <u>2</u>, 625

D'Oliveira, J.J.G. & Torres, F.O. (1972) Kaposi's sarcoma in the Bantu of Mozambique. <u>Cancer</u>, <u>30</u>, 353-361

Dörffel, J. (1932) Histogenesis of multiple idiopathic hemorrhagic sarcoma of Kaposi. <u>Arch. Dermatol. Syph.</u>, <u>26</u>, 608-634

Dupont, A., Chabeuf, R. & Vanbreuseghem, R. (1948) Angiosarcomatose de Kaposi chez des Noirs. <u>Arch. belges Dermatol. Syph.</u>, <u>4</u>

Durack, D.T. (1981) Opportunistic infections and Kaposi's sarcoma in homosexual men. <u>New Engl. J. Med.</u>, <u>305</u>, 1465-1567

Dutz, M. & Stout, A.P. (1960) Kaposi's sarcoma in infants and children. Cancer, 13, 684-694

Ecklund, R.E. & Valaitis, J. (1962) Kaposi's sarcoma of lymph nodes: a case report. Arch. Pathol., 74, 224-229

Essex, M., McLane, M.F., Lee, T.H., Falk, L., Howe, C.W.S. & Mullins, J.I. (1983) Antibodies to cell membrane antigens associated with human T-cell leukemia virus in patients with acquired immunodeficiency syndrome. Science, 220, 859-863

Fauci, A.S. (1982) The syndrome of Kaposi's sarcoma and opportunistic infections: an epidemiologically restricted disorder of immunoregulation. Ann. intern. Med., 96, 777-779

Fauci, S.A., Macher, A.M., Longo, D.L., Lane, H.C., Rook, A.H., Masur, H. & Gelmann, E.P. (1984) Acquired immunodeficiency syndrome: epidemiologic, clinical, immunologic and therapeutic considerations. Ann. intern. Med., 100, 92-106

Friedman-Kien, A.E., Laubenstein, L.J., Rubinstein, P., Buimovici-Klein, E., Marmor, H., Stahl, R., Spigland, I., Kim, K.S. & Zolla-Pazner, S. (1982) Disseminated Kaposi's sarcoma in homosexual men. Ann. intern. Med., 96, 693-700

Gallo, R.C., Sarin, P.S., Gelmann, E.P., Robert-Guroff, M., Richardson, E., Kalyanaraman, V.S., Mann, D., Sidhu, G.D., Stahl, R.E., Zolla-Pazner, S., Leibowitch, J. & Popovic, M. (1983) Isolation of human T-cell leukemia virus in acquired immune deficiency syndrome (AIDS). Science, 220, 865-867

Gange, R.W. & Jones, W.-E. (1978) Kaposi's sarcoma and immunosuppressive therapy: an appraisal. Clin. exp. Dermatol., 3, 135-146

Gigase, P.L. (1965) Quelques considérations du sarcoma de Kaposi en Afrique. Ann. Soc. belge Méd. trop., 45, 195-210

Giraldo, G., Beth, E. & Haguenau, F. (1972) Herpes-type particles in tissue culture of Kaposi's sarcoma from different geographical regions. J. natl Cancer Inst., 49, 1509-1513

Giraldo, G., Beth, E., Kourilsky, F.M., Henle, W., Henle, G., Miké, V., Huraux, J.M., Andersen, H.K., Gharbi, M.R., Kyalwazi, S.K. & Puissant, A. (1975) Antibody patterns to herpesviruses in Kaposi's sarcoma: serological association of European Kaposi's sarcoma with cytomegalovirus. Int. J. Cancer, 15, 839-848

Giraldo, G., Beth, E., Henle, W., Henle, G., Miké, V., Safai, B., Huraux, J.M., McHardy, J. & de-Thé, G. (1978) Antibody patterns to herpesviruses in Kaposi's sarcoma. II. Serological association of American Kaposi's sarcoma with cytomegalovirus. Int. J. Cancer, 22, 126-131

Giraldo, G., Beth, E. & Huang, E.S. (1980a) Kaposi's sarcoma and its relationship to cytomegalovirus (CMV). III. CMV DNA and CMV early antigens in African Kaposi's sarcoma. Int. J. Cancer, 26, 23-29

Giraldo, G. & Beth, E. (1980b) The relationship of cytomegalovirus to certain human cancers, particularly to Kaposi's sarcoma. In: Giraldo, G. & Beth, E., eds, The Role of Viruses in Human Cancer, Amsterdam, Elsevier-North Holland, pp. 57-73

Gottlieb, G.J., Ragaz, A., Vogel, J.V., Friedman-Kien, A.E., Rywlin, A.M., Weiner, E.A. & Ackerman, A.B. (1981) A preliminary communication on extensively disseminated Kaposi's sarcoma in young homosexual men. Am. J. Dermatopathol., 3, 111-114

Gottlieb, G.J., Groopman, J.E., Weinstein, W.M., Fahey, J.L. & Detels, R. (1983) The acquired immunodeficiency syndrome. Ann. intern. Med., 99, 208-220

Guillet, G., Chouvet, B., Thivolet, J. & Perrot, H. (1980) Traitements immunosuppresseurs et maladie de Kaposi. A propos de 2 observations. Ann. Dermatol. Vénéréol., 107, 907-919

Hallenberger (1914) Multiple Angiosarkome der Haut bei einen Kamerunneger. Arch. Schiffs.-u. Tropenhyg., 18, 647-651

Harwood, A.R., Osoba, D., Hofstader, S.L., Goldstein, M.A., Cardella, C.J., Holecek, M.J., Kunyenetz, R. & Giammarco, R.A. (1979) Kaposi's sarcoma in recipients of renal transplants. Am. J. Med., 67, 759-765

Hoshaw, R.A. & Schwartz, R.A. (1980) Kaposi's sarcoma after immunosuppressive therapy with prednisone. Arch. Dermatol., 116, 280-282

Hurlbut, W.B. & Lincoln, C.S., Jr (1949) Multiple hemorrhagic sarcoma and diabetes mellitus. Arch. intern. Med., 84, 738-750

Kaposi, M. (1872) Idiopatisches multiples Pigmentsarkom der Haut. Arch. Dermatol. Syph., 4, 265-273

Klein, M.B., Perreira, F.A. & Kantor, I. (1974) Kaposi's sarcoma complicating lupus erythematosus treated with immunosuppression. Arch. Dermatol., 110, 602-604

Klepp, O., Dahl, O. & Stenwig, J.T. (1978) Association of Kaposi's sarcoma with prior immunosuppressive therapy: a 5-year material of Kaposi's sarcoma in Norway. Cancer, 42, 2626-2630

Kreiss, J.K., Lawrence, D.N., Kasper, C.K., Goldstein, A.L., Naylor, P.H., McLane, M.F., Lee, T.N. & Essex, N. (1984) Antibody to human T-cell leukemia virus membrane antigens, beta-2-microglobulin levels, and thymosine alpha 1 levels in hemophiliacs and their spouses. Ann. intern. Med., 100, 178-182

Kungu, A. & Gatei, D.G. (1981) Kaposi's sarcoma in Kenya: a retrospective clinicopathological study. Antibiot. Chemother., 29, 38-55

Leung, F., Fam, A.G. & Osoba, D. (1981) Kaposi's sarcoma complicating corticosteroid therapy for temporal arteritis. Am. J. Med., 71, 320-322

Lever, W.F. (1969) Maladie de Kaposi. In: Lever, W.F., ed., Histopathologie de la Peau, Paris, Masson et Cie, pp. 616-620

Lothe, F. (1960) Multiple idiopathic hemorrhagic sarcoma of Kaposi in Uganda. <u>Un. Int. Cancr. Acta</u>, <u>16</u>, 1447-1451

Lothe, F. (1963) Kaposi's sarcoma in Uganda Africans. <u>Acta Pathol. Microbiol. Scand.</u>, <u>161</u>, 1-70

Maclean, C.M.U. (1963) Kaposi's sarcoma in Nigeria. <u>Br. J. Cancer</u>, <u>17</u>, 195-205

Master, J.P., Taylor, J.F., Kyalwazi, S.K. & Ziegler, J. (1970) Immunological studies in Kaposi's sarcoma in Uganda. <u>Br. med. J.</u>, <u>1</u>, 600-602

Mathieu, J. (1948) Un cas d'angiosarcomatose de Kaposi chez un Noir du Congo belge. <u>Ann. Soc. belge Méd. trop.</u>, <u>28</u>, 445-450

Meynadier, J., Guilhou, J.J., Peyron, J.L. & Guillot, B. (1981) Maladie de Kaposi chez un psoriasique soumis à une cortico-thérapie locale et prolongée. <u>Dermatologica</u>, <u>162</u>, 417-423

Moe, N. (1966) Hodgkin's disease and Kaposi's sarcoma. Report of a case. <u>Acta Pathol. Microbiol. Scand.</u>, <u>68</u>, 189-193

Moertel, C.G. (1966) Multiple primary malignant neoplasms, their incidence and significance. <u>Recent Results Cancer Res.</u>, <u>7</u>, 34-37

Montgomery, H. (1967) <u>Kaposi's sarcoma (Multiple idiopathic hemorrhagic sarcoma of Kaposi)</u>. In: Montgomery, H., ed., <u>Dermatopathology</u>, 2, New York, Hoeber Medical Division, Harper & Row Publishers, pp. 1110-1120

Myers, B.D., Kessler, E., Levi, J., Pick, A. & Rosenfeld, J.B. (1974) Kaposi's sarcoma in kidney transplant recipients. <u>Arch. intern. Med.</u>, <u>133</u>, 307-311

Oettlé, A.G. (1962) Geographical and racial differences in the
    frequency of Kaposi's sarcoma as evidence of environmental
    or genetic causes. Un. Int. Cancr. Acta, 18, 330-363

Offenstadt, G., Pinta, P., Hericord, P., Jagveux, M., Jean, F.,
    Amstutz, P., Valade, S. & Legavre, P. (1983) Multiple
    opportunistic infections due to AIDS in a previously healthy
    black woman from Zaire. New Engl. J. Med., 308, 775

Oluwasanmi, J.O., Williams, A.O. & Alli, A.F. (1969) Superficial
    cancer in Nigeria. Br. J. Cancer, 23, 714-728

Penn, I. (1979) Kaposi's sarcoma in organ transplant recipients:
    report of 20 cases. Transplantation, 27, 8-11

Pitchenic, A.E., Fischl, M.A., Dickinson, G.N., Becker, D.M.,
    Fournier, A.M., O'Connel, M.T., Colton, R.M. & Spira, J.T.
    (1983) Opportunistic infections and Kaposi's sarcoma among
    Haitians. Ann. intern. Med., 98, 277-284

Quenum, A. & Camain, R. (1958) Les aspects africains de la
    maladie de Kaposi, réticulopathie maligne systématisée.
    Ann. Anat. Pathol., 3, 337-368

Reynolds, W.A., Winkelmann, R.K. & Soule, E.H. (1965) Kaposi's
    sarcoma: a clinicopathological study with particular
    reference to its relationship to the reticuloendothelial
    system. Medicine, 44, 419-443

Rothman, S. (1962a) Some clinical aspects of Kaposi's sarcoma in
    the European and North American population. Un. Int. Cancr.
    Acta, 18, 364-371

Rothman, S. (1962b) Remarks on sex, age and racial distribution
    of Kaposi's sarcoma and on possible etiopathogenic factors.
    Un. Int. Cancr. Acta, 18, 326-329

Rudolf, R.I. (1977) Kaposi's sarcoma after renal transplanta-
    tion. Arch. Dermatol., 113, 1307

Safai, B., Miké, V., Giraldo, G., Beth, E. & Good, R.A. (1980)
    Association of Kaposi's sarcoma with second primary mali-
    gnancies: possible etiopathogenic implications. Cancer,
    45, 1472-1479

Siegal, J.H., Janis, R., Alper, J.C., Schutte, H., Robbins, L. & Blaufox, M.D. (1969) Disseminated visceral Kaposi's. Appearance after human renal homograft operation. J. Am. med. Assoc., 207, 1493-1496

Slavin, G., Cameron, H.M. & Singh, H. (1969) Kaposi's sarcoma in mainland Tanzania: A report of 117 cases. Br. J. Cancer, 23, 349-367

Slavin, G., Cameron, H.M., Forbes, C. & Morton-Mitchell, R. (1970) Kaposi's sarcoma in East African children. A report of 51 cases. J. Pathol., 100, 187-199

Sonnet, J. & De Bruyère, M. (1983) Syndrome de déficit acquis de l'immunité. Acquired immunodeficiency syndrome (AIDS). Etat de la question. Données personnelles de la pathologie observée chez des Zairois. Louvain Méd., 102, 297-307

Stribling, J., Weitzner, S. & Smith, G.V. (1978) Kaposi's sarcoma in renal allograft recipients. Cancer, 42, 442-446

Symmers, D. (1948) Kaposi's disease. Arch. Pathol., 32, 764-786

Taelman, H., Dasnoy, J., Van Merck, E. & Eyckmans, L. (1983) Syndrome d'immunodéficience acquise chez trois malades du Zaïre. Ann. Soc. belge Méd. trop., 63, 73-74

Taylor, J.F. (1973) Lymphocyte transformation in Kaposi's sarcoma. Lancet, 1, 883-884

Taylor, J.F. & Ziegler, J.L. (1974) Delayed cutaneous hypersensitivity reactions in patients with Kaposi's sarcoma. Br. J. Cancer, 30, 312-318

Taylor, J.F., Templeton, A.C., Kyalwazi, S.K. & Lubega, A. (1971a) Kaposi's sarcoma in pregnancy. Br. J. Surg., 58, 577-579

Taylor, J.F., Templeton, A.C., Vogel, C.L., Ziegler, J.L. & Kyalwazi, S.K. (1971b) Kaposi's sarcoma in Uganda: A clinicopathological study. Int. J. Cancer, 8, 122-135

Tedeschi, C.G. (1958) Some considerations concerning the nature of the so-called Kaposi's sarcoma. Arch. Pathol., 66, 656-684

Templeton, A.C. (1972) Studies in Kaposi's sarcoma. Post-mortem findings and disease patterns in women. Cancer, 30, 854-867

Templeton, A.C. (1973) Soft tissue tumors. Recent Results Cancer Res., 41, 262-268

Templeton, A.C. (1981) Kaposi's sarcoma. Pathol. Annu., 16, 315-336

Templeton, A.C. & Bhana, D. (1975) Prognosis in Kaposi's sarcoma. J. natl Cancer Inst., 55, 1301-1304

Ten Seldam, R.F.J., Helwig, E.B., Sobin, L.H. & Torloni, H. (1975) Histological Typing of Skin Tumours (International Histological Classification of Tumours, No. 12), Geneva, World Health Organization, p. 79

Thijs, A. (1957) L'angiosarcomatose de Kaposi au Congo belge et au Ruanda-Urundi. Ann. Soc. belge Méd. trop., 37, 295-307

Thomsen, H.K., Jacobsen, M. & Machova-Moler, A. (1981) Kaposi's sarcoma among homosexual men in Europe. Lancet, 2, 688

Weschler, Z., Leviatan, A. & Kranokuki, D. (1979) Primary Kaposi's sarcoma in lymph nodes concurrent with chronic lymphatic leukemia. Am. J. clin. Pathol., 71, 234-236

Zisbrod, E., Haimov, M., Schanzer, H., Ambinder, E. & Burrows, L. (1980) Kaposi's sarcoma after kidney transplantation. Report of complete cutaneous and visceral involvement. Transplantation, 30, 383-384

ROLE OF CYTOMEGALOVIRUS IN KAPOSI'S SARCOMA

G. Giraldo & E. Beth

Division of Viral Oncology
G. Pascale Foundation National Tumour Institute
Naples, Italy

S.K. Kyalwazi

Department of Surgery
New Mulago Hospital
Makerere University
Kampala, Uganda

RESUME

Des études antérieures ont montré une association entre le cytomégalovirus (CMV) et les formes classiques et endémiques, et même par extension les formes épidémiques du sarcome de Kaposi (SK). Cette association est basée:

- sur l'identification de séquences d'acide nucléique homologues à celles du CMV dans des biopsies tumorales et/ou des cultures primaires établies à partir de ces tumeurs. Par contre, aucune homologie n'a été retrouvée avec le virus d'Epstein-Barr (EBV), ni avec le virus Herpes simplex de type 1 (HSV-1) ou de type 2 (HSV-2).

- sur la détection, dans ces échantillons tumoraux, des produits des gènes du CMV, en particulier des antigènes précoces. Il n'a pas été possible de mettre en évidence les antigènes tardifs du CMV, ni la présence de particules virales, ce qui élimine la possibilité que le CMV soit simplement "de passage", ou que le tissu tumoral soit un site préférentiel de réplication virale.

Les sujets atteints de syndrome immuno-déficitaire acquis (SIDA), les transplantés rénaux sous thérapie immunosuppressive et les sujets immunosupprimés de façon iatrogène constituent les trois principaux groupes dans lesquels le SK est le plus souvent observé. Les oncogènes du CMV, dont au moins deux ont été identifiés dans des systèmes expérimentaux, pourraient être impliqués dans le développement du SK chez ces sujets. De plus, les études de transformation in vitro indiquent clairement que le virus est impliqué dans l'initiation de la transformation tandis que d'autres facteurs (agents co-cancérogènes, activation d'oncogènes cellulaires ?) pourraient être nécessaires au maintien du phénotype transformé. Les cellules endothéliales, permissives pour l'infection CMV, pourraient être la cible initiale de ces évènements, puisqu'on a montré qu'elles constituent la plus grande partie du tissu malin.

Les données obtenues pendant 14 années de recherche sur le SK sont exposées et les mécanismes étiopathogéniques possibles de ce type de tumeur sont discutés.

SUMMARY

Previous studies have established an association between cytomegalovirus (CMV) and classic and endemic Kaposi's sarcoma (KS) which can be extended to include the epidemic form of KS. The identification of nucleic acid sequences homologous to CMV but not to Epstein-Barr virus (EBV) and Herpes simplex virus type 1 (HSV-1) and type 2 (HSV-2) as well as the detection of CMV gene products, particularly early antigens, in tumour biopsies and/or early cultures derived from them is an important criterion in the establishment of the type of association. Detection of CMV early antigens but not late antigens as well as the failure to demonstrate virus particles in primary tumour biopsies rule out a simple passenger role of this virus or a preferential site for virus replication in neoplastic tissue.

In the setting of a profound immune dysfunction, as in the case of acquired immune deficiency syndrome (AIDS), renal transplant recipients under immunosuppressive therapy, and other iatrogenically immunosuppressed patients (the three groups in which KS has been most frequently observed), the specific involvement of CMV oncogenes, of which at least two have been so far identified in experimental systems, is strongly indicated. Moreover, in vitro transformation experiments indicate that the virus is clearly involved in the initiation of transformation, while other factors (co-carcinogens, activation of cellular onco- genes?) might be required for the maintenance of the transformed phenotype. Endothelial cells, permissive for CMV infection, might be the prime target for these events, since there is evidence that they are a main constituent of KS tissue.

Data obtained during 14 years of research on KS are reviewed and possible etiopathogenetic mechanisms giving rise to this type of tumour are discussed.

INTRODUCTION

Kaposi's sarcoma (KS), a haemangiosarcoma which is frequent- ly localized to the skin, became of interest to many physicians and biologists when Quenum and Camain (1958) reported a high incidence of this tumour - considered to be rare since its first description by Kaposi (1872) - in indigenous populations of equatorial Africa. In addition, they noted that the symptomato- logy of KS was much more varied in Africa. No further develop- ments took place until 1972, when two papers were published by our group suggesting, on the basis of the results obtained, that KS was an important natural model in the search for viruses and co-factors associated with human cancer (Giraldo et al., 1972a,- b). It appeared to us that KS was an interesting tumour and worthy of study for the following reasons: (1) Its peculiar geographical distribution among the native populations of equa- torial African countries is strongly reminiscent of that of Burkitt's lymphoma in Africa, another human cancer associated with a virus, the Epstein-Barr virus (EBV) (Epstein & Achong, 1979). In this connection, it is of interest that a high incidence of KS has been found in particular tribes, as well as cluster-like occurrences (Rogoff, 1968; Templeton & Hutt, 1973; McHardy et al., 1984). (2) KS evolves rapidly in children, but follows a protracted course in adults, and in some cases spon- taneous regressions have been observed. This biological behaviour, when considered together with the histological findings, suggests an immunological response of the host, similar to that seen with virus-induced tumours in animals. (3) A second primary neoplasm, and particularly Hodgkin's disease, is not uncommon in patients with KS and this is considered to be more than coincidental, thus indicating the possible persistence of a tumour inducer (Safai et al., 1980). (4) The multiplicity of lesions suggests a multifocal origin of KS, consistent with virus infection.

It was impossible in 1972 to foresee that this tumour would arouse world-wide attention some 10 years later due to an epidemic resulting from profound cultural changes in a particular population group in our society. Indeed, the current epidemic of KS associated with acquired immune deficiency syndrome (AIDS) (Centers for Disease Control, 1981; Haverkos & Curran, 1982), affecting mainly homosexual men, provides a unique natural model whereby vital information can be obtained on crucial interrelationships between oncogenes and immune responses, immunosuppressive genes and viruses, genetics and life-style (Giraldo & Beth, 1984a).

The purpose of this communication is to summarize the results obtained in our laboratory during 13 years of studies on KS and its association with cytomegalovirus (CMV), to focus on KS in its epidemic form and analyse the data for the various types of KS, and finally to hypothesize as to the etiopathogenic mechanisms giving rise to this type of tumour (Giraldo & Beth, 1980, 1984a,b; Giraldo et al., 1981). For the sake of clarity it may be worthwhile identifying at least three main forms of KS, which will subsequently be referred to as: (1) the classic form, with a relatively low frequency in European and American populations (male/female ratio 3:1, mean age: 68 years); (2) the endemic form, with a relatively high frequency in equatorial Africa, mainly in males (male/female ratio 14:1, mean age: 35 years) and in children (male/female ratio 3:1); and (3) the epidemic form of KS identified in 1981, mainly in homosexual men (mean age: 35 years), first described in the United States of America (Centers for Disease Control, 1981), then in Europe (Biggar et al., 1984) and now also reported in patients from various parts of Central Africa. Moreover, an additional form of KS, known since the 1970s, is represented by that seen in renal transplant recipients under immunosuppressive therapy (Stribling et al., 1978; Harwood et al., 1979; Penn, 1979) and other iatrogenically immunosuppressed individuals (Klein et al., 1974; Kapadia & Krause, 1977; Klepp et al., 1978).

Between 1971 and the present time, 210 patients with KS from Zaire, Uganda, Cameroon and Senegal (endemic KS), from Tunisia, France, Italy and the United States (classic KS) and recently from France and the United States (epidemic KS) have been and/or are being studied in our laboratory (Table 1).

Table 1. KS patients studied during 1971-1984

Form of Kaposi's sarcoma	Geographical location	No. of patients	Mean age (years)	Sex	
				M	F
Classic	France	18	67.4	14	4
	Italy	9	60.3	8	1
	United States	42	69.8	31	11
	Algeria	2	63.0	2	0
	Morocco	3	48.5	3	0
	Tunisia	13	54.4	12	1
Endemic	Cameroon	9	44.0	9	0
	Uganda	79	43.0	78	1
	Zaire	4	46.7	4	0
	Senegal	6	38.3	6	0
Epidemic	France	6	38.0	5	0
	United States	20	35.0	20	0
Total		210		192	18

ASSOCIATION OF CMV WITH KAPOSI'S SARCOMA

Accumulating serological and molecular epidemiological evidence points to a specific association between CMV and KS, whether in its classic, endemic or epidemic form, as well as probably in kidney transplant recipients and other iatrogenically immunosuppressed patients (Table 2).

Table 2.   Findings supporting the association of CMV with Kaposi's sarcoma

---

All patients with KS are CMV seropositive (Drew et al., 1981; Giraldo et al., 1975,1978)

Specific serological association with CMV but not with EBV, HSV-1 or HSV-2 (Giraldo et al., 1975,1978)

Identification of CMV DNA in KS biopsies (endemic and epidemic form) (Giraldo et al., 1980; Boldogh et al., 1981; Shaw et al., 1983; McDougall et al., unpublished data)

Identification of CMV-determined early antigens in KS biopsies and/or early KS cell cultures (classic, endemic and epidemic form) (Giraldo et al., 1980; Boldogh et al., 1981; Drew et al., 1982)

Failure to demonstrate CMV or CMV-determined late antigens in KS biopsies (Giraldo et al., 1980; Civantos et al., 1982)

Growth properties in vitro of CMV strain K9V are reminiscent of those of the oncogenic CMV strain Mj (Glaser et al., 1977)

Induction of fatal lymphoproliferative disease in infant baboons (Papio cynocephalus) (Giraldo et al., 1981) by CMV strain K9V, isolated from endemic KS of Zaire (Giraldo et al., 1972a,b)

CMV can be isolated from urine, semen, liver, lung tissue (epidemic form); on rare occasions from tumour biopsy in tissue culture (lymph-node involvement, endemic form) (Giraldo et al., 1972a,b; Drew et al., 1981,1982; Gyorkey et al., 1982)

CMV infections and/or reactivation of endogenous virus is most common and severe in renal transplant patients, who develop KS with high frequency (Fiala et al., 1975; Stribling et al., 1978; Harwood et al., 1979; Penn, 1979)

In order to determine whether an association existed with high titres of antibodies either to CMV, EBV, herpes simplex virus type 1 (HSV-1) or type-2 (HSV-2) in patients with classic and endemic KS, extensive serological analyses were undertaken (Giraldo et al., 1975,1978). Briefly, it was possible to demonstrate a specific serological association of CMV with KS in patients, whether from America or Europe, with the classical form. All patients' sera contained CMV antibodies, and the geometric mean titres were significantly higher than those in sera from age- and sex-matched melanoma patients, as well as in sera from age- and sex-matched healthy blood bank donors. In contrast, no association was found with EBV, HSV-1 or HSV-2. No serological association with CMV could be found in patients with endemic KS. However, viral infections and/or activation of latent viruses occur frequently in subjects living in endemic and epidemic areas so that specific viral associations to a particular disease (syndrome) cannot be easily established, since control subjects matched by geographical and socioepidemiological criteria are equally exposed to the agents concerned.

In order to strengthen the serological association of CMV with KS, nucleic acid hybridization studies were undertaken on cell DNA and RNA of KS biopsy specimens, mainly from endemic areas but also from one patient with classic KS, and a search was made for CMV-determined early antigens. The results have been published elsewhere (Giraldo et al., 1980; Boldogh et al., 1981) and are summarized in Table 3. The amount of CMV DNA in sarcoma tissue was calculated to be in the range 0.7-1 genome equivalent per diploid cell. The presence of virus-specific RNA was demonstrated in 5 of 10 tumour biopsies. No EBV- or HSV-2-specific nucleic acid homologies could be detected. It was recently demonstrated that the CMV genome contains regions of DNA sequences which can hybridize with normal human DNA (Rüger & Fleckenstein, 1984). For this reason, emphasis is currently being placed on analyses of CMV sequences in tumour tissue, using as hybridizing probe cloned viral DNA subfragments, free of cellular DNA, which contain the region(s) responsible for transformation, in order to determine whether CMV DNA is present in KS. At the same time, transfection experiments are in progress using high-molecular-weight DNA from KS tissue and NIH 3T3 cells as well as primary rat cells. Transformants will be analysed for human repetitive Alu sequences, known cellular oncogenes (c-onc) and CMV nucleic acid sequences. A third line of investigation is aimed at determining, in cell clones obtained by transfection with subfragments of CMV, whether flanking cellular sequences of

GIRALDO ET AL.

the integrated sites of viral fragments become activated or their expression altered (McDougall et al., unpublished data).

Table 3. Detection of CMV DNA, CMV RNA, and CMV early antigens in KS biopsies and/or early cell lines derived from them

KS code	Geographical location	CMV DNA[a]	CMV RNA[a]	CMV-determined early antigen(s)[a]	
				Biopsy	Cultured cells
KS-22	Uganda	NT	NT	NT	+
KS-32	Uganda	NT	NT	+	+
KS-38	Uganda	NT	NT	+	NT
KS-55	Senegal	NT	NT	+	NT
KS-71	Senegal	NT	NT	+	NT
KS-80	Uganda	+	NT	+	NT
KS-82	Uganda	NT	NT	NT	+
KS-86	Uganda	−	−	+	NT
KS-87	Uganda	+	+	+	NT
KS-93	Uganda	+	+	+	NT
KS-94	Uganda	−	+	+	NT
KS-95	Uganda	−	−	+	NT
KS-97	Uganda	−	−	−	NT
KS-102	Uganda	+	NT	NT	NT
KS-103	Uganda	−	−	−	NT
KS-107	Uganda	+	+	+	NT
KS-111	Uganda	+	NT	NT	+
KS-114	United States	−	+	+	NT
KS-120	Uganda	−	−	+	NT

[a] NT = Not tested

BIOLOGICAL PROPERTIES OF CMV

CMV has biological properties reminiscent of those of other oncogenic DNA viruses, e.g., ability to stimulate host-cell DNA and RNA synthesis, production of high levels of the oncogenic marker ornithine decarboxylase, and transforming potential in vitro for hamster and human embryo fibroblasts (Huang et al., 1984; Rapp, 1984). CMV-determined antigens can be demonstrated in the cytoplasm and on the cell surface of transformed cells in vitro, and cell cultures derived from them induce fibrosarcomas when injected into newborn hamsters. However, after long periods of subculturing, DNA-DNA reassociation experiments with a sensitivity as high as 0.1 viral genome equivalent per cell failed to detect CMV DNA sequence homologies in such cells (Huang et al., 1984). It is possible, therefore, that CMV is involved in the initiation of transformation but is not necessarily needed for the maintenance of the transformed state. Experimental data using CMV DNA transforming fragments confirm this possibility (Huang et al., 1984).

The transforming ability of CMV at subgenomic levels was first demonstrated by Nelson et al. (1982), using the strain AD169. They showed that the transforming region is located in the 2.9 Kb HindIII fragment E between map units 0.123 and 0.14 on the viral DNA molecule. The possible involvement of such a small piece of viral DNA in cell transformation points to a hit-and-run mechanism. Moreover, CMV DNA contains more than one transforming region. Clanton et al. (1983) identified a second distinct transforming region in CMV DNA (Towne strain XbaI fragment E). It is homologous to the HSV-2 DNA fragment BglII fragment C, known to induce neoplastic transformation of diploid cells. Morphological transformation of NIH 3T3 cells could be produced by transfection with this viral DNA fragment and neoplastic growth occurred when it was injected into nude mice.

KAPOSI'S SARCOMA IN AIDS

United States and Europe

As in endemic and classical KS, males predominate among cases of the epidemic form of KS. Table 4 shows that, of all cases of KS observed in the on-going epidemic of AIDS, 98.5% occur in males and that, when divided by sex preference, 93% of all KS patients are homo- or bisexual men (Giraldo & Beth,

1984b). In addition, as far as sexual orientation and disease
category are concerned, 41% of homosexual men with AIDS have KS
compared to only 7% of heterosexual patients. Although the
Centers for Disease Control have by now received more than 4000
reports of AIDS, no changes in the proportion with KS have been
noted. It should be pointed out that most of the malignancies in
the epidemic of AIDS are KS, which accounts for more than 90% of
all reported cancers, but non-Hodgkin's lymphomas of the
Burkitt's type and, rarely, squamous-cell carcinomas are also
seen (Conant et al., 1982; Ziegler et al., 1982). This epidemic
of AIDS and its association with an otherwise rare tumour, namely
KS, is unusual, therefore, and poses a great challenge to viral
oncologists, immunologists and epidemiologists. Particular environmental and host factors specific to sex and sexually associated life-styles would seem relevant to the development of KS in
this striking outbreak (Table 5). Possible clues to the causes
of this syndrome, which must certainly be multifactorial in
etiology, are derived from studies of the socioepidemiological
aspects. A national case-control study on homosexual men with
epidemic KS supports this view (Jaffe et al., 1983). The
variables most strongly associated with AIDS were: (1) a large
number of male sex partners per year (median 61); (2) promiscuity; and (3) the use of illicit substances, known to be immunosuppressive. Moreover, a cluster of cases has been discovered
in the epidemic of AIDS and KS (Auerbach et al., 1984), reminiscent of the endemic situation of KS (McHardy et al., 1984). The
cluster comprises 40 sexually related homosexual AIDS patients,
24 of whom had KS alone, 8 had KS and Pneumocystis carinii
pneumonia, 1 had disseminated CMV infection and 1 toxoplasmosis
of the central nervous system. The mean latency period between
sexual contact and onset of symptoms was estimated at 10.5 months
(range 7-14 months), which is similar to the estimated mean
latency period for the development of KS in immunosuppressed
kidney transplant recipients (Harwood et al., 1979; Penn, 1979).
A cluster of cases among individuals in close contact with one
another is usually taken as evidence of the infectious nature of
a condition. If a transmissible agent does exist, this would
mean that, in the epidemic of AIDS and KS, the latter would be
the first transmissible malignancy with a short incubation period
discovered in humans.

Table 4. Kaposi's sarcoma in AIDS patients (epidemic form)a

Patients	No. with KS	Total No.	Proportion with KS (%)
Men[b]	611	620	98.5
Homo- and bisexual men[b]	579	620	93.0
All AIDS patients	620	1972	31.0
Homo- and bisexual men with AIDS	579	1393	41.0
Heterosexual patients with AIDS	41	574	7.0

[a] Source: Centers for Disease Control, 15 July 1983, personal communication

[b] The comparison is with all KS patients.

Table 5. Risk factors for Kaposi's sarcoma (epidemic form)

Environment and lifestyle
    Multiple sex partners (homosexual males)
    Certain sexual practices (semen ingestion; oral, rectal)
    Multiple sexually transmitted infections
       (parasitic, bacterial, fungal, viral: CMV, EBV, HSV-1,
       HSV-2, HBV, adeno- and papovaviruses, HTLV)
    Use of inhalants (nitrites), intravenous drug abuse
       (cocaine, heroin)
    Use of steroid creams (oestrogen)

Host characteristics
    Predominance of males (homosexual males; hormones;
       sex-linked?)
    Immunogenetics (HLA-DR5, HLA-DR3)
    History of mononucleosis (EBV) or mononucleosis-like
       syndrome (CMV)
    Immunosuppression - immunodeficiency
    Activation of cellular oncogenes

AIDS has been increasingly reported in various European countries, with the highest incidence in France, followed by the Federal Republic of Germany and Belgium, and again more than 70% of cases occur in the highest risk group found in the United States, namely homosexual men (Biggar et al., 1984). A new feature of the outbreak in Europe is the link with Africa, 22% of reported cases, particularly from France and Belgium, having been born or lived for several years in Central Africa (including Zaire, Congo, Mali, Gabon, Rwanda, Burundi, Chad and Cameroon.

Central Africa

KS is endemic in various equatorial African countries but, in addition to the recent findings in Sardinia (Cottoni et al., 1980), the epidemic of AIDS is also developing in Central Africa, and there are now more than 100 cases, mainly reported in residents of Kinshasa, Zaire. No definite risk groups have been identified. The male/female ratio is 3:2, which is clearly different from what is found in the United States and Europe. In October-November 1983, 49 cases alone were observed in two large hospitals in Kinshasa; 21% of the men and 90% of the women affected were unmarried. Homosexuality is virtually unknown in equatorial African populations (McHardy et al., 1984). However, heterosexual promiscuity, particularly in crowded urban areas, cannot be ruled out. This might therefore explain a mode of transmission reminiscent of that of an infectious agent, as suggested for the epidemic in the West, transmitted by intimate sexual contact. That AIDS can be transmitted between heterosexual men and women has been reported (Harris et al., 1983). The incidence of KS in African AIDS (Biggar et al., 1984), as compared to that in the epidemic in the United States (Table 4), appears somewhat lower (about 17% versus 31%, respectively). Since male/female ratios are significantly different (the male/-female ratio in the United States is 16:1), this may merely be a biased observation and more specific data are needed for purposes of the comparison. It is obvious, however, that more female subjects are contracting AIDS. This might mean that AIDS is caused by one agent and KS by another, in combination with various other environmental and host factors. In support of this view is the fact that, in the United States, 41% of homosexual men with AIDS develop KS while only 7% of heterosexual AIDS patients do so. A two-agent theory is therefore favoured: AIDS could be mainly due to an apparently new agent, e.g., lymphadeno-pathy associated virus (LAV-1) (Barré-Sinoussi et al., 1983) or human T-cell leukaemia virus (HTLV-3) (Popovic et al., 1984), with a specific lytic T4-cell tropism, while the development of KS depends on intensive exposure to a second virus in a particular subpopulation of men with the appropriate genetic and immuno-genetic predisposition. CMV is a leading candidate for the second agent, based on the high prevalence of CMV excretion among promiscuous homosexual men (epidemic KS); it is ubiquitous in Central Africa (endemic KS); kidney transplant recipients and other iatrogenically immunosuppressed patients have a high incidence of CMV infection/reactivation, and KS is now developing frequently among them. Moreover, the molecular epidemiological findings associate this virus with KS.

Currently, consideration is being given to the possibility that T-cell-tropic retroviruses might have originated in Africa (Brun-Vézinet et al., 1984), where an undiagnosed AIDS syndrome might have existed for a long time. It did not cause an epidemic because the indigenous rural population in Equatorial Africa is widely scattered and because of traditional life-styles. As a result of the recent tendency for rural people to migrate to crowded urban areas associated with poor socioeconomic living conditions and increased promiscuity, the virus has spread, with a consequent epidemic in a population with no immunological resistance to such an agent. Moreover, some of the endemic KS seen in the past, and particularly the progressive type of disease, which is more frequently seen in Africa and is associated with immunodysfunction, might have been preceded by what is now called AIDS. In fact, on analysing sera from KS patients from Kinshasa, bled in 1972, retrospectively, we found in 2 out of 4 sera high titres of antibodies against HTLV (Giraldo & Beth, unpublished data). Both patients had the progressive form of the disease.

The AIDS agent might have been brought to Europe by Europeans who had lived in Central Africa, as well as by African residents working in France and in Belgium (Belgium has links with Zaire and France with the Congo, the two countries with the highest incidence so far in Africa of generalized lymphadenopathy and AIDS as well as HTLV infections). The disease might have been carried to Haiti and the Caribbean by Haitians who went to Zaire in the 1960s and by Cubans who went to Angola, which borders on Zaire, in the 1970s. Homosexual men from the United States, who frequently vacation in Haiti, might have introduced the virus to the United States. Moreover, thousands of Haitians and Cubans, including some homosexual men, have left their islands to live in the United States in the last 10 years. The virus might also have been taken from the United States to Europe and vice versa by infected vacationing homosexual men.

CMV, IMMUNOSUPPRESSION AND KAPOSI'S SARCOMA

It would be surprising if CMV did not contribute substantially to the immune defects observed in the various forms of KS. CMV, together with EBV, is the pathogen most frequently found in equatorial Africans and among AIDS patients, particularly homosexual men, and viral antibodies are present in high titres in such populations (Giraldo et al., 1975,1978; Drew et al., 1982; Friedman-Kien et al., 1982). CMV infections induce immunosuppression and cause abnormal T-cell subsets (Hirsch & Felsenstein, unpublished data). Promiscuous homosexual men have shown a reduced T4/T8 radio due to a high frequency of sexually transmitted infections (Kornfeld et al., 1982). That homosexual men experience multiple episodes of CMV infections was shown by the high prevalence in such men of IgM antibodies and the frequent isolation of the virus from their semen (Drew et al., 1981,1982). It is possible that a combined T-cell assault launched by CMV and other T-cell-tropic pathogens, e.g., HTLV or HTLV-like agents, or a combined assault against both T- and B-cells by CMV and EBV takes place. The use of immunosuppressive drugs, such as amyl nitrite, might also enhance CMV-induced hyporesponsiveness in patients with AIDS, as may other frequent microbial infections in equatorial Africans (e.g., holoendemic malaria), immunosuppressive therapy or increased age; all these conditions are frequently associated with the various forms of KS.

ASSOCIATION OF HLA-DR WITH KAPOSI'S SARCOMA

There appears to be a genetic link between a particular HLA phenotype and a subset of AIDS patients, predisposing them to the development of lymphadenopathies with progression to KS. In fact, a higher frequency of the HLA-DR5 phenotype has been repeatedly found in these patients (Enlov et al., 1983; Metroka et al., 1983). Similarly, epidemic and classic KS patients have a significantly higher frequency of HLA-DR5 (Friedman-Kien et al., 1982; Pollack et al., 1983; Rubinstein et al., 1984), and it would not be surprising if this also applies to patients with the endemic form of KS, since the highest known frequency of HLA-DR5 occurs in the native population of equatorial Africa (Friedman-Kien et al., 1982). It is of interest that HLA-DR3 is reduced in KS patients, as convincingly shown by the recent findings of Leone et al. (1984) and Contu (1984) in an immunogenetic analysis of 'classic' KS patients in Sardinia. Their results strongly support the hypothesis that the development and evolution of KS is genetically determined. Susceptibility and resistance to the disease seem to be linked with the HLA-DR5 and HLA-DR3 alleles, respectively. The immunological status of the same patients was determined, and revealed profound abnormalities, particularly in respect of cell-mediated immunity, in both the localized and progressive forms of the disease. It is thought that HLA-DR5-associated factors can confer a genetic predisposition to T-cell impairment, perhaps due to a mutant I_R gene. The finding of a similar immunological dysfunction, combined with an increased frequency of HLA-DR5, in patients with generalized lymphadeno-pathy in a group of drug abusers in Sardinia (Contu, 1984), supports the hypothesis that HLA-DR5-linked susceptibility plays a role in the development of the immune impairment.

DISCUSSION

Molecular epidemiological studies have established a specific association between CMV and KS, first demonstrated in the classic and endemic forms, but which can be extended to the epidemic form of the disease. The identification of nucleic acid sequences homologous to CMV but not to EBV or HSV-2, as well as the detection of CMV gene products, particularly early antigens, in tumour biopsies and/or early cell cultures derived from them, is an important factor in the establishment of the type of asso-ciation. Detection of CMV early, but not late antigens, as well as the failure to demonstrate virus particles in primary biopsies, rule out a simple passenger role of this virus or a preferential site for virus replication in neoplastic tissue. Positive results were also obtained recently at subgenomic level, using as hybridization probe the cloned CMV DNA fragment EcoRI J, which does not hybridize to human cellular DNA and contains sequences coding for the major immediate early CMV-determined protein IE 72K (McDougall et al., 1984).

In patients with profound immune dysfunction, e.g., AIDS patients, renal transplant recipients under immunosuppressive therapy, and other iatrogenically immunosuppressed patients (the three groups in which KS has been frequently observed), there is a strong case for the specific involvement of CMV since, in experimental systems at least, two different transforming regions of the genome have been so far identified. Moreover, the fact that immunosuppressed patients have frequent CMV infections does not rule out the oncogenic potential of this virus, since a close association of the virus with host cells, and particularly with endothelial cells in this case (Guarda et al., 1981; Nadji et al., 1981), may provide a perfect opportunity for it to induce neoplastic transformation during long-term viral persistence.

If AIDS is seen as an accelerated model for immunosuppression, the following etiopathogenic mechanisms leading to KS can be hypothesized. In subjects developing AIDS, a breakdown of cell-mediated immunity, probably caused by a T-cell-tropic virus (LAV-1 or HTLV-3), results in chronic inflammation due to persistent infection(s), often by CMV and EBV, which in turn leads frequently to generalized lymphadenopathy. As a consequence, increased amounts of angiogenesis factors (Taylor & Folkman, 1982) are produced, resulting in an activation of endothelial cells. Immunogenetic control (HLA-DR5 versus HLA-DR3) might at this point influence the outcome of the disease. If the patient is HLA-DR5-positive but HLA-DR3-negative there is a high probability that the syndrome will progress to KS. The HLA-DR antigen function might be at the level of the immune-response genes mainly controlling cell-mediated immunity and/or at the receptor level of activated endothelial cells in CMV infection.

In vitro transformation experiments indicate that the virus is involved in the initiation of transformation, while other factors (co-carcinogens, activation of cellular oncogenes, e.g., c-myc, c-sis) might be required for the maintenance of the transformed phenotype. In KS, endothelial cells which are permissive for CMV infection are the prime target for these events, since they are the main constituent of the tumour tissue. How does CMV act in transformation? Does the virus act as a mutagen, and is transformation the result of a hit-and-run mechanism? The failure consistently to detect specific viral nucleic acid sequences or proteins in KS points in that direction. Moreover, transforming CMV DNA fragment(s) contain sequences similar in structure to that of insertion sequence (IS)-like elements (McDougall et al., unpublished data). Hit and run or permanent insertion into the cell genome could provide a promoter/insertion type of activation of endogenous viral oncogenes and/or flanking cellular oncogenes. Another possibility, based on the finding of HVS-2 and human papilloma virus (HPV) DNA sequences in the same tumour

(cervical carcinoma) (McDougall et al., 1984), is that CMV and
another common virus could interact in an initiation/promotion
relationship to bring about transformation.

The importance of the on-going epidemic of AIDS in Central
Africa may be far greater than is now realised. It is known that
the indigenous populations of Equatorial Africa have a high prevalence of viral infections and viral carrier states, the viruses
concerned including oncogenic viruses (herpesviruses, hepatitis B
virus and possibly also retroviruses), as well as a high incidence of cancer, which often progresses very rapidly. An epidemic
of LAV-1 or HTLV-3 infection, resulting in immunosuppression and
finally in AIDS, could therefore generate a dramatic upsurge of
KS and various other types of oncogenic-virus-associated cancers
in this region, where they would be much less easy to control
than in the West.

ACKNOWLEDGEMENTS

This study was supported by a grant from the Comitato
Nazionale delle Ricerche (CNR) and the Associazione Italiana per
la Ricerca sul Cancro.

REFERENCES

Auerbach, D.M., Darrow, W.W., Jaffe, H.W. & Curran, J.W. (1984)
    Cluster of cases of the acquired immune deficiency syndrome.
    Patients linked by sexual contact. Am. J. Med., 76, 467-492

Barré-Sinoussi, F., Chermann, J.C., Rey, F., Nugeyre, M.T.,
    Chamaret, S., Gruest, J., Dauguet, C., Axler-Blin, C.,
    Vezinet-Brun, F., Rouzioux, C., Rozenbaum, W. & Montagnier,
    L. (1983) Isolation of a T-lymphotropic retrovirus from a
    patient at risk for acquired immune deficiency syndrome
    (AIDS). Science, 220, 868-871

Biggar, R.J., Bouvet, E., Ebbesen, P., Faber, V., Koch, M.,
    Melbye, M. & Velimirovic, B. (1984) AIDS in Europe, status
    quo 1983. Eur. J. Cancer clin. Oncol., 20, 155-173

Boldogh, I., Beth, E., Huang, E.S., Kyalwazi, S.K. & Giraldo, G. (1981) Kaposi's sarcoma. IV. Detection of CMV DNA, CMV RNA and CMNA in tumor biopsies. Int. J. Cancer, 28, 469-474

Brun-Vézinet, F., Rouzioux, C., Charamet, S., Gruest, J., Barré-Sinoussi, F., Géroldi, D., Chermann, J.C., Piot, P., Taelman, H., Bridts, C., Stevens, W., McCormick, J.B., Mitchell, S., Kapita, B., Wobin, O., Mbendi, N., Mazebo, P., Kayember, N.N., Desmyter, J., Feinsod, F.M., Quinn, T.C. & Montagnier, L. (1984) Prevalence of antibodies to lymphade-nopathy associated retrovirus in African patients with acquired immune deficiency syndrome. Science (submitted for publication)

Centers for Disease Control (1981) Kaposi's sarcoma and Pneumo-cystis pneumonia among homosexual men - New York City and California. Morb. Mortal. Wkly Rep., 30, 305-308

Civantos, F., Penneys, N.S. & Haines, H. (1982) Kaposi's sarcoma: absence of cytomegalovirus. J. invest. Dermatol., 79, 79-80

Clanton, D.J., Jariwalla, R.J., Kress, C. & Rosenthal, L.J. (1983) Neoplastic transformation by a cloned human cyto-megalovirus DNA fragment uniquely homologous to one of the transforming regions of herpes simplex virus. Proc. natl Acad. Sci. USA, 80, 3826-3830

Conant, M.A., Volberding, P., Fletcher, V., Lozada, F.I. & Silverman, S., Jr (1982) Squamous cell carcinoma in sexual partner of Kaposi's sarcoma patient. Lancet, 1, 286

Contu, L. (1984) Immunogenetic factors of classic Kaposi's sarcoma in Sardinia. In: Giraldo, G. & Beth, E., eds, Proceedings of International Meeting on AIDS, Cagliari, 1-3 May, Basle, Karger

Cottoni, F., Ena, P. & Cerimele, D. (1980) Kaposi's sarcoma in North Sardinia from 1977 to 1979. Ital. gen. Rev. Derm., 17, 13-22

Drew, W.L., Mintz, L., Miner, R.C., Sands, M. & Ketterer, B. (1981) Prevalence of CMV infection in homosexual men. J. infect. Dis., 143, 188-192

Drew, W.L., Miner, R.C., Ziegler, J.L., Gullett, J.H., Abrams, D.L., Conant, M.A., Huang, E.-S., Groundwater, J.R., Voldberding, P. & Mintz, L. (1982) Cytomegalovirus and Kaposi's sarcoma in young homosexual men. Lancet, 2, 125-127

Enlov, R.W., Roldan, A.N., LoGalbo, P., Mildvan, D., Mathur, U. & Winchester, R.J. (1983) Increased frequency of HLA-DR4 in lymphadenopathy stage of AIDS. Lancet, 2, 51-52

Epstein, M.A. & Achong, B.G. (1979) The relationship of the Epstein-Barr virus to Burkitt's lymphoma. In: Epstein, M.A. & Achong, B.G., eds, The Epstein-Barr Virus, Berlin, Heidelberg, New York, Springer Verlag, pp. 321-329

Fenoglio, C.M., Oster, M.W., Gerfo, P.L., Reynolds, T., Edelson, R., Patterson, J.A.K., Madeiros, E. & McDougall, J.K. (1982) Kaposi's sarcoma following chemotherapy of testicular carcinoma in a homosexual man: demonstration of CMV RNA in sarcoma cells. Hum. Pathol., 13, 955-959

Fiala, M., Payne, J.E., Berne, T.V., Moore, T.C., Henle, W., Montgomerie, J.Z., Chatterjee, S.N. & Guze, L.B. (1975) Epidemiology of cytomegalovirus infection after transplantation and immunosuppression. J. infect. Dis., 132, 421-433

Friedman-Kien, A.E., Laubenstein, L.J., Rubenstein, P., Buimovici-Klein, E., Marmor, M., Stahl, R., Spigland, I., Kim, K.S. & Zolla-Panzer, S. (1982) Disseminated Kaposi's sarcoma in homosexual men. Ann. Intern. Med., 96, 693-700

Giraldo, G. & Beth, E. (1980) The relationship of cytomegalovirus to certain human cancers, particularly to Kaposi's sarcoma. In: Giraldo, G. & Beth, E., eds, The Role of Viruses in Human Cancer, New York, Amsterdam, Elsevier-North Holland, Vol. 1, pp. 57-73

Giraldo, G. & Beth, E. (1984a) Kaposi's sarcoma: a natural model of interrelationships between viruses, immunologic responses, genetics and oncogenesis. Antibiot. Chemother., 32, 1-11

Giraldo, G. & Beth, E. (1984b) Kaposi's sarcoma today. In:
    Stone, J., ed., Dermatologic Immunology and Allergy, St.
    Louis, The C.V. Mosby Co., Medical and Dental Division (in
    press)

Giraldo, G., Beth, E., Coeur, P., Vogel, C.L. & Dhru, D.S.
    (1972a) Kaposi's sarcoma: a new model in the search for
    viruses associated with human malignancies. J. natl Cancer
    Inst., 49, 1495-1507

Giraldo, G., Beth, E. & Haguenau, F. (1972b) Herpes-type virus
    particles in tissue culture of Kaposi's sarcoma from
    different geographic regions. J. natl Cancer Inst., 49,
    1509-1526

Giraldo, G., Beth, E., Kourilsky, F.M., Henle, W., Henle, G.,
    Miké, V., Huraux, J.M., Andersen, H.K., Gharbi, M.R.,
    Kyalwazi, S.K. & Puissant, A. (1975) Antibody patterns of
    herpesviruses in Kaposi's sarcoma: Serologic association of
    European Kaposi's sarcoma with cytomegalovirus. Int. J.
    Cancer, 15, 839-848

Giraldo, G., Beth, E., Henle, W., Henle, G., Miké, V., Safai, B.,
    Huraux, J.M., McHardy, J. & de-Thé, G. (1978) Antibody
    patterns to herpesviruses in Kaposi's sarcoma. II. Sero-
    logic association of American Kaposi's sarcoma with cyto-
    megalovirus. Int. J. Cancer, 22, 126-131

Giraldo, G., Beth, E. & Huang, E.-S. (1980) Kaposi's sarcoma and
    its relationship to cytomegalovirus (CMV). III. CMV DNA and
    CMV early antigens in Kaposi's sarcoma. Int. J. Cancer, 26,
    23-29

Giraldo, G., Beth, E. & Kyalwazi, S.K. (1981) Etiologic implica-
    tions on Kaposi's sarcoma. Antibiot. Chemother., 29, 12-31

Glaser, R., Geder, L., St. Jeor, S., Michelson-Fiske, S. &
    Haguenau, R. (1977) Partial characterization of a herpes-
    type virus (K9V) derived from Kaposi's sarcoma. J. natl
    Cancer Inst., 59, 55-59

Guarda, L.G., Silva, E.G., Ordonez, N.G. & Smith, J.L. (1981)
    Factor VIII in Kaposi's sarcoma. Am. J. clin. Pathol., 76,
    197-200

Gyorkey, F., Sinkovics, J.G., Luchi, R.J., Small, S.D., Craig, P., Rossen, R., Gyorkey, P. & Melnick, J.L. (1982) Kaposi's sarcoma (KS) in lymph nodes of a patient with cytomegalovirus (CMV) viremia. Proc. Am. Assoc. Cancer Res., 23, 280

Harris, C., Small, C.B., Klein, R.S., Friedland, G.H., Moll, B., Emeson, E.E., Spigland, I. & Steigbigel, N.H. (1983) Immunodeficiency in female sexual partners of men with the acquired immune deficiency syndrome. New Engl. J. Med., 308, 1181-1184

Harwood, A.R., Osoba, D., Hofstader, S.L., Goldstein, M.B., Cardella, C.J., Holecek, M.J.,Kunynetz, R. & Giammarco, R.A. (1979) Kaposi's sarcoma in renal transplants. Am. J. Med., 67, 759-765

Haverkos, H.W. & Curran, J.W. (1982) The current outbreak of Kaposi's sarcoma and opportunistic infections. Ca (NY), 32, 330-339

Huang, E.-S., Boldogh, I., Baskar, J.F. & Mar, E.-C. (1984) The molecular biology of human cytomegalovirus and its relationship to various human cancers. In: Giraldo, G. & Beth, E., eds, The Role of Viruses in Human Cancer, Vol. 2, Amsterdam, New York, Elsevier-North-Holland, pp. 169-194

Jaffe, H.W., Choi, K., Thomas, P.A., Haverkos, H.W., Auerbach, D.M., Guinan, M.E., Rogers, M.F., spira, T.J., Darrow, W.W., Kramer, M.A., Friedman, S.M., Monroe, J.M., Friedman-Kien, A.E., Laubenstein, L.J., Marmor, M., Safai, B., Dritz, S.K., Crispi, S.J., Fannin, S.L., Orkwis, J.P., Kelter, A., Rushing, W.R., Thacker, S.B. & Curran, J.W. (1983) National case-control study of Kaposi's sarcoma and Pneumocystis carinii pneumonia in homosexual men. I. Epidemiologic results. Ann. intern. Med., 99, 145-151

Kapadia, S.B. & Krause, J.R. (1977) Kaposi's sarcoma after long-term alkylating agent therapy for multiple myeloma. South. med. J., 70, 1011-1013

Kaposi, M. (1872) Idiopathisches multiples Pigmentsarkom der Haut. Arch. Dermatol. Syph., 4, 265-273

Klein, M.B., Pereira, F.A. & Kantor, I. (1974) Kaposi's sarcoma complicating systemic lupus erythematosus treated with immunosuppression. Arch. Dermatol., 110, 602-604

Klepp, O., Dahl, O. & Stenwig, J.T. (1978) Association of Kaposi's sarcoma and prior immunosuppressive therapy. Cancer, 42, 2626-2630

Kornfeld, H., Vande Stouwe, R.A., Lange, M., Reddy, M.M. & Grieco, M.H. (1982) T-lymphocyte subpopulations in homosexual men. New Engl. J. Med., 307, 729-731

Leone, A.L., La Nasa, G., Carcassi, C., Pintus, A., Tanchis, A., Cerimele, D., Eonu, G., Ferrari, L. & Contu, L. (1984) HLA phenotypes and classic Kaposi's sarcoma in Sardinia. In: Giraldo, G. & Beth, E., eds, Proceedings of International Meeting on AIDS, Cagliari, 1-3 May Basle, Karger

McDougall, J.K., Smith, P., Tamini, H.K., Tolentino, E. & Galloway, D.A. (1984) Molecular biology of the relationship between herpes simplex virus-II and cervical cancer. In: Giraldo, G. & Beth, E., eds, The Role of Viruses in Human Cancer, Vol. 2, Amsterdam, New York, Elsevier-North Holland, pp. 59-71

McHardy, J., Williams, E.H., Geser, A., de-Thé, G., Beth, E. & Giraldo, G. (1984) Endemic Kaposi's sarcoma: incidence and risk factors in the West Nile District of Uganda. Int. J. Cancer, 33, 203-212

Metroka, C.E., Cunningham-Rundles, S., Pollack, M.S., Sonnabend, J.A., Davis, J.M., Gordon, B., Fernandez, R.D. & Mouradian, J. (1983) Generalized lymphadenopathy in homosexual men. Ann. intern. Med., 99, 585-591

Nadji, M., Morales, A.R. & Ziegles-Weissman, J. (1981) Kaposi's sarcoma: immunohistologic evidence for an endothelial origin. Arch. Pathol. lab. Med., 105, 274-275

Nelson, J.A., Fleckenstein, B., Galloway, D.A. & McDougall, J.K. (1982) NIH 3T3 cells with cloned fragments of human cytomegalovirus strain AD169. J. Virol., 43, 83-91

Penn, I. (1979) Kaposi's sarcoma in organ transplant recipients. Transplantation, 27, 8-11

Pollack, M.S., Safai, B., Myskowski, P.L., Gold, J.W.M., Pandey, J. & Dupont, P. (1983) Frequencies of HLA and Gm immuno-genetic markers in Kaposi's sarcoma. Tissue antigens, 21, 1-8

Popovic, M., Sarngadharan, M.G., Read, E. & Gallo, R.C. (1984) Detection, isolation, and continuous production of cyto-pathic retrovirus (HTLV-III) from patients with AIDS and pre-AIDS. Science, 224, 497-500

Quenum, A. & Camain, R. (1958) Les aspects africains de la maladie de Kaposi, réticulopathie maligne systématisée. Ann. Anat. Pathol., 3, 337-368

Rapp, F. (1984) Cytomegalovirus and carcinogenesis. J. natl Cancer Inst., 72, 783-787

Rogoff, M.G. (1968) Kaposi's sarcoma. Age, sex and tribal incidence in Kenya. In: Clifford, P., Linsell, C.A. & Timms, G.L., eds, Cancer in Africa, Nairobi, East African Medical Journal, pp. 445-448

Rubinstein, P., Rothman, W.M. & Friedman-Kien, A. (1984) Immu-nologic and immunogenetic findings in patients with epidemic Kaposi's sarcoma. Antibiot. Chemother., 32, 87-98

Rüger, R. & Fleckenstein, B. (1984) Search for DNA sequences of human cytomegalovirus in Kaposi's sarcoma. Antibiot. Chemo-ther., 32, 43-47

Safai, B., Miké, V., Giraldo, G., Beth, E. & Good, R.A. (1980) Association of Kaposi's sarcoma with second primary malig-nancies: possible etiopathogenic implications. Cancer, 45, 1472-1479

Shaw, S., Spector, D., Abrams, D. & Gottlieb, M.S. (1983) Characterization of HCMV sequences in Kaposi's sarcoma tissues from AIDs patients. In: Plotkin, S.A., Mishaelson, S., Pagano, J.S., Rapp, F., eds, Proceedings of the Conference on Pathogenesis and Prevention of Human Cytomegalovirus Infections, Philadelphia, 20-22 April, New York, A.R. Liss

Stribling, J., Weitzner, S. & Smith, G.V. (1978) Kaposi's sarcoma in renal allograft recipients. Cancer, 42, 442-446

Taylor, S. & Folkman, J. (1982) Protamine is an inhibitor of angiogenesis. Nature, 297, 307-312

Templeton, A.C. & Hutt, M.S.R. (1973) Distribution of tumors in Africa. Recent Results Cancer Res., 41, 1-22

Ziegler, J.L., Miner, R.C., Rosenbaum, E., Lennette, E.T., Shillitoe, E., Casavant, C., Drew, W.L., Mintz, L., Gershow, J., Greenspan, J., Beckstead, J. & Yamamoto, K. (1982) Outbreak of Burkitt's-like lymphoma in homosexual men. Lancet, 2, 631-633

PAPILLOMAVIRUSES AND SKIN CANCER IN AFRICA

M.A. Lutzner

National Cancer Institute
Bethesda, MD, USA
and
Unité des Papillomavirus
Institut Pasteur
Paris, France

RESUME

Bien que l'origine virale de certains cancers épithéliaux précédés de papillomes ait été suggérée depuis longtemps, la première preuve de l'association entre les papillomavirus et le cancer a été apportée en 1934 par les études de Shope et Rose chez le lapin.

L'introduction de la technique d'hybridation moléculaire a permis dans les années 1970 à l'équipe de Gérard Orth (Institut Pasteur, Paris), de montrer la présence de l'ADN du papilloma - virus humain de type 5 (HPV-5) - dans les cancers humains succédant à l'épidermodysplasie verruciforme de Lutz-Lewandovsky.

Quelques années plus tard, il a été possible de démontrer la présence d'ADN du même HPV-5 dans le cancer cutané d'un transplanté rénal immunosupprimé. L'équipe de l'Institut Pasteur a récemment augmenté le nombre des papillomavirus potentiellement oncogènes en montrant la présence d'ADN de l'HPV-8 et de l'HPV-14 dans des cancers cutanés de malades atteints d'épidermodysplasie verruciforme.

Ces dernières années trois autres équipes ont montré l'association des HPV-6, -10, -11, -16 et -18 avec les cancers verruqueux de la peau et des muqueuses, les papules Bowenoïdes, les maladies de Bowen cutanées et les cancers du col utérin.

Ces cancers de la peau et des muqueuses sont généralement traités chirurgicalement, mais il a été montré que l'administration orale de rétinoïdes (dérivés synthétiques de la vitamine A) ou l'apport intralésionnel d'interféron leucocytaire sont efficaces dans le traitement des cancers _in situ_ consécutifs aux épidermodysplasies verruciformes.

SUMMARY

Although it was suggested long ago that certain epithelial cancers preceded by papillomas might be caused by viruses, the first proof that papillomaviruses were associated with cancer dates from the work on rabbits in 1934 by Shope and Rose. In the 1970s, the introduction of the blot hybridization technique enabled Orth and his co-workers at the Institut Pasteur, Paris, to demonstrate the presence in man of the DNA of human papillomavirus type 5 (HPV-5) in cancers following Lutz-Lewandovsky epidermodysplasia verruciformis.

Some years later, it was possible to demonstrate the presence of the same HPV-5 DNA in the skin cancer of an immunosuppressed recipient of a renal transplant. The number of potentially oncogenic papillomaviruses has recently been increased by the demonstration at the Institut Pasteur of the presence of the DNAs of HPV-8 and HPV-14 in the skin cancers of patients with epidermodysplasia verruciformis. In recent years, an association has been demonstrated between HPV-6, -10, -11, -16, and -18 with verrucous cancers of the skin and mucous membranes, Bowenoid papules, Bowenoid skin diseases and cervical cancer.

Such cancers of the skin and mucous membranes are usually treated by surgery, but it has been shown that oral administration of retinoids (synthetic derivatives of vitamin A) or the use of leucocyte interferon intralesionally are effective in cancers _in situ_ following epidermodysplasia verruciformis.

INTRODUCTION

Sunlight is known to be a major factor in the production of skin cancer in light-skinned peoples living in tropical climates (reviewed by Urbach, 1969). As reported in a review by Stoll (1979), the incidence of squamous-cell carcinoma of the skin in regions such as Australia and New Zealand, populated primarily by peoples of the Celtic race (Irish and Scots) who freckle but cannot tan, has been estimated at 38 per 100 000. The average incidence among Caucasians in eight American cities is estimated at 12 per 100 000, whereas it is only between 1 to 2 per 100 000 in dark-skinned peoples of India, Africa, and the United States. Further support for the role of skin pigment in protection against ultraviolet-induced cancer comes from the observation by Oettle in 1963 that all African albinos who are non-pigmented, because of a genetic disorder of melanin formation, eventually develop skin cancer.

Another major advance in understanding the role of sunlight in skin cancer came from the observation by Cleaver in 1968 that patients with the genetic disorder xeroderma pigmentosum, who are particularly susceptible to skin cancer (reviewed by Robbins et al., 1974), have an impaired DNA-repair system, resulting in inability to repair sunlight-damaged DNA, leading to mutations and skin cancer. Dark skin pigmentation offers little protection in this disease.

ROLE OF PAPILLOMAVIRUSES

Still another major advance in understanding skin cancer came from studies by Orth et al. (1980) of yet another genetic disorder, epidermodysplasia verruciformis (EV), characterized by widespread, long-lasting papillomavirus-induced warty lesions in childhood (Figs 1-4), progressing in young adulthood to cancers localized to sun-exposed areas of skin (Figs 5-8) (reviewed by Lutzner, 1978; Lutzner et al., 1984). Orth and his colleagues discovered that human papillomavirus type 5 (HPV-5) DNA could be found in EV cancers, strongly suggesting a causative role for papillomavirus in these skin cancers. A co-factor role for ultraviolet light in the pathogenesis of papillomavirus-induced EV cancers is indicated by the report of Jacyk (1979), who found that black Africans suffering from EV do not develop skin cancers, apparently protected by their skin pigment. Lutzner et al. (1984) have reported one black African with EV who did develop skin cancers, but these were on non-sun-exposed skin areas (Fig. 9), suggesting that a co-factor other than sunlight was involved in this instance. A series of other observations suggesting synergism between papillomaviruses and ultraviolet light in production of skin cancers has been reviewed by Lutzner et al. (1983).

FIG. 1. BACK OF AN AFRICAN MAN SUFFERING FROM HUMAN
PAPILLOMAVIRUS-INDUCED (HPV-5) EPIDERMODYSPLASIA
VERRUCIFORMIS (EV)

His lesions are scaly, depigmented macules, which coalesce to
form figurate patterns.

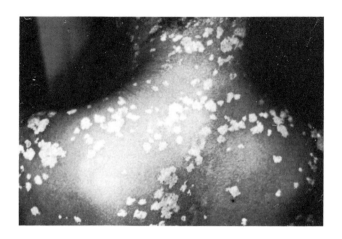

FIG. 2. A CLUSTER OF BENIGN, PIGMENTED MACULES
ON THE PALM OF THE SAME AFRICAN MAN

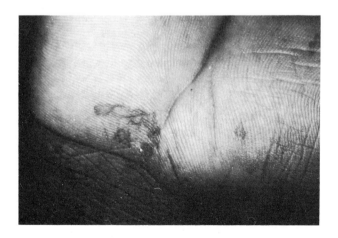

FIG. 3. THE SAME CLUSTER 18 MONTHS LATER

Note that the lesion on the lower right is nodular and exuberant; it proved to be an invasive squamous-cell carcinoma, and obviously developed at the site of a previously benign macule.

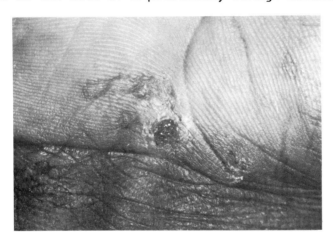

FIG. 4. TYPICAL CYTOLOGICAL FEATURES OF AN HPV-5-INDUCED EV BENIGN LESION FROM AN IMMUNOSUPPRESSED RENAL ALLOGRAFT RECIPIENT, SHOWING CHARACTERISTIC ENLARGED CLEAR CELLS

Note the homogeneous clear spaces in both the cytoplasm and nuclei.

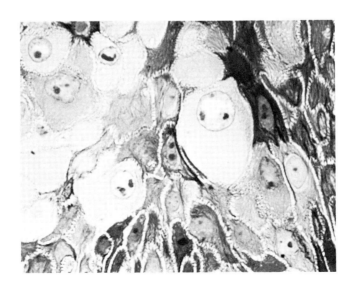

FIG. 5. A NORTH AFRICAN PATIENT SUFFERING FROM EV

Note the invasive squamous-cell carcinomas on his forehead, the
Bowenoid carcinomas <u>in situ</u> of his preauricular skin, and the
benign, depigmented macules on his neck and upper back.

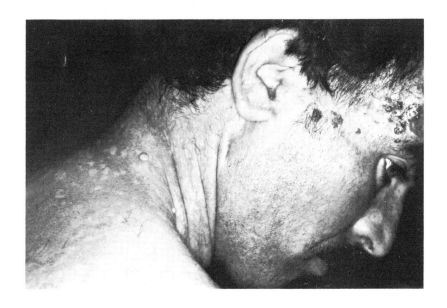

FIG. 6.   A CLOSE-UP VIEW OF THE SAME PATIENT SHOWING AN INVASIVE
SQUAMOUS-CELL CARCINOMA OF HIS FOREHEAD AND MULTIPLE BOWENOID
<u>IN SITU</u> CARCINOMAS ON THE REST OF HIS FACE

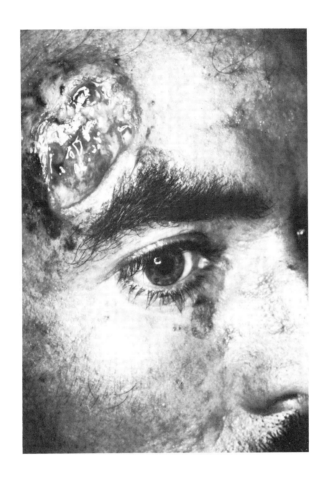

FIG. 7.   CHARACTERISTIC HISTOLOGICAL FEATURES OF A BOWENOID
IN SITU CARCINOMA FROM AN EV PATIENT

Note the dyskeratotic cells, the multinucleated cells, hyper-
chromatic nuclei, and loss of normal cell polarization.

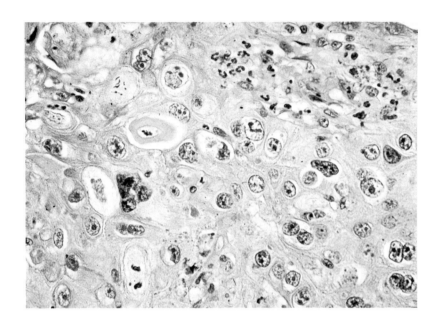

FIG. 8.   HISTOLOGICAL FEATURES OF AN INVASIVE SQUAMOUS-CELL
CARCINOMA FROM AN EV PATIENT

Note that the dermis is filled with islands of invasive epidermal
cells.

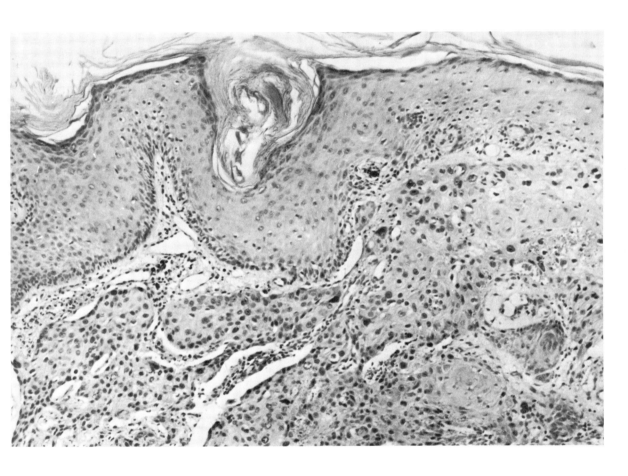

FIG. 9. THE PALM OF THE AFRICAN MAN ILLUSTRATED IN FIGS 1-3

The large tumour on his thenar eminence proved to be a squamous-cell carcinoma invading into the tendons, and requiring amputation of the thumb. An earlier lesion at this site had been treated with X-rays, after which it paradoxically increased in size. X-ray therapy appears to be contraindicated in papilloma-virus-induced lesions.

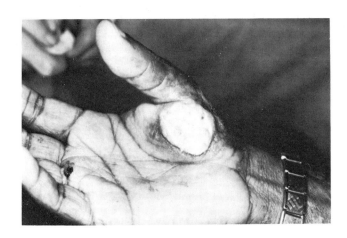

Evidence that papillomaviruses and immunosuppression or immunodepression and sunlight may serve as co-factors leading to a high incidence of warts and skin cancers, as observed by Penn (1980), in immunosuppressed renal allograft recipients, comes from the work of Lutzner et al. (1980, 1983) who found HPV-5 in benign warts of immunosuppressed renal allograft recipients (Fig. 10) and genome copies of HPV-5 in skin cancers developing preferentially in sun-exposed skin in one of these patients (Figs 11 & 12). Other evidence for the co-factor effects of sunlight, immunosuppression, and papillomavirus infection have been reviewed by Lutzner (1982).

FIG. 10. IMMUNOFLUORESCENCE MICROGRAPH SHOWING THE PRESENCE OF
EV-HPV STRUCTURAL ANTIGENS IN THE NUCLEI OF A BENIGN LESION OF
AN IMMUNOSUPPRESSED RENAL ALLOGRAFT RECIPIENT (RAR)

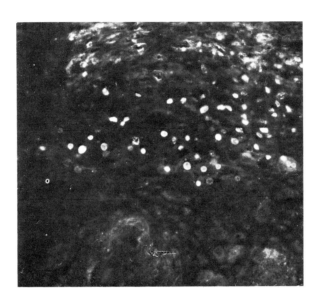

FIG. 11. SECTION OF AN EARLY INVASIVE SQUAMOUS-CELL CARCINOMA
FROM THE CHEEK OF THE SAME RAR AS IN FIGURE 10

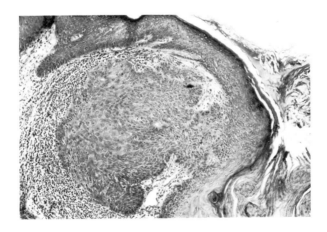

FIG. 12.   DETECTION OF HPV-5 DNA IN BENIGN LESIONS
AND SKIN CANCERS (AS SHOWN IN FIGS 10 & 11 ABOVE)
FROM THE SAME RAR, USING THE SOUTHERN BLOT TECHNIQUE

Lane a contains uncleaved DNA extracted from the patient's benign
lesions and lanes c-f contain this DNA cleaved with SacI, BamHI,
EcoRI, and PstI endonucleases, respectively.   Lane b contains
uncleaved DNA extracted from benign lesions of an HPV-5-infected
patient with EV and lanes g-j contain this DNA cleaved with the
same four restriction endonucleases.   Lanes k and l contain DNA
from the RAR's in situ cancer, cleaved with BamHI and PstI respectively, while lanes m and n contain DNA from the patient's
early invasive carcinoma, cleaved with the same restriction
endonucleases.   Arabic numerals indicate weights of fragments in
megadaltons;   Roman numerals indicate DNA forms: I (circular,
supercoiled molecules);   II (circular, relaxed molecules);   and
III (linear molecules).   The smallest HPV-5 PstI fragment (lane
j) ran off the gel.

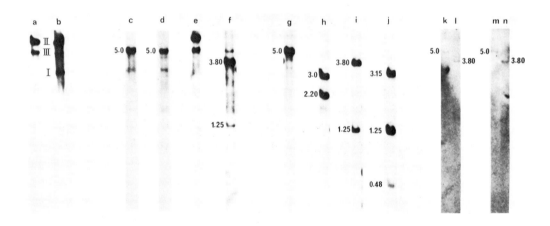

As discussed above, skin carcinomas occurring on sun-exposed
skin are common in light-skinned, but rare in dark-skinned
peoples. However, many dark-skinned populations of the world are
prone to develop squamous-cell carcinomas in chronic leg ulcers,
an extremely common disease in some parts of the world (see

Elmes & Baldwin, 1947; Oettle, 1963; Oluwasanmi et al., 1969;
Stoll, 1979).   Of relevance might be the observation by
Srinivasan & Desikan (1971) that verrucous carcinomas may also
develop in lepromatous neurotrophic plantar ulcers.   Such
carcinomas resemble a disorder of the foot known as epithelioma
cuniculatum (Aird et al., 1954) (Figs 13 & 14), a disease suspected to be papilloma-virus induced.

FIG. 13. VERRUCOUS SQUAMOUS-CELL CARCINOMA DEVELOPING
IN A NEUROTROPHIC FOOT ULCER IN A BLACK LEPROMATOUS PATIENT
BORN IN MARTINIQUE.

It resembles an epithelioma cuniculatum.

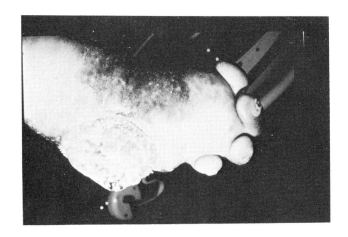

As reviewed by Gissmann[1], human papillomaviruses types 6 and
11 infect both laryngeal papillomas and genital condylomas, and
HPV-16 and -18 genomes have been found in cervical carcinomas.
Gissmann and his co-workers have also found HPV-16-related DNA in
Bowenoid papulosis of the glans penis or the vulva. Kremsdorf et
al. (1983a,b) have found HPV-5, -8, -12, -14, -15, -17, and
-19-24 infecting benign lesions of patients with epidermodysplasia verruciformis, and HPV-5, -8 and -14 genomes have been found
in EV skin cancers (Orth, 1980; Lutzner et al., 1984). HPV-1 is
associated with plantar warts, HPV-2, -4 and -7 with common skin
warts, HPV-3 and -10 with flat warts, and HPV-13 with oral

---

[1] This volume

mucosal warts, known as focal epithelial hyperplasia (see review
by Lutzner, 1983). It would be of interest to explore verrucous
carcinomas of the oral cavity for this oral papillomavirus or
others that might be discovered.

FIG. 14. HISTOLOGICAL FEATURES OF THE LESION SHOWN IN FIGURE 13

These are characteristic of an invasive carcinoma of the epithelioma cuniculatum type, with marked hyperkeratosis and papillomatosis, and large nests of well differentiated squamous cells and
horny cysts in the dermis.

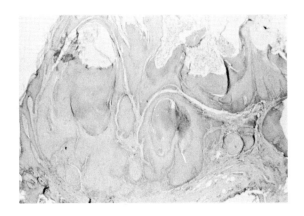

Since it appears that penile and cervical condylomas, and
possibly penile and cervical cancers, diseases so common in
Africa, are probably sexually transmitted, it would be of
interest to explore penile lesions as well as cervical lesions in
greater depth, to determine the causative HPV types. Papilloma-
virus-infected urethral condylomas in the male and Bowenoid papulosis lesions of the foreskin, shaft, and glans of the penis are
good candidates for such studies[1].

---

[1] This volume

Two recent advances in the therapy of papillomavirus-induced diseases are the oral administration of the synthetic retinoids and the use of leucocyte interferon intralesionally, both of which have had beneficial, although temporary, effects in these diseases (Lutzner & Blanchet-Bardon, 1980; Blanchet-Bardon et al., 1981).

Armed with this new information about HPV types and the results of on-going molecular biological studies of the papillomaviruses (for review, see Howley, 1983), it is hoped that the future will bring specific virucidal drugs effective against these viruses and perhaps also preventive vaccines.

REFERENCES

Aird, I., Johnson, H.D., Lennox, B. & Stansfeld, A.G. (1954) Epithelioma cuniculatum. A variety of squamous cell carcinoma peculiar to the foot. Br. J. Surg., 42, 245-250

Blanchet-Bardon, C., Puissant, A., Lutzner, M., Orth, G., Nutini, M.T. & Guesry, P. (1981) Interferon treatment of skin cancer in patients with epidermodysplasia verruciformis. Lancet, 1, 274

Cleaver, J.F. (1968) Defective repair replication of DNA in xeroderma pigmentosum. Nature, 218, 652-656

Elmes, G.T. & Baldwin, R.B.T. (1947) Malignant disease in Nigeria: an analysis of a thousand tumours. Ann. trop. Med. Parasitol., 41, 321-330

Howley, P.M. (1983) The molecular biology of papillomavirus transformation. Am. J. Pathol., 113, 414-421

Jacyk, W.K. (1979) Epidermodysplasia in Nigerians. Dermatologica, 159, 256-265

Kremsdorf, D., Jablonska, S., Favre, M. & Orth, G. (1983a) Biochemical characterization of human papillomaviruses associated with epidermodysplasia verruciformis. J. Virol., 43, 436-447

Kremsdorf, D., Jablonska, S., Favre, M. & Orth, G. (1983b) Human
    papillomaviruses associated with epidermodysplasia verruci-
    formis II. Molecular cloning and biochemical characteriza-
    tion of HPV-3a, -8, -10, -12 genomes. J. Virol., 48, 340-
    351

Lutzner, M.A. (1978) Epidermodysplasia verruciformis. An auto-
    somal recessive disease characterized by viral warts and
    skin cancer. A model for viral oncogenesis. Bull. Cancer
    (Paris), 65, 169-182

Lutzner, M.A. (1982) Immunopathology of papillomavirus-induced
    warts and skin cancers in immunodepressed and immunosup-
    pressed patients. Springer Semin. Immunopathol., 5, 53-62

Lutzner, M.A. (1983) The human papillomaviruses. A review.
    Arch. Derm., 119, 631-635

Lutzner, M.A. & Blanchet-Bardon, C. (1980) Oral aromatic reti-
    noid (Ro 10-9359) treatment of human papillomavirus type-5-
    induced epidermodysplasia verruciformis. N. Engl. J. Med.,
    302, 1091

Lutzner, M.A., Croissant, O., Ducasse, M.-F., Kreis, H. &
    Crosnier, J. (1980) A potentially oncogenic human papillo-
    mavirus (HBV-5) found in two renal allograft recipients. J.
    invest. Dermatol., 75, 353-356

Lutzner, M.A., Orth, G., Dutronquay, V., Ducasse, M.-F., Kreis,
    H. & Crosnier, J. (1983) Detection of human papillomavirus
    type 5 DNA in skin cancers of an immunosuppressed renal
    allograft recipient. Lancet, 2, 422-424

Lutzner, M.A., Blanchet-Bardon, C. & Orth, G. (1984) Clinical
    observations, virological studies, and treatment trials in
    patients with epidermodysplasia verruciformis, a disease
    induced by specific human papillomaviruses. J. invest.
    Dermatol. (in press)

Oettle, A.G. (1963) Skin cancer in Africa. Natl Cancer Inst.
    Monogr., 10, 197-214

Oluwasanmi, J., Williams, A.O. & Alli, A.F. (1969) Superficial
    cancer in Nigeria. Brit. J. Cancer, 23, 714-728

Orth, G., Favre, M., Breitburd, F., Croissant, O., Jablonska, S., Obalek, S., Jarzabek-Chorzelska, M. & Rzesa, G. (1980) Epidermodysplasia verruciformis; a model for the role of papillomaviruses in human cancer. Cold Spring Harbor Conf. Cell Prolif., 7, 259-282

Penn, I. (1980) Immunosuppression and skin cancer. Clin. plast. Surg., 7, 361-368

Robbins, J.H., Kraemer, K.H., Lutzner, M.A., Festoff, B.W. & Coon, H.G. (1974) Xeroderma pigmentosum, an inherited disease with sun sensitivity, multiple cutaneous neoplasias and abnormal DNA repair. Ann. intern. Med., 80, 221-248

Srinivasan, H. & Desikan, K.V. (1971) Cauliflower growths in neuropathic plantar ulcers in leprosy patients. J. Bone Jt Surg., 53-A, 123-132

Stoll, H.L. (1979) Squamous cell carcinoma. In: Fitzpatrick, T.B., Eisen, A., Wolff, K., Freedberg, I.M. & Austen, K.F., eds, Dermatology in General Medicine, New York, McGraw-Hill, pp. 362-377

Urbach, F. (1969) Geographic pathology of skin cancer. In: Urbach, F., ed., Biologic Effects of Ultraviolet Radiation, Oxford, Pergamon Press

SHORT COMMUNICATION: A RETROSPECTIVE REVIEW OF PATIENTS WITH KAPOSI'S SARCOMA TREATED IN THE RADIOTHERAPY DEPARTMENT, KENYATTA NATIONAL HOSPITAL 1973–1983

K. Muhombe

Nairobi, Kenya

A total of 126 patients were referred for treatment to the Radiotherapy Department of the Kenyatta National Hospital, Nairobi, with a confirmed diagnosis of Kaposi's sarcoma. This was less than the number of patients diagnosed annually histo-pathologically. The geographical distribution of the patients coincided with that of the endemic malaria and Burkitt's lymphoma zones, and the high-incidence areas of nasopharyngeal carcinoma in Kenya.

Immunological studies were not done on these particular patients, but one patient had hairy-cell leukaemia, for which he had been given cytotoxic chemotherapy prior to developing Kaposi's sarcoma.

Radiotherapy was found to be the best method of treatment, the patients treated in this way having longer periods of remission. Unfortunately, most of the patients were lost to follow-up 36 months after treatment.

LYMPHOMAS, LEUKAEMIAS AND IMMUNODEFICIENCIES

OPPORTUNITIES FOR STUDY OF LYMPHOID NEOPLASIA IN AFRICA

G.T. O'Conor

International Agency for Research on Cancer
Lyon, France

RESUME

Les modèles animaux ont fortement suggéré que les leucémies lymphoïdes et les lymphomes malins pourraient avoir une étiologie virale. A la suite de la première description par Ludwig Gross, en 1951, de la transmission de la leucémie murine par l'inoculation de filtrats acellulaires à des souriceaux nouveaux-nés, et de l'identification subséquente de nombreux virus de type C induisant des tumeurs chez les animaux, l'attention s'est concentrée sur les rétrovirus à ARN. Cependant, c'est grâce aux études menées en Afrique que le lymphome de Burkitt a été reconnu comme une entité, et que le virus d'Epstein-Barr a été découvert. Beaucoup considèrent ce virus comme le premier virus cancérogène pour l'homme identifié. Les recherches que ces premières études ont suscitées ont permis des progrès énormes dans la compréhension de la cancérogenèse humaine, et un développement significatif de la thérapeutique.

Plus récemment, le premier rétrovirus humain a été identifié et caractérisé dans le laboratoire du Dr Robert Gallo. Il est de plus en plus évident que ce virus, isolé à partir d'un patient atteint de lymphome T, est étiologiquement associé à un type spécifique de néoplasme des cellules T, décrit tout d'abord au Japon.

L'Afrique peut être considérée comme le berceau de la pathologie géographique et elle détient encore d'énormes possibilités d'informations uniques sur l'étiologie et la prévention du cancer. Les néoplasmes du système lymphoïde constituent d'excellents modèles pour l'étude du cancer humain, particulièrement en Afrique, puisque, en tant que tumeurs du système immunitaire, leur induction et leur évolution sont fortement influencées par les facteurs de l'environnement, tels que l'infection et la nutrition, qui ont un effet profond sur la réponse immune. De plus, il a été montré que quelques-unes au moins des tumeurs de ce groupe sont associées à des virus transformants spécifiques.

Il est nécessaire dans l'immédiat de collecter des données précises, reproductibles et comparables, sur l'incidence et les caractéristiques des différents types de tumeurs lymphoïdes et sur les populations chez qui elles surviennent dans les différents pays d'Afrique. De telles données fourniront la base de nouvelles études étiologiques et thérapeutiques qui pourraient être menées de façon simultanée ou consécutive.

Des approches réalistes de ces objectifs sont envisagées ici, et des études spécifiques concernant les questions posées par l'information disponible sont discutées.

SUMMARY

Animal models have strongly suggested that lymphoid leukaemias and malignant lymphomas might have a viral etiology. Following the first report by Ludwig Gross in 1951 of the transmission of mouse leukaemia by cell-free filtrates inoculated into newborn mice and the subsequent identification of many tumour-inducing type-C viruses in animals, attention was focused on the RNA retroviruses. However, it was work in Africa which led to the recognition of Burkitt's lymphoma as an entity and to the discovery of the Epstein-Barr virus. Many refer to this DNA virus as the first recognized human tumour virus. The research that these early studies stimulated has resulted in enormous progress in our understanding of human carcinogenesis and in highly significant advances in therapy.

More recently, the first human retrovirus was identified and characterized in the laboratory of Dr Robert Gallo. There is increasing evidence that this virus, isolated from a patient with a T-cell lymphoma, is etiologically associated with a specific type of T-cell neoplasm first described in Japan.

Africa may be considered the cradle of geographical pathology and the potential for generating unique information on cancer etiology and cancer control is still enormous. Lymphoid neoplasms are excellent models for the study of human cancer, particularly in Africa, since as tumours of the immune system, their induction and evolution is strongly influenced by those environmental factors, such as infection and nutrition, which have a profound effect on the immune response. In addition, there is good evidence that at least some of the tumours in this group are associated with specific transforming viruses.

There is an immediate need to collect accurate, reproducible and comparable data on the incidence and characteristics of the different types of lymphoid neoplasia and on the populations in which they occur in the various African countries. Such data will provide the basis for undertaking simultaneous or subsequent etiological and therapeutic studies.

Realistic approaches to these goals are considered and specific studies relating to questions posed by available information discussed.

INTRODUCTION

The suggestion that viruses may be important in the etiology and pathogenesis of lymphoid leukaemias and malignant lymphomas in man was strongly supported by experience with animal models. Following the first report, by Ludwig Gross in 1951 (Gross, 1951), of transmission of mouse leukaemias by cell filtrates inoculated into newborn mice and the subsequent identification of tumour-inducing type-C viruses in many animal species, attention was primarily focused on the RNA retroviruses. It was almost 30 years later, however, before a human counterpart of this group of viruses was finally isolated in the laboratory of Dr Robert Gallo and proven to be of human origin (Poiesz et al., 1981). There is increasing evidence that this virus, isolated from a patient with a T-cell lymphoma, and thus called human T-cell leukaemia virus (HTLV), is etiologically associated with a T-cell neoplasm, adult T-cell leukaemia/lymphoma (ATL/L), first described by Takatsuki in Japan (Blattner et al., 1984; Takutsuki et al., 1976).

Meanwhile, work in Africa in the late 1950s and early 1960s led to the recognition and description of Burkitt's lymphoma (BL) (Burkitt, 1958; Burkitt & O'Conor, 1961; O'Conor, 1961) and to the discovery of the Epstein-Barr virus (Epstein et al., 1964), a DNA virus considered by many to be the first human tumour virus. The early studies on BL in Africa undoubtedly provided the stimulus for world-wide research which has led to significant advances in cancer therapy and which continues to have an enormous impact on our understanding of human carcinogenesis.

BL and ATL/L are, thus far, the only lymphoid neoplasms in man which have been shown to have an association with specific transforming viruses, but the mechanisms by which these viruses may act to induce oncogenesis remain unclear.   More detailed discussions of both these tumour types is presented elsewhere. This   paper   is   concerned   primarily   with   some   suggestions, approaches and recommendations for the study of lymphoid neoplasms generally, on the supposition that many are indeed virus-associated and with the expectation that scientists and clinicians in Africa will continue to make significant contributions in this field of oncology.

GEOGRAPHICAL PATHOLOGY

Historically, clues to etiology and the identification of risk factors for specific types of cancer have come largely from clinical   observations   and   relevant   laboratory   studies   in different population groups and from the appropriate analyses of accurately recorded data.   The application of this combination of disciplines to the study of disease may be defined as geographical pathology.

Africa can perhaps be called the cradle of geographical pathology and this approach has led to many discoveries that pointed the way ahead at a time when laboratory studies were for the most part limited to histopathology, data were recorded using punched cards, and these data were analysed without benefit of sophisticated computer programming.   Advances in clinical and laboratory diagnostic techniques and the availability of rapid data processing have made it possible to greatly extend the potential of geographical pathology, and there is still an enormous opportunity to generate unique information relative to cancer etiology and to cancer control.

Lymphoid neoplasms, as mentioned above, have proven to be excellent models for the study of human cancer.   This is particularly true in Africa since the induction and evolution of these tumours of the immune system are strongly influenced by environmental factors prevalent in African countries, such as infection and malnutrition, which are known to have a profound effect on immune response.

Based on data from a variety of sources, but mainly from established cancer registries, some important geographical differences in the occurrence and natural history of lymphoid neoplasia have been revealed. These include differences in: (1) total incidence or relative frequency; (2) incidence and/or relative frequency of specific subtypes; (3) time trends; (4) prevalence of lymphoma and leukaemia in children; and (5) prevalence of extranodal lymphomas. All of these parameters are believed to be of significance in relation to etiology and to associated environmental and host risk factors. Although available information of this type is incomplete, so that definitive conclusions are precluded, it does provide a basis for developing some testable hypotheses and for planning more detailed studies directed towards answering specific questions.

The overall incidence of malignant lymphomas and lymphoid leukaemias is relatively low in all countries, but clear differences do exist. In Table 1 some comparative rates for the major broad groups of lymphoid tumours from representative countries or continents are shown, and it will be seen that the highest rates for all types are found in the United States. This reflects, in large part, the age structure of the population, since these figures are for total incidence and the occurrence of most lymphomas and lymphoid leukaemias increases with age. The rates in Latin American countries, however, are also relatively high as compared with Japan and India. Senegal is currently the only African country for which data have been published and numbers of cases are small. The cancer registries in Kampala, Uganda, and in Ibadan, Nigeria, are not among those included in the most recent edition of Cancer Incidence in Five Continents (Waterhouse et al., 1982). This is unfortunate, since these two registries have been the source of much of the knowledge currently available about cancer in Africa.

There is a striking deficit of Hodgkin;s disease (HD) as well as of lymphoid leukaemia in the data recorded from Japan and from India. In contrast, but not shown here, non-Hodgkin's lymphomas (NHL) and HD account for a substantial proportion of all cancer in some of the Middle Eastern and North African countries (Godwin, personal communication; Aboul-Nasr, 1979; Omar, 1984).

Table 1.   Comparative incidence rates of lymphoid neoplasms
(males)a

Country	NHL[b]	HD	Lymphoid leukaemia	Myeloma
Colombia	6.0	3.0	2.0	2.0
Denmark	5.0	3.0	4.5	3.0
India	3.0	1.0	1.0	1.0
Japan	4.0	0.5	1.0	1.0
Senegal	3.5	1.5	0.5	0.2
Singapore:				
Chinese	4.0	1.0	1.5	1.0
Malays	3.0	0.5	0.5	0.5
Indians	2.0	1.5	1.0	1.0
USA	8.0	4.0	4.5	3.5

[a] Based on Waterhouse et al., 1982

[b] Lymphosarcoma and other reticuloses (ICD 200 and 202)

These very limited data, as well as other data on age and
sex distribution provided by participating registries and
published in Cancer Incidence in Five Continents, do illustrate
important regional differences, but are limited by the broad
categorization imposed by the rubrics of the International
Classification of Diseases (ICD) (World Health Organization,
1975), which do not recognize the lymphoma and leukaemia subtypes
that are distinct biological entities and have known relevance in
relation to both etiology and therapy.

The Surveillance Epidemiology and End Results (SEER) Programme of the US National Cancer Institute (Young et al., 1981) records data from 10 population-based registries in the USA and Puerto Rico. Most diagnoses are histologically confirmed and coded according to the International Classification of Disease for Oncology (ICD-O) (World Health Organization, 1976), which permits a division by histological type. Some data for the years 1973-1977 (Puerto Rico excluded) are shown in Tables 2-4. This additional detail is useful for many purposes and the quality of the data may be expected to improve with time, but important deficiencies nevertheless remain. The distribution of NHL by histological type is shown in Table 2 and a high percentage of NHL cases are seen to be unclassified. The nodular or follicular lymphomas are clearly under-represented, since it is known from other studies (National Cancer Institute, 1982), that this group constitutes 30% or more of NHL in the USA. BL, on the other hand, is now widely recognized and accurately reported. It represents, of course, a much higher percentage in children (30-40% of NHL). In Table 3, the histological types of HD are listed and the predominance of nodular sclerosis in the USA is confirmed. Again, however, the data suffer from the inclusion of a large number of cases in which subtype was not recorded. In Table 4 the frequency of acute and chronic lymphocytic leukaemia is compared. Some obvious differences in the age-distribution curves for NHL and HD and for the acute and chronic lymphocytic leukaemias are illustrated in Figs 1 and 2 respectively. The shapes of these curves are characteristic for the United States, but again important differences may be seen when they are compared with similar curves for other population groups.

Table 2. Non-Hodgkin's lymphoma: distribution by histological
typea

Type	No.	%
Lymphosarcoma[b]	2236	25.7
Reticulosarcoma[c]	2702	31.0
Well differentiated lymphocytic	1323	15.2
Nodular	786	9.0
Undifferentiated	59	0.7
Burkitt's lymphoma	50	0.6
Not otherwise specified	1367	15.7
Total	8707	100.0

SEER 1973-1977

[a] Source: Young et al., 1981

[b] Includes poorly differentiated lymphocytic

[c] Includes 'histiocytic'

Table 3. Hodgkin's disease: distribution by histological type[a]

Type	No.	%
Nodular sclerosis	1057	35.8
Mixed cellularity	666	22.5
Lymphocyte-predominant	203	6.9
Lymphocyte-depleted	185	6.3
Not otherwise specified	844	28.5
Total	2955	100.5

[a] Source: Young et al., 1981

Table 4. Frequency of acute and chronic lymphocytic leukaemia[a]

Type	No.	%
Acute	1061	28.6
Chronic	2653	71.4
Total	3714	100.0

[a] Source: Young et al., 1981. Not otherwise specified and 'lymphosarcoma cell' leukaemia have been omitted. Hairy-cell leukaemia has been included with chronic lymphocytic leukaemia

FIG. 1. AGE-DISTRIBUTION CURVES FOR NON-HODGKIN'S LYMPHOMA (●)
AND HODGKIN'S DISEASE (▲) IN THE USA (FROM YOUNG <u>et al.</u>, 1981)

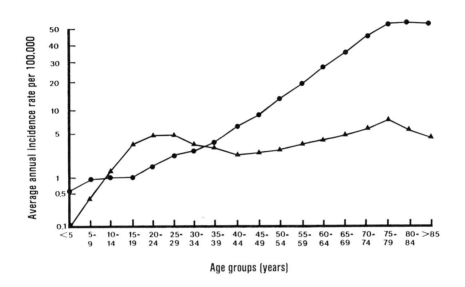

SUGGESTED RESEARCH TOPICS AND DATA REQUIREMENTS

Many questions posed by the existing information on the
geographical pathology of lymphoid neoplasms lend themselves to
study in Africa as well as to international collaborative
research. Specific tumour types or tumour groups to which these
questions relate are discussed below.

Burkitt's lymphoma

BL has proven to be the prototype of a human cancer model
and discoveries stemming from research on this predominantly
'African tumour' have had a profound effect on many scientific
disciplines. It continues to be an important model, there are
many unanswered questions, and more information and more precise
definitions are needed, as follows:

(<u>a</u>) There is a need for new or updated information on the
incidence and/or frequency of BL and its association with EBV,
particularly in North African countries and in other non-endemic
regions of Africa.

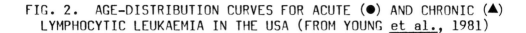

FIG. 2. AGE-DISTRIBUTION CURVES FOR ACUTE (●) AND CHRONIC (▲)
LYMPHOCYTIC LEUKAEMIA IN THE USA (FROM YOUNG et al., 1981)

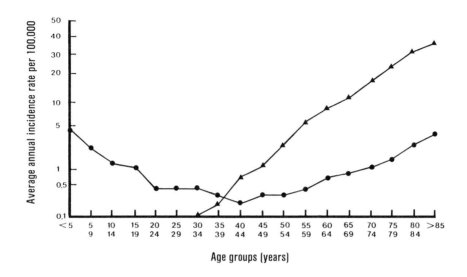

(b) Clinical epidemiological and laboratory differences between endemic and non-endemic BL must be more clearly defined.

(c) The distinction between BL and so called undifferentiated lymphoma, non-Burkitt type, should be clarified.

(d) Reports that there has been a decrease in the prevalence of BL in some countries of high incidence need well documented confirmation (Geser & Brubaker, 1984; Owor, 1984). Time trends for BL should be kept under continued surveillance and should be related, if possible, to specific environmental factors.

Follicle centre-cell (FCC) lymphomas

This subtype is by far the most common lymphoma of adults in Western countries, accounting for 40% or more of all NHL. It is believed that it is much less frequent in other areas of the world and that the nodular or follicular form may be quite rare in some countries (National Cancer Institute, 1982; O'Conor, 1984).

The relative frequency of FCC lymphomas, particularly the nodular or follicular form, should be determined and explanations sought for any deficit. Are the reported deficits due to the age structure of the population, to the growth rate of the tumour or to specific environmental or host factors?

Diffuse large-cell (DLC) lymphomas

In African countries, as well as in other countries of the so-called developing world, DLC tumours of high grade are relatively common.

A better definition and characterization of the subtypes within this presumed heterogeneous group of tumours is required. There is a need for objective criteria for the identification of distinct biological and/or etiological entities, if indeed they do exist.

Extranodal lymphomas

Again, in Africa and in many of the less developed countries, it is thought that there is an excess of extranodal lymphomas.

The percentage of extranodal tumours within the overall NHL should be documented, along with site distribution and subtype.

Immunoproliferative small intestinal disease (IPSID)

This is a rare condition on a world-wide basis but endemic foci exist, particularly in countries of the Mediterranean region.

A precise clinical, epidemiological and laboratory characterization of IPSID in the various phases of its evolution is required.

Acute lymphocytic leukaemia (ALL)

Leukaemia of all types has been thought to be relatively uncommon in Africa, but whether this is really so remains a subject of controversy.

The clinical and laboratory definition of subtypes with reproducible accuracy is now possible with the use of histo-chemical and immunological markers and should be a priority in the major African countries.

The age-specific incidence and distribution of all subtypes in different African countries and ethnic groups should be documented.

Chronic lymphocytic leukaemia (CLL)

This disease, one of the most common in the West, is rare in the East.

The incidence and age distribution of CLL in African countries should be determined, and a clinical definition and confirmation of the reported increased prevalence of CLL in young women in some African countries (Williams et al., 1984) is of particular interest.

Adult T-cell leukaemia/lymphoma (ATL/L)

'Endemic' foci of ATL/L have so far been reported only from parts of Japan and from the Caribbean basin. There is a need for:

(a) The incidence and relative frequency of this condition in Africa to be determined.

(b) The prevalence of HTLV antibodies and the frequency of association of positive serology with ATL/L and other haemato-poetic diseases to be studied.

(c) The clinical characteristics of HTLV-associated diseases in Africa to be described.

Other requirements

The above list of topics is, of course, not exhaustive but does cover subjects of great current interest. There is an immediate need to collect accurate, reproducible and comparable data on the characteristics of the different types of lymphoid neoplasia and on the populations in which they occur in the various countries of Africa. The collection of this type of information is a necessary first step and provides the basis for planning and implementing concurrent or subsequent etiological studies and for conducting clinical trials directed towards intervention and therapy.

SOME RECOMMENDATIONS

Cancer registries

Cancer registries should be established, continued or upgraded as the case may be in selected strategic centres. The registries may be population- or hospital-based, but every effort must be made to ensure that the data are of high quality. This should not be an impossible task and in itself will have a favourable effect on the local health care system. Good medical records are an essential part of high-quality medical care and cancer registration is really no more than an accurate description of the patient and of his tumour.

Classification

Lymphoid neoplasms must be classified histologically and cytologically, with care, precision and objectivity. There continues to be much confusion and controversy relating to classification schemes. It is, however, less important which scheme is used than how it is used, since there is a reasonable degree of translateability between all classification systems. The essential task is to identify as accurately as possible the known clinical entities and to maintain appropriate record-linkage with the relevant clinical departments. This linkage is best achieved through multidisciplinary conferences - tumour boards, staging conferences, etc. - which once again are an integral component of effective cancer patient management.

The possible existence of clinical or etiological entities not yet recognized or described should also be kept in mind. The current lymphoma and leukaemia classifications were largely designed on the basis of experience in Western countries, and are not necessarily relevant or applicable elsewhere. One need only recall that prior to 1960 Burkitt's lymphoma as an entity was not known and has only recently been included in the classification of malignant lymphoma. Likewise, adult T-cell leukaemia/lymphoma was first described in 1976 and does not fit readily into most classification systems currently in wide use.

Laboratory studies

Biochemical and immunological tumour markers and the techniques for their application to the study of lymphoid tumours are now available to most pathology laboratories. The introduction of such studies into the routine examination of lymphomas and leukaemias allows these tumours to be more objectively defined and classified. Cytogenetic characterization of lymphoid neoplasms is also of increasing importance but may currently be outside the scope of many routine laboratories.

Perhaps, the most important point to be made in this context is that an adequate laboratory description or classification of lymphoid neoplasms, be it based on morphological, immunohistochemical, cytogenetic or ultimately molecular studies, requires meticulous attention to the collection, handling and processing of the tumour tissue. Specimens must be properly fixed and/or rapidly frozen as soon as possible after surgical removal or biopsy. It is recommended that the pathologist or laboratory specialist be on hand to receive the fresh specimen. When sufficient material is available, a portion should also be stored at -80°C for future studies, when indicated.

DISCUSSION

The opportunities in Africa for applied research and for making significant scientific contributions to the study of lymphoid neoplasms are truly without limits. The clinical material is abundant and the necessary scientific competence exists in many centres. The pace of basic research or the level of funding available in highly developed countries should not be a deterrent. Africa has in the past played a key role in the geographical pathology of cancer as well as in numerous other areas of biomedical research. The many African countries and their scientific institutions clearly have a continuing role of great importance. Most of the studies which have been suggested in this presentation relate to the generation of information of a type which does not currently exist and which is of crucial importance for the conduct of both laboratory and clinical research now and in the immediate future.

REFERENCES

Aboul-Nasr, A.L. (1979) The Cancer registry for the Metropolitan Cairo Area, Progress Report 5, Cairo, Cairo University Press

Blattner, W.A., Robert-Guroff, M., Kalyanaraman, U.S., Sarin, P., Jaffe, E.S., Blayney, D.W., Zener, K.A. & Gallo, R.C. (1984) Preliminary epidemiologic observations on a virus associated with T-cell neoplasia in man. In: Magrath, I.A., O'Conor, G.T. & Ramot, B., eds, Pathogenesis of Leukaemias and Lymphomas: Environmental Influences, New York, Raven Press, pp. 339-348

Burkitt, D.P. (1958) A sarcoma involving the jaws in African children. Br. J. Surg., 197, 218-223

Burkitt, D.P. & O'Conor, G.T. (1961) Malignant lymphoma in African children: I. A clinical syndrome. Cancer, 14, 258-269

Epstein, M.A., Achong, B.G. & Barr, Y.M. (1964) Virus particles in cultured lymphoblasts in Burkitt's lymphoma. Lancet, 1, 702-703

Geser, A. & Brubaker, G. (1984) A preliminary report of epidemiological studies of Burkitt's lymphoma, EBV infection and malaria in North Mara, Tanzania. In: Lenoir, G. & O'Conor, G., eds, Burkitt's Lymphoma: A Human Cancer Model (IARC Scientific Publications No. 60), Lyon, International Agency for Research on Cancer (in press)

Gross, L. (1951) "Spontaneous" leukaemia developing in C_3H mice following inoculation, in infancy, with AK-leukaemic extracts, or AK embryos. Proc. Soc. exp. Biol. Med., 76, 27-32

National Cancer Institute (1982) National Cancer Institute sponsored study of classifications on non-Hodgkin's lymphomas. The Non-Hodgkin's Lymphoma Pathologic Classification Project. Summary and description of a working formulation for clinical usage. Cancer, 49, 2112-2135

Omar, Y. (1982) Cancer incidence in Kuwait. In: Aoki, K. et al., eds, Cancer Prevention in Developing Countries, Nagoya University Press, pp. 145-149

O'Conor, G.T. (1961) Malignant lymphoma in African children: II. A pathological entitity. Cancer, 14, 270-283

O'Conor, G.T. (1984) Geographical variations in the occurrence of leukaemias and lymphomas: Summary and comments. In: Magrath, I.A., O'Conor, G.T. & Ramot, B., eds, Pathogenesis of Leukaemias and Lymphomas: Environmental Influences, New York, Raven Press, pp. 123-127

Owor, R. (1984) Geographic distribution of malignant lymphomas and leukaemias in Uganda. In: Magrath, I.A., O'Conor, G.T. & Ramot, B., eds, Pathogenesis of Leukaemias and Lymphomas: Environmental Influences, New York, Raven Press, pp. 29-33

Poiesz, B.J., Ruscetti, F.W., Reitz, J.S., Kalyanaraman, V.S. & Gallo, R.C. (1981) Isolation of a new type C retrovirus (HTLV) in primary uncultured cells of a patient with Sezary T-cell leukaemia. Nature, 294, 286-271

Takutsuki, K., Uchiyama, T., Sagawa, K. & Xodoli, J. (1976) Adult T-cell leukemia in Japan. In: Topics in Hematology, Proceedings of the 16th International Congress of Hematology, Amsterdam, Oxford, Excerpta Medica, pp. 73-77,

Waterhouse, J., Muir, C., Shanmugaratnam, K. & Powell, J., eds (1982) Cancer Incidence in Five Continents, Vol. IV (IARC Scientific Publications No. 42), Lyon, International Agency for Research on Cancer

Williams, C.K.O., Essien, E.M. & Bamgboye, E.A. (1984) Trends in leukaemia incidence in Ibadan, Nigeria. In: Magrath, I.A., O'Conor, G.T. & Ramat, B., eds, Pathogenesis of Leukaemias and Lymphomas: Environmental Influences, New York, Raven Press, pp. 17-27

World Health Organization (1975) International Classification of Diseases, Geneva

World Health Organization (1976) International Classification of Diseases for Oncology, Geneva

Young, J.L. Jr., Percy, C.L. & Asire, A.J., eds (1981) Surveil-
    lance, Epidemiology and End Results: Incidence and mortal-
    ity data, 1973-1977. <u>Natl Cancer Inst. Monogr.</u>, <u>57</u>

ETIOLOGY OF ENDEMIC BURKITT'S LYMPHOMA

C.L.M. Olweny

Harare, Zimbabwe

RESUME

De nombreuses preuves démontrent le rôle étiologique du virus d'Epstein-Barr (EBV) dans le lymphome de Burkitt (LB). Le LB répond aux critères de Henle-Koch. Les malades atteints de LB ont un taux d'anticorps anti-EBV considérablement plus élevé que les témoins normaux ou présentant d'autres tumeurs. On retrouve l'ADN et l'antigène nucléaire d'EBV dans une proportion élevée (90%) des tissus de LB des régions d'endémie. L'EBV peut transformer et immortaliser les lymphocytes B humains; il est reconnu comme responsable de tumeurs lympho-réticulaires chez les jeunes singes.

Le fait que le LB endémique soit presque invariablement associé à l'EBV tandis que le LB non endémique ne l'est pas, met en évidence l'hétérogénéité de la maladie en dépit d'une uniformité morphologique.

Le rôle du paludisme en tant que co-facteur induisant une immuno-suppression et favorisant la prolifération des cellules transformées par l'EBV est discuté. L'identification d'anomalies chromosomiques spécifiques, aussi bien dans les cas de LB endémique que de LB non endémique, souligne l'importance des facteurs génétiques.

SUMMARY

There is a considerable volume of evidence linking Epstein-Barr virus (EBV) etiologically with Burkitt's lymphoma (BL). BL has satisfied the Henle-Koch criteria. Thus BL patients have significantly higher EBV antibody titres than normal or tumour controls. EBV DNA and EBV-determined nuclear antigen (EBNA) have been demonstrated in a high proportion (>90%) of endemic BL tissues. EBV can transform and immortalize human B-lymphocytes and is known to cause lymphoreticular tumours in New World monkeys.

The fact that endemic BL is almost invariably associated with EBV while this is rarely true of the non-endemic form suggests disease heterogeneity in spite of morphological uniformity.

The role of malaria as a co-factor in causing immunosuppression and promoting proliferation of EBV-transformed cell is discussed. The identification of specific chromosomal abnormalities in both endemic and non-endemic BL underscores the importance of a suitable genetic background.

INTRODUCTION

Burkitt's lymphoma (BL) is the commonest lymphoreticular tumour in most of tropical Africa. In Uganda it accounts for about 40% of all lymphoreticular tumours, followed by the large-cell lymphomas (21%), small-cell lymphomas (17%) and Hodgkin's disease (16%). Because of this order of frequency, practitioners in tropical Africa ought perhaps to talk of Burkitt and non-Burkitt lymphomas instead of the traditional Hodgkin's and non-Hodgkin's lymphomas. Recent observations in East and West Africa have indicated a steady decline in the number of cases admitted for treatment. At the Uganda Cancer Institute, for instance, about 42 new cases were admitted in 1972, while in 1975 the total numbers seen were about 30 and in 1977 less than 10. Similar trends have been reported from Ghana[1]. The explanation for this decline in the number of new cases reporting for treatment is not immediately clear, but it has been suggested as being indicative of the absence or removal of one or more of the environmental factors causing BL.

A human tumour can be suspected of having a viral etiology either because similar tumours are known to be caused by a virus or because the epidemiological characteristics favour a virus as the etiological agent. In 1971, four criteria were put forward which a virus must satisfy before it can be regarded as an oncogenic virus in man (Henle et al., 1971). The Henle-Koch criteria, as they are currently known, include:

---

[1] Nkrumah, this volume

(1) A significant immune response to viral products must be found in patients as compared to controls;

(2) Viral tumour markers, namely viral genomes and viral products, must be detected in the tumour;

(3) The candidate virus must be able to transform in vitro;

(4) The candidate virus must be able to cause malignant tumours in vivo.

EPSTEIN-BARR VIRUS

Epstein-Barr virus (EBV) is a lymphotrophic virus whose main target is human B-lymphocytes which have specific EBV receptors. In vitro, EBV can convert normal lymphocytes into permanently growing cell lines. Cells that are transformed by EBV carry multiple copies of the viral genome per cell and express EBV-specific nuclear antigen (EBNA). Some EBV-DNA-carrying immortalized cell lines can grow as malignant tumours after heterotransplantation into immunologically deficient animals (e.g., nude mice). EBV can also transform the B-lymphocytes of some simian hosts and these transformed cells can grow progressively after reimplantation and kill the original autochthonous host. In New World monkeys (marmosets and owl monkeys), EBV is directly oncogenic, causing lymphoma, and the tumours carry the EBV genome and contain EBNA.

Studies in man carried out in many laboratories but notably in Stockholm and Philadelphia by Klein and Henle, respectively, reveal a significant elevation of EBV antibodies in patients with BL when compared with controls. In Uganda the geometric mean titre for viral capsid antigen (VCA) and early antigen were significantly higher in BL patients than in non-BL controls (patients with Hodgkin's disease, lymphocytic and histocytic lymphomas) (Table 1) (Olweny et al., 1977). In addition, EBNA and EBV DNA were found only in patients and not in controls (Table 2). The prospective seroepidemiological study carried out in the West Nile District of Uganda (de-Thé et al., 1978) was designed to determine:

(a) whether BL is due to delayed EBV infection, as is the case with infectious mononucleosis;

(b) whether BL developed in children heavily and chronically
infected with EBV;

(c) whether EBV is just a passenger virus in BL.

Table 1. EBV serology in BL and non-BL patients in Uganda[a]

Item	VCA	EA		EBNA
		D	R	
BL patients:				
Geometric mean titre	294.5	13.9	37.6	22.6
Variance	3.235	1.760	7.124	3.345
Non-BL patients:				
Geometric mean titre	90.1	11.3	10.0	29.7
Variance	3.227	1.290	0.0	2.995
Level of significance (p)	< 0.01	>0.05	<0.01	>0.05

[a] VCA, viral capsid antigen; EA, early antigen; D, diffuse; R, restricted; EBNA, EBV-specific nuclear antigen

The study, initiated in 1973 and completed in 1976, identified 14 children with BL for whom pretumour sera were available.
It was evident that children seroconverted 6-24 months before the
tumour developed. High VCA titres did not protect children
against BL; if anything, they favoured its development (de-Thé
et al., 1978). Antibody levels to other viruses, such as herpes
simplex virus, cytomegalovirus, measles virus, and adenovirus
type 5, did not differ significantly from those of controls
(Geser et al., 1979).

Table 2. EBV genome studies in BL and non-BL patients in Uganda

Item	BL patients	Non-BL patients
Number studied	34	25
Sex ratio (M/F)	2:1	1.8:1
Mean age (years)	7.2	16.3
Range	2 - 15	4 -60
EBNA-positive	27 (79%)	0
EBV-DNA-positive	14/15 (93%)	0/15 (0%)
Mean number of genome equivalents per cell	39	< 2
Range	8 - 86	< 2

For the association between the ubiquitous EBV and the geo-graphically restricted BL to be a causal one therefore calls for special circumstances at the time of primary EBV infection. In Equatorial Africa such special circumstances include:

(a) an early, unrecognized EBV infection in childhood;

(b) a massive EBV infection, reflected by a high EBV/VCA titre in children who will later develop BL (de-Thé et al., 1978).

There is no evidence that, following early and massive EBV infection, chronic EBV infection develops, similar to what is observed with hepatitis B virus and hepatocellular carcinoma. However, BL in endemic areas is known to carry multiple copies of the EBV genome, often 30-40 per cell in 95% of cases (Olweny et al., 1977). Thus, the Henle-Koch criteria have all been satis-fied in the case of EBV and BL. There are obvious difficulties in conducting the ultimate test of oncogenicity in man so that the question whether the circumstantial evidence so far accumulated is strong enough to establish a causal relationship will remain unanswered for some time.

ROLE OF MALARIA

African BL is also associated with endemic malaria (Williams, 1966). The evidence for this association is mainly epidemiological and includes:

(a) The close correlation between the intensity of Plasmodium falciparum transmission and the distribution of BL;

(b) The fact that urban dwellers in areas where there is a low level of malaria transmission are relatively protected against BL;

(c) The decline in BL incidence where death rates due to malaria are also on the decline;

(d) The older age of onset of BL in patients who have migrated from malaria hypoendemic regions to malaria hyperendemic areas.

The role of malaria appears to be that of immunosuppression, which promotes proliferation of EBV-transformed cells. EBV-infected cells are probably target cells for non-EBV-related events, such as malaria-induced impaired T-cell-mediated cytotoxicity and later chromosomal translocation and abnormal gene expression.

CYTOGENETIC ASPECTS

Lymphomatous cell lines derived from both EBV-genome-positive and -negative BL tumours have all been shown to exhibit characteristic karyotypic anomalies, either t(8;14), t(8;22) or t(2;8) (Lenoir et al., 1982). These chromosomal abnormalities may be related to rearrangements of DNA sequences coding for immunoglobulin and the c-myc oncogene.

It would thus appear that the pathogenesis of African BL involves EBV, which initiates a multistep process leading to chromosomal translocation and abnormal expression of the c-myc oncogene. Stated differently, EBV appears to be the initiator causing immortalization of B-lymphocytes. Malaria acts as the promoter facilitating the proliferation of the transformed cells and this increase in transformed cells provides a much higher statistical opportunity for the emergence and proliferation of cytogenetically abnormal BL cells.

REFERENCES

de-Thé, G., Geser, A., Day, N.E., Tukei, P.M., Williams, E.H., Beri, D.P., Smith, P.G., Dean, A.G., Bronkamm, G.K., Feorino, P. & Henle, W. (1978) Epidemiological evidence for causal relationship between Epstein-Barr virus and Burkitt's lymphoma from Ugandan prospective study. Nature, 274, 756-761

Geser, A., Feorino, P.M. & Sohier, R. (1979) Further studies of antibody levels to herpes simplex virus, cytomegalovirus, measles virus and adenovirus type 5 in Burkitt's lymphoma patients. Med. Microbiol. Immunol., 167, 175-180

Henle, G., Henle, W., Klein, G., Günven, P., Clifford, P., Morrow, R.H. & Ziegler, J.L. (1971) Antibodies to early Epstein-Barr virus induced antigens in Burkitt's lymphoma. J. natl Cancer Inst., 46, 861-871

Lenoir, G.M., Preud'homme, J.L., Bernheim, A. & Berger, R. (1982) Correlation between immunoglobulin light chain expression and variant translocation in Burkitt's lymphoma. Nature, 298, 474-476

Olweny, C.L.M., Atine, I., Kaddu-Mukasa, A., Owor, R., Andersson-Anvret, M., Klein, G., Henle, W. & de-Thé, G. (1977) Epstein-Barr virus genome studies in Burkitt's and non-Burkitt's lymphomas in Uganda. J. natl Cancer Inst., 58, 1191-1196

Williams, A.O. (1966) Haemoglobin electrophoresis and Burkitt's lymphoma. Br. J. Genet.

PATHOLOGY OF BURKITT'S LYMPHOMA IN ZAIRE

M.M.R. Kalengayi & L. Mubikayi

Department of Pathology, Medical Faculty,
and Kinshasa University Hospital, University of Kinshasa,
Kinshasa, Zaire

RESUME

Une étude a été réalisée sur 527 cas de lymphome diagnostiqués durant la période 1960-1980 dans le Département de Pathologie de l'Université de Kinshasa. Parmi ces cas, 115 se sont avérés être des lymphomes de Burkitt (LB), et le maxillaire le site le plus fréquemment affecté. La plupart des cas (74%) ont été diagnostiqués durant la première décade de la vie et la majorité (75%) des cas de LB à localisation maxillaire ont été observés chez de jeunes enfants. Les résultats montrent que la maladie est très commune au Zaïre et survient dans toutes les Provinces du pays et dans tous les groupes ethniques.

SUMMARY

A study was made of 527 cases of lymphoma diagnosed over the period 1960-1980 in the Department of Pathology of the University of Kinshasa. Of these cases, 115 were found to be Burkitt's lymphoma, the maxilla being the most frequently affected site. Most of the cases (74%) were diagnosed during the first decade of life and the majority (75%) of the cases of maxillary BL occurred in young children. The results show that the disease is quite common in Zaire and occurs in all the Provinces of the country and among all ethnic groups.

INTRODUCTION

Since the appearance of the papers on cancer in Zaire by De Smet (1956) and Thys (1957), no other general studies have been carried out on the disease in this country.

In contrast with the abundant literature available on Burkitt's lymphoma (BL) in several other African countries (see extensive reviews in Burkitt and Wright, 1970), only two brief reports describing four (de Scoville & Parmentier, 1968) and 15 (Olson et al., 1969) cases respectively have been published dealing with this tumour in Zaire.

In order to make good these shortcomings, work was undertaken in the Department of Pathology, Kinshasa University Hospital, with the aim of obtaining an accurate profile of cancer in Zaire, including all types of malignant lymphomas[1].

The present paper is one of a series devoted to the profile of cancer in Zaire and aims particularly to depict the pathological patterns of a large number of BL cases observed in the Department of Pathology of the University of Kinshasa, which has the advantage of being able to examine pathological specimens originating from almost the entire country, namely seven of the eight Provinces of Zaire and Kinshasa City.

MATERIALS AND METHODS

Selection of cases

The study covers the 20-year period from 1960 to 1980. All cases diagnosed as lymphomas during this period and all biopsies for which there was a problem of differential diagnosis with lymphoma in general and with BL in particular were revised as described in detail elsewhere[1]. Furthermore, to increase the likelihood of detecting undiagnosed cases of BL, all biopsies of lymph-nodes and other organs liable to be affected by BL were re-evaluated.

---

[1] Mubikayi & Kalengayi, this volume

Biopsy specimens were usually fixed in formaldehyde solution (10%) or in Bouin's fluid. They were then embedded in paraffin and stained with haematoxylin and eosin in the usual manner. If necessary, supplementary serial and thinner sections were prepared and re-examined with particular attention to the margins of the slices in order to identify more accurately the characteristic 'starry sky' pattern of BL (Wright, 1970).

Parameters considered

For each case of histologically confirmed BL, the following parameters were systematically considered: histopathological features, relative frequency as compared to other lymphomas, anatomical site, age and sex distribution, and geographical distribution throughout the country.

RESULTS

Histologically, all the lesions diagnosed as BL showed homogeneous proliferation of variably mature lymphocytes - sometimes showing mitotic figures - with the characteristic 'starry sky' appearance throughout the proliferation (Fig. 1). However, as mentioned above, it was sometimes necessary to prepare additional, serial and thinner sections and to examine particularly the margins of the slide to find evidence of this almost pathognomonic appearance.

In the present study, a total of 527 cases of lymphoma were investigated and were found to be made up as follows:

Hodgkin's disease   139 (26.6%)

Poorly differentiated
  lymphocytic lymphoma   119 (23%)

Burkitt's lymphoma   115 (21.3%)

Of the remainder, histiocytic lymphoma accounted for 14%, well differentiated lymphocytic lymphoma for 9%, undifferentiated lymphocytic lymphoma for 5%, nodular lymphoma for 1% and mycosis fungoides for 0.1%.

FIG. 1. BURKITT'S LYMPHOMA IN THE OVARY

Homogeneous proliferation of variably immature lymphocytes;
throughout the tumour very numerous clear macrophages are seen
resulting in the characteristic 'starry sky' pattern; H & E

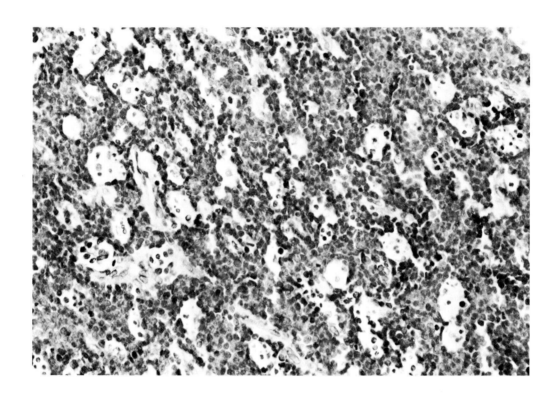

With regard to the anatomical localization of the cases of BL, the following results were obtained:

Maxilla	37 (32.17%)
Gastrointestinal tract	18 (15.65%)
Lymph-nodes:	
cervical	5 (4.34%)
others	11 (9.56%)
Ovaries	8 (6.95%)
Miscellaneous organs	
or tissues	21 (18.26%)
Not specified	15 (13.04%)

As concerns age, most of the cases (74%) were diagnosed during the first decade of life, 14% in the course of the second decade and only 12% between 20 and 70 years of age, in contrast with the age curve of other lymphomas encountered in the same study (Fig. 2). Furthermore, the majority (75%) of the cases of maxillary BL occurred in young children.

Males were found to be more affected (57.30% of cases) by BL than females (43.70%), i.e., a M/F ratio of 1.31/1. Moreover, 16% of the 46 female cases were located in the ovaries and 75% of the ovarian cases (6) were bilateral.

Geographically, the study clearly showed that BL occurs in all the provinces and ethnic groups of Zaire, albeit with quite variable frequencies. Table 1 shows the distribution throughout the country.

FIG. 2.   AGE CURVES OF DIFFERENT LYMPHOMAS IN ZAIRE

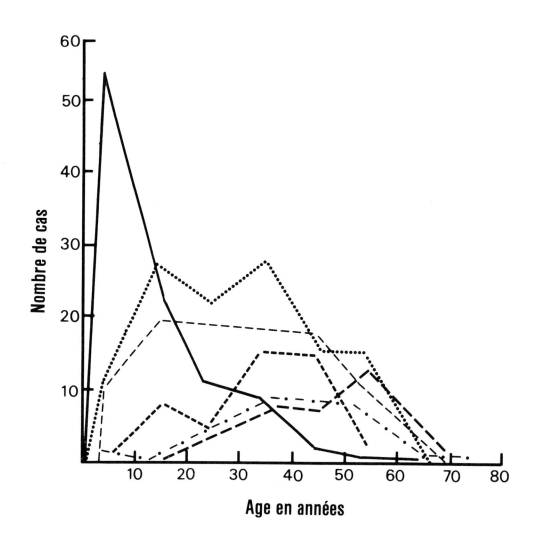

Table 1. Geographical distribution

Area	No. of cases	Frequency (%)
Kinshasa City	47	40.80
Lower Zaire	23	20.00
Equator	12	10.40
Eastern Kasai	11	9.50
Bandundu	6	5.20
Kivu	6	5.20
Western Kasai	5	4.45
Upper Zaire	5	4.45
Shaba[a]	0	0.00

[a] No requests for pathologist's reports received from this province, but several cases were observed by one of the authors (Kalengayi).

DISCUSSION

This retrospective study of BL in Zaire shows that this disease is quite common in the country. In contrast with several early reports on BL in other African countries such as Uganda (Burkitt, 1958; Burkitt & O'Conor, 1961; O'Conor, 1961), Nigeria (Brew & Jackson, 1960), it was only later that this lymphoma was described in Zaire by de Scoville and Parmentier (1968) and by Olson et al. (1969). However, BL was apparently encountered earlier among the multivisceral and multifocal lymphosarcomas described by De Smet (1956) and by Thys (1957), as pointed out by Hutt (1970). The present study, covering the period from 1960 to 1980, definitely demonstrates the occurrence of BL in Zairians as early as 1962-1963.

With regard to histopathology, the features were the same as those described in the original reports (see review by Wright, 1970b), and are shown in Figure 1.

In the present study, BL was found to be third in frequency amongst the lymphomas, while it is the most frequent lymphoma encountered in Uganda (Wright, 1973). This discrepancy may be explained by the fact that BL has been extensively studied in Uganda both in biopsies and in autopsies, while in this study it was investigated almost exclusively in biopsy material. When the frequency of BL was compared with that of Kaposi's sarcoma over the same period, Kalengayi and Kashala found that Kaposi's sarcoma was 2.6 times more frequent than BL in the general population[1].

The most frequently affected organs in this study in order of decreasing frequency are exactly the same as those described by Wright (1970) in Uganda in a larger series including autopsies (Table 2). In Zaire, Olson et al. (1969) found that males were markedly more affected by BL than females (M/F = 4/1), while Burkitt (1970), in a larger series in Uganda, reported a M/F ratio of 2.1/1. This latter figure is similar to our finding of an M/F ratio of 1.31/1. The small size of the series studied by Olsen et al. probably explains their widely differing results.

As reported elsewhere (Burkitt, 1958, 1970; Burkitt & O'Conor, 1961; Brew & Jackson, 1960; Wright, 1970a), BL was found predominantly in young children under 10 years of age (74% of the cases). Furthermore, it is worthwhile noting that the majority of maxillary localizations (75%) occurred in those young children. The predominance of BL in childhood and in the maxilla, when compared to all other lymphomas and other malignancies are the characteristics that led to this lymphoma being regarded as a specific clinicopathological entity (Hutt, 1970).

If this broader study of BL in Zaire is combined with the two previous reports (de Scoville & Parmentier, 1968; Olson et al., 1969), it is clear that this disease is encountered in all the provinces and ethnic groups of this country. The apparent absence of BL in Shaba province in the present study (Table 1) is due only to the fact that this province has had its own pathology laboratory for several years so that hospitals of this area send hardly any requests for pathologist's reports to the Department of Pathology in Kinshasa.

---

[1] See Kalengayi & Kashala, this volume

Indeed, the four early cases reported by de Scoville and Parmentier (1968) were observed in Shaba province and one of the authors (Kalengayi) has diagnosed at least six cases of BL when travelling as consultant pathologist in this area. Thus BL appears to be ubiquitous in Zaire, in the same way as Kaposi's sarcoma, although with very variable frequency. Further investigations are needed in order to provide a more accurate profile of this epidemiological parameter[1].

In connection with the possible role of malaria in the etiology of BL (Burkitt, 1970; Haddow, 1970; Ziegler, 1981), it should be noted that malaria is hyperendemic throughout Zaire. However, superposition of BL and malaria maps in Zaire as well as in other African countries requires further epidemiological studies before definite conclusions can be reached on the etiological relationships between these two diseases. Furthermore, the epidemiobiochemical marker of BL, i.e., Epstein-Barr virus antigen, has apparently not been studied in Zaire. Surveys of the prevalence of Epstein-Barr virus in Zaire, as carried out in other African countries, are needed in order to evaluate possible links between the virus and the causation of BL.

REFERENCES

Brew, D.P. St.J. & Jackson, J.G. Quoted by Hutt, M.S.R. (1970)

Burkitt, D.P. (1958) A sarcoma involving the jaws in African children. Br. J. Surg., 46, 218-223

Burkitt, D.P. & O'Conor, G.T. (1961) Malignant lymphoma in African children. I. A clinical syndrome. Cancer, 14, 258-269

Burkitt, D.P. (1970) Geographical distribution. In: Burkitt, D.P. & Wright, D.H., eds, Burkitt's lymphoma, London, Livingstone, pp. 186-197

Burkitt, D.P. & Wright, D.H., eds (1970) Burkitt's Lymphoma, London, Livingstone

---

[1] See Kalengayi & Kashala, this volume

Haddow, A.J. (1970) Epidemiological evidence suggesting an infective element in the etiology. In: Burkitt, D.P. & Wright, D.H., eds, Burkitt's Lymphoma, London, Livingstone, pp. 198-214

Hutt, M.S.R. (1970) Introduction and historical background. In: Burkitt, D.P. & Wright, D.H., eds, Burkitt's Lymphoma, London, Livingstone, pp. 1-5

O'Conor, G.T. (1961) Malignant lymphoma in African children. Cancer, 14, 270-283

Olson, C.W., Smith, J.H., Testerman, N., Bastin, J.P. & Frazer, H. (1969) Burkitt's tumors in the Democratic Republic of the Congo. Cancer, 23, 740-746

de Scoville, A. & Parmentier, R. (1968) Contribution à l'étude de la pathologie géographique de la maladie de Burkitt. Bull. Acad. roy. Méd. belg., 8, 613-642

de Smet, M.P. (1956) Observations cliniques de tumeurs malignes des tissus réticuloendothéliaux et des tissus hématopoiétiques au Congo. Ann. Soc. belge Méd. trop., 36, 56-70

Thys, A. (1957) Considérations sur les tumeurs malignes des indigènes du Congo Belge et du Rwanda Urundi. A propos de 2.536 cas. Ann. Soc. belge Méd. trop., 37, 483-514

Wright, D.H. (1970a) Gross distribution and haematology. In: Burkitt, D.P. & Wright, D.H., eds, Burkitt's Lymphoma, London, Livingstone, pp. 64-81

Wright, D.H. (1970b) Microscopic features, histochemistry, histogenesis. In: Burkitt, D.P. & Wright, D.H., eds, Burkitt's Lymphoma, London, Livingstone, pp. 82-102

Wright, D.H. (1973) Lymphoreticular neoplasms. In: Templeton, ed., Tumors in a Tropical Country, Berlin, Springer-Verlag, pp. 270-297

Ziegler, J.L. (1981) Burkitt's lymphoma. New Engl. J. Med., 305, 735-745

CHANGES IN THE PRESENTATION OF BURKITT'S LYMPHOMA IN GHANA OVER A 15-YEAR PERIOD (1969–1982)

F.K. Nkrumah

Department of Paediatrics and Child Health
University of Zimbabwe
Harare, Zimbabwe

RESUME

Au cours d'une période de 15 ans, 485 cas de lymphome de Burkitt provenant pour la plupart de la moitié sud du Ghana ont été enregistrés au Burkitt's Tumour Project d'Accra. L'analyse des cas, de la localisation des tumeurs, de leur répartition selon l'âge et le sexe a permis de conclure que: (i) le nombre de cas de LB diagnostiqués au Ghana a progressivement diminué au cours des 15 dernières années; à présent, le nombre de nouveaux cas n'est plus que de la moitié environ de ce qu'il était il y a dix ans; (ii) la répartition des cas selon le sexe est pratiquement demeurée inchangée durant cette période; (iii) il y a eu une augmentation significative du nombre de patients présentant une localisation abdominale de la maladie et une diminution du nombre de ceux présentant une localisation faciale. Ce changement a été particulièrement manifeste chez les hommes, chez qui la proportion de cas à localisation abdominale a plus que doublé; (iv) l'âge des patients, hommes et femmes, lors de l'apparition de la maladie a augmenté progressivement au cours de cette période de 15 années.

Les implications et interprétations possibles des résultats ci-dessus sont discutées.

SUMMARY

Over a 15-year period, 485 cases of Burkitt's lymphoma (BL) mainly from the southern half of Ghana, were referred to the Burkitt's Tumour Project in Accra, Ghana. From an analysis of the numbers of cases referred each year, the sites of tumour involvement, and the age and sex frequencies, it was concluded that: (i) the number of cases of BL diagnosed in Ghana has decreased progressively over the last 15 years; the number of newly diagnosed cases is now only about one half of what it was 10 years ago; (ii) the male/female ratio has remained practically unchanged over this period; (iii) there has been an overall increase in patients presenting with abdominal disease and a decrease in those presenting with facial disease. This change was particularly apparent in males, in whom the proportion of cases with abdominal disease has more than doubled; (iv) there has been a progressive increase in age at presentation for both males and females over the 15-year period.

The possible implications of, and reasons for the above findings are discussed.

INTRODUCTION

It is now over two and a half decades since Burkitt drew the attention of the medical world to a distinctive malignancy occurring in African children, which predominantly involved facial structures and abdominal viscera. This malignant tumour of childhood was subsequently histologically defined as a lymphoma and later further morphologically classified as malignant lymphoma, Burkitt's type, or simply Burkitt's lymphoma (BL), named appropriately after the original describer of the disease entity. Over the last decade and a half or so, a considerable body of information relating to the epidemiology, pathology, clinical presentation, response to chemotherapy and possible pathogenesis of so-called African or endemic BL has been collected in many African countries, but principally in centres in East and West Africa where the disease appears to occur with the highest frequency.

In the so-called endemic areas for BL in tropical Africa, this malignancy has been shown to be the most common malignancy of childhood. Indeed in the few centres in tropical Africa where cancer registers have been established, BL has been shown to account for over 50% of all childhood malignancies. In Ghana, West Africa, where BL is endemic and also constitutes the commonest childhood malignancy, the Burkitt's Tumour Project

(BTP) was established in 1966 within the Department of Child Health of the University of Ghana Medical School, Accra, as a centre for data collection, research and treatment of this malignancy.

RESULTS

This paper will confine itself to a review of changes in the presentation of BL in Ghana as documented by the BTP over a 15-year period from 1968 to 1982. A review of the data was necessitated by the fact, that over the last few years, it became apparent to those closely associated with the Project in Accra that fewer and fewer BL patients were being referred to the centre for diagnosis and treatment (in spite of an active policy of encouraging such referral) and also that the clinical presentation of the disease had changed somewhat over the years.

Over the 15-year period (1968-1982) a total of 485 patients with BL were diagnosed and treated at the BTP centre in Accra. The overall age and sex distribution is shown in Figure 1. The patients were aged from 2 to 20 years, with a progressive increase in the ages affected from age 3 years to a peak at 6-8 years. A sudden drop in numbers is noticeable after 12-14 years, above which the disease occurs infrequently.

The overall male/female ratio for the 485 patients over the 15-year period was 1.7:1, as shown by Table 1, which also gives the break-down, by year, of the number of confirmed BL cases referred to the BTP from 1968 to 1982, and the break-down by sex. This shows a remarkable and progressive decrease in the numbers of BL cases referred to the BTP over the 15-year period.

FIG. 1.   AGE AND SEX DISTRIBUTION OF 485 BURKITT'S LYMPHOMA
PATIENTS FROM GHANA, WEST AFRICA.   □, MALE; ▨, FEMALE

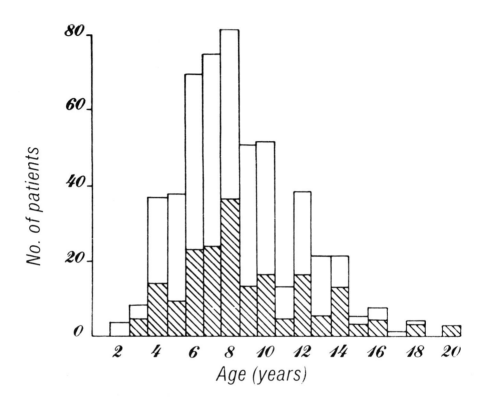

Table 2 shows the number of BL cases referred from the
Eastern Region of Ghana, a province close to the capital, Accra.
This Region has an excellent health infrastructure and, because
of its proximity to the Project centre in Accra, referral of
cases of BL was felt to be optimal and possibly close to the true
incidence of the disease in the Region.   A declining rate of
referral over the years is again confirmed for this Region, which
would indicate an overall decrease in BL over the years.

Table 1. Annual number of cases of BL in Ghana over a 15-year period (1968-1982)

Year	Male		Female		Total
	No.	%	No.	%	
1968	8	50	8	50	16
1969	21	58	15	48	36
1970	21	51	20	49	41
1971	24	59	17	41	41
1972	25	66	13	34	38
1973	19	76	6	24	25
1974	31	69	12	31	45
1975	31	62	19	38	50
1976	27	69	12	31	39
1977	24	60	16	40	40
1978	21	68	10	32	31
1979	11	65	6	35	17
1980	12	50	12	50	24
1981	12	67	6	33	18
1982	17	65	9	35	26
Total	304	63	181	37	485

Sites of involvement on initial presentation by 5-year periods are presented in Table 3. The most significant finding is a relative increase in patients presenting with abdominal disease towards the end of the period. If the proportion of patients presenting with any facial or abdominal involvement is broken down by year and sex, there is a striking increase in males presenting with abdominal tumour over the years (Fig. 2). A trend analysis gives a highly significant x^2 trend value of $p = 0.01$. This increase was particularly apparent in those males presenting with abdominal disease only. At the same time, a less consistent but equally significant decine in males presenting with facial tumours can be seen (x^2 trend $p = 0.01$). No significant change in the number of females with abdominal or facial disease was discernable over the 15-year period.

Table 2. Number of BL patients referred to the Burkitt's Tumour
Project from the Eastern Region of Ghana, 1971-1981

Year	No. of BL cases
1971	6
1972	9
1973	2
1974	9
1975	11
1976	10
1977	8
1978	7
1979	5
1980	4
1981	3

Table 3. Sites of involvement on initial presentation of BL in
Ghana over a 15-year period (1968-1982)

Site	1968-1972[a]	1973-1977[b]	1978-1982[c]
Face	120 (68.9%)	93 (46.7%)	65 (57.5%)
Abdomen	82 (47.1%)	141 (71%)	67 (59.3%)
CNS (meninges)	11 (6.3%)	9 (4.5%)	14 (12.4%)
Paraplegia	7 (4.0%)	10 (5.0%)	9 (8.0%)
Cranial neuropathy	4 (2.3%)	5 (2.5%)	4 (3.5%)
Pleura	3 (1.7%)	8 (4.0%)	4 (3.5%)
P. lymph-nodes	3 (1.7%)	15 (7.5%)	4 (3.5%)
Skin	6 (3.4%)	7 (3.5%)	7 (6.2%)
Thyroid	3 (1.7%)	7 (3.5%)	2 (1.7%)
Salivary glands	2 (1.2%)	5 (2.5%)	9 (8.0%)
Bone marrow	-	9 (4.5%)	8 (7.1%)
Bone (other than facial)	7 (4.0%)	3 (1.5%)	1 (0.8%)
Testes	2 (1.2%)	2 (1%)	1 (0.8%)
Breast	-	1 (0.5%)	2 (1.6%)

[a] 174 patients; [b] 199 patients; [c] 113 patients

FIG. 2.   PERCENTAGE OF CASES WITH ANY ABDOMINAL OR FACIAL TUMOUR
          BY YEAR OF PRESENTATION. ●, MALE; ○, FEMALE

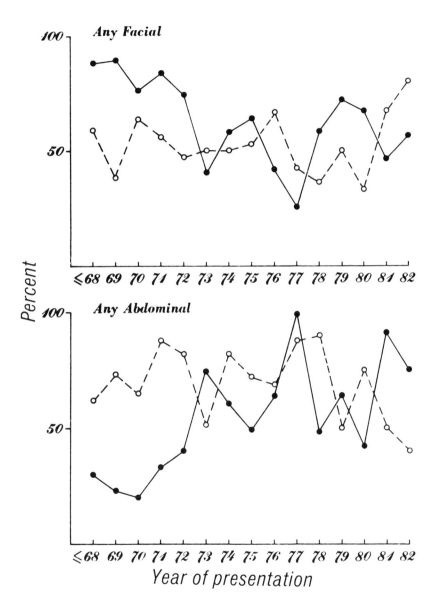

Another interesting observation arising from the analysis of
the data is the gradually progressive increase in the average age
at presentation for both males and females over the 15-year
period (see Fig. 3).

FIG. 3. AVERAGE AGE OF ONSET BY YEAR
●, MALE; ○, FEMALE; ■, TOTAL

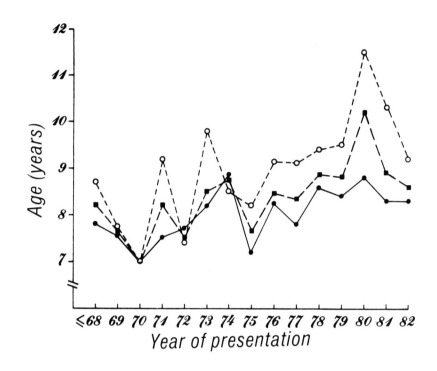

DISCUSSION

The most striking observation is the marked increase in the
proportion of males with abdominal involvement and the declining
incidence of BL in Ghana over the study period. No satisfactory
explanation of these changes can be suggested but it is possible
that they may be interrelated. In high-incidence areas, BL has a
younger age of onset and a higher proportion of facial tumours
than in low-incidence ones (Morrow et al., 1974). In the analysis, a trend can be seen towards increasing age and falling
proportion of facial disease that is consistent with the observed
declining incidence.

It is believed that incidence rates of BL in Ghana are
falling as it now requires increased attention to surveillance
and encouragement of the referral of cases to maintain a steady
referral rate. A similar experience has been reported from the
North Mara District of Tanzania (Siemiatychi et al., 1980). It

will be of interest to see whether this decline has also been accompanied by a shift in presenting sites as well as in age and whether similar trends have been observed in other endemic areas.

A measurable decline in BL incidence immediately raises the question whether such a change could have been initiated by corresponding changes in epidemiology or in transmission of the two strongly incriminated environmental etiologically associated factors - Epstein-Barr virus (EBV) and endemic malaria. It is tantalizing to speculate that possible changes in endemicity, transmission or host response to EBV or malaria infection may be related to or account for the observed trends in Ghana. There are no available data in Ghana on EBV infection to suggest significant changes in its transmission or its seroepidemiology. Studies by the centre in Accra, done 5 years ago, documented an almost universal seroconversion by the age of 2 years to this virus (Biggar et al., 1978). Another longitudinal or even cross-sectional study of infants and young children may possibly again be necessary to ascertain whether there has been any shift in EBV transmission patterns. With regard to malaria, data have recently been assembled that would suggest a shift in transmission pattern and seroepidemiology, at least in sampled populations from urban and rural Ghana. A marked decline in malaria transmission has been documented in urban Accra but a much smaller one in a rural area (Gardiner et al., 1984).

This was associated with an expected decline in, and late acquisition of antibody to malaria in an urban population of children, but with smaller changes in the rural population. The changes have been attributed to the increasingly widespread use of antimalarial drugs in Ghana. Whether such changes in malaria transmission could account for the observed changes in BL incidence and the presenting pattern in Ghana, is still highly speculative. Documentation of similar trends in other BL endemic areas is needed to confirm the above observations.

REFERENCES

Biggar, R.J., Henle, W., Fleisher, G., Böcker, J., Lennette, E.T. & Henle, G. (1978) Primary Epstein-Barr virus infections in African infants. Int. J. Cancer, 22, 239-243

Gardiner, C., Biggar, R.J., Collins, W.E. & Nkrumah, F.K. (1984)
    Malaria in urban and rural areas of southern Ghana: a
    survey of parasitaemia, antibodies and anti-malarial practi-
    ces. Bull. World Health Org., 62, 607-613

Morrow, R.H., Levine, P.H., Ziegler, J.L. & Berrad, C. (1974)
    What is Burkitt's lymphoma? Lancet, 2, 1268-1269

Siemiatychi, J., Brubaker, G. & Geser, A. (1980)   Space-time
    clustering of Burkitt's lymphoma in East Africa: Analysis
    of recent data and a new look at old data. Int. J. Cancer,
    25, 197-203

LA MALADIE DE HODGKIN AU ZAÏRE:
PROFIL HISTOLOGIQUE ET ANATOMOCLINIQUE

L. Mubikayi & M.M.R. Kalengayi[1]

Département d'Anatomie Pathologique
Faculté de Médecine et Cliniques Universitaires de Kinshasa
Université de Kinshasa
Kinshasa, Zaïre

SUMMARY

A total of 139 cases of Hodgkin's disease diagnosed over a 20-year period in the Department of Pathology, Kinshasa University Hospital, have been analysed with regard to relative frequency, histological type, anatomical site and age and sex of patients.

Hodgkin's disease was found to be the most frequent of all lymphomas diagnosed, i.e., 139/527 cases or 26.37%. Histological forms reputed to be of poorer prognosis - mixed cellular and lymphocyte depleted - predominate and represent 31.5% and 31%, respectively, while the lymphocyte-predominant and scleronodular forms account for only 26.5% and.11%, respectively. Lymph nodes were the most frequent site affected (84%). More males are affected than females (ratio, 2.56:1); and the majority (49%) of people suffering from this lymphoma range from 18 to 40 years of age.

These findings do not provide a complete pathological pro-file of Hodgkin's lymphoma in Zaïre. Nevertheless they indicate the main features that require further similar investigations in other areas of the country, before any definitive conclusions can be reached.

---

[1] A qui toute correspondance doit être adressée

RESUME

Cent trente neuf cas de maladie de Hodgkin diagnostiqués de
1960 à 1980 dans le Département d'Anatomie Pathologique de
l'Hôpital Universitaire de Kinshasa, ont été analysés.

Il en ressort que cette maladie constitue le lymphome le
plus fréquent: 139 cas pour 527 lymphomes, soit 26,37%. Son
profil histopathologique est caractérisé par la prédominance des
formes à mauvais pronostic, formes à cellularité mixte (31,5%) et
à déplétion lymphocytaire (31%), suivies par la forme à prédominance lymphocytaire (26,5%), tandis que la forme à sclérose nodulaire se révèle rare. Les ganglions lymphatiques se sont avérés
être le site préférentiel (84%) de la survenue de ce lymphome.
Les hommes sont plus affectés que les femmes dans un rapport de
2,56:1. L'affection a été retrouvée en majeure partie chez des
gens âgés de 18 à 40 ans (49%).

Ces résultats ne reflètent certes pas le profil complet de
la pathologie du lymphome de Hodgkin au Zaïre. Néanmoins, ils en
offrent les traits les plus intéressants qui devront être complé-
tés par des études similaires dans d'autres régions du pays avant
d'être généralisés.

INTRODUCTION

S'il existe quelques études d'ensemble sur le profil du
cancer en Afrique (Doll et coll., 1966, 1970; Templeton, 1973),
il n'y en a guère sur le Zaïre où l'on retrouve seulement quelques travaux fragmentaires datant déjà de plusieurs dizaines
d'années (De Smet, 1956; Thys, 1957). C'est le cas en particulier pour les lymphomes qui, dans d'autres pays d'Afrique, ont
déjà été l'objet de plusieurs travaux (Wright, 1973).

En ce qui concerne la maladie de Hodgkin, elle n'a guère été
étudiée au Zaïre, si ce n'est trois cas signalés par De Smet
(1956) sur 24 tumeurs du système réticulo-endothélial (SRE) et 55
autres cas mentionnés par Thys (1957) sur 318 cancers du SRE.

Par ailleurs, deux des cas rapportés par De Smet (1956)
étaient de diagnostic douteux et ces auteurs utilisaient la classification histologique de Jackson & Parker (1947) aujourd'hui
abandonnée. Une comparaison de leurs travaux avec ceux publiés
dans d'autres pays s'avère donc hasardeuse sinon impossible.

Ces différents écueils ont motivé la présente étude qui se propose donc d'analyser rétrospectivement la maladie de Hodgkin au Zaïre en la situant par rapport aux autres lymphomes étiquetés selon une des classifications modernes les plus répandues et en recensant certains aspects de son profil anatomoclinique. Cet article s'insère dans un travail d'ensemble en cours dans le Département d'Anatomie Pathologique des Cliniques Universitaires de Kinshasa sur le profil du cancer au Zaïre.

MATERIEL ET METHODES

Sélection des cas

L'étude porte sur tous les cas de lymphomes diagnostiqués dans ce Département sur une période de 20 ans, de 1960 à 1980.

Tous les cas diagnostiqués comme lymphomes sous diverses nomenclatures ont été réexaminés histologiquement. Ainsi ont été réanalysées toutes les biopsies portant ces diagnostics: lymphome malin, lymphosarcome, lymphocytosarcome, hématosarcome, maladie de Hodgkin, histiocytosarcome, lymphoblastome, tumeur de Burkitt, réticulosarcome, lymphome gigantofolliculaire, mycosis fungoïdes.

Toutes les biopsies pour lesquelles se posait un problème de diagnostic différentiel avec un lymphome ont été également revues histologiquement. Ainsi, nous avons réévalué toutes les lames qui portaient le diagnostic de leucémie, tumeur ou sarcome anaplasique, sarcome à cellules rondes, carcinome lymphoépithélial, hyperplasie folliculaire et cellules atypiques au niveau des ganglions lymphatiques.

En outre, pour augmenter les chances de découvrir des lymphomes qui seraient passés inaperçus, toutes les biopsies ganglionnaires ont été revues.

Le matériel ainsi sélectionné et révisé histologiquement a permis d'exclure des diagnostics erronés de lymphomes et d'en découvrir d'autres ignorés. Les autres lymphomes font l'objet d'un article à part.

Les biopsies examinées avaient été fixées dans une solution de formol à 10% ou dans le liquide de Bouin et colorées à l'hématoxyline-éosine. Lorsque c'était nécessaire, des recoupes supplémentaires dans les blocs de paraffine et la coloration à la réticuline ont été effectuées.

Paramètres étudiés

Les paramètres suivants ont été analysés pour chaque cas:

- Type histologique.- La maladie de Hodgkin a été étiquetée histologiquement selon la classification de Lukes & Butler (1966) tandis que les autres lymphomes ont été classés selon celle de Rappaport (1966). Le recours à d'autres classifications n'était pas possible pour ce matériel analysé rétrospectivement.

- Age, sexe et localisations anatomiques.- Ces paramètres ont été repris dans les renseignements fournis dans les réquisitions anatomopathologiques.

La répartition géographique n'a pas été étudiée ici car la plus grande partie des échantillons analysés provient essentiellement des régions proches des Cliniques Universitaires de Kinshasa.

RESULTATS

Cette étude a permis de recenser ainsi 527 lymphomes répartis comme suit (Tableau 1):

Tableau 1. Distribution des différents types de lymphomes étudiés

Type du lymphome	No. de cas	%
Lymphome indifférencié	27	5,1
Lymphome de Burkitt	115	21,8
Lymphome histiocytaire (réticulosarcome)	69	13,0
Lymphome lymphocytaire peu différencié	119	22,6
Lymphome lymphocytaire bien différencié	51	9,7
Lymphome nodulaire	6	1,2
Lymphome de Hodgkin	139	26,4
Mycosis fungoïdes	1	0,2

La réévaluation histopathologique des 139 cas de la maladie de Hodgkin a donné la répartition suivante:

- type à prédominance lymphocytaire (PL):   37 cas, soit 26,6%
- type à sclérose nodulaire (SN)   : 15 cas, soit 10,8%
- type à cellularité mixte (CM)   : 44 cas, soit 31,6%
- type à déplétion lymphocytaire (DL)   : 43 cas, soit 30,9%

La distribution générale selon l'âge est illustrée dans la Figure 1 (article en préparation), tandis que le Tableau 2 présente la répartition des différents types histologiques de la maladie de Hodgkin selon l'âge. Les Tableaux 3 et 4 montrent la répartition des différents types histologiques selon le sexe et selon la localisation.

Tableau 2. Répartition des différents types histologiques de la maladie de Hodgkin selon l'âge

Age	PL	SN	CM	DL	Total
0 - 10 ans	4	1	7	2	14
10 - 20 ans	9	4	5	15	33
20 - 30 ans	7	5	9	8	29
30 - 40 ans	11	4	13	11	39
40 - 50 ans	3	1	6	2	12
50 - 60 ans	3	0	3	3	9
60 - 70 ans	0	0	1	2	3
Total	37	15	44	43	139

PL = type à prédominance lymphocytaire; SN = type à sclérose nodulaire; CM = type à cellularité mixte; DL = type à déplétion lymphocytaire

FIG. 1. DISTRIBUTION DE PRINCIPAUX LYMPHOMES SELON L'AGE

Lymphome de Burkitt (——); lymphome de Hodgkin (...); lymphome lymphocytaire peu différencié (---);lymphome histiocytaire (- ■ ■); lymphome indifférencié (-·-); lymphome lymphocytaire bien diffé-rencié (x)

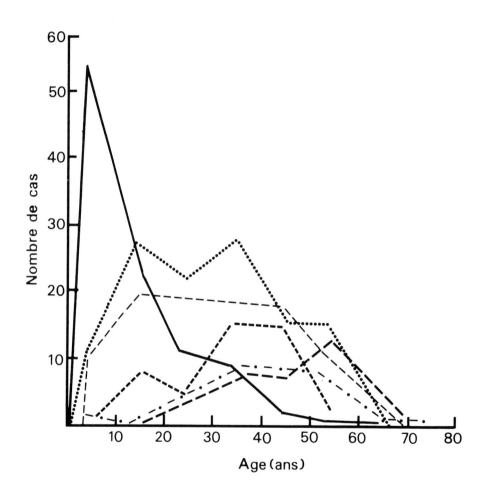

Tableau 3. Distribution de la maladie de Hodgkin selon le type histologique et selon le sexe

Type	Sexe		Total
	M	F	
PL	30	7	37
SN	9	6	15
CM	29	15	44
DL	32	11	43
Total	100	39	139

PL = type à prédominance lymphocytaire; SN = type à sclérose nodulaire; CM = type à cellularité mixte; DL = type à déplétion lymphocytaire

Tableau 4. Etude de différents type histologiques de la maladie de Hodgkin selon le site

Type	GlC	AGl	TD	R	NP	Total
PL	13	17	2	0	5	37
SN	4	10	1	0	0	15
CM	16	18	0	0	10	44
DL	19	20	1	1	2	43
Total	52	65	4	1	17	139

GlC = ganglions cervicaux; AGl = autres ganglions; TD = tube digestif; R = rate; NP = site non précisé

DISCUSSION

La maladie de Hodgkin est le lymphome le plus fréquent dans cette étude: 139 cas sur 527, soit 26,4%. En Grande-Bretagne et aux Etats-Unis d'Amérique, c'est également le lymphome le plus communément rencontré (Anderson et coll. 1970).

Sur le plan histologique, ce sont les types à cellularité mixte et à déplétion lymphocytaire qui sont les plus fréquents dans notre étude. Le Tableau 5 compare les types histologiques de la maladie de Hodgkin dans divers pays à nos observations au Zaïre.

Tableau 5. Fréquence des types histologique de la maladie de Hodgkin dans divers pays (tous âges)

Auteurs	Pays	No. de cas	PL %	SN %	CM %	DL %
Wright (1973)	Uganda	128	18	12	50	20
Lukes & Butler (1966)	USA	377	16	40	26	28
Kadin et coll. (1971)	USA	117	11	73	16	0
Baroni & Malchiodi (1980)	Italie	184	13,5	32	39,1	15,2
Présente étude	Zaïre	139	26,5	11	31,5	31

En Ouganda (Wright, 1973) comme au Zaïre, on observe une faible proportion de lymphomes Hodgkiniens de type à sclérose nodulaire et une forte proportion à cellularité mixte et à déplétion lymphocytaire. Ces deux derniers types représentent ensemble 70% des cas de la maladie de Hodgkin dans le travail de Wright (1973) et 61% des cas de la présente étude. Aux Etats-Unis (Lukes & Butler, 1966; Kadin et coll., 1971) et en Italie (Baroni & Malchiodi, 1980), il existe une forte proportion du type à sclérose nodulaire (respectivement, 40%, 73% et 32% pour chacune des études) et moins de formes à cellularité mixte (respectivement, 26%, 16% et 39,1%) et à déplétion lymphocytaire (respectivement, 28%, 0% et 15,2%).   Une étude sud-africaine (Cohen & Hamilton, 1980) montre également la prédominance de la forme à sclérose nodulaire chez les blancs.

La prédominance des formes graves de la maladie dans les milieux sous-développés pourrait s'expliquer par les mauvaises conditions socio-économiques et la faiblesse de l'immunité due aux fréquentes maladies infectieuses et parasitaires et à la malnutrition.   En outre, les consultations tardives du fait d'une infrastructure sanitaire déficiente donnent rarement au médecin l'occasion d'observer les formes précoces de la maladie.   Aussi, l'hypothèse selon laquelle ces différences seraient dues à un facteur racial plutôt qu'aux conditions de vie demeure purement spéculative.

La répartition générale selon l'âge montre une courbe bimodale dont les pics sont situés au cours de la deuxième et de la quatrième décades.   Cette bimodalité a été décrite par d'autres auteurs (Baroni & Malchiodi, 1980;   Cohen & Hamilton, 1980).   Mac Mahon (1966) a vu dans cette bimodalité la preuve que la maladie de Hodgkin recouvre non pas une mais deux entités.   Cette hypothèse est controversée (Smithers, 1970).

L'étude des différents types histologiques de la maladie de Hodgkin en fonction de l'âge (Tableau 1) ne montre pas de corrélation.

La répartition selon le sexe montre une prédominance des hommes sur les femmes avec un sex-ratio de 1,56:1.   Comme pour l'âge, il n'existe pas une corrélation entre un type histologique donné et le sexe (Tableau 3).

La distribution selon le site anatomique (Tableau 4) montre que le lymphome de Hodgkin est essentiellement une maladie des ganglions.   Les localisations en dehors de ces territoires sont rares: 5 cas seulement sur 139.   Il n'y a pas de rapport entre le site anatomique et le type histologique.

Des études complémentaires dans d'autres zones du Zaïre sont nécessaires avant d'étendre définitivement ces résultats à l'ensemble du pays, car notre Laboratoire ne dessert environ que les deux tiers du pays.   La région du Shaba lui échappe complètement.   La plus grande partie du matériel biopsique provient de Kinshasa et du Bas-Zaïre à cause de leur proximité avec les Cliniques Universitaires.   Néanmoins, les résultats présentés ici

offrent aux médecins praticiens du Zaïre un profil de la pathologie de la maladie de Hodgkin et situent cette maladie par rapport
aux autres lymphomes. Ces cancers ne sont pas rares dans la
pratique médicale courante de ce pays.

REMERCIEMENTS

Les auteurs remercient Mr M. Mazhunda et Mme M. Diyoyo pour
la dactylographie, Mr. M. Mawaba et Mr M. Roseleers pour les
microphotographies et les figures.

REFERENCES

Anderson, R.E., Ishida, K., Li, Y., Ishimaru, T. & Nishiyama, H.
    (1970) Geographic aspects of malignant lymphomas and multi-
    ple myeloma. Amer. J. Path., 61, 58-98

Baroni, C.D. & Malchiodi, F. (1980) Histology, age and sex dis-
    tribution, and pathologic correlations of Hodgkin's disease.
    A study of 184 cases observed in Rome, Italy. Cancer, 45,
    1549-1555

Cohen, C. & Hamilton, D.G. (1980) Epidemiologic and histologic
    patterns of Hodgkin's disease. Comparison of the black and
    white populations of Johannesburg, South Africa. Cancer,
    46, 186-189

De Smet, M.P. (1956) Observations cliniques de tumeurs malignes
    des tissus réticuloendothéliaux et des tissus hémolympho-
    poïétiques au Congo. Ann. Soc. belge Méd. Trop., 36, 56-70

Doll, R., Payne, P. & Waterhouse, J.A.H., eds (1966) Cancer
    Incidence in Five Continents, Vol. 1, UICC, Berlin, Springer

Doll, R., Muir, C.S., Waterhouse, J.A.H., eds (1970) Cancer
    Incidence in Five Continents, Vol. II, UICC, Genève,
    Springer

Jackson, H., Jr & Parker, F., Jr (1947) Hodgkin's Disease and
    Allied Disorders, New York, Oxford University Press

Kadin, M.E., Glastein, E. & Dorfman, R.F. (1971) Clinicopatho-
    logic studies of 117 untreated patients subjected to laparo-
    tomy for the staging of Hodgkin's disease. Cancer, 27,
    1277-1294

Lukes, R.J. & Butler, J.J. (1966) The pathology and nomenclature
    of Hodgkin's disease. Cancer Res., 26, 1063-1081

Mac Mahon, B. (1966) Epidemiology of Hodgkin's disease. Cancer
    Res., 26, 1189-1200

Rappaport, H. (1966) Malignant lymphomas. In: Tumors of the
    Hematopoietic System, Washington DC, Amer. Forces Institute
    of Pathology, pp. 91-155

Smithers, D.W. (1970) Hodgkin's disease: one entity or two?
    Lancet, ii, 1285-1287

Templeton, A.C., ed. (1973) Tumors in a Tropical Country,
    Berlin, Springer-Verlag

Thys, A. (1957) Considérations sur les tumeurs malignes des
    indigènes du Congo Belge et du Ruanda-Burundi. A propos de
    2 546 cas. Ann. Soc. belge Med. Trop., 37, 483-514

Wright, D.H. (1973) Lymphoreticular neoplasms. In: A.C.
    Templeton, ed., Tumors in Tropical Country, Berlin,
    Springer-Verlag, pp. 270-291

SOME BIOLOGICAL AND EPIDEMIOLOGICAL CHARACTERISTICS OF HUMAN LEUKAEMIA IN AFRICANS

C.K.O. Williams

Department of Haematology
College of Medicine
University of Ibadan
Ibadan, Nigeria

RESUME

Des rapports provenant de différentes parties d'Afrique ont permis de définir les caractères épidémiologiques de la leucémie: (1) le diagnostic de leucémie aiguë lymphoblastique (LAL) est peu fréquent avant l'âge de 5 ans; (2) la leucémie aiguë myéloblastique (LAM) est fréquemment associée à la présence de chloromes; (3) l'apparition de leucémie lymphoïde chronique (LLC) est fréquente avant l'âge de 50 ans, en particulier chez les femmes.

Les caractères biologiques et épidémiologiques des sous-types de leucémies ont été déterminés chez 146 patients qui ont été suivis prospectivement de juillet 1978 à juin 1982. Il y avait 44 cas de leucémie myéloïde chronique (LMC), 34 cas de LAL, 33 de LAM et 31 de LLC. L'incidence et la distribution des LMC selon l'âge sont similaires à Ibadan et dans les populations noires et blanches des Etats-Unis. L'incidence des LAL chez les enfants de 0 à 4 ans d'Ibadan est inférieure respectivement à un tiers et à un dixième de celles observées chez les enfants noirs et chez les enfants blancs des Etats-Unis; mais entre 10 et 14 ans, l'incidence de la maladie est la même dans les trois populations. La LAM semble être plus fréquente chez les enfants Nigérians de 5 à 9 ans que chez les enfants des Etats-Unis; chez cinq des neuf enfants de ce groupe d'âge (55,6%), elle était associée à un chlorome. Les enfants atteints de LAL ont globalement un statut socio-économique significativement plus élevé que ceux atteints de LAM. Avant 50 ans, la LLC survient de façon prédominante chez les femmes (ratio homme:femme = 1:6) qui ont un

statut socio-économique significativement plus bas que celles qui
ont une LMC. A 50 ans ou plus, la maladie prédomine chez les
sujets de sexe masculin (ratio homme:femme = 5:3).

Tous les patients atteints de LAL possédaient de nombreux
facteurs associés à un pronostic défavorable parmi lesquels le
sexe masculin (25/34) une leucocytose > 10^{10}/litre (31/34),
>10^{11}/litre (10/34), une morphologie L-2 ou L-3 (21/25), une
réaction négative à l'acide périodique de Schiff (15/19) et une
invasion tissulaire (15/34), ce qui donne l'impression que chez
les jeunes Nigérians, la LAL est essentiellement de type agressif
et hyperprolifératif. Les caractères épidémiologiques de la LAL
et de la LLC observés chez les Africains suggèrent que le style
de vie joue un rôle dans la leucémogenèse tandis que les traits
cliniques de ces maladies suggèrent que les caractéristiques
biologiques sont différentes de celles observées pour les mêmes
maladies dans les pays développés.

SUMMARY

Reports from various parts of Africa have documented the
epidemiological features of leukaemia as including: (1) infrequent diagnosis of acute lymphoblastic leukaemia (ALL) below
the age of 5 years;   (2) frequent association of acute myelogenous leukaemia (AML) with chloromas;   (3) frequent occurrence,
predominantly in women, of chronic lymphocytic leukaemia (CLL)
below the age of 50 years.   The biological and epidemiological
features of leukaemia subtypes were determined in 146 patients
who were seen prospectively between July 1978 and June 1982.
There were 44 cases of chronic myelocytic leukaemia (CML), 34 of
ALL, 33 of AML and 31 of CLL. The age distribution and incidence
of CML in Ibadan was similar to those of the Black and White
populations of the United States.   The incidence of ALL in 0-4
year-old Ibadan children was estimated to be less than one-third
and one-tenth of those of Black and White children in the United
States, respectively, but the incidence of the disease was
similar for the 3 populations in the third quinquennium.   AML
appeared to be more prevalent in 5-9-year-old Nigerian children
than in children in the United States and was associated with
chloroma in 5 of 9 (55.6%) children in the age-group.   As a
group, children with ALL were of significantly higher socioeconomic status than those with AML. CLL occurred below 50 years
predominantly in women (male:female = 1:6) who were significantly
of lower socioeconomic status than their CML counterparts.   Male

patients predominated (male:female = 5.3) at and above 50 years. Numerous factors indicating a poor prognosis co-existed in all ALL_1 patients, including male sex (25/34), WBC $>10^{10}$/litre (31/34, $>10^{11}$/litre (10/34), L2 or L3 morphology (21/25), periodic acid Schiff (PAS) negativity (15/19) and tissue invasion (15/34), thus giving the impression that ALL in young Nigerians is predominantly of an aggressive and hyperproliferative type. The epidemiological features of ALL and CLL in Africans suggest a role for the influence of life-style in leukaemognesis while the clinical patterns of these disorders suggest that the biological characteristics differ from those of similar diseases in developed countries.

INTRODUCTION

Epidemiological characteristics recognizable from descriptions of human leukaemias from various parts of Africa include infrequent diagnosis of acute lymphoblastic leukaemia (ALL) in the first quinquennium (Table 1) (O'Conor & Davies, 1960; Allan & Watson-Williams, 1963; Sonnet et al., 1966; Gelfand, 1967; Haddock, 1967; Lothe, 1967; Kasili & Taylor, 1970; Edington & Hendrickse, 1972; Essien, 1972; Jeffrey & Gelfand, 1972; Amsel & Nabembezi, 1974; Lowe, 1974; Williams, 1975; Fleming, 1979; Williams et al., 1982, 1984), frequent association of childhood acute myelogenous leukaemia (AML) with chloromas (Davies & Owor, 1965; Essien, 1972; Templeton, 1973; Williams et al., 1982, 1984) and frequent occurrence of chronic lymphocytic leukaemia (CLL) below the age of 50 years, especially in women (Table 2) (Sonnet et al., 1966; Haddock, 1967, Lothe, 1967; Kasili & Taylor, 1970; Jeffrey & Gelfand, 1972; Essien, 1976; Kela-We, 1977; Fleming, 1979; Williams & Bamgboye, 1983; Williams et al., 1984). Unlike the situation reported from developed Western countries, where acute leukaemia represents about 60% of all leukaemia subtypes, the chronic leukaemias make up between 50 and 70% of all leukaemia subtypes in series from various African countries (Table 3). For unknown reasons, the East African series appear to have a higher percentage of acute, and a lower percentage of chronic leukaemias than the West African ones and vice versa (Table 3). While the observation of a lower percentage of acute leukaemia in all African series vis-a-vis the experience in developed countries would ordinarily suggest under-diagnosis of the disease due to the rapid demise of the patients with this

type of leukaemia, it has been suggested that the situation may
be due, at least in part, to unknown environmental factors (Allan
& Watson-Williams, 1963; Davies, 1965; Williams et al., 1982).

Table 1. Acute leukaemia in Africa[a]

Countries	Study period	Total No.		% ALL ≼ 5 years	% AML with chloroma	ALL/AML ratio	Reference
		ALL	AML				
Central Africa							
Zaire	1958-1963	?10	7	0	1/7	10:7	Sonnet et al., 1966
East Africa							
Kenya	1967-1969	6	12	16.7	NG	1:2	Kasili & Taylor, 1970
Uganda	1952-1958[b]	2	5	NG	NG	2:5	O'Conor & Davies, 1960
Uganda	1965-1966	NG	NG	?10.8	11	NG	Lothe, 1967
Southern Africa							
Harare, Zimbabwe	1959-1964	? 5	?10	0	NG	?1:2	Gelfand, 1964
Harare, Zimbabwe	1967-1969	11	10	?14.2	0	1:2	Jeffrey & Gelfand, 1972
Harare, Zimbabwe	1967-1972	25[c]	21	8.5	?	1:1	Lowe, 1974
West Africa							
Ibadan, Nigeria	1958-1962	NG	NG	?2.8	NG	NG	Allan & Watson-Williams 1963
Ibadan, Nigeria	1958-1968	26	57	3.3	3.5	1:2	Essien, 1972
Ibadan, Nigeria	1978-1982	30	31	12.9	22.6	1:1	Williams et al., 1984
Zaria/Kaduna, Nigeria	1970-1976	21	28	9.5	NG	3:4	Fleming, 1979

[a] NG = not given

[b] Childhood leukaemias only

[c] Including cases of undifferentiated leukaemia

     Apart from those clinical features that can be explained on
the basis of late presentation, chronic myeloid leukaemia (CML)
in the African appears to have biological features similar to
those observed and reported in Caucasians in developed countries.
The same appears to be true for the myeloproliferative syndromes
in general (C.K.O. Williams, unpublished data). The lymphoproliferative syndromes, however including ALL, CLL and the
lymphomas, show unique biological characteristics in Africans.
The biological characteristics of childhood ALL, as observed in
Ibadan, Nigeria, and in the Black children of Johannesburg, South
Africa (Kusman et al., 1980; Williams, 1984; MacDougall &
Janowitz, unpublished data) are more like those of T-ALL than
those of 'common ALL' (c-ALL) (Greaves et al., 1981). In fact,
it has been suggested on clinical grounds that c-ALL is a very
infrequent disease in Ibadan (Williams et al., 1982) and this is

Table 2. Sex-ratios among patients with chronic lymphocytic leukaemia in various African countries[a]

Countries	Study period	No. of cases	< 50 years Male:Female	> 50 years Male:Female	All ages Male:Female	Reference
Central Africa						
Zaire	1958-1963	9	0:1	3:1	2:1	Sonnet et al., 1966
East Africa						
Uganda	1963-1966	16	5:3	5:3	5:3	Lothe, 1967
Southern Africa						
Harare, Zimbabwe	1959-1964	6	NG	NG	NG	Gelfand, 1962
Harare, Zimbabwe	1967-1968	12	2:1	2:3	3:1	Jeffrey & Gelfand, 1972
Harare, Zimbabwe	1967-1972	16	6:1	5:4	2:1	Lowe, 1974
West Africa						
Accra, Ghana	1956-1966	25	NG	NG	16:9	Haddock, 1967
Ibadan, Nigeria	1958-1968	85	NG	NG	1:1	Essien, 1976
Ibadan, Nigeria	1978-1982	31	1:6	2:1	??	Williams et al., 1984
Zaria/Kaduna, Nigeria	1970-1976	47	3:7	2:1	..1:1	Fleming, 1979

[a] NG = not given

Table 3. Distribution of leukaemia subtypes in various African countries

Location	Period	No. of cases	Leukaemia subtypes (%)						Reference
			ALL	AML	AL	CML	CLL	CL	
Central Africa									
Zaire	1958-1963	35	?28.5	25.8	54.3	20.0	25.7	45.7	Sonnet et al., 1966
East Africa									
Nairobi, Kenya	1967-1969	105	27.8	24.6	52.4	25.4	16.2	41.6	Kasili & Taylor, 1970
Kampala, Uganda	1963-1967	88	20.8	31.2	52.3	29.5	18.2	47.7	Lothe, 1967
Southern Africa									
Harare, Zimbabwe	1967-1969	58	29.3	19.0	48.3	27.6	20.7	48.3	Jeffrey & Gelfand, 1972
Harare, Zimbabwe	1962-1972	95	26.3	22.1	48.4	34.7	16.8	51.6	Lowe, 1974
West Africa									
Accra, Ghana	1956-1966	53	NG	NG	29	25.5	45.5	71.0	Haddock, 1967
Ibadan, Nigeria	1958-1962	108	NG	NG	33.3	28.7	38.0	66.7	Allan & Watson-Williams, 1963
Ibadan, Nigeria	1958-1968	262	9.9	21.8	31.7	34.4	31.6	66.0	Essien, 1972, 1976
Ibadan, Nigeria	1978-1982	137	21.9	22.6	44.5	32.8	22.6	55.5	Williams et al., 1984
Kaduna/Zaria, Nigeria	1970-1976	136	15.4	20.5	36.0	29.4	34.6	64	Fleming, 1979

consistent with the views of Ramot and Magrath (1982) that it is predominantly a disease of affluent societies.

Not only does the frequent occurrence before the age of 50 years distinguish CLL as seen in Africa from its mode of manifestation elsewhere, but the disease also usually presents in Africa with marked splenomegaly and lymphadenopathy (Haddock, 1967; Gelfand, 1967; Essien, 1976), thereby resembling the less common European 'forme splénique pure' of French authors (Payet et al., 1960).

The earlier suggestion that the deviant biological and epidemiological features of childhood ALL in Ibadan, Nigeria, could be attributed to unknown environmental factors (Williams et al., 1982) has been supported by the views of Ramot and Magrath (1982) as well as by further analysis of the relationships between leukaemia subtypes and the life-style of the people in the area (Williams et al., 1984). In this report the biological and epidemiological features of human leukaemias in Africa are again described and the relationship between the life-style of the people and the patterns of human leukaemia subtypes is examined.

MATERIALS AND METHODS

A prospective study of patients diagnosed as suffering from various forms of leukaemia was undertaken at the Department of Haematology, University College Hospital (UCH), Ibadan, Nigeria, between 1 July 1978 and 30 June 1982. The diagnosis of leukaemia was based on clinical findings and the results of haematological investigations including full blood counts (FBC), peripheral blood cell morphology by a Romanovsky stain and bone marrow morphology by May-Gruenwald-Giemsa stain. Of the other special cytochemical stains in use for differentiating between the various leukaemia subtypes, only the periodic acid-Schiff (PAS) stain was regularly available.

Since recent census figures for the Nigerian population were not available, a rough estimate of leukaemia incidence for Ibadan city was made, based on a projection of the population sizes of the various age-groups of males and females derived from the last reliable census held in 1963 in Nigeria. For this purpose, a number of guide-lines recommended by national Nigerian and international bodies were taken into consideration. These included an assumption of a constant growth-rate of between 2.5% (Federal Office of Statistics, 1968) and 5.0% (Onibokun et al., 1981) for Ibadan since 1963, and a recent report (World Bank, 1981) that 47.2%, 50.3% and 2.5% of the Nigerian population were within the age-groups 0-14, 15-64 and 65 years and above, respectively. A fuller description of the methods used in the estimation of leukaemia incidence in these patients has recently been published (Williams & Bamgboye, 1983).

In order to evaluate the probable influence of life-style on the patterns of subtypes as observed among our patients, the socioeconomic status of the patients was characterized on a scale ranging from 1 to 5 according to their level of education and their occupation. In socioeconomic status (SES) class 1 were grouped highly educated individuals, senior public officers and business executives; SES 2: post-secondary-school educated, middle-level public officers; SES 3: post-primary-school educated, lower-level public officers and skilled hand-workers; SES 4: primary-school-educated and unskilled hand-workers; SES 5: illiterates, peasant farmers and petty traders. Applying these criteria to the socioeconomic characteristics of the population of Ibadan, as described in the works of Odebiyi (1980) and Onibokun et al. (1981), it appears that 20-30% of the Ibadan population can be categorized as SES 1, 2 or 3, respectively, and the remaining 70-80% as SES 4 or 5.

The biological nature of the leukaemias as observed in the present series has also been characterized by their response to standard chemotherapy programmes. Thus, cases of ALL were managed with vincristine, 2.0 mg/m^2 per week x 4 doses and prednisolone 40 mg/m^2 per day x 28 days. To these was added either doxorubicin hydrochloride 20-30 mg/m^2 per day x 3 doses or a combination of cyclophosphamide 600 mg/m^2 per week x 2 doses and cytosine arabinoside 50 mg/m^2, 12-hourly x 14 doses. Remission was maintained with 6 mercaptopurine 100 mg/m^2 daily and methotrexate 12.5 mg/m^2 orally twice weekly. Courses of consolidation chemotherapy were given at 3-monthly intervals using the same agents administered at remission induction at the same doses and schedules, except that prednisolone was given only for 14 days. AML was treated with cytosine arabinoside 50 mg/m^2 12-hourly x 14 doses, to which was added either doxorubicin hydrochloride alone or a combination of cyclophosphamide, vincristine and prednisolone at the same doses and schedules as described earlier, except that only 2 doses of vincristine were given and prednisolone was given for 14 days. CLL was treated with chlorambucil, 5 mg daily, while CML was treated with busulphan, 4-6 mg daily. Blastic crises of CML were managed in the same way as acute leukaemias.

RESULTS

Age and sex distribution

A total of 34 (25 male, 9 female) ALL, 33 (22 male, 11 female) AML, 33 (12 male, 21 female) CLL and 44 (26 male, 18 female) CML patients were seen at the University College Hospital (UCH), Ibadan, Nigeria, from 1 July 1978 to 30 June 1982.   The age and sex distribution of these patients are shown in Figure 1. Of the ALL patients, 8 (23.5%) were below the age of 5 years. The ratio ALL:AML below the age of 15 years was approximately 4:3.   there was a male/female ratio of 2:15 among CLL patients who were less than 50 years old, while among those who were 50 years old or more, the ratio was 5:3.   Among males, AML was predominantly a disease of childhood (median age: 9 years) while among females, the median age was 33 (9-55) years (Table 4).

FIG. 1.   AGE AND SEX DISTRIBUTION OF 144 LEUKAEMIA PATIENTS
SEEN AT UNIVERSITY COLLEGE HOSPITAL, IBADAN, NIGERIA
FROM 1 JULY 1978 TO 30 JUNE 1982

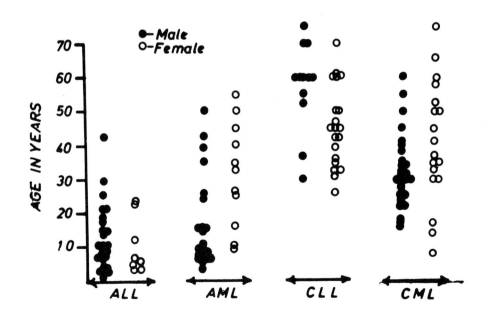

Table 4. Clinical and laboratory features of acute myelogenous leukemia (AML) in Ibadan[a]

Feature	Male	Female	Total
No. of patients	22	11	33
Median age (years)			
All age-groups	9 (3-50)	33 (9-55)	15 (3-55
Childhood	7 (3-14)	9 (9-10)	7.5 (3-14)
Chloroma-associated variant	7 (3-24)	10	7.5 (3-24)
Tissue invasion			
Median size of liver (cm below RCM)[b]	2 (0-11)	2 (0-8)	0 (0-11)
Median size of spleen (cm below LCM)[c]	2 (0-16)	3 (0-8)	2 (0-16)
Solid tumours (chloroma)	9	2	11
CNS involvement	2	0	2
Lymphadenopathy	0-+	0-+	0-+
Laboratory			
Median PCV[d] (%)	15 (8-41)	17 (8-24)	16.5 (8-41)
Median WBC x 10^9/litre	14.4 (1.0-213.0)	45.9 (16.6-160)	22.8 (1.0-213)
Myeloblastic morphology	14	9	23
Promyelocytic morphology	3	1	4
Myelomonocytic morphology	5	1	6

[a] Figures in parentheses are ranges.

[b] RCM = right costal margin

[c] LCM = left costal margin

[d] PCV = packed cell volume

Clinical and laboratory features of acute leukaemia

As shown in Table 5 and Figure 2, tissue invasion, as manifested by hepatosplenomegaly, mediastinal and testicular masses as well as infiltration of the central nervous system, occurred frequently among ALL patients. Leucocytosis in excess of 10^{10}/litre was found in all but 5 (85.3%) while 10 (29.4%) had WBC > 10^{11}/litre. There was a correlation between leucocyte count and the presence of tissue invasion; above a WBC of 10^{11}/litre and below 10^{10}/litre, 9 out of 10 and 2 out of 5, respectively, had evidence of tissue invasion (Fig. 2). Among AML patients, tissue invasion was less common and leucocytosis was less marked than in ALL. There was no correlation between tissue invasion and the degree of leucocytosis. Where they occurred, the chloromas (Fig. 3) were associated with childhood

AML (30%);   5 out of 9 (55.6%) AML cases observed in the second quinquennium were associated with chloromas.

Table 5. clinical and laboratory features of acute lymphoblastic leukemia (ALL) in Ibadan[a]

Feature	Male	Female	Total
No. of patients	25	9	34
Median age (years)			
All age-groups	10 (0.6-42)	6.0 (5.5-23)	9.5 (0.6-42)
Childhood	7 (0.6-14)	5.5 (4-12)	6 (0.6-14)
Tissue invasion			
Median size of liver (cm below RCM)[b]	6 (0-16)	5 (0-9)	5 (0-16)
Median size of spleen (cm below LCM)[c]	9 (0-15)	8 (0-17)	9 (0-17)
Mediastinal mass	6	0	6
CNS invasion	4	0	4
Testicular mass	5	0	5
Laboratory			
Median PCV[d]	18 (11-43)	18 (9-40)	18 (9-43)
Median WBC x 10^9/litre	120.0 (3.4-683)	20.1 (3.4-51)	75 (3.4-683)
FAB classification:			
L-1	2	2	4
L-2	15	5	20
L-3	1	0	1
Cytochemistry:			
PAS-positive[e]	3	1	4
PAS-negative[f]	11	4	15

[a] Figures in parentheses are ranges.

[b] RCM = right costal margin

[c] LCM = left costal margin

[d] PCV = packed cell volume

[e] 0-10% cells positive

[f] ≥20% cells positive

FIG. 2.   CLINICAL FEATURES OF ALL AND AML

Dots represent cases of tissue invasion in ALL, while closed
squares represent cases of chloroma in patients with AML.

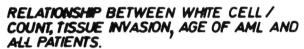

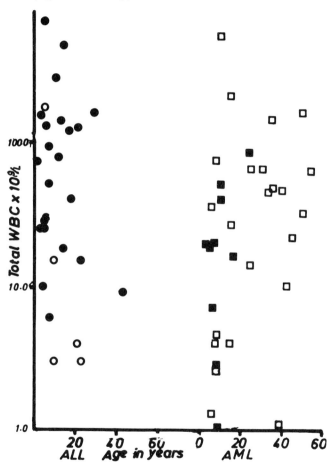

FIG. 3. ORBITAL CHLOROMAS IN A 9-YEAR OLD NIGERIAN BOY

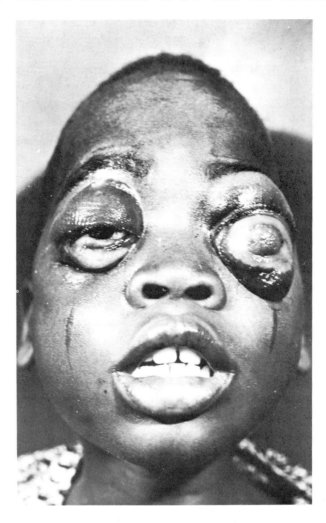

The most common morphological variant in ALL was L-2, and
this was observed in 20 (80%) out of 25 cases, while in 15 (79%)
out of 19 cases the PAS cytochemical test was negative.   The
myeloblastic variant with 23 (69.7%) out of 33 cases, was the
most common morphological variant of AML, followed by the myelo-
monocytic variant, which occurred in 6 (18.2%) out of 33 cases
(Table 4).

Treatment response and survival of 65 acute leukaemia patients (33 ALL and 32 AML) are shown in terms of remission rate in Table 6 and the life-table plot in Figure 4. Four (16%) of 25 ALL and 14 (48.3%) of 29 of AML patients died early, either before or shortly after commencement of chemotherapy, usually from infection or haemorrhage or both. The two longest surviving ALL and AML patients died around days 600 and 350, respectively (Fig. 4).

Table 6. Outcome of chemotherapy in acute leukemia

Outcome	ALL	AML
Complete remission	12	6
Partial remission	3	2
No remission	6	7
Early death	4	14
Total evaluable patients	25	29

Chronic leukaemias

The clinical and laboratory features of CLL, as observed in 15 patients below the age of 50 years and 16 older patients, are shown in Table 7. There appear to be a few differences in the nature of the disease as seen in the two groups; the median leucocyte count is lower in the younger age-group (53.4×10^9/litre versus 37.0×10^9/litre), while the disease appears to be less lethal in the younger, as compared with the older age-group. Furthermore, 4 (25%) of the 16 older patients had skin manifestations, unlike the younger group, where none of the 15 patients had such manifestations.

FIG. 4.   SURVIVAL OF PATIENTS WITH ALL AND AML
SEEN AT UNIVERSITY COLLEGE HOSPITAL, IBADAN, NIGERIA
1979-1982

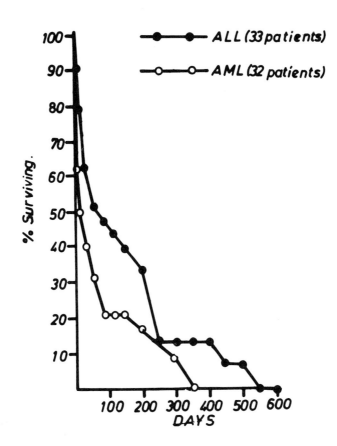

Massive hepato- and/or splenomegaly was present in all CML patients. About 30% of these patients presented either in a state of blastic crisis or transformed into that state within 3 months of initial presentation. A history of chronic illness with an abdominal mass of 1-3 years duration was usually obtained from CML patients at the time of first presentation. If deaths within the first 3-4 months are excluded, the median survival of CML patients was 2-3 years in this series.

Table 7. Clinical and laboratory features of chronic lymphocytic leukaemia seen at the UCH, Ibadan, Nigeria, 1978-1982[a]

Feature	$\leq$ 50 years	$\geq$ 50 years
Number of cases	15	16
Median age (years)	37 (26-47)	60 (50-75)
Male:female ratio	2:13	5:3
Lymphadenopathy	+ (4) - ++ (1)	+ (1) - +++ (8)
Liver (cm below costal margin)	5 (0-10)	7 (0-17)
Spleen (cm below costal margin)	20 (0-25)	17 (0-29)
Cutaneous manifestation	0	4
Median PCV[b]	28 (18-49)	32.5 (20-45)
Median lymphocyte count (x 10^9/litre)	53.5 (11.0-640.0)	37.0 (10.0-458.0)
Bone marrow involvement	4/4	4/4
Response to treatment:		
Good	8	3
poor	1	5
Unavailable	6	8
Survival:		
Died	3	8
Defaulted	7	8
Lived > 1 year after diagnosis	5	0

[a] Figures in parentheses are ranges

[b] PCV = packed cell volume

The socioeconomic status of the patients with various leukaemia subtypes is given in Table 8 in the form of mean scores on a socioeconomic scale (SES) ranging from 1 to 5 (see Materials and Methods). Childhood ALL was associated with a significantly lower mean score than that for comparable AML patients ($p <$ 0.05), thus suggesting that this disease was associated with a higher socioeconomic status than childhood AML. Furthermore, there was a trend towards a lower mean score from the third to the first quinquennium among children with ALL, although the trend was not statistically significant. Thus, the younger the child with ALL the greater the likelihood of his being of higher socioeconomic status. CLL occurring in patients under 50 years of age was significantly associated with a lower socioeconomic status than that of their CML counterparts ($p <$ 0.05) and this

was particularly so among women with CLL, who were all scored as
SES 5.

Table 8.   Characteristics of patients with various leukaemia
subtypes, as measured on a socioeconomic scale (SES) (mean
score), University College Hospital, Ibadan, Nigeria, 1978-1982[a]

Age-groups	ALL	AML	CLL	CML
0-4	3.8 (3-5)	-	-	-
5-9	4.25 (3-5)	4.6 (4-6)[b]	-	-
10-14	4.43 (1-5)	5.0[c]	-	5.0
15-19	4.5 (4.5)	4.0	-	4.0 (4.4)
20-24	3.75 (2-5)	5[d]	-	2.7 (2-4)
25-29	4 (4-5)	3.3 (2-4)	5.0	4.5 (4-5)
30-34	-	5.0	5.0 (5x3)	3.6 (1-5)
35-39	-	3.6 (2-5)	4.0 (2-5)	5.0
40-44	-	1.0	5.0	4.7 (4-5)
45-49	-	-	5.0	4.0
50-54	-	4.5 (4-5)	5.0	5.0
55-59	-	4	5.0	5.0
60-64	-	-	5.0	5.0
65-69	-	-	-	-
70-74	-	-	5.0	-
75-79	-	-	3.0	2.5
All age-groups	4.19 (1-5)	4.19 (1-5)	4.82 (2-5)	4.18 (1-5)

[a] Figures in parentheses are ranges.

[b] Including 5 cases of chloroma associated AML (CA-AML) with a mean
SES of 4.8 (4-5)

[c] Including 2 cases of CA-AML with a SES of 5

[d] Including a case of CA-AML with a SES of 5

DISCUSSION

From the numerous publications describing the biological and epidemiological features of the leukaemias in Africa (O'Conor & Davies, 1960; Allan & Watson-Williams, 1963; Davies & Owor, 1965; Sonnet et al., 1966; Gelfand, 1967; Haddock, 1967; Lothe, 1967; Kasili & Taylor, 1970; Edington & Hendrickse, 1972; Essien, 1972; Jeffrey & Gelfand, 1972; Templeton, 1973; Amsel & Nabembezi, 1974; Lowe, 1974; Williams, 1975; Essien, 1976; Kela-We, 1977; Fleming, 1979; Williams et al., 1979, 1984; Williams & Bamgboye, 1983) a number of unique features of this group of diseases which have previously been recognized, have been further confirmed in the analysis of the cases evaluated in the present series. A comparison of the incidence rates for acute leukaemia in Ibadan and in Black and White patients in the USA is shown in Table 9. The most striking differences occurred in the first quinquennium, in which ALL was at least 10 times as common in White and at least twice as common in Black children in the USA as in Ibadan children. AML, however, was at least twice as common in Ibadan as in the Black and White children in the USA. ALL in Ibadan children was frequently associated with biological characteristics indicating a poor prognosis, including high WBC at presentation, negative reaction to PAS, L-2 morphology, male sex and evidence of tissue invasion at presentation. It is therefore not surprising that the treatment response in these patients was poorer than would have been expected in Caucasian children in the USA treated with a comparable chemotherapeutic regimen (C.K.O. Williams, unpublished data). The most striking biological characteristic of AML in parts of Africa is its frequent association, especially in childhood, with chloromas (Davies & Owor, 1965; Williams et al., 1982). Using routine techniques it did not appear in the present series of patients that a particular cytological variant of AML was associated with chloroma formation.

Table 9. Comparison of leukemia incidence rates[a] in patients in Ibadan, Nigeria, and the USA

Type of leukaemia and age-group	Ibadan	USA	
		Blacks[b]	Whites[b]
ALL			
0–4	<0.35–0.69	1.5	4.7
5–9	<0.41–0.82	1.2	2.2
10–14	<0.80–1.6	0.9	1.3
0–14	0.3–1.0	1.3	2.46
0–74	~0.18–0.37	?	0.1
AML			
0–4	<0.11–0.23	0.5	0.8
5–9	<1.0–2.2	0.6	0.6
10–14	<0.16–0.32	0.5	0.5
0–14	0.27–0.90	0.47	0.74
0–74	~0.28–0.58	0.2	0.4
All leukaemia variants			
0–74	0.89–1.8	0.7	0.8

[a] Per 100 000

[b] Source: Young et al. (1981)

By its presentation with minimal lymphadenopathy and massive splenomegaly, CLL appears to mimic the classical presentation of CML, as described in the Caucasian by Wintrobe (1967) and, with the possible exception of the variant of the disease occurring below 50 years, CLL in Nigerians does not appear to be as indolent a disease as described in Caucasians of similar age. Thus there may be some biological differences between CLL in Africans and in the Caucasians of Western Europe and the USA.

The most striking epidemiological feature of acute leukaemia in Africans is the deficit of ALL in the first quinquennium. While this observation has been attributed to underdiagnosis by some authors (Lothe, 1967; Vanier & Pike, 1967), others have suggested that the deficit may be real and may reflect a unique feature of ALL in Africa (Davies, 1965; Williams et al., 1982, 1984; Williams & Bamgboye, 1983). Of particular interest are the differential rates of change in the incidence of the leukaemias in the various age-groups. For example in Ibadan, Nigeria, the incidence of ALL appears to have increased two-fold between 1958-1968 and 1978-1982, unlike the incidence of AML, CLL and CML, which showed much smaller changes (Williams et al., 1984). The most marked change was observed in the incidence rate of childhood ALL, especially in the first quinquennium.

Children with ALL as a group are of higher socioeconomic status as compared to those with AML, and this appears to be particularly so in the 0-4 year age-group (Table 8). Thus, the Ibadan experience suggests an association between increasing affluence and increasing incidence of ALL in the first quinquennium. There appear to be several ways of explaining this association: (1) mortality in the first quinquennium may be lowest among people of higher socioeconomic status, thus making it possible for ALL, a typical neoplastic disease of the first 4 years of life, to emerge at a higher incidence rate; (2) it is possible that the life-style of those of higher socioeconomic status is associated with exposure of the child (and probably also of the mother) to the causative agent(s) of ALL; (3) the life-style of those of higher socioeconomic status may lead to an alteration in the biology of the lymphoid system and consequently in the pattern of neoplastic lymphoproliferative diseases occurring in this group of people; (4) various combinations of these causes may be operative at different degrees.

There is evidence in the literature associating the early-peak pattern of childhood leukaemia with improvements in the life-style of people in various parts of the developed world, and although this association is now so characteristic of childhood ALL in developed societies, it emerged at different times in these societies (Magrath & Ramot, 1982). Similarly, chloroma formation used to be a more frequent complication of AML in the past in Europe (Davies & Hayhoe, quoted by Fleming, 1979), although it was recently estimated that this complication now occurs about 30 times more frequently in Ibadan than in British children (Williams et al., 1982).

Apart from its association with the female sex (male:female = 1:6), CLL occurring before 50 years of age also appears to be associated with the lowest socioeconomic status (Fleming, 1979; Williams et al., 1984). However, poor education of women above 30 years of age is a very common feature in the Ibadan area, so that it is not clear what role, if any, illiteracy may play in the pathogenesis of CLL in women before the age of 50 years.

Preliminary investigations of the immunological phenotypic characteristics of peripheral blood and/or bone marrow leucocytes of 17 consecutive previously untreated ALL patients in Ibadan revealed 2 cases of c-ALL, 1 of null-ALL, 13 of T-ALL and 2 of B-ALL. There were 8 children among these patients, of whom 1 had c-ALL (a 20-month-old girl), 1 had null-ALL, 6 had T-ALL and none had B-ALL (C.K.O. Williams, unpublished data). Thus, although the number of the phenotyped cases of ALL is very small, in comparison to patterns of leukaemia subtype in British children, among whom c-ALL has been estimated to account for almost 75% of cases (Greaves et al., 1981), there appears to be a severe deficit of c-ALL among Ibadan patients, especially in childhood, as well as a relative excess of T-ALL. The excess of T-ALL among our paediatric cases of ALL is consistent with the impression of the aggressive nature of ALL in Ibadan children. Characterization of 19 cases of CLL revealed that they were of B-lymphocyte phenotype, and this is consistent with experience in Caucasians in Western Europe (Preud'homme & Seligman, 1974).

The differences between the biological and epidemiological features of leukaemia in Africa and in the developed societies of Europe and the USA cannot be explained by genetic differences but rather by the marked differences in life-style and socioeconomic situation. There is a need to explain all the major features of leukaemia in Africans, if possible, in terms of the environmental and socioeconomic factors prevalent in African countries today; these include malnutrition, parasitic and other opportunistic infections and poor sanitation. Studies in both experimental animals and humans have now established that severe atrophic changes of the thymolymphatic system are a constant feature in malnutrition, and that these changes are most pronounced and least reversible when they occur during the intrauterine period or very early in infancy. The mechanism underlying these changes is believed to be related to the increased up-take of free circulating adrenocorticosteroids as well as to a deficiency of certain nutrients required for the development of the thymolymphatic system. Consequently, there is a depletion of circulating T-lymphocytes, and this is manifested in the form of an impairment of cell-mediated immunity and increased susceptibility to infection (McFarlane & Hamid, 1973; McFarlane et al., 1977; Smythe et al., 1971).

The epidemiology of human leukaemias in Africans, with the delayed childhood peak in incidence, the reduction in the lymphocytic variant, the apparent increase (at least in childhood) in the myeloid variant and the association of the latter with chloroma formation, are reminiscent of the observations of Gross (1970) on the influence of environmental factors in leukaemogneesis. Following underfeeding of Ak mice, Gross observed a delay in the onset and in the rate of occurrence of virus-induced and spontaneously occurring leukaemia. Although splenectomy of C3H mice did not alter the incidence or latency of virus-induced leukaemia, thymectomy inhibited or considerably delayed the development of lymphatic leukaemia, and frequently caused the myelogenous forms to appear later in life, often in the form of 'chloroleukaemia'. The pattern of leukaemia in Africans may thus be nature's equivalent of Gross' observations (Fig. 5).

The female excess observed in some African countries among CLL patients below the age of 50 years led to the suggestion that this might be due to pregnancy-associated immune-suppression and the additive influence of an oncogenic virus (Fleming, 1979). With the discovery of the human T-cell leukaemia virus (HTLV), Fleming (1983) speculated that this virus might be involved in the pathogenesis of CLL in middle-aged African women, apparently based on an analogy with the observation that cases of adult T-cell leukaemia/lymphoma (ATL) described by Catovsky et al. (1982) occurred mainly in Black West Indian women. From the observation that all typical cases of CLL phenotyped in Ibadan (including women under 50 years) were of B-cell type (C.K.O. Williams, unpublished data), it appears unlikely that the variant of CLL in African women under 50 years of age is HTLV-associated ATL. However, a role for HTLV in the pathogenesis of CLL can still not be ruled out, especially in view of the observation of Blattner and his colleagues (personal communication) that all but one case of CLL in Jamaicans who were positive for HTLV was of B-cell phenotype. Other environmental factors, like malaria, cannot be excluded in the relatively early emergence of CLL in these patients.

FIG. 5. DIAGRAM ILLUSTRATING THE EFFECT OF MALNUTRITION
AND INFECTION ON THE THYMOLYMPHATIC TISSUE AND ITS HYPOTHETICAL
INFLUENCE ON THE INCIDENCE OF CHILDHOOD LEUKAEMIA

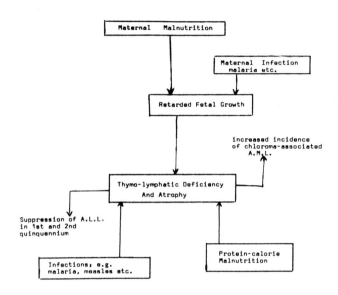

The study of the patterns of leukaemia and lymphoma in Africans promises to aid in elucidating the mechanisms of the influence of the environment in leukaemogenesis.

ACKNOWLEDGEMENTS

I am grateful to my colleagues at University College Hospital, Ibadan, Nigeria, for referring their patients, allowing them to be studied and for helping in their management; to Dr M.F. Greaves, for allowing a preliminary report to be made, in part, on an on-going international study of leukaemia phenotypes; to Professor B.O. Osunkoya of the Postgraduate Institute of Medical Research and Training, College of Medicine, University of Ibadan, Nigeria, and Professor J.F. Holland, Mount Sinai School of Medicine, New York, NY, USA, for useful discussions; and to Mrs Funmi Esan for secretarial assistance.

REFERENCES

Amsel, S. & Nabembezi, J.S. (1974)   Two years survey of hemato-
    logic malignancies in Uganda.   J. natl Cancer Inst., 52,
    1397-1401

Allan, N.C. & Watson-Williams, E.G. (1963)   A study of leukaemias
    among Nigerians in Ibadan.   In: Proceedings of the 9th
    Congress of the European Society of Haematology, Basel,
    Karger, pp. 906-915

Catovsky, D., Greaves, M.F., Rose, M., Galton, D.A.G., Golden,
    A.W.G., McCluskey, D.R., White, J.M., Lampert, I., Counikas,
    G., Ireland, R., Brownell, A.I., Bridges, J.M., Blattner,
    W.A. & Gallo, R.C. (1982)   Adult T-cell lymphoma-leukaemia
    in Blacks from the West Indies.   Lancet, 1, 639-643

Davies, J.N.P. (1965)   Leukemia in children in tropical Africa.
    Lancet, 2, 65-67

Davies, J.N.P. & Owor, R. (1965)   Chloromatous tumours in African
    children in Uganda.   Br. med. J., 11, 405-407

Edington, G.M. & Hendrickse, M. (1972)   The geographical patho-
    logy of cancer in Africa with special reference to the
    Western State of Nigeria and tumours of the lymphoreticular
    tissue.   Dokita, 4, 1-9

Essien, E.M. (1972)   Leukaemia in the African - Part I. The acute
    leukaemias.   Afr. J. med. Sci., 3, 117-130

Essien, E.M. (1976)   Leukaemia in Nigerians: the chronic leukae-
    mias.   East Afr. med. J., 53, 96-103

Federal Office of Statistics, Nigeria (1968)   Rural Demographic
    Sample Survey (1965-66)

Fleming, A.F. (1979)   Epidemiology of the leukaemias in Africa.
    Leuk. Res., 3, 51-59

Fleming, A.F. (1983)   HTLV: Try Africa.   Lancet, 1, 69

Gelfand, M. (1967) Leukaemia in the African. J. trop. Med. Hyg., 70, 85-87

Greaves, M.F., Janossy, G., Peto, J. & Kay, H. (1981) Immuno- logically defined subclasses of acute lymphoblastic leukae- mia in children: their relationship to presentation features and prognosis. Br. J. Haematol., 48, 179-197

Gross, L. (1970) Oncogenic Viruses, 2nd Ed., Oxford, Pergamon Press, pp. 298-302 and 415-420

Haddock, D.R.W. (1967) The pattern of leukaemia in Accra, Ghana. J. trop. Med. Hyg., 70, 60-62

Jeffrey, C. & Gelfand, M. (1972) Leukaemia in the Rhodesian African. J. trop. Med. Hyg., 75, 176-179

Kasili, E.G. & Taylor, J.R. (1970) Leukaemia in Kenya. East Afr. med. J., 47, 461-468

Kela-We, I. (1977) Les leucémies lymphoides chroniques au Zaïre: à propos de 39 cas. Méd. Afr. noire, 24, 255-259

Kusman, B., Jacobson, R.J. & MacDougall, L.G. (1980) A two year study of acute leukaemia in the South African Black in Johannesburg. In: Neiburge, H.E., ed., Prevention and Detection of Cancer, Part II, Detection, Vol. 2, Cancer Detection in Specific Sites, New York, Marcel Dekker, pp. 2329-2337

Lothe, F. (1967) Leukaemia in Uganda. Trop. geogr. Med., 19, 163-170

Lowe, R.F. (1974) The incidence of leukaemia in the Rhodesian African - a five year hospital survey. Cent. Afr. J. Med., 20, 80-84

McDougall, L.G. & Jankowitz, P. (1980) Differences in the inci- dence, type of leukaemia and survival in Black and White children with acute leukaemia in Johannesburg (Abstract). Proc. Intern. Soc. Haemat. Eur-Afric. Division, Aug. 30- Sept. 4, 1980, Athens, Greece, pp. 239

McFarlane, H. & Hamid, J. (1973) Cell-mediated immune response in malnutrition. Clin. exp. Immunol., 13, 153-164

McFarlane, H., Olusi, S.O., Adeshina, H.A., Ade-Serrano, M.A. & Osunkoya, B.O. (1977) Evidence of impaired immunological response in malnourished human population. In: Proceedings, XIII Symposium of the Swedish Nutrition Foundation, pp. 23-41

O'Conor, G.T. & Davies, J.N.P. (1960) Malignant tumours in African children with special reference to malignant lymphoma. J. Pediat., 56, 526-535

Odebiyi, A.I. (1980) Socio-economic status, illness, behaviour and attitude towards disease aetiology in Ibadan. Niger. behav. Sci. J., 3, 172-186

Onibokun, P., Adesokan, R.B. & Bello, I. (1981) Oyo State: A Survey of Resources for Development, Ibadan, Nigerian Institute of Social and Economic Research, University of Ibadan

Payet, M., Camain, R., Sankale, M. & Pene, P. (1960) Les hémopathies malignes chez l'African. Bull. Soc. Méd. Afr. noire Lang. fr., 5, 205-222

Preud'homme, K.L. & Seligman, M. (1974) Surface immunoglobulins on human lymphoid cell. Prog. clin. Immunol., 2, 121-174

Ramot, B. & Magrath, I.T. (1982) Hypothesis: the environment is a major determinant of the immunological sub-type of lymphoma and acute lymphoblastic leukaemia in children. Br. J. Haematol., 52, 183-189

Smythe, P.M., Breton-Stiles, G.G., Grace, H.J., Mafoyane, A., Schonland, M., Coovadia, H.M., Loening, W.E.K., Parent, M.A. & Vos, C.H. (1971) Thymolymphatic immunity in protein-calorie malnutrition. Lancet, 2, 939-943

Sonnet, J., Michaux, J.L. & Hekster, C. (1966) Incidence and forms of leukaemia among Congolese Bantus. Trop. geogr. Med., 18, 272-286

Templeton, A.C. (1973) Leukaemia. Recent Results Cancer Res., 41, 298-301

Vanier, T.M. & Pike, M.C. (1967) Leukaemia incidence in tropical Africa. Lancet, 5, 512-513

Williams, A.O. (1975) Tumours of childhood in Ibadan, Nigeria. Cancer, 36, 370-378

Williams, C.K.O. (1984) Clinical manifestations of lymphoid leukaemias in Ibadan. Niger. med. J. (in press)

Williams, C.K.O. & Bamgboye, E.A. (1983) Estimation of incidence of human leukaemia subtypes in an urban African population. Oncology, 40, 381-386

Williams, C.K.O., Folami, A.O., Laditan, A.A.O. & Ukaejiofo, E.O. (1982) Childhood acute leukaemia in a tropical population. Br. J. Cancer, 46, 89-94

Williams, C.K.O., Essien, E.M. & Bamgboye, E.A. (1984) Trends in leukaemia incidence in Ibadan, Nigeria. In: Magrath, I., O'Conor, G.T. & Ramot, B., eds, Environmental Influences in the Pathogenesis of Leukaemias and Lymphomas, Vol. 27, New York, Raven Press, pp. 17-27

Wintrobe, M.M. (1967) Clinical Haematology, London, Henry Kimpton, pp. 995-998

World Bank (1981) Nigeria - Country Economic Memorandum (Report 3279), Washington, DC

Young, J.L., Percy, C.L., & Asire, A.J., eds (1981) Surveillance, Epidemiology and End Results: Incidence and Mortality Data, 1973-1977, National Cancer Inst. Monogr. 57, Bethesda, MD, National Cancer Institute

HUMAN T-CELL LEUKAEMIA VIRUS IN AFRICA: POSSIBLE ROLES IN HEALTH AND DISEASE

C.K.O. Williams

Department of Haematology, College of Medicine,
University of Ibadan
Ibadan, Nigeria

A.O.K. Johnson

Department of Paediatrics, College of Medicine,
University of Ibadan
Ibadan, Nigeria

W.A. Blattner

Environmental Epidemiology Branch
National Cancer Institute
Bethesda, MD, USA

RESUME

L'observation d'une concentration de cas de leucémies-/lymphomes T de l'adulte (ATL) dans les régions côtières du Japon méridional a conduit à soupçonner leur association à un agent de l'environnement. Le virus des leucémies/lymphomes T humains (HTLV) a été identifié ensuite comme l'agent causal probable de ces cas de lymphomes et leucémies et de ceux qui ont été observés par la suite dans la première génération d'émigrés Noirs Antillais vivant en Angleterre et aux Etats-Unis, dans les zones forestières d'Amérique du Sud et dans certains Etats du sud-est des Etats-Unis. On a également identifié des anticorps anti-HTLV dans des cas de maladies lympho-prolifératives malignes, à Ibadan et à Zaria au Nigéria, et dans le sérum de malades cancéreux provenant de différentes parties d'Afrique; cela indique que l'Afrique est une région majeure pour l'infection HTLV. On montre ici que l'infection HTLV en Afrique est associée à des néoplasmes non seulement des cellules T, mais aussi des cellules B, tels que le lymphome de Burkitt et la leucémie lymphoide chronique (LLC). Les taux de prévalence de l'infection chez les donneurs de sang normaux semblent se situer entre 3,7% dans le

Nigéria septentrional sub-sahélien et 10-15% dans la zone de
forêt vierge du sud-ouest du Nigéria.

SUMMARY

Observation of clustering of adult T-cell leukaemia/lymphoma
(ATL) in the coastal areas of southern Japan led to speculations
about its association with an environmental agent. Human T-cell
lymphoma/leukaemia virus (HTLV) was later identified as the
probable causal agent in these and similar cases of lympho-
ma/leukaemia, which were subsequently observed in first-genera-
tion West Indian Black emigrants living in England and the USA,
in the forest areas of South America and in some south-eastern
states of the USA. HTLV antibodies have also been identified in
cases of malignant lymphoproliferative diseases (MLPD) in Ibadan
and Zaria in Nigeria and in the sera of cancer patients from
various parts of Africa, thus indicating that Africa is a major
region for HTLV infection. Evidence is presented of the association of HTLV infection in Africa not only with T-cell but also
B-cell neoplasia, such as Burkitt's lymphoma and chronic lymphocytic leukaemia (CLL). The prevalence rates of infection in
normal blood donors appear to range from 3.7% in sub-Sahelian
northern Nigeria to 10-15% in the south-western rain-forest area
of Nigeria.

INTRODUCTION

Although an association between animal leukaemia and retroviruses was established by virologists many years ago (Wong-Staal
& Gallo, 1982), only recently was it possible to demonstrate a
link between a representative of this group of viruses, human
T-cell leukaemia virus (HTLV), and human disease. The observation, first made in sporadic cases of adult T-cell lymphoid
malignancies in the United States (Poiesz et al., 1980a), was
made possible as a result of the discovery of a growth factor
that stimulated the proliferation in vitro of T-lymphocytes
(Morgan et al., 1976; Mier & Gallo, 1980; Poiesz et al., 1980b).
Clinical and epidemiological studies have shown that the prototype disease associated with HTLV is adult T-leukaemia/lymphoma
(ATL) (Blattner et al., 1982). This clinicopathological entity
is characterized as a malignancy with aggressive course and poor
prognosis (Uchiyama et al., 1977; Blattner et al., 1982)
involving the proliferation of lymphocytes with the phenotypic

characteristics of relatively mature lymphocytes (Takatsuchi et al., 1982; Blayney et al., 1983b). Other characteristics of this entity include a diffuse histological pattern with frequent pleomorphic cytology, stage-IV presentation with visceral involvement, and hypercalcaemia and opportunistic infection in one-third to one-half of the cases (Blayney et al., 1983a). Clusters of this disease (when it was not known that it was virally associated) were originally described in the southern islands of Japan, Kyushu and Shikoku (Uchiyama et al., 1977; Robert-Guroff et al., 1982). The virus from such cases was shown to be HTLV type-1 (Robert-Guroff et al., 1982). Subsequently, a form of lymphoma/leukaemia with features similar to those of Japanese ATL were described in Black Caribbean emigrants in the United Kingdom (Catovsky et al., 1982). These cases were later shown to be positive for HTLV virus and/or antibody (Blattner et al., 1982). More recently, 69% of Jamaican patients presenting with non-Hodgkin's lymphoma (NHL) were seropositive for HTLV (Blattner et al., 1983b).

Other cases of HTLV-associated lymphoma/leukaemia have been reported in Caucasians either resident in underdeveloped countries or resident in a developed country but having travelled widely in HTLV endemic areas (Blattner et al., 1983a; Blayney et al., 1983a), or in Blacks resident in some south-eastern states of the USA (Blayney et al., 1983a). Thus, the disease appears to be prevalent among non-Caucasians, socioeconomically deprived individuals, and residents of underdeveloped tropical regions of the world. The high prevalence in the endemic area of antibodies to the virus, especially among close associates of ATL patients, supports a horizontal mode of infectivity of the virus (Blattner et al., 1982, 1983a). So far, all virus isolates from cases of ATL have been of one type, HTLV-1, including the so-called Japanese adult T-cell leukaemia virus (ATLV) (Popovic et al., 1982).

Recently, high titres of HTLV antibodies were found in sera obtained from various parts of Africa from patients with diverse neoplastic disorders (Saxinger & Gallo, 1984). This finding, at the least, suggests that the prevalence rate of HTLV infection is probably quite considerable in the African continent, unlike its low prevalence rate in Europe and some other parts of the world (Blattner et al., 1983a,b). Two cases of HTLV-associated lymphoproliferative disorders (LPD) were recently identified in Ibadan, Nigeria, among 9 appropriately screened cases of LPD (Williams et al., 1984). One of the 2 HTLV seropositive cases had clinical and

laboratory features of ATL, including the immunological phenotypic characteristics of mature T-cells, while the other presented as an aggressive form of chronic lymphocytic leukaemia (CLL)
(Williams et al., 1984). In another study done in the savanna-
/sub-Sahelian region of Nigeria, HTLV-seropositive cases
occurring in association with various types of LPD have also
recently been described (Fleming et al., 1983).

Other reports indicating that HTLV infection may be widespread in parts of Africa include that of Yamamoto et al. (1983)
demonstrating that ATLV (HTLV) and its antibody were present in
over 80% of African green monkeys captured in Kenya and studied
after 2 years of captivity in the Federal Republic of Germany.
While this would suggest that the African green monkey is, at the
least, one of the natural reservoirs for the virus in Africa, as
has similarly been established for Japanese macacques (Miyoshi et
al., 1982), there is no evidence of horizontal monkey-to-man
transmission, unlike the male-to-female horizontal transmission
pattern that has been found among Japanese monkeys (Miyoshi et
al., 1983). Thus, although only a very limited epidemiological
study of HTLV infection has so far been undertaken in Africa,
there appears to be enough reason to speculate that the African
continent represents a major cluster area for the virus. It has
recently been suggested that the virus might have been brought to
Japan by the 16th century Portuguese seamen who had contacts with
Africa and lived in regions of Japan now endemic for HTLV (Gallo
et al., 1983). HTLV epidemiology appears to be explainable on
the basis of transmission of the virus from Old World primates to
man through an insect vector, or from man to man through personal
contact.

MATERIALS AND METHODS

Beginning in 1982, patients at the Department of Haematology, University College Hospital (UCH), Ibadan, Nigeria,
referred for haematological assessment were screened for clinical
and laboratory features of adult T-cell lymphoma/leukaemia. Subsequently, the search for evidence of HTLV infection was expanded
to include evidence of HTLV seropositivity in all forms of malignant LPD. This paper reports the preliminary findings of the
study, which is still in progress.

Blood was obtained from patients with haematopoietic and
lymphoreticular malignancies, usually at the time of diagnosis
and prior to chemotherapy. The sera from these samples were

stored at $-20^{\circ}C$ in plastic shipment containers and were shipped
in dry ice at intervals of 2-6 months to the laboratory of Dr
R.G. Gallo, National Cancer Institute, Bethesda, MD, USA, for
assay of antibodies to HTLV whole-virus antigen. This was done
in two stages. The serum samples were first screened with an
indirect enzyme-linked immunoabsorbent assay (ELISA) (Saxinger &
Gallo, 1984). Samples found positive at this stage were subjected to specificity-competition assays whereby the titre of the
antibodies was determined. Immunological phenotypic characterization of mononuclear cells of appropriate diseased tissue
(peripheral blood, bone marrow, lymph-node or skin biopsy) was
undertaken, using the technique of rosette formation with neur-
aminidase (treated or untreated sheep red blood cells and
untreated mouse red blood cells), as well as the indirect immunofluorescence technique, using murine monoclonal antibodies,
including DA-2 (an anti-HLA-DR antibody), S-33, WT 1 and OKTILA
(pan-T-antibodies), AL-2 and J-5 (anti-CALLA antibodies), OKT3,
OKT4, OKT6 and OKT8 (anti-T-'Subtype' antibodies) and antibody to
terminal deoxynucleotidyl transferase (anti-Tdt).

RESULTS

Table 1 shows the results of the two-stage assay for HTLV in
the first 9 Ibadan patients whose sera were assayed at the
National Cancer Institute in 1983. One case each of ATL and CLL
were found to be HTLV-positive. To date, 165 serum samples from
Ibadan patients have been analysed. Table 2 shows the preliminary results of the screening assays in the various categories of
study subjects, expressed as ratios of tests to controls; ratios
of less than 2.0 rarely give a positive reaction, while about 10%
of ratios in the range 2.0-5.0 and 90% of those over 5 eventually
do so in confirmatory tests on sera of American and Japanese
origin (Jeffrey Clark, personal communication). It is, however,
reasonable to predict that, after the confirmatory assays have
been done, about 10-15% of normal blood donors in Ibadan would be
found to be seropositive for HTLV. Diseases in which HTLV sero-
sensitivity would be demonstrable in this series would include
non-Hodgkin's (non-Burkitt's) lymphoma as well as cases of
lymphoma-like states, such as gross splenomegalies and autoimmune
haemolytic anaemias, Burkitt's lymphoma (BL) and CLL.

WILLIAMS ET AL.

Table 1. Results of two-stage assay for HTLV in Ibadan patients with lymphoreticular neoplasia[a]

Subject/initials	Age/sex	Diagnosis	HTLV antibodies	Titre
NGR 577523/MA	25/M	CTCL	1.0	-
NGR 605782/OB	11/M	ALL	0.86	-
NGR 612459/BA	10/F	ALL	1.60	-
NGR 622222/AF	19/F	ATL	16.05	4000
NGR 622224/BLS	21/M	HD	0.63	-
NGR 622626/IL	63/M	TSS	1.92	-
NGR 622963/AA	25/M	NHL	1.06	-
NGR 623297/MAR	57/F	CLL	11.32	1700
NGR 623560/FA	15/F	BL	1.71	-

[a] Expressed as test:control ratios. CTCL = cutaneous T-cell lymphoma; NHL = non-Hodgkin's lymphoma; ALL = acute lymphoblastic leukaemia; ATL = adult T-cell leukaemia; HD = Hodgkin's disease; TSS = tropical splenomegaly syndrome; CLL = chronic lymphocytic leukaemia; BL = Burkitt's lymphoma

Table 3 shows the immunological phenotypic characteristics of mononuclear cells in 3 Ibadan patients with clinical features of ATL. In all 3, features of mature T-cells were demonstrated while in 2 the typical suppressor T-lymphocyte phenotype of ATL cells was also observed. Figure 1 shows a patient believed to be the first African case of ATL to be appropriately documented.

Table 2.   HTLV antibody screening test results in 157 Ibadan
patients[a]

Category of study subjects	No. of cases	Test:control ratios[b]		
		< 2	2-5	> 5
NBNHL	16	5 (31.3)	9 (56.3)	2 (12.5)
Lymphoma-like disorders[c]	8	3 (37.5)	2 (25)	3 (37.5)
BL	29	15 (51.7)	11 (37.9)	3 (10.3)
HD	10	6 (60)	4 (40)	0
CLL	14	8 (57.1)	2 (14.3)	4 (28.6)
ALL	15	10 (66.7)	5 (33.3)	0
CML	6	3 (50.0)	3 (50.0)	0
AM1	6	3 (50.0)	2 (33.3)	1 (16.7)
Non-haematopoietic malignancies	10	4 (40.0)	6 (60.0)	0
Non-neoplastic disorders	12	9 (75.0)	2 (16.7)	1 (8.7)
Haemophilia	6	2 (33.3)	4 (66.7)	0
Normal blood donors	27	6 (22.2)	18 (66.7)	3 (11.1)

[a] Abbreviations as in Table 1. In addition: NBNHL =
non-Burkitt's non-Hodgkin's lymphoma

[b] Figures in parentheses are percentages of the total number

[c] Unexplained splenomegaly and idiopathic immune haemolytic
anaemias

Table 3. Immunological phenotypic characteristics in 3 Ibadan patients with clinical features of adult T-cell lymphoma/leukaemia[a]

Initials	Age/sex	Tissue sampled[b]	ER[c]	Pan T	T-subtypes	Tdt[d]	HTLV titre
AF	19/M	SB	–	+	ND[e]	–	4000
AJ	50/F	PB	+	++	T3+++, T4++, T6⁻, T8+	±	NA[f]
OS	40/M	PB	+++	++	T4++, others ND[d]	–	NA[f]

[a] – = negative; + = 10-30% positive; ++ = 31-60% positive; +++ = > 60% positive

[b] SB = skin biopsy; PB = peripheral blood

[c] ER = E-rosettes (see Methods)

[d] Tdt = terminal deoxynucleotidyl transferase

[e] ND = Not done

[f] NA = Not available

DISCUSSION

The highest prevalence rates for HTLV infection have been observed in the endemic areas of Japan and were as high as 16% in apparently normal individuals in the Nagasaki area (Robert-Guroff et al., 1983) and as high as 30% in relations of Japanese patients with ATL (Blattner et al., 1983a,b). With prevalence rates of up to 4% demonstrable in certain areas among apparently normal individuals, the Caribbean has proved to be the second most important area for HTLV infection so far. The preliminary results (Table 2) of screening tests done on 27 normal blood donors (among a total of 165 study subjects) suggest that a 10-15% seropositivity rate is quite possible in the Ibadan area of Nigeria. If this initial impression is proved right by confirmatory tests, the rain-forest region of south-western Nigeria would have been shown to be a major cluster area for HTLV. Fleming et al. (1983) reported a prevalence rate of 3.7% among normal blood

FIG. 1.   NINETEEN-YEAR-OLD NIGERIAN WITH CUTANEOUS LESIONS
OF ADULT T-CELL LYMPHOMA LEUKAEMIA

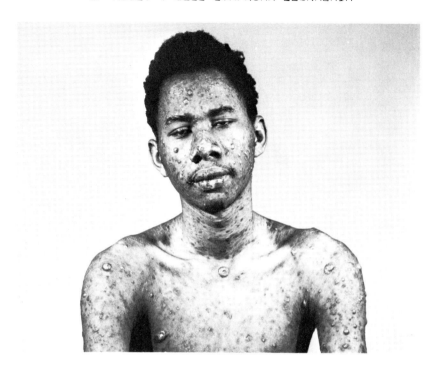

donors in the savanna/sub-Sahelian region of northern Nigeria.
The difference may be due to differences in the ecological
characteristics of the two regions. If prevalence rates for HTLV
infection are found in other parts of Black Africa similar to
those in Ibadan, Africa could then be considered as harbouring
the largest population of people at risk for infection by the
virus.

     With its well-established, characteristic T-lymphocyte
tropism (Gallo et al., 1982), it is understandable that HTLV
should be associated with neoplasia originating from, at the
least, a subset of T-lymphocytes (Blattner et al., 1983a,b). We
have characterized the mononuclear cells in 3 out of 8 cases of
non-Hdogkin's lymphoma as mature T-cells (Table 3), thereby
suggesting that these were cases of ATL. This was proved in the
only case in which HTLV antibody was found. Thus, ATL occurs in
Africans but its prevalence rate among cases of lymphoid neoplasia in them is yet to be determined. The results of HTLV
screening assays shown in Table 2 suggest that HTLV infection

occurred in at least 10% of BL patients in Ibadan. A similar observation was made by Saxinger and his colleagues (unpublished data). CLL, which in Ibadan has been shown to have the characteristic phenotype of B-lymphocytes (C.K.O. Williams, unpublished data), also appears to be associated with HTLV infection (Table 2). These observations would appear to confirm a recent finding that HTLV may infect B-lymphocytes. Studies in Japan and the Caribbean have suggested increasing HTLV infection with advancing age. However, the association of HTLV with an African childhood neoplasia would tend to suggest an earlier exposure in African children to the source of infection than elsewhere.

The acquired immunodeficiency syndrome (AIDS), a disease that has been associated in the USA and Europe with homosexuals, drug addicts, haemophiliacs, and Haitian emigrants, has also been linked to HTLV infection (Gelmann et al., 1983). Recently, a series of African patients from Zaire have been diagnosed as suffering from this disease; they were not known to be homosexuals (Clumeck et al., 1984). This report, and others indicating a high prevalence of Kaposi's sarcoma in Central Africa (Olweny, 1983), suggest a role for HTLV in various forms of disease in Africa.

The anticipated rate of 10-15% seropositivity for HTLV among blood donors in Ibadan should serve as a warning of the problems that loom ahead in blood transfusion services in Africa in the near future. The lymphocytes of seropositive individuals are known to contain the viral genome of HTLV (Gallo et al., 1982). If HTLV can be transmitted horizontally in primates, from male to female (Miyoshi et al., 1983), and if horizontal spread from ATL patients to their close relations is thought to be responsible for the high prevalence rate of HTLV seropositivity in the latter (Robert-Guroff et al., 1983), it is to be expected that blood transfusion will be capable of effecting the transmission of the virus from an infected donor to a recipient.

The story of HTLV is just beginning to unfold. It appears that Africa may turn out to be the focal point in many ways for the study of this virus and, perhaps, the continent of origin, from where it has been disseminated to other parts of the world (Gallo et al., 1983). It seems almost certain, however, that with time this newly discovered virus will come to be associated with a variety of medical problems in Africa, some of which may so far be unrecognized.

ACKNOWLEDGEMENTS

We are grateful to Dr R.C. Gallo, in whose laboratory all the HTLV serological assays were done; to Dr M.F. Greaves, who provided the monoclonal antibodies for the characterization of the lymphoid neoplasia; to the consultants of the Departments of Medicine, Paediatrics and Haematology, University College Hospital, Ibadan, for referring patients for study; and finally to Mrs C.O. Kayode and Mrs O.A. Adebiyi for typing the manuscript.

REFERENCES

Blattner, W.A., Kalynaraman, V.S., Robert-Guroff, M., Lister, T.A., Galton, D.A.G., Sarin, P.S., Crawford, M.H., Catovsky, D.I., Greaves, M. & Gallo, R.C. (1982) The human type-C retrovirus, HTLV, in blacks from the Caribbean region, and relationship to adult T-cell leukaemia/lymphoma. Int. J. Cancer, 30, 257-264

Blattner, W.A., Blayney, D.W., Robert-Guroff, M., Sarnghadharan, M.G., Sarin, P.S., Jaffe, E.S. & Gallo, R.C. (1983a) Epidemiology of human T-cell leukemia/lymphoma virus. J. infect. Dis., 147, 406-416

Blattner, W.A., Gibbs, W.N., Saxinger, C., Robert-Guroff, M., Clark, J., Lofter, W., Hanchard, B., Campbell, M. & Gallo, R.C. (1983b) Human T-cell leukaemia/lymphoma virus-associated lymphoreticular neoplasia in Jamaica. Lancet, 2, 61-64

Blayney, D.W., Blattner, W.A., Robert-Guroff, M., Jaffe, E.S., fisher, R.I., Bunn, P.A., Patton, M.G., Rarick, H.R. & Gallo, R.C. (1983a) The human T-cell leukemia-lymphoma virus in the south-eastern United States. J. Am. Med. Assoc., 25, 1048-1052

Blayney, D.W., Jaffe, E.S., Blattner, W.A., Cossman, J., Robert-Guroff, M., Longo, D., Bunn, P.A. & Gallo, R.C. (1983b) The human T-cell leukaemia/lymphoma virus (HTLV) associated American adult T-cell leukaemia/lymphoma (ATL). Blood, 62, 401-405

Catovsky, D., Greaves, M.F., Rose, M., Gaston, D.A.G., Golden, A.W.G., McCluskey, D.R., White, J.M., Lampert, I., Bourikas, G., Ireland, R., Brownell, A.I., Bridges, J.M., Blattner, W.A. & Gallo, R.C. (1982) Adult T-cell lymphoma-leukaemia in Blacks from the West Indies. Lancet, 1, 639-643

Clumeck, N., Sonnet, J., Taelman, H., Mascart-Lemone, F., De Bruyere, M., Vandeperre, P., Dasnoy, J., Marcelis, L., Lamy, M., Jonas, C., Eyckmans, L., Noel, H., Vanhaeverbeek, M. & Buteler, J. (1984) Acquired immunodeficiency syndrome in African patients. New Engl. J. Med., 310, 492-497

Fleming, A.F., Yamamoto, N., Bhusnurmath, S.R., Maharajan, R., Schneider, J. & Hunsmann, G. (1983) Antibodies to ATLV (HTLV) in Nigerian blood donors and patients with chronic lymphocytic leukaemia or lymphoma. Lancet, 2, 334-335

Gallo, R.C., Mann, D., Broder, S., Ruscetti, F., Maeda, M., Kalyanaraman, V., Robert-Guroff, M. & Reitz, M. (1982) Human T-cell leukemia-lymphoma virus (HTLV) is in T- but not B-lymphocytes from a patient with cutaneous T-cell lymphoma. Proc. natl Acad. Sci. USA, 79, 5680-5683

Gallo, R.C., Sliski, A. & Wong-Staal, F. (1983) Origin of human T-cell leukaemia-lymphoma virus. Lancet, 2, 962-963

Gelman, E.P., Popovic, M., Blayney, D., Masur, H., Sidhu, G., Stehl, R.E. & Gallo, R.C. (1983) Viral DNA of a retrovirus, human T-cell leukemia virus, in two patients with AIDS. Science, 220, 862-865

Mier, J.W. & Gallo, R.C. (1980) Purification and some characteristics of human T-cell growth factor from phytohemagglutinin-stimulated lymphocyte conditioned media. Proc. natl Acad. Sci. USA, 77, 6134-6138

Miyoshi, I., Yoshimoto, S., Fujishita, M., Taguchi, H., Kubonishi, I. & Niiya, K. (1982) Natural adult T-cell leukaemia virus infection in Japanese monkeys. Lancet, 2, 658

Miyoshi, I., Fujishita, M., Taguchi, H., Niiya, K., Kobayashi, M., Matsubayashi, K. & Miwa, N. (1983) Horizontal transmission of adult T-cell leukaemia virus from male to female Japanese monkey. Lancet, 1, 241

Morgan, D.A., Ruscetti, F.W. & Gallo, R.C. (1976) Selective in vitro growth of T lymphocytes from normal human bone marrow. Science, 193, 1007-1008

Olweny, C.L.M. (1983) Cancer patterns in Nigeria and Uganda. In: Solanke, T.F., Osunkoya, B.O., Williams, C.K.O. & Agboola, O., eds, Cancer in Nigeria, Ibadan, Ibadan University Press, pp. 233-249

Poiesz, B.J., Ruscetti, F.W., Gasdar, A.F., Bunn, P., Minna, J. & Gallo, R.C. (1980a) Detection and isolation of type C retrovirus particles from fresh and cultured lymphocytes of a patient with cutaneous T-cell lymphoma. Proc. natl Acad. Sci. USA, 77, 7415-7419

Poiesz, B.J., Ruscetti, F.W., Mier, J.W., Woods, A.M. & Gallo, R.C. (1980b) T-cell lines established from human T-lymphocytic neoplasias by direct responses to T-cell growth factor. Proc. natl Acad. Sci. USA, 77, 6815-6819

Popovic, M., Reitz, M.S., Sarngadharan, M.G., Robert-Guroff, M., Kalyanaraman, V.S.S., Nakao, Y., Miyoshi, I., Minowada, J., Yoshida, M., Ito, Y. & Gallo, R.C. (1982) The virus of Japanese adult T-cell leukaemia is a member of the human T-cell leukaemia virus group. Nature, 300, 63-66

Robert-Guroff, M., Nakao, Y., Notake, K., Ito, Y., Sliski, A. & Gallo, R.C. (1982) Natural antibodies to human retrovirus HTLV in a cluster of Japanese patients with adult T-cell leukemia. Science, 215, 975-978

Saxinger, C. & Gallo, R.C. (1984) Application of the indirect ELISA microtest to the detection and surveillance of human T-cell leukaemia-lymphoma virus (HTLV). Lab. Invest. (in press)

Takatsuchi, K., Uchiyama, T., Yeshima, T., Hattori, T., Toibana,
    T., Tsudo, M., Wano, Y. & Yodoi, J. (1982) Adult T-cell
    leukemia: proposal as a new disease and cytogenetic, pheno-
    typic and functional studies of leukemic cells. Gann
    Monogr. Cancer Res., 28, 13-21

Uchiyama, T., Yodoi, J., Sagawa, K., Takatsuki, K. & Uchino, U.
    (1977) Adult T-cell leukemia: clinical and hematologic
    features of 16 cases. Blood, 50, 481-492

Williams, C.K.O., Saxinger, C., Alabi, G.O., Junaid, T.A.,
    Blayney, D.W., Greaves, M.F., Gallo, R.C. & Blattner, W.A.
    (1984)   HTLV-associated lymphoproliferative disorder:
    Report of two cases in Nigeria. Br. med. J. (in press)

Wong-Staal, F. & Gallo, R.C. (1982) Retroviruses and leukemia.
    In: Gunz, F. & Henderson, E.S., eds, Leukemia, New York,
    Grune and Stratton, pp. 329-358

Yamamoto, N., Hinuma, Y., zur Hausen, H., Schneider, J. &
    Hunsmann, G. (1983) African green monkeys are infected with
    adult T-cell leukemia virus or a closely related agent.
    Lancet, 1, 240-241

VIRUS-ASSOCIATED LYMPHOMAS, LEUKAEMIAS AND IMMUNODEFICIENCIES IN AFRICA

G. de-Thé

CNRS Laboratory of Epidemiology and Tumour Immunovirology
Faculty of Medicine Alexis Carrel
Lyon, France

RESUME

Les relations entre virus et cancers, tels que le cancer primitif du foie et les cancers génitaux, sont d'une grande importance pour l'Afrique. D'autre part, les lymphomes, les leucémies et les déficits immunitaires, bien que moins importants sur le plan de la santé publique, constituent un domaine d'un intérêt particulier pour la recherche, et leur association avec d'une part le virus d'Epstein-Barr (EBV) et d'autre part les rétrovirus humains découverts récemment mérite une attention particulière.

Les cancers liés à l'EBV observés en Afrique couvrent le lymphome de Burkitt (BL) et le cancer du nasopharynx (NPC). Existe-t-il des lympho-proliférations polyclonales liées au chromosome X en Afrique ? La question reste ouverte. L'inter-relation entre le virus EB, le paludisme holo-endémique et les facteurs génétiques (oncogènes) a été déchiffrée durant ces dernières années de sorte que le lymphome de Burkitt constitue aujourd'hui une pierre de Rosette dans la compréhension de la cancérogenèse multifactorielle. Le rôle du virus EB dans l'étiologie du cancer du nasopharynx (NPC) n'est pas encore établi, bien qu'hautement probable. Déjà le dosage des IgA dirigées contre l'antigène de la capside virale (VCA) permet la détection précoce du NPC dans les zones de haute incidence, et le diagnostic différentiel dans les régions de faible incidence. Un vaccin contre le virus EB pourrait-il aider les pays africains dans la prévention des cancers associés à l'EBV ? La question reste ouverte.

Les maladies associées aux rétrovirus humains découverts
récemment (les virus des leucémies T humaines: les HTLV) représentent un nouveau domaine aussi bien pour la recherche que pour
l'évaluation de la santé publique. On dispose aujourd'hui pour
l'Afrique d'une information limitée sur la distribution géographique, la prévalence selon l'âge et l'association à des maladies des différents membres de la famille des rétrovirus (HTLV-1,
HTLV-2, LAV/HTLV-3). Il reste encore à déterminer la proportion
de maladies malignes de la lignée T liées au HTLV dans les différentes régions d'Afrique aussi bien que l'importance des immuno-
déficiences causées par les différents membres de la famille des
rétrovirus. Le syndrome typique d'immunodéficience acquise
(SIDA) semble exister en Afrique centrale, spécialement au Zaïre,
où les virus HTLV pourraient représenter un problème de santé
publique important s'ils s'avèrent être responsables d'immunodé-
ficiences sub-cliniques favorisant des formes sévères de maladies
virales, bactériennes ou parasitaires, secondaires à l'altération
de l'immunité à médiation cellulaire.

L'Afrique est, et restera longtemps, un continent d'une
importance déterminante pour saisir le rôle des virus dans les
proliférations malignes humaines, et en paticulier les proliférations hématopoïétiques.

SUMMARY

The relationship between viruses and naturally occurring
cancers, such as hepatocellular carcinoma and genital cancers, is
of great importance to Africa. On the other hand, lymphomas,
leukaemias and immunodeficiencies, although of less immediate
public health importance, constitute an area of outstanding
interest for research and their association with the Epstein-Barr
virus (EBV) and the newly discovered human retroviruses merits
world-wide attention.

EBV-related malignancies in Africa include both Burkitt's
lymphoma (BL) and nasopharyngeal carcinoma (NPC). Whether X-
linked polyclonal lymphoproliferations exist in Africa remains an
open question. The interrelationship between EBV, holoendemic
malaria and genetic factors (oncogenes) has been deciphered in
recent years, to make BL a kind of Rosetta stone for the understanding of multistage carcinogenesis. Although the role of EBV
in the causation of NPC is not well understood, the viral capsid
antigen (VCA) IgA test already allows both early detection of NPC

in high-incidence areas and differential diagnosis in low-incidence areas. The question whether an EBV vaccine would be of value in African countries, in relation to EBV-associated malignancies, remains an open one.

The diseases associated with the recently discovered human retroviruses (human T-lymphocyte leukaemia viruses: HTLVs) represent a new area for both research and public health assessment. Limited information is available today on the geographical distribution, age prevalence and association with disease in Africa of the different members of the retrovirus family (HTLV-1, HTLV-2, LAV/HTLV-3). The proportion of HTLV-related T-cell malignancies in different parts of Africa as well as the importance of immunodeficiencies caused by the different members of the retrovirus family remain to be determined. Typical acquired immunodeficiency syndrome (AIDS) appears to exist in Central Africa, especially Zaire, and HTLVs could be of public health importance if they cause severe forms of viral, bacterial or parasitic diseases through impairment of cell-mediated immunity.

Africa, is and will long remain a continent of crucial importance with regard to the role of viruses in human malignancies and especially in haematopoietic proliferative disorders.

INTRODUCTION

"Ex Africa semper aliquid novi" wrote Pliny some 2500 years ago. This still holds good today from the view-point of medical research. While in the previous century Africa was considered to be a cancer-free continent but a privileged area for research on parasitic diseases, it has in recent years been the scene of developments of vital importance in the study of the role of viruses in human cancers. The childhood lymphoma discovered by Denis Burkitt in East Africa has proved to be the cornerstone for the understanding of the relationship between environment and human tumours. Africa has also witnessed the first attempt to prevent hepatocellular carcinoma by vaccination against hepatitis B, thanks to the pioneering work of Maupas and the medical school in Senegal. Last, but not least, Africa appears to be the probable reservoir of the human retrovirus family. This last subject may well constitute one of the most fascinating developments in medical research at the end of the 20th century.

This Symposium is devoted to the problem of viruses and cancers in Africa. If one looks outside Africa and considers the problem from a world view-point, the role of biological environmental factors in the development of human cancers is of vital importance to all tropical and developing countries. The number of virus-associated cancer cases in the world, arising each year, can be estimated at around half a million for genital cancers associated with human papillomaviruses (HPV), at a quarter of a million for hepatocellular carcinoma (HCC) associated with hepatitis B virus (HBV), and at nearly one-tenth of a million for EBV-associated proliferative disorders. The number of cancer cases associated with the HTLV group of viruses cannot be estimated at present.

For Africa, the two main cancer killers are genital cancers and HCC, both of which are associated with DNA viruses (HPV and HBV, respectively). While the control of HCC through vaccination is in sight, progress in the control of genital cancers lies in easier early detection through HPV markers. Cancers related to Epstein-Barr virus (EBV), namely Burkitt's lymphoma and nasopharyngeal carcinoma, represent major cancer localizations in some areas in Africa, the former being the major tumour among children between 0 and 14 years in Equatorial Africa and the latter being the main ENT cancer in North and East Africa. Similarly, Kaposi's sarcoma is a very frequent tumour in some areas of Central Africa, especially Zaire. Its association with viruses is not yet established although there are some interesting data concerning the relation between it and cytomegalovirus (CMV)[1]. The question of HTLV-related diseases and malignancies remains completely open in Africa. The problem of human retroviruses in Africa will first be considered, after which the African tumours associated with EBV will be reviewed.

---

[1] See Giraldo et al., this volume

HUMAN RETROVIRUSES AND AFRICA

The recent discovery by Gallo and colleagues of a new family of human retroviruses (Gallo, 1984a) is of great interest for Africa. The detection and isolation of the etiological agent of the epidemics of acquired immunodeficiency syndrome (AIDS) in the USA and Europe are important for Africa, since this continent may well represent the original reservoir of these retroviruses. Three questions should be considered at this point: What is the prevalence of these viruses in Africa ? Are HTLVs of pathological importance for Africa ? What are the priorities of HTLV-related research in Africa ?

Before an attempt is made to answer these questions, it is worth recalling that three subtypes of the human retrovirus family have been identified and that each subtype has a number of variants (Gallo, 1984b). The first HTLV was isolated in a Black American with Sezary syndrome (Poiesz et al., 1980). Simultaneously, an identical virus, called adult T-cell leukaemia virus (ATLV), was isolated by Japanese workers in clinically aggressive T-cell leukaemias occurring among adults in epidemic form in south-west Japan (Miyoshi et al., 1981; Hinuma et al., 1982). A second subtype, called HTLV-2, differing somewhat at the DNA level, was isolated from a hairy-cell leukaemia in north-west America (Kalyanaraman et al., 1982). The third subtype was discovered in the laboratory of Montagnier in France (Barré-Sinoussi et al., 1983) and later by the Gallo group in the United States (Popovic et al., 1984), from AIDS patients. This subtype, HTLV-3/LAV, is cytopathic for T-lymphocytes, while HTLV-1 and HTLV-2 are able to transform these cells.

Prevalence of human retroviruses in Africa

C.K.O. Williams and W.A. Blattner have reported[1] that HTLV-1 and associated T-cell malignancies exist in Nigeria. Central Africa may thus be a third area of the world in which HTLV-1 related T-cell malignancies occur, the other two being south-west Japan (Hinuma et al., 1982) and the Caribbean (Blattner et al., 1982; Catovsky et al., 1982). The Centers for Disease Control in the United States together with the Institute of Tropical Medicine in Antwerp have shown that AIDS syndromes do

---

[1] This volume

exist in Central Africa (Clumeck et al., 1984; Piot et al., 1984; Van de Perre et al., 1984). Moreover, antibodies to LAV are present in up to 10% of normal populations (Montagnier et al., personal communication).

It has been shown by studying sera from different African countries that the prevalence of HTLV-1 in Africa increases in going from North to Equatorial Africa, where it reaches 10% of the population (see Table 1). Sera have been tested for HTLV-3 antibodies and evidence found of HTLV-3 infection in both Uganda and the Ivory Coast (de-Thé, unpublished data).

Are HTLVs important for health in Africa ?

Very limited information is available with which to answer this question (Fleming et al., 1983; Hunsmann et al., 1983; Saxinger et al., 1984). African health authorities may initially be inclined to consider such viruses as irrelevant to their list of priorities, since infection by HTLVs has probably long existed and been controlled in the populations concerned. The question whether AIDS is a new disease in Central Africa or not cannot be answered because of the difficulty, until recently, of diagnosing such syndromes. Among the Black Bonis, an isolated group of African origin living in French Guiana, a high prevalence of HTLV-1 antibodies has been found, which indicates that HTLV is not new and came to the Caribbean from Africa around three centuries ago (Gessain et al., 1984). The epidemic of AIDS in the United States is due in part to the lack of antibodies in the population, in contrast to the situation in the Caribbean and in Africa.

In view of the increasing interchange of people between the African countries and Europe, the United States, etc., HTLV-related diseases may become important health problems in Africa.

HTLVs may also be of importance in relation to parasitic, bacterial and viral diseases in Africa if, as seems likely, HTLV-1, -2 or -3 specifically depress the subgroups of T-cells responsible for the T-cell immunity that controls infections by certain infectious agents. If this were to be the case, vaccination against HTLV would be of great interest to the populations in areas where infection by this type of virus is endemic.

Table 1. HTLV-1 ELISAa antibodies in normal populations[b]

Population	No. of sera tested	ELISA biotech $5<R^c<8$	ELISA biotech $R>8$	Total + ve (%)	High titres (%)
France					
Mont de Marsan	318	1	0	0.3	0
French West Indians (Paris)	279	0	1	0.3	0.3
Malaria patients (Lyon)	269	4	13	6.3	4.8
Drug abusers (Toulouse)	45	0	0	0	0
Africa					
Morocco	297	1	0	0.3	0
Upper Volta	43	2	0	4.6	0
Ivory Coast	100	9	7	16	7
Uganda	57	5	1	10	2
Indian Ocean					
Reunion	242	0	0	0	0
South-East Asia					
Macao	299	0	0	0	0

[a] Enzyme linked immunosorbent assay

[b] Source: de-Thé et al., unpublished data

[c] R = Ratio of reading at 492 nm of the test serum as compared to HTLV-negative serum

Future research on HTLV in Africa

The first step in assessing the situation in Africa must be to investigate the prevalence of the different viral subtypes in different parts of Africa, from north to south and from east to west. This could be done by a team of researchers and techni-cians who, under the auspices of WHO, would collect blood specimens from different areas of each country and from the

various ethnic groups. The aims of such a 'HTLV safari' would be
first, to assess the geographical distribution of infection by
HTLV-1, -2 and -3, and second, to investigate the mode of spread
of this virus and the age prevalence rate. The mode of infection
in the United States, believed to be mainly sexual, may not be
that prevailing in the endemic areas of Africa. The age prevalence rate would provide an answer to that important question.
The third aim of such an investigation would be to collect data
on the diseases associated with each subtype of HTLV. Collection
of blood in different hospital wards and by disease categories
might give some idea of such associations with retroviruses. The
next step would be to measure immunodeficiencies (T4/T8 ratios)
and other indicators of cell-mediated immune status versus the
level of HTLV antibodies. The question as to whether HTLV infections are or are not associated with severe forms of parasitic,
bacterial or viral infections is of prime interest for Africa.

EBV-RELATED CANCERS IN AFRICA

EBV, discovered in 1964, is the fifth human herpesvirus and
is associated with three types of proliferations. The first is a
polyclonal B-cell proliferation, usually caused by a primary
infection by this agent, the second a monoclonal B-cell proliferation named Burkitt's lymphoma, discovered in Africa, and the
third a carcinoma of the nasopharynx prevalent in East and North
Africa, but also and to a greater extent in South-east Asia.

X-linked lymphoproliferations

Primary infection by EBV occurs very early in life in the
African continent, especially in the equatorial areas (de-Thé,
1977). Such infection usually induces a polyclonal B-cell proliferation, which is soon controlled by specific cell-mediated
immunity involving EBV-specific cytotoxic T-cells. Such cell-
mediated immunity, in turn, is controlled by genetic factors and
certain immunogenetic defects therefore result in polyclonal
B-cell proliferations, discovered and studied over the last 10
years by Purtillo[1]. Since Africa is an area where EBV infection
occurs very early and massively, a search should be made for such
polyclonal lymphoproliferations associated with primary infection. Glandular fevers, which are known to exist in African

---

[1] This volume

children, may well represent the clinical symptoms associated with primary EBV infection, but this still remains to be proved. The only data available on the consequences of primary infection are those obtained in Ghana by Biggar et al. (1978) showing that, in fact, as in the rest of the world, primary infection by EBV is mainly clinically silent. The relationship between sickle-cell trait and diseases associated with primary EBV infection should also be studied.

African B-cell lymphoma in children

This tumour, originally described by Burkitt (1958), accounts for up to 80% of all childhood malignancies in children between 0 and 14 years of age in Equatorial Africa. With regard to the natural history of this type of tumour in Africa today, Nkrumah[1] has drawn attention to the progressive decrease in incidence, and the changes in age prevalence and in clinical presentation in Ghana, and these observation have been confirmed by Brubaker[1]. It appears as if Burkitt's lymphoma now occurs later in life, with more frequent abdominal and less frequent facial localization. These changes are associated with a decrease in incidence in both West and East Africa. This is of interest with regard to the role of EBV and malaria in the development of this tumour.

Socioeconomic development is known to be associated with changes in hygienic habits, with delayed infection by common viruses, such as polio, measles and herpesviruses, and with a decrease in the malaria burden. It is probable that delayed primary infection by EBV is becoming increasingly common in Equatorial Africa, which in turn decreases the risk or delays the development of Burkitt's lymphoma.

The etiology of Burkitt's lymphoma has been discussed by Olweny[1]. Pathogenesis can be divided into three stages (see Fig. 1).

---

[1] This volume

FIG. 1.   MULTISTAGE DEVELOPMENT OF BURKITT'S LYMPHOMA

LYDMA: lymphocyte-defined membrane antigen

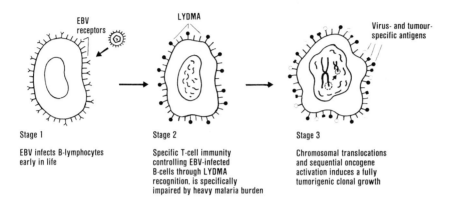

Stage 1

EBV infects B-lymphocytes
early in life

Stage 2

Specific T-cell immunity
controlling EBV-infected
B-cells through LYDMA
recognition, is specifically
impaired by heavy malaria burden

Stage 3

Chromosomal translocations
and sequential oncogene
activation induces a fully
tumorigenic clonal growth

The first appears to be an early and massive infection by
EBV in African children, possibly associated with the fact that
more than two-thirds of mothers have transforming EBV in their
saliva and that most of them premasticate adult food for their
newborns. Such a cultural habit may well be modified by socioeconomic development with consequent delayed EBV primary infection. Massive EBV infection in immunologically immature
children results in polyclonal B-cell proliferation, poorly
controlled by their immature immunological systems and involving
T-cell subsets. The second stage is associated with a heavy
malaria burden, as discussed by Olweny[1] and by Brubaker[1]. The
specific impairment of cell-mediated immunity by a heavy malaria
burden, as shown by Moss et al. (1983), is probably the first
example of a highly specific defect in cell-mediated immunity
leading to a malignant proliferation, and supports the concept of
the key role of immunological surveillance in cancer. The third
stage, associated with a genetic event at the cellular and
molecular level, has been discussed by Lenoir[1]. If the oncogene
activation hypothesis is confirmed, the aim of cancer research in
the future will be to determine how the environmental oncogenic

---

[1] This volume

factors (biological, chemical or physical) sequentially activate cellular oncogenes, leading to monoclonal independent growth.

What are the prospects for the control of Burkitt's lymphoma in Africa ? Is vaccination, as proposed by Epstein (1979), realistic? Even though this tumour is the major cause of deaths from cancer among children, its control is not a high priority from a public health view-point. In contrast, the control of malaria, which is a major lethal disease among African children, should be reconsidered. Brubaker[1] has reported the interesting results of malaria control activities in Tanzania, carried out in collaboration with IARC.

The role of environmental factors associated with certain life-styles should also be studied in relation to Burkitt's lymphoma. Ito et al. (1981) have suggested that the habit of children of eating Euphorbiaceae might be associated with the presence of promoting factors in the vicinity of the developing teeth, where the tumour originates.

The relative importance of both EBV and malaria in the etiology of Burkitt's lymphoma has been assessed by comparing the incidence of EBV-associated tumours in different parts of the world (de-Thé, 1984). Lymphomas of the same histopathological type, but sometimes clinically different from the African form, exist all over the world but with low incidence. Table 2 shows the incidence of non-Hodgkin's lymphomas and, within this group, the proportion of the Burkitt's lymphoma type and EBV-associated tumours. The final column shows the estimated incidence of EBV-associated Burkitt's lymphoma in Europe, North Africa and East Africa, from which it can be seen that there is a 20-fold difference between Europe and North Africa and a further 10-fold difference between North and East Africa. EBV by itself appears to be responsible for the 20-fold difference between Europe and Africa, whereas malaria appears to be responsible for the further 10-fold increase between North and East Africa. Thus the relative importance of environmental factors, and especially of biological environmental factors, in the varying incidence (up to 200-fold) of a given tumour all over the world can be assessed.

---

[1] This volume

Table 2. Incidence of EBV-associated Burkitt's lymphoma in children aged 4-14 years in different geographical areas[a]

Area	NHML incidence per 100 000 per year (% of childhood tumours)	BL/NHML (%)	EBV-associated BL/all BL (%)	Incidence of EBV-associated BL per 100 000 per year
East Africa (Uganda)	9-15 (~80)	95	97	~8-12
North Africa (Algeria)	2-4 (30)	47	85	~1-2
Industrialized countries (France, USA)	1-2 (9)	30	10-15	~0.04-0.08

[a] BL = Burkitt's lymphoma; NHML = non-Hodgkin's malignant lymphoma.

Source: de-Thé, 1984

Nasopharyngeal carcinoma

Undifferentiated carcinoma of the nasopharynx is the main ENT tumour among North and East African males. It should be noted here that the distribution of this cancer probably depends more on ethnic than on geographical factors and that chemical environmental factors associated with life-style probably play a role analogous to that of EBV. The association between EBV and nasopharyngeal carcinoma (NPC), in contrast to Burkitt's lymphoma, is consistent, regular and specific all over the world for the undifferentiated type of NPC. The gradient described above for Burkitt's lymphoma is not seen with NPC. Chinese, North African or Caucasian patients with NPC all have the same high level of antibodies to EBV, as well as EBV genomes present in their epithelial tumour cells. Such a consistent and regular association implies that EBV plays a role in the development of this carcinoma, although the mechanism by which it contributes to the transformation of the nasopharyngeal epithelial cells is still unknown. The close association between the lymphoid element and the epithelial mucosa in the nasopharynx should be stressed at this point. Such cellular interaction is probably of crucial importance, since this type of tumour exists only in the lympho-epithelium part of the nasopharynx.

As discussed at this Symposium by Zeng, the association between EBV and NPC, and particularly the viral capsid antigen (VCA) and early antigen (EA) antibodies of the IgA class, permits the early detection of this tumour in high-incidence areas. For intermediate areas, such as North and East Africa, EBV serology assists in the differential diagnosis.

Another environmental factor, probably of a chemical nature, appears to play a role in the development of this tumour. Chemical factors, such as promoters belonging to the phorbol ester family, may be involved. This is the working hypothesis of both Zeng (1983) and Ito et al. (1983), who feel that certain Euphorbiaceae present in the environment of the high-incidence areas may well play a role.

Another possible explanation of the ethnic distribution of NPC (which cannot be explained by the ubiquitous EBV), is the possibility that the food habits of certain ethnic groups are associated with a reactivating agent(s) that plays(s) a role in the development of this tumour. This is the working hypothesis of the anthropologist, A. Hubert, who has compared the food habits of North Africans, Cantonese Chinese and Eskimos, the three groups at highest risk for this tumour. She came to the conclusion that certain methods of preserving food may lead to the presence of mycotoxins in it, although this remains to be proved (Hubert & de-Thé, 1982).

As far as the control of NPC is concerned, it is possible that vaccination against EBV might be of value (Epstein et al., 1983). The situation in North and East Africa, where 25% of the tumours develop before the age of 20, would favour vaccination, since the time necessary to assess the results would be shorter than in China, where NPC develops 20 years later. Is EBV vaccination soon after birth feasible in Africa ? The situation with regard to hepatis B vaccination is totally different, since the impact on hepatocellular carcinoma is only of secondary importance as compared with the prevention of acute and chronic hepatitis. Since it is not known whether any other diseases are associated with EBV, the question as to the value of EBV vaccination may remain unanswered. Population-based detection of NPC through the detection of IgA/VCA remains an immediate possibility, if the target populations are carefully selected among males in the specific age-group concerned, e.g., above 40 or in North African families with multiple cases of this tumour.

CONCLUSIONS

Collaboration between African clinicians and researchers in hospitals with their European and American counterparts should be further strengthened. The role of the Technical Secretariat of the OAU and of the International Association for Research and Control of Virus Associated Cancers will be of crucial importance in promoting such collaboration. Once again, the words of Pliny will come true: "Semper novi ex Africa".

REFERENCES

Barré-Sinoussi, F., Chermann, J.C., Rey, F., Nugeyre, M.T., Chamaret, S., Gruest, J., Dauget, C., Axler-Blin, C., Vézinet-Brun, F., Rouzioux, C., Rozenbaum, W. & Montagnier, L. (1983) Isolation of a T-lymphotropic retrovirus from a patient at risk for acquired immune deficiency syndrome (AIDS). Science, 220, 868-871

Biggar, R.J., Henle, W., Fleisher, G., Bocker, J., Lennette, E.T. & Henle, G. (1978) Primary Epstein-Barr virus infection in African infants. I. Decline of maternal antibodies and time of infection. Int. J. Cancer, 22, 239-243

Blattner, W.A., Kalyanaraman, V.S., Robert-Guroff, M., Lister, R.A., Galton, D.A.G., Sarin, P.S., Crawford, M.G., Catovsky, D., Greaves, M. & Gallo, R.C. (1982) The human type-C retrovirus, HTLV, in Blacks from the Caribbean region and relationship to adult T-cell leukemia-lymphoma. Int. J. Cancer, 30, 257-264

Burkitt, D.P. (1958) A sarcoma involving the jaws in African children. Br. J. Surq., 46, 218

Catovsky, D., Greaves, M.F., Rose, M., Galton, D.A.G., Goolden, A.W.G., McCluskey, D.R., White, J.M., Lampert, I., Bourikas, G., Ireland, R., Brownell, A.J., Bridges, M.M., Blattner, W.A. & Gallo, R.C. (1982) Adult T-cell lymphoma-leukemia in Blacks from the West Indies. Lancet, 1, 639-643

Clumeck, N., Sonnet, J., Taelman, H., Mascart-Lemoine, F., de Bruyère, M., Vandeperre, P., Dasnoy, J., Margelis, L., Lamy, M., Jonas, C., Eyckmans, L., Noel, H., Vanhaeverbeek, M. & Butzler, J.P. (1984) Acquired immunodeficiency syndrome in African patients. New Engl. J. Med., 310, 492-497

de-Thé, G. (1977) Is Burkitt's lymphoma related to a perinatal infection by Epstein-Barr virus? Lancet, 1, 335-338

de-Thé, G. (1984) Epstein-Barr virus and Burkitt's lymphoma world-wide: the causal relationship revisited. In: Lenoir, G.M., O'Conor, G.T. & Olweny, C.L.M., eds, Burkitt's Lymphoma: A Human Cancer Model (IARC Scientific Publications No. 60), Lyon, International Agency for Research on Cancer (in press)

Epstein, M.A. (1979) Vaccine control of EB-virus associated tumors. In: Epstein, M.A. & Achong, B.G., eds, The Epstein-Barr Virus, Berlin, Heidelberg & New York, Springer, pp. 440-448

Epstein, M.A., North, J.R. & Morgan, A.J. (1983) Possibilities for antiviral vaccine intervention in nasopharyngeal carcinoma. In: Prasad, ed., Nasopharyngeal Carcinoma: Current Concepts, Kuala Lumpur, University of Malaya, pp. 375-386

Fleming, A.F., Yamamoto, N., Bhusnurmath, S.R., Maharajan, R., Schneider, J. & Hunsmann, G. (1983) Antibodies to ATLV (HTLV) in Nigerian blood donors and patients with chronic lymphatic leukaemia or lymphoma. Lancet, 2, 334-335

Gallo, R.C. (1984a) Human T-lymphotropic retroviruses. In: Gallo, R.C., Essex, M.E. & Gross, L., eds, Human T-Cell Leukemia/Lymphoma Virus, Cold Spring Harbor, Cold Spring Harbor Laboratory, pp. 1-8

Gallo, R.C. (1984b) Human T-cell leukemia-lymphoma virus and T-cell malignancies in adults. Cancer surveys (in press)

Gessain, A., Calender, A., Strobel, M., Lefait-Robin, R. & de-Thé, G. (1984) Haute prévalence d'anticorps anti-HTLV1 chez les Boni, groupe d'origine africaine, isolé depuis le 18ème siècle en Guyane Française. C.R. Acad. Sci. Paris (in press)

Hinuma, Y., Komoda, H., Chosa, T., Kondo, T., Kohakura, M., Takenaka, T., Kiruchi, M., Ichimaru, M., Yunoki, K., Sato, I., Matsuo, R., Takiuchhi, Y., Uchino, H. & Hanaoka, M. (1982) Antibodies to adult T-cell leukemia virus associated antigen (ATLA) in sera from patients with ATL and controls in Japan: a nation-wide sero epidemiologic study. Int. J. Cancer, 29, 631-635

Hubert, A. & de-Thé, G. (1982) Comportement alimentaire, modes de vie et cancer du rhinopharynx (NPC). Bull. Cancer (Paris), 69, 476-482

Hunsmann, G., Schneider, J., Schmitt, J. & Yamamoto, N. (1983) Detection of serum antibodies to adult T-cell leukemia virus in non human primates and in people from Africa. Int. J. Cancer, 32, 329-332

Ito, Y., Kishishita, M., Morigaki, T., Yanase, S. & Hirayama, T. (1981) Induction and intervention of Epstein-Barr virus expression in human lymphoblastoid cell lines: a stimulation model for study of cause and prevention of nasopharyngeal carcinoma and Burkitt's lymphoma. In: Grundmann, E., Krueger, G.R.F. & Ablashi, D.V., eds, Nasopharyngeal Carcinoma, Stuttgart & New York, Gustav Fischer Verlag, pp. 255-262

Ito, Y., Yanase, S., Kishishita, M., Hirayama, T., Hirota, M., Oohigashi, H. & Koshinizu, K. (1983) The roles of Epstein-Barr virus, normal bacterial flora and promoter plant diterpene esters in causation of nasopharyngeal carcinoma. In: Prasad, Nasopharyngeal Carcinoma: Current Concepts, Kuala Lumpur, University of Malaya, pp. 321-327

Kalyanaraman, V.S., Sarngadharan, M.G., Robert-Guroff, M., Miyoshi, I., Blayney, D., Golde, D. & Gallo, R.C. (1982) A new subtype of human T cell leukemia virus (HTLV-II) associated with a T-cell variant of hairy cell leukemia. Science, 218, 571-573

Miyoshi, I., Kubonishi, I., Yoshimoto, S., Akagi, T., Ohtaiki, Y., Shiraishi, Y. & Hinuma, Y. (1981) Type C virus particles in a cord T-cell line derived by co-cultivating normal human cord leukocytes and human leukaemia T-cells. Nature, 294, 770-771

Moss, D.J., Burrows, S.R., Castelino, D.J., Kane, G., Pope, J.H., Rickinson, A.B., Alpers, M.P. & Heywood, P.F. (1983) A comparison of Epstein-Barr virus-specific T-cell-immunity in malaria endemic and non-endemic regions of Papua New-Guinea. Int. J. Cancer, 31, 727-732

Piot, P., Taelman, H., Minilangu, K.B., Mbendi, N., Ndangi, K., Kalambayi, K., Bridts, C., Quinn, T.C., Feinsod, F.M., Wobin, O., Mazebo, P., Stevens, P., Mitchell, S. & McCormick, J.B. (1984) Acquired immunodeficiency syndrome in a heterosexual population in Zaire. Lancet, 2, 65-69

Poiesz, P.J., Ruscetti, F.W., Gazdar, A.F., Bunn, P.A., Minna, J.D. & Gallo, R.C. (1980) Detection and isolation of type C retrovirus particles from fresh and cultured lymphocytes of a patient with cutaneous T cell lymphoma. Proc. natl Acad. Sci. USA, 77, 7415-7419

Popovic, M., Sarngadharan, M.G., Read, E. & Gallo, R.C. (1984) Detection, isolation and continuous production of cytopathic retroviruses (HTLV-III) from patients with AIDS and pre-AIDS. Science, 224, 497-500

Saxinger, W.C., Lange-Wantzin, G., Thomsen, K., Lapin, B., Yakovleva, L., Li, Y.W., Guo, H.G., Robert-Guroff, M., Blattner, W.A., Ito, Y. & Gallo, R.C. (1984) Human T-cell leukemia virus: a diverse family of related exogenous retroviruses of humans and old world primates. In: Gallo, R.C., Essex, M.E. & Gross, L., eds, Human T-Cell Leukemia-/Lymphoma Virus, Cold Spring Harbor, Cold Spring Harbor Laboratory, pp. 323-330

Van De Perre, P., Lepage, P., Kestelyn, P., Hekker, A.C., Rouvroy, D., Bogaerts, J., Kayhigi, J., Butzler, J.P. & Clumeck, N. (1984) Acquired immunodeficiency syndrome in Rwanda. Lancet, 2, 62-65

Zeng, Y., Zhong, J.M., Mo, Y.K., Miao, X.C. (1983) EB virus EA
    induction of Raji cells by Chinese medicinal herbs. _Inter-
    virology_, _19_, 201-204

POSSIBLE VIRAL ETIOLOGY OF CHILDHOOD ACUTE
LYMPHOSARCOMA-CELL LEUKAEMIA IN KENYA

E.G. Kasili

Department of Pathology
College of Health Sciences
University of Nairobi
Nairobi, Kenya

RESUME

Les leucémies aiguës avec aspect lymphosarcomateux représentent au Kenya 13-14% de toutes les leucémies de l'enfance. Elles
surviennent par périodes chez des enfants âgés de 5 à 9 ans, et
on peut de ce fait soupçonner un facteur leucémogène de l'environnement. Une étude des enfants atteints de leucémie aiguë a
été réalisée; elle confirme que la leucémie aiguë avec aspect
lymphosarcomateux constitue une entité clinique spécifique au
sein des leucémies lymphocytaires aiguës. Le virus des leucémies
T humaines (HTLV) joue-t-il un rôle dans son étiologie? Cela
reste à déterminer.

SUMMARY

Childhood acute lymphosarcoma-cell leukaemia (CALSCL)
accounts for 13-14% of all childhood leukaemias in Kenya. It
occurs in temporal clusters in children aged 5-9 years, and an
environmental leukaemogenic factor is therefore suspected. A
study of children with acute leukaemia was carried out, and
suggested that CALSCL is a specific clinical entity amongst the
acute lymphocytic leukaemias. Whether human T-cell leukaemia
virus (HTLV) may play a role in its etiology remains to be
determined.

INTRODUCTION

Childhood acute lymphosarcoma-cell leukaemia (CALSCL), a leukaemic transformation of the non-Hodgkin's lymphomas, is common among childhood acute leukaemias in sub-Saharan Africa (Kasili, 1978, 1980), accounting for 13-14% of all childhood leukaemias in Kenya. It mainly affects children aged 5-9 years, among whom temporal clusters occur, suggesting an environmental etiological factor.

MATERIALS AND METHODS

A total of 198 cases of childhood acute leukaemia (CAL), diagnosed at the Kenyatta National Hospital, Nairobi, over the period 1975-1983 were analysed for:

(1)   The monthly variation in acute lymphoblastic leukaemia (ALL), acute non-lymphocytic leukaemia (ANLL) and CALSCL.

(2)   The age distribution of these three subtypes of CAL.

(3)   The differences at presentation in the frequency of occurrence of splenomegaly, mediastinal mass, generalized lymphadenopathy and bone pain in ALL and CALSCL.

(4)   The differences in initial total leucocyte count in ALL and CALSCL.

(5)   Remission induction rates and duration of survival after complete remission, in all three subtypes.

RESULTS

A seasonal variation was found in CALSCL, with peaks in March, June and December, while the peaks for ALL were in January and October. ANLL occurred more or less uniformly throughout the year. The difference in age distribution was particularly marked as between ALL (56% of cases occur in the 0-4-year age-group) and CALSCL (67.8% of cases in the 5-9 year age-group). With regard to presenting features, generalized lymphadenopathy occurred more frequently in CALSCL than in ALL, and a mediastinal mass was invariably found in the former but rarely in the latter. Spleno-megaly occurred in 76% of cases of CALSCL but only in 52% of cases of ALL. Bone pain was not found to be an important discriminating feature. Initial total leucocyte counts were elevated in 40% of CALSCL patients but only in 18% of ALl patients. Remission induction rates in CALSCL were slightly lower than those for ALL, but survival is significantly inferior in the former.

DISCUSSION

The study confirmed that CALSCL is a specific clinical entity amongst the acute lymphocytic leukaemias because of its distinct clinicopathological features. The occurrence of clusters of the disease at certain times of the year suggests that it is caused by an environmental leukaemogenic agent, possibly human T-cell leukaemia virus (HTLV), which is found with high frequency in Kenyan green monkeys (Yamamoto et al., 1983). Although HTLV has so far been reported only in association with adult haematological malignancies, the clinical characteristics and behaviour of CALSCL are very similar to those of adult T-cell leukaemia in Jamaican Blacks (Catovsky et al., 1982). A number of further studies on CALSCL are therefore planned.

REFERENCES

Catovsky, D., Greaves, M.F., Rose, M., Galton, D.A., Goolden, A.W., McCluskey, D.R., White, J.M., Lampert, I., Bourikas, G., Ireland, R., Brownell, A.I., Bridges, J.M., Blattner, W.A. & Gallo, R.C. (1982) Adult T-cell lymphoma-leukaemia in Blacks from the West Indies. Lancet, 1, 639-643

Kasili, E.G. (1978) Acute lymphosarcoma cell leukaemia of childhood. Nairobi J. Med., 10, 20

Kasili, E.G. (1980) Leukaemia in Kenya, MD Thesis, University of Nairobi

Yamamoto, N., Hinuma, Y., zur Hausen, H., Schneider, J., Hunsmann, G. (1983) African green monkeys are infected with adult T-cell leukaemia virus or closely related agent. Lancet, 1, 240-241

SQUAMOUS-CELL CARCINOMA, KAPOSI'S SARCOMA AND BURKITT'S LYMPHOMA ARE CONSEQUENCES OF IMPAIRED IMMUNE SURVEILLANCE OF UBIQUITOUS VIRUSES IN ACQUIRED IMMUNE DEFICIENCY SYNDROME, ALLOGRAFT RECIPIENTS AND TROPICAL AFRICAN PATIENTS

D.T. Purtilo, G. Manolov, Y. Manolova, S. Harada & H. Lipscomb
Departments of Pathology and Laboratory Medicine and Pediatrics,
and the Eppley Institute for Research in Cancer and
Allied Diseases
University of Nebraska Medical Center
Omaha, NE, USA

RESUME

Le système immunitaire a évolué sous l'action des pressions sélectives darwiniennes comme moyen de défense contre les virus ubiquitaires. La surveillance immunitaire contre les antigènes viraux protège les sujets normaux. Les individus atteints de déficits immunitaires congénitaux ou acquis deviennent vulnérables aux virus ubiquitaires et cela peut entraîner l'apparition de néoplasmes tels que des lymphomes B, des cancers primitifs du foie, des épithéliomas spinocellulaires, des sarcomes de Kaposi, des cancers du col utérin et du pénis.

Le déficit immunitaire permet au virus Epstein-Barr, au virus de l'hépatite B, au papillomavirus, au virus Herpes simplex et au cytomégalovirus d'induire la prolifération des cellules-cibles. A chaque virus correspond une cellule-cible spécifique, portant des récepteurs pour le virus, et l'infection entraîne la prolifération des cellules-cibles plutôt que leur lyse. Divers cofacteurs tels que l'alimentation, l'exposition à des agents promoteurs, les parasitoses, l'exposition à la lumière ultraviolette peuvent favoriser le développement de cancers. Selon le type et la gravité du déficit immunitaire, une prolifération graduelle peut aboutir à l'évolution d'un clone malin. Le passage d'une prolifération polyclonale de cellules infectées par un virus à une tumeur maligne monoclonale est vraisemblablement dû à des remaniements chromosomiques spécifiques, qui permettent l'activation d'un oncogène et qui confèrent à la cellule altérée un avantage de croissance sélectif sur les cellules diploïdes normales. La prévention de l'oncogénèse virale est peut être

possible grâce au traitement des individus immunodéficients
atteints de troubles précancéreux. L'immunothérapie et la
thérapie antivirale peuvent prévenir la progression de la prolifération induite par le virus.

SUMMARY

The immune system has evolved under Darwinian pressures as a
defence against ubiquitous viruses. Immune surveillance against
viral antigens protects the normal host. Individuals with inherited or acquired immune-deficiency disorders can become vulnerable to ubiquitous viruses and neoplasms can ensue, such as
B-cell lymphoma, hepatocellular carcinoma, squamous-cell carcinoma, Kaposi's sarcoma, and carcinoma of the penis and uterine
cervix. Immunodeficiency permits Epstein-Barr virus, hepatitis B
virus, papillomavirus, herpes simplex virus, and cytomegalovirus
to induce sustained target-cell proliferation. Each virus
selects specific cellular targets bearing viral receptors and the
infection leads to proliferation of the target cells rather than
lysis. Various co-factors, including nutrition, exposure to
tumour-promoting agents, parasitic infection, and ultraviolet
light, may promote carcinogenesis. Depending on the type and
severity of the immune deficiency, gradual proliferation may lead
to evolution of a malignant clone. Conversion of polyclonal
virally infected proliferating cells to give monoclonal malignancy is probably due to specific cytogenetic rearrangements
which allow oncogene activation and endow an altered tumour cell
with selective growth advantages over normal diploid cells.
Prevention of viral oncogenesis may be possible by treatment of
immune-deficient individuals with premalignant disorders.
Immunotherapy and antiviral therapy may prevent progression of
viral-induced proliferation to malignancy.

The purpose of this paper is to discuss and evaluate the
role of immune deficiency and viruses in the induction of
malignancies commonly occurring in Africans residing in sub-
Saharan Africa (Purtilo, 1976). The types of malignancies
commonly occurring in this region are believed to be due to
ubiquitous viruses. A failure of immune surveillance mechanisms
to recognize viral antigens and abrogate proliferation of
infected target cells predisposes to malignancy by increasing the

chance of a proliferating cell undergoing a cytogenetic or molecular alteration which endows it with malignant characteristics.

The immunological surveillance hypothesis has been elaborated during this century by Ehrlich, Thomas, Burnet, and Schwartz (reviewed by Purtilo & Linder, 1983). This hypothesis rests on several assumptions: (1) that neoplastic cells possess unique tumour antigens: (2) tumour antigens provoke an immune response in the host; and (3) the immune response is protective and eliminates the tumour. Evidence supporting this view has come from the reports of Starzl and Penn and Gatti and Good that there is a markedly increased occurrence of certain malignancies, especially malignant lymphomas, in renal allograft recipients and children with congenital immune deficiency (reviewed in Purtilo et al., 1984a). However attractive this hypothesis may be in explaining the occurrence of all types of malignancies, it is clear that only a limited number of neoplasms occur in immune-deficient patients.

Table 1 shows the malignant neoplasms occurring in increased frequency in immune-deficient patients. The unifying biological theme present in the groups of patients with immune deficiency is the possibility that the malignancies could be associated with ubiquitous viruses. Given these clinical observations, this hypothesis is being tested by studying 'experiments of nature' with inherited immune-deficiency disorders and also in patients with acquired immune deficiency. The study of Epstein-Barr virus (EBV) and its role as an oncogenic virus in immune-deficient patients will be discussed in detail as a model for testing this hypothesis. In addition, etiological factors responsible for squamous-cell carcinoma, Kaposi's sarcoma, and hepatocellular carcinoma will be considered. Immune surveillance is not responsive to tumour-specific antigens, but to virus-specific antigens. Failure to control proliferation of cellular targets infected by ubiquitous viruses may lead to malignancy in Africans who are immunosuppressed.

Table 1. Malignant neoplasms in immune-deficient patients[a]

Group	Malignancies	Virus or other factor
Inherited immune deficiency	B-cell lymphoma	EBV
	Leukaemia	Chromosome breakage
	Hepatocellular carcinoma	HBV, anabolic steroids
Renal transplant recipients	Squamous-cell carcinoma	HBV, ultraviolet light
	B-cell lymphoma	EBV
	Kaposi's sarcoma	CMV
	Cervical carcinoma	HPV, HSV
	Kaposi's sarcoma	CMV
	B-cell lymphoma	EBV, chromosome breakage
Male homosexuals	Oral squamous-cell carcinoma	HPB, HSV
	Cloagenic carcinoma	HSV, HPB
	Hepatocellular carcinoma	HBV
Africans	Hepatocellular carcinoma	HBV, aflatoxin
	Kaposi's sarcoma	CMV
	Burkitt's lymphoma	EBV
	Squamous-cell carcinoma	HPV, HSV

[a] EBV, Epstein-Barr virus; HPB, human papillomavirus; CMV, cytomegalovirus; HBV, hepatitis B virus; HSV, herpes simplex virus. Source: Purtilo et al. (1984b). Published by permission of Grune & Stratton

EBV-ASSOCIATED DISEASES IN IMMUNE-DEFICIENT PATIENTS

Burkitt's (1958) seminal observation of malignant B-cell lymphoma in African children residing in holoendemic malarial regions continues to serve as a model for investigating the etiology of malignancies in Africa and elsewhere. Recognition of EBV (Epstein et al., 1964) through collaborative studies with Burkitt (Fig. 1) led in turn to the recognition that infectious mononucleosis is caused by this virus (Henle et al., 1966). Immunological studies of patients with infectious mononucleosis and more recently in those with immune deficiency have uncovered some of the mechanisms of immunological surveillance against this virus (reviewed in Purtilo et al., 1984a).

Individuals with acute infectious mononucleosis have pharyngitis, fever, lymphadenomegaly, and malaise. The atypical lymphocytes found in the peripheral blood of these patients reflect an immunological struggle occurring in the patient. The virus has a tropism for B-cells since they contain receptors. A polyclonal B-cell proliferation is initiated by the virus and is subdued by an explosive T-cell and natural killer cell (NK) response which abrogates this potentially lethal B-cell proliferation (Purtilo et al., 1984a). In vitro interferon prevents the outgrowth of B-cells infected by the virus (Garner et al., 1984) and a similar phenomenon presumably occurs in vivo. Concurrently, antibodies to viral capsid antigen (VCA) of IgM class and antibodies to early antigen (EA) emerge in the patient's serum. Later, IgG antibodies against VCA and anti-EBV nuclear-associated antigen (EBNA) appear (Henle et al., 1979). EBV-specific cytotoxic T-cells, which may serve to maintain the latency of the virus, appear late.

Uncommonly, infectious mononucleosis results from primary infection by EBV. Nearly 95% of African children are seropositive by age 5. Studies performed by Klein and others have revealed the presence of the EBV genome in approximately 97% of Burkitt's lymphomas (Klein, 1975). The debate regarding the role of EBV in the etiology of Burkitt's lymphoma has continued during the past 25 years (Purtilo et al., 1984c). A hypothesis to explain the mechanism permitting this ubiquitous and usually non-life-threatening viral infection to produce Burkitt's lymphoma is that immune deficiency enables the virus to produce a chronic B-cell proliferation, which eventually converts to a malignant B-cell neoplasm. This view has resulted from studies of individuals with immune deficiency.

FIG. 1.   ELECTRON MICROGRAPH OF A LYMPHOBLASTOID LINE
DISPLAYING EPSTEIN-BARR VIRUS PARTICLES
(PUBLISHED BY PERMISSION OF <u>THE LANCET</u>)

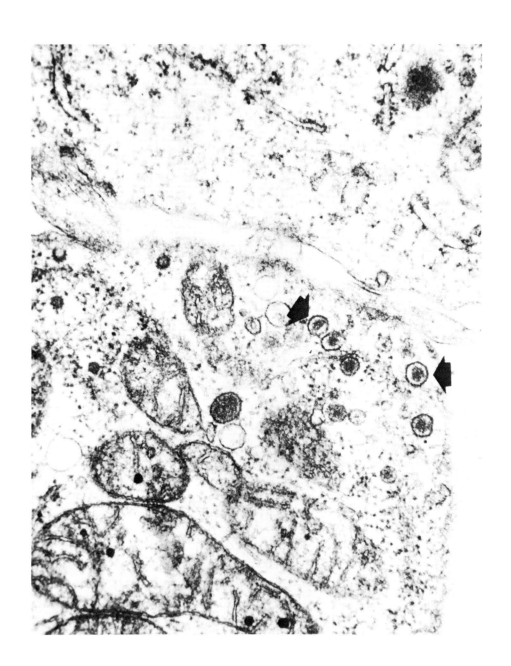

In 1975, Purtilo et al. (1975) described the X-linked lymphoproliferative (XLP) syndrome in the Duncan kindred. In this family, three brothers had died of infectious mononucleosis, two maternally related male cousins succumbed to malignant lymphoma, one following 10 months of chronic infectious mononucleosis, and a sixth male died of agammaglobulinaemia following infectious mononucleosis. At autopsy, destruction and depletion of the thymus gland was seen and T-cell dependent regions of lymph-node and spleen were found to be depleted. The registry of cases of X-linked lymphoproliferative syndrome (Purtilo et al., 1982) contains more than 100 patients, of whom two-thirds have died of infectious mononucleosis and one-third have developed malignant lymphoma. Approximately 20% of the patients have developed hypo- or agammaglobulinaemia and a slightly smaller number of males have developed aplastic anaemia. The expression of this genetic disorder following EBV infection has been 100% and the mortality has been approximately 85%.

Immunological studies of the surviving boys with XLP and males at risk for the syndrome reveal their inability to mount a full spectrum of antibodies against EBV. In particular, the affected males lack antibodies against EBNA (Sakamoto et al., 1980). In addition, they lack T-cell-specific killing of autologous B-cells, as measured in the regression assay (Harada et al., 1982). Non-specific immunity, as assessed by NK activity against the erythroleukaemia cell line K562, is reduced in the majority of affected males. The NK cell is thought to provide a first line of defence against both malignancy and viruses. No previous sensitization or memory for the antigen is required for NK activity. However, in XLP, males at risk for the syndrome show normal NK function (Seeley et al., 1982), as do male homosexuals prior to developing acquired immune deficiency syndrome (AIDS). In males with XLP, NK defects occur after infection by EBV. It is postulated that destruction of thymus epithelium is, in part, responsible for the progression of the immune deficiency in XLP and male homosexuals with AIDS following infection by EBV (Purtilo et al., 1984c).

A variety of life-threatening EBV-induced lymphoproliferative diseases, including malignant lymphomas, have also been demonstrated in other patients with primary immune deficiency, such as severe combined immune deficiency, ataxia telangiectasia, and common variable immune deficiency (Purtilo & Klein, 1981).

Immune deficiency is believed to be an important factor in permitting EBV to induce Burkitt's lymphoma in African children (Purtilo et al., 1984c). the following may be cited in support of this notion. EBV infects early in life at a time when the immune system is immature. Males are predominantly affected by Burkitt's lymphoma and show inferior immune responses to EBV as compared to females. Malnutrition is common in African children and Burkitt's lymphoma is known to occur mainly in the lower socioeconomic strata. Nutritional thymectomy occurs in children with kwashiorkor and may also occur, to a lesser extent, in those with borderline malnutrition. Exposure to toxins which may be immunosuppressive, such as cyanide in cassava and aflatoxin contaminating maize, may contribute to immune deficiency. Chronic measles infection is known to occur in malnourished individuals and such viruses can be associated with chromosomal breakage. Finally, malaria is known to suppress T-cell immunity (reviewed in Purtilo et al., 1983). Supporting this view are the findings by investigators studying children in areas endemic for Burkitt's lymphoma in New Guinea (Moss et al., 1983), who have demonstrated that individuals with malaria show defective recognition of EBV antigens in the autologous B-cell regression assay.

The view that immune deficiency is permissive of lymphomagenesis in immune-deficient patients is further supported by studies of individuals undergoing renal transplantation. Collaborative studies with Hanto and Klein (Saemundsen et al., 1981; Hanto et al., 1981, 1984) have shown that EBV produces B-cell lesions which are life-threatening in renal transplant recipients. It has been demonstrated by molecular hybridization that the EBV genome is present in virtually every case where tissue has been examined. Two patterns of disease appear, depending on the age of the individual. Patients less than 20 years of age show an infectious-mononucleosis-like disorder, low EBV-specific antibody titres, a brief incubation period from time of transplantation to appearance of tumour, widespread disease, and death within 3 months. In contrast, individuals older than 45 years of age show localized tumour masses associated with elevated EBV-specific antibody titres, an incubation period of several years, and survival for approximately 9 months (Hanto et al., 1984). The development of these lymphoproliferative lesions is probably due to suppression of the cytotoxic EBV-specific and natural killer cells against viral antigens. This allows infected B-cells to continue proliferating unabated, leading to polyclonal infiltrative lesions. If the immune suppression is less severe, a gradual transformation to monoclonal malignancy may occur

(Hanto et al., 1982). Reactivation of EBV is probably the more common pattern in these patients. Moreover, withdrawal of immune suppression leads to regression of the transplant lymphomas (Starzl et al., 1984).

The use of immunosuppressive agents, such as antithymocyte globulin and especially cyclosporins, can lead to a high frequency of malignant lymphomas in renal and cardiac transplant patients (Penn, 1984). Cyclosporin is a metabolite of a fungus (Borel, 1983). Hence it seems reasonable to suppose that ingestion of fungal contaminants could cause immunosuppression in certain Africans eating mouldy foods.

Ubiquitous viruses are responsible for malignancies seen in male homosexuals with AIDS, which appeared in the United States in 1981 in large urban areas (Morbidity and Mortality Weekly Report, 1981). Diagnostic criteria for AIDS developed by the Centers for Communicable Diseases in Atlanta, Georgia, include: (1) the presence of reliably diagnosed disease at least moderately indicative of an underlying cellular immune deficiency, such as Kaposi's sarcoma in a patient less than 60 years of age, Pneumocystis pneumonia or other opportunistic infections; and (2) the absence of known causes of underlying immunodeficiency and of any other reduced resistance reported to be associated with the disease (immunosuppressive therapy, lymphoreticular malignancy). To date, the major risk groups in the United States have been male homosexuals, intravenous heroin abusers, Haitians, and haemophiliacs. More than two-thirds of the patients have been male homosexuals from large urban areas such as New York City, San Francisco, and Los Angeles. It is apparent that a number of highly promiscuous male homosexuals show prodromal AIDS, which has been described as the wasting-lymph-node syndrome. These indivuals variously show chronic lymphadeno-megaly, recurrent flu-like symptoms, fatigue, malaise, weight loss, anorexia, fever, night sweats, diarrhoea, and opportunistic infections. They may also show immune thrombocytopenia purpura.

The etiological basis of AIDS continues to be a vexing problem. The hypothesis receiving most attention during the past 3 years is that a single agent is responsible for the disorder (Fauci, 1983). Postulates of a new virus, a mutated old virus, or a retrovirus, such as human T-cell leukaemia virus, have all been explored. However, HTLV-I is a transforming and not a lytic virus. The rationale behind such postulates is that the hypothetical virus would destroy helper T-cells, leading to immune dys-

function and susceptibility to opportunistic infections and
malignancies. HTLV-III has been incriminated as the cause of
AIDS (Montagnier, 1984).

It is more probable, however, that changes in life-style and
medical practices have led to an overloading of the immune system
with repeated bombardment by viral antigens and other immunosuppressive agents (Sonnabend et al., 1983) (Fig. 2). Under
usual environmental conditions, the immune system combats but one
or at most two pathogens simultaneously, and multiple infections
over a sustained period of time lead to a collapse of the immune
system. Highly promiscuous male homosexuals are repeatedly
exposed to cytomegalovirus, HTLV-III, and other viral, bacterial,
fungal, and parasitic infections, which also contribute to overwhelming the immune system. Moreover, men who are recipients of
sperm per rectum or per os often develop antibodies which may
cross-react with human NK and cytotoxic T-cells and thereby
suppress immunity. A reversible phase of acquisition termed
pre-AIDS is characterized by hyperplasia of the immune system and
immune regulatory disturbances. Occasionally, a second phase,
AIDS, occurs which is irreversible and fatal within a few years.
It is suggested that destruction of thymic epithelium in these
patients leads to progressive loss of immune regulation (Purtilo
et al., 1984b). Defective immune surveillance permits increasing
viral burdens. Individuals with severe immune deficiency succumb
to opportunistic infections, especially with Pneumocystis
carinii. Those with slightly better immune competence may
develop Kaposi's sarcoma, malignant lymphomas (carrying EBV) or
squamous-cell carcinomas (Table 1). Hundreds of the initial 3000
patients with AIDS have developed Kaposi's sarcoma and 90
patients with malignant lymphoma (predominantly B-cell type) have
recently been studied.

ETIOLOGY OF KAPOSI'S SARCOMA

Immune suppression as a major factor in the induction of
Kaposi's sarcoma (KS) has been recognized for many years
(reviewed in Penn, 1983). KS is also found commonly associated
with malignant lymphomas. This malignancy is common among native
Africans residing in rain forests, where it accounts for 3-9% of
all malignancies. In contrast, it is rare in the United States.

FIG. 2. DIAGRAM SHOWING SUGGESTED PROCESS OF DEVELOPMENT
OF ACQUIRED IMMUNE DEFICIENCY SYNDROME (AIDS) IN MALE HOMOSEXUALS

Frequent sexual encounters expose these men to repeated cytomegalovirus (CMV) infections and contact with allogeneic semen.
Immune responses to these agents are deleterious and lead to the
acquisition of immunodeficiency. Formation of cross-reacting
antibodies and immune complexes impairs immune regulation and
surveillance. If exposure is sustained, disease progresses.
Opportunistic infections and viral-induced malignant neoplasms
can then develop.
EBV, Epstein-Barr virus; INF, interferon
From Sonnabend et al., 1983. Published by permission of the
Journal of the American Medical Association

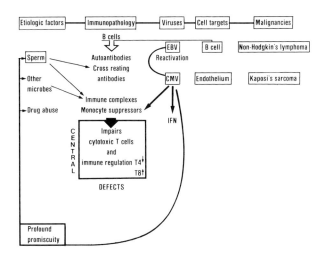

However, among elderly individuals of Mediterranean ancestry,
especially Italians and Jews, the incidence is higher. A 400-
500-fold increased occurrence of KS is found in renal transplant
recipients and the tumour is the major type of malignancy in AIDS
patients. The common feature of all the populations at high risk
for this malignancy is depression of cellular immunity.

An additional factor associated with immune deficiency is the marked male predominance (10:1). HLA-DR5 has been found as the genetic marker of KS in AIDS patients and in the Mediterranean populations with a higher incidence of the tumour. Spontaneous regression of KS has been reported (Costa & Rabson, 1983), and this finding has led to the postulate that it is not a true tumour, but is polyclonal and will regress when cellular immunity against the lesion is restored.

Cytomegalovirus (CMV) has been the candidate virus in the etiology of KS (Giraldo et al., 1972). A herpesvirus has been isolated from an African KS cell line, serological studies have revealed elevated antibody titres to the virus in patients, and molecular hybridization studies have revealed CMV DNA in KS (Drew et al., 1982). A recent study of 15 Zambian men and 1 woman with KS (Downing et al., 1984) has revealed features similar to those of AIDS: the average age was 39 years, inverted T-helper-to-suppressor ratios were found and polymicrobial infection, including seropositivity for CMV, was documented.

SQUAMOUS-CELL CARCINOMA AND IMMUNE DEFICIENCY TO PAPILLOMAVIRUSES

Cutaneous squamous-cell carcinomas are common in renal transplant allograft recipients (Walder et al., 1971; Penn, 1984) and are occurring in the oral and anal mucosa of male homosexuals (Sonnabend et al., 1983). Carcinoma of the uterine cervix and penis are common in Africans (Oettle, 1962; Templeton, 1973). Substantial evidence associates papillomaviruses with these malignancies.

The human papillomaviruses (HPVs) have long been recognized as the causative agent of benign cutaneous and mucosal proliferative lesions. Currently, more than 20 distinct HPVs have been described. Individual types are associated with particular lesions (Howley, 1982; Jablonska et al., 1982). For example, HPV type 5 (HPV-5) DNA has been identified in skin cancers of renal allograft recipients (Lutzner et al., 1983). HPV-6 and -11 have been found in genital and laryngeal papillomas and cervical carcinoma (Gissman et al., 1983). Herpes simplex infection has been proposed to act as a promoter in carcinogenesis of uterine cervix cells (already) infected by papillomavirus (zur Hausen, 1982).

It is highly likely that various promoting agents, such as simultaneous viral infections, tumour-promoting chemicals or ultraviolet light (Walder et al., 1971), may be involved in the development of squamous-cell carcinomas. Failure of immune surveillance against viral antigens probably permits these malignancies to develop. Oesophageal carcinoma, another squamous-cell carcinoma common in certain regions of Africa and China, should be investigated for the presence of HPV and immune deficiency.

HEPATOCELLULAR CARCINOMA

Hepatocellular carcinoma (HCC) is a major form of cancer in several areas of Africa and portions of South-east Asia. During the past decade, substantial evidence has accrued suggesting that hepatitis B virus (HBV) is an etiological agent of HCC (London, 1981; Prince & Alcabes, 1982). The infection leading to HCC probably arises early in life form a seropositive mother. Persistent infection may lead to chronic active hepatitis or integration of the virus into the cellular DNA of the hepatocyte and this integration converts the hepatocyte into HCC (London, 1981). Alternatively, the individual with chronic active hepatitis may go on to develop postnecrotic cirrhosis and show integrated viral genome in the cellular DNA of the tumour cells. However, viral DNA is not integrated in the tumour DNA in all cases.

The association between aflatoxin and HBV is an important epidemiological finding in HCC (Lutwick, 1979). In the United States, Purtilo and Gottlieb (1974) have associated another hepatotoxin, namely ethanol, with cirrhosis and HCC. Thus a hepatotoxin as well as a persistent virus infection in immune-deficient persons are probably requirements for the development of HCC. Rarely, HCC has occurred in renal graft recipients (Dalgleish et al., 1983) and rarely in male homosexuals. Possibly the rare occurrence of HCC in renal allograft recipients and AIDS patients is due to insufficient hepatoxicity. In other words, the immune suppression could be so profound that the cytotoxic T-cells fail to destroy the infected hepatocytes. This destruction, which is followed by an enhanced proliferation of hepatocytes, could be a necessary step in hepatic carcinogenesis. A cytogenetic or molecular alteration of the genetic apparatus is probably needed for the malignant conversion.

A marked male predominance is observed in HCC. A relative immune deficiency is noted when comparing gender differences in chronic HBV infection and HCC. Chu et al. (1983), in their study of Taiwanese, found a marked male-to-female difference in the carriage rate of HBV and in antibody response to the HBV e antigen and antibody. The male-to-female ratio increased from 1.2 in asymptomatic carriers to 6.3 in chronic liver disease, and to 9.8 in HCC. Previously, Purtilo and Sullivan (1979) had noted that there was an immunological basis for superior survival of females. For each infectious disease morbidity and mortality are higher among males than females. It is also noteworthy that Burkitt's lymphoma, KS and HCC occur predominantly in males. The superior immune responses of females provide competent immune surveillance against the ubiquitous viruses which may, in immune-deficient persons, induce Burkitt's lymphoma, KS, cutaneous squamous-cell carcinoma, and HCC.

Life-style and environmental factors could contribute to the immune suppression of a large number of Africans. Malnutrition, for example, leads to thymolymphatic atrophy and acquired immune deficiency (Smythe et al., 1971; Purtilo & Connor, 1975). As mentioned earlier, holoendemic malaria suppresses cellular immunity. Similarly, gastrointestinal parasites and other infectious diseases, especially those caused by viruses, suppress immunity. Fungal metabolites contaminating food may also contribute to suppression. Immune suppression and persistent viral infections among certain Africans may thus be responsible for the high frequency of the malignancies described here.

CONDITIONS PERMITTING UBIQUITOUS VIRUSES TO INDUCE MALIGNANCIES

How can ubiquitous viruses induce neoplasia? It is probable that this takes place as follows:

(1) Each virus selects specific cellular targets according to the presence or absence of viral receptors, e.g., EBV selects B-cells; CMV - endothelial cells; HPV - squamous cells; herpes simplex virus - squamous cells; and HBV - hepatocytes.

(2) The virus acts in part as a mutagen in the target cells.

(3) The virus provokes proliferation of target cells rather than lysis.

(4)   Various co-factors, including nutrition, exposure to tumour-promoting agents, ultraviolet light, etc., act synergistically to promote carcinogenesis.

(5)   The immune defect is of a type and degree which allows gradual proliferation. The host survives for months, so that an adequate incubation period allows a malignant clone to evolve.

(6)   A final common pathway in the evolution of these malignancies may be a conversion from polyclonality to monoclonality due to specific cytogenetic rearrangements allowing activation of oncogenes in the target cell. The genetically altered cell has a selective growth advantage over normal diploid cells.

(7)   The proliferation is reversible during the polyclonal phase when immune competence is increased or viral burden decreased (Purtilo & Linder, 1983).

The reversibility of KS (Costa & Rabson, 1983) and of EBV-carrying malignant lymphomas (Starzl et al., 1984) substantiates the view that immune deficiency permits viral induced malignancies to develop. Of importance to both clinicians and basic scientists is the way in which the polyclonal proliferation develops into a monoclonal malignancy.

CONVERSION FROM POLYCLONAL TO MONOCLONAL PROLIFERATION

Klein (1979) has hypothesized that three steps occur in the development of African Burkitt's lymphoma: (1) EBV transforms B-cells and immortalizes them; (2) holoendemic malaria promotes proliferation of B-cells; and (3) a cytogenetic translocation involving chromosomes 8 and 14 endows a cell with survival advantages. In addition to these factors, it is suggested that immune suppression allows the infected target cell to proliferate unabated. This increases the chances for the cell to undergo a cytogenetic rearrangement.

Manolov and Manolova (1971) have described a specific 14q+ cytogenetic alteration in an African Burkitt's lymphoma cell line. An identical marker chromosome has been observed in a Burkitt-like lymphoma from a patient with AIDS (Fig. 3). Subsequently, other investigators have confirmed that a reciprocal translocation occurs at a break-point in chromosome 14 involving

the heavy chain gene loci and in chromosome 8 at the point where
the oncogene c-myc resides. The reciprocal translocation resulting in the approximation of the c-myc oncogene to the activated
heavy chain immunoglobulin locus promotes the c-myc oncogene and
thereby changes the characteristics of the cell (Leder et al.,
1983).

FIG. 3. BURKITT'S LYMPHOMA KARYOTYPE SHOWING
8;14 TRANSLOCATION FROM A PATIENT WITH AIDS
From Petersen et al., 1984
Published by permission of Yorke Publishers

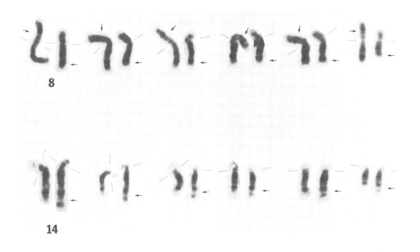

The hypothesis that the cytogenetic alteration endows the
altered cell with survival advantages is supported by cellular
immune studies which demonstrate that the cytogenetically altered
Burkitt's lymphoma cell is more resistant to NK and EBV-specific
cytotoxic killing than the autologous, diploid lymphoblastoid
cell line (Rooney et al., 1984). It seems likely that similar
cytogenetic or molecular alterations occur in other proliferating
target cells driven by the viruses discussed in this review.

The hope of controlling virus-associated malignancies in
Africa resides in prevention of immune deficiency by improved
nutrition, sanitation, and medical care. Such prevention or
early detection could lead to intervention strategies. The use
of vaccines and antiviral agents may abrogate chronic persistent
viral infections which lead to sustained polyclonal proliferation

of target cells. Finally, since these malignancies may be determined by ubiquitous viruses, the development of new intervention strategies using monoclonal antibodies to viral antigens, interferon, or other immune modulating substances is possible.

REFERENCES

Borel, J.F. (1983) Cyclosporine: historical perspectives. Transplant. Proc., 15, 2219-2229

Burkitt, D. (1958) A sarcoma involving the jaws in African children. Br. J. Surg., 46, 218-223

Chu, C.M., Liaw, Y.F., Sheen, I.S., Lin, D.-Y. & Huang, M.-J. (1983) Sex difference in chronic hepatitis B virus infection: an appraisal based on the status of hepatitis B e antigen and antibody. Hepatology, 3, 947-950

Costa, J. & Rabson, A.S. (1983) Generalized Kaposi's sarcoma is not a neoplasm (Letter). Lancet, 1, 58

Dalgleish, A.G., Tiller, D.J., Horvath, J. & Tattersall, M.H.N. (1983) Hepatocellular carcinoma associated with hepatitis B in a renal graft recipient. Med. J. Aust., 2, 240-241

Downing, R.G., Eglin, R.P. & Bayley, A.C. (1984) African Kaposi's sarcoma and AIDS. Lancet, 1, 478-480

Drew, W.L., Miner, R.C., Ziegler, J.L., Gullett, J.H., Abrams, D.I., Conant, M.A., Huang, E.-S., Groundwater, J.R., Volberding, P. & Mintz, L. (1982) Cytomegalovirus and Kaposi's sarcoma in young homosexual men. Lancet, 2, 125-127

Epstein, M.A., Achong, B.G. & Barr, Y.M. (1964) Virus particles in cultured lymphoblasts from Burkitt's lymphoma. Lancet, 1, 702-703

Fauci, A.S. (1983) Editorial: the acquired immune deficiency syndrome. The ever-broadening clinical spectrum. J. Am. med. Assoc., 249, 2375-2376

Garner, J.G., Hirsch, M.S. & Schooley, R.T. (1984) Prevention of Epstein-Barr virus-induced B-cell outgrowth by interferon alpha. Infect. Immun., 43, 920-924

Giraldo, G., Beth, E. & Haguenau, F. (1972) Herpes-type virus particles in tissue culture of Kaposi's sarcoma from different geographic regions. J. natl Cancer Inst., 49, 1509-1513

Gissmann, L., Wolnik, L., Ikenberg, H., Koldovsky, U., Schnurch, H.G. & zur Hausen, H. (1983) Human papillomavirus types 6 and 11 DNA sequences in genital and laryngeal papillomas and in some cervical cancers. Proc. natl Acad. Sci. USA, 80, 560-563

Hanto, D.W., Frizzera, G., Purtilo, D.T., Sakamoto, K., Sullivan, J.L., Saemundsen, A.K., Klein, G., Simmons, R.L. & Najarian, J.S. (1981) Clinical spectrum of lymphoproliferative disorders in renal transplant recipients and evidence for the role of Epstein-Barr virus. Cancer Res., 41, 4253-4261

Hanto, D.W., Frizzera, G., Gajl-Peczalska, K.J., Purtilo, D.T. & Simmons, R.L. (1984) Lymphoproliferative diseases in renal allograft recipients. In: Purtilo, D.T., ed., Immune Deficiency and Cancer: Epstein-Barr Virus and Lymphoproliferative Malignancies, New York, Plenum Press, pp. 321-347

Harada, S., Sakamoto, K., Seeley, J.K., Lindsten, T., Bechtold, T., Yetz, J., Rogers, G., Pearson, G. & Purtilo, D.T. (1982) Immune deficiency in the X-linked lymphoproliferative syndrome. I. Epstein-Barr virus-specific defects. J. Immunol., 129, 2532-2540

Henle, G. & Henle, W. (1966) Immunofluorescence in cells derived from Burkitt's lymphoma. J. Bacteriol., 91, 1248-1256

Henle, G., Lennette, E.T., Alspaugh, M.A. & Henle, W. (1979) Rheumatoid factor as a cause of positive reactions in tests for Epstein-Barr virus-specific IgM antibodies. Clin. exp. Immunol, 36, 415-422

Howley, P.M. (1982) The human papillomaviruses. Arch. Pathol. lab. Med., 106, 429-432

Jablonska, S., Orth, G. & Lutzner, M.A. (1982) Immunopathology of papillomavirus-induced tumors in different tissues. Springer Semin. Immunopathol., 5, 33-62

Klein, G. (1975) the Epstein-Barr virus and neoplasia. N. Engl. J. Med., 293, 1353-1357

Klein, G. (1979) Lymphoma development in mice and humans: diversity of initiation is followed by convergent cytogenetic evolution. Proc. natl Acad. Sci. USA, 76, 2442-2446

Leder, P., Battey, J., Lenoir, G., Moulding, C., Murphy, W., Potter, H., Stewart, T. & Taub, R. (1983) Translocation among antibody genes in human cancer. Science, 222, 765-771

London, W.T. (1981) Primary hepatocellular carcinoma - etiology, pathogenesis, and prevention. Hum. Pathol., 12, 1085-1097

Lutwick, L.I. (1979) Relation between aflatoxin, hepatitis-B virus, and hepatocellular carcinoma. Lancet, 2, 755-757

Lutzner, M.A., Orth, G., Dutronquay, V., Ducasse, M.-F., Kreis, H. & Crosnier, J. (1983) Detection of human papillomavirus type 5 DNA in skin cancers of an immunosuppressed renal allograft recipient. Lancet, 2, 422-424

Manolov, G. & Manolova, Y. (1971) A marker band in one chromosome No. 14 in Burkitt lymphomas. Hereditas, 69, 300-303

Montagnier, L., Guest, J., Chamaret, S., Dauguet, C., Axler, C., Guetard, D., Nugeyre, M.T., Bare-Sinoussi, F., Chermann, J.-C., Brunet, J.B., Klatzmann, D. & Gluckman, J.C. (1984) Adaptation of lymphadenopathy associated virus (LAV) to replication in EBV-transformed B lymphoblastoid cell lines. Science, 225, 63-66

Morbidity and Mortality Weekly Report (1981) Kaposi's sarcoma and Pneumocystis pneumonia among homosexual men - New York city and California. 30, 303-308

Oettle, A.G. (1962) Cancer and environmental influences. South Afr. Cancer Bull., 6, 110

Penn, I. (1983) Kaposi's sarcoma in immunosuppressed patients.
    J. clin. lab. Immunol., 12, 1-10

Penn, I. (1984) Allograft transplant cancer registry. In:
    Purtilo, D.T., ed., Immune Deficiency and Cancer: Epstein-
    Barr Virus and Lymphoproliferative Malignancies, New York,
    Plenum Press, pp. 201-308

Peterson, J.M., Tubbs, R.R., Savage, R.A., Calabrese, L.C.,
    Proffitt, M.R., Manolova, Y., Manolov, G., Schumaker, A.,
    Tatsumi, E., McClain, K. & Purtilo, D.T. (1984) Small non-
    cleaved B cell Burkitt-type lymphoma with chromosome t(8;14)
    translocation and carrying Epstein-Barr virus in a male
    homosexual with the acquired immune deficiency syndrome.
    Am. J. Med. (in press)

Prince, A.M. & Alcabes, P. (1982) The risk of development of
    hepatocellular carcinoma in hepatitis B virus carriers in
    New York. A preliminary estimate using death-records
    matching. Hepatology, 2, 15S-20S

Purtilo, D.T. (1976) Malignancies in the tropics. In: Conor,
    D.H. & Binford, C., eds, Pathology of Tropical and Extra-
    ordinary Diseases, Washington, DC, Armed Forces Institute of
    Pathology, pp. 647-660

Purtilo, D.T. (1983) Nutritional considerations in the epidemio-
    logy of lymphoma. In: Butterworth, C.E. Jr & Hutchinson,
    M., eds, Nutritional Factors in Induction and Maintenance of
    Malignancy, New York, Academic Press, pp. 11-30

Purtilo, D.T., ed. (1984)   Immune Deficiency and Cancer:
    Epstein-Barr Virus and Lymphoproliferative Malignancies, New
    York, Plenum Press

Purtilo, D.T. & Conor, D.H. (1975) Fatal infections in protein-
    calorie malnourished children with thymolymphatic atrophy.
    Arch. Dis. Child., 50, 149-152

Purtilo, D.T. & Gottlieb, L.S. (1973) Cirrhosis and hepatoma
    occurring in Boston City Hospital 1917-1968. Cancer, 32,
    458-462

Purtilo, D.T. & Klein, G. (1981) Introduction to Epstein-Barr virus and lymphoproliferative diseases in immunodeficient individuals. Cancer Res., 41, 4209

Purtilo, D.T. & Linder, J. (1983) Oncological consequences of impaired immune surveillance against ubiquitous viruses. J. clin. Immunol., 3, 197-206

Purtilo, D.T., Harada, S., Meuwissen, H., Lipscomb, H., Ochs, H., Sonnabend, J., Manolov, G. & Manolova, Y. (1984a) Epstein-Barr virus-induced diseases in immune deficient patients. In: Rapp, F., ed., Herpesvirus, New York, Alan R. Liss

Purtilo, D.T., Lipscomb, H., Harada, S., Hayes, J., Manolov, G., Manolova, Y., Witkin, S. & Sonnabend, J. (1984b) Etiological factors in the induction of acquired immune deficiency syndrome (AIDS). In: Nakamura, R., ed., Clinical Laboratory Molecular Analyses: New Strategies in Autoimmunity, Cancer and Virology, Grune & Stratton

Purtilo, D.T., Manolov, G., Manolova, Y., Harada, S. & Lipscomb, H. (1984c) Role of Epstein-Barr virus in the etiology of Burkitt's lymphoma. In: Lenoir, G., O'Conor, G. & Olweny, C., eds, Burkitt's Lymphoma: A Human Cancer Model, Lyon, International Agency for Research on Cancer (in press)

Purtilo, D.T. & Sullivan, J.L. (1979) Immunological bases for superior survival of females. Am. J. Dis. Child., 133, 1251-1253

Rooney, C.M., Rickinson, A.B., Moss, D.J., Lenoir, G.M. & Epstein, M.A. (1984) Cell-mediated surveillance mechanisms and the pathogenesis of Burkitt's lymphoma. In: Lenoir, G., O'Conor, G. & Olweny, C., eds, Burkitt's Lymphoma: A Human Cancer Model, Lyon, International Agency for Research on Cancer (in press)

Saemundsen, A.K., Purtilo, D.T., Sakamoto, K., Sullivan, J.L., Synnerholm, A.C., Hanto, D., Simmons, R., Anvret, M., Collins, R. & Klein, G. (1981) Documentation of Epstein-Barr virus infection in immunodeficient patients with life-threatening lymphoproliferative diseases by Epstein-Barr virus complementary RNA/DNA and viral DNA/DNA hybridization. Cancer Res., 41, 4237-4242

Sakamoto, K., Freed, H. & Purtilo, D.T. (1980) Antibody
    responses to Epstein-Barr virus in families with the
    X-linked lymphoproliferative syndrome. J. Immunol., 125,
    921-925

Smythe, P.M., Schonland, M., Brereton-Stiles, G.G., Coovadia,
    H.M., Grace, H.J., Leoning, W.E.K., Foyane, M.A., Parent,
    M.A. & Vos, G.H. (1971) Thymolymphatic deficiency and
    depression of cell-mediated immunity in protein-calorie mal-
    nutrition. Lancet, 2, 939

Sonnabend, J., Witkin, S.S. & Purtilo, D.T. (1983) Acquired
    immunodeficiency syndrome, opportunistic infections, and
    malignancies in male homosexuals. A hypothesis of etiologic
    factors in pathogenesis. J. Am. Med. Assoc., 249, 2370-2374

Starzl, T.E., Nalesnik, M.A., Porter, H.A., Ho, M., Iwatsuki, S.,
    Griffith, B.P., Rosenthal, J.T., Hakala, T.R., Shaw, B.W.,
    Hardesty, R.L., Atchison, R.W., Jaffe, R. & Bahnson, H.T.
    (1984) Reversibility of lymphomas and lymphoproliferative
    lesions developing under cyclosporine-steroid therapy.
    Lancet, 1, 583-587

Templeton, A.C., ed. (1973) Tumours in a Tropical Country; A
    Survey of Uganda 1964-68, Berlin, New York, Springer-Verlag

Walder, B.K., Robertson, M.R. & Jeremy, D. (1971) Skin cancer
    and immunosuppression. Lancet, 1, 1282-1283

zur Hausen, H. (1982) Human genital cancer: synergism between
    two virus infections or synergism and initiating events.
    Lancet, 2, 1370-1372

SHORT COMMUNICATION: MALARIA AND BURKITT'S LYMPHOMA IN NORTH MARA, TANZANIA

G. Brubaker

Shirati Mission Hospital
Musoma, Tanzania

The similarity in the geographical distribution of malaria and Burkitt's lymphoma (BL) suggests that there may be a causal relationship. This relationship was found to hold true in the North Mara District of Tanzania, where the prevalence of malaria was 40-50% in the lowland area with a high incidence of BL and 10-20% in a neighbouring highland area where BL was virtually absent.

To test this hypothesis, a malaria control trial was conducted on a population of 100 000 children aged 0-10 years who were at risk of BL. The trial was carried out from 1977 to 1982 and the incidence of BL was recorded.

The trial succeeded in reducing the prevalence of malaria to 10% for the first 2 years, but it then rose slowly over the next few years to nearly its former level. Three years after the reduction in malaria prevalence there was a dramatic reduction in BL to 1 case per year for 2 years. During the last half of 1983 there were 4 new cases of BL in the study area and in the first 3 months of 1984 there have already been 5 new cases. If this relationship holds, we would expect to see an unprecedented number of new cases over the next few years, since malaria has returned to its former level, or even higher, following the discontinuation of malaria control in 1982.

INDEX OF AUTHORS

INDEX OF AUTHORS

IARC SCIENTIFIC PUBLICATIONS

Available from Oxford University Press, Walton Street, Oxford OX2 6DP, UK and in London,
New York, Toronto, Delhi, Bombay, Calcutta, Madras, Karachi, Kuala Lumpur, Singapore,
Hong Kong, Tokyo, Nairobi, Dar es Salaam, Cape Town, Melbourne, Auckland
and associated companies in Beirut, Berlin, Ibadan, Mexico City, Nicosia.

Laboratory Decontamination and Destruction of Carcinogens in Laboratory Wastes: Some N-Nitrosamines	No. 43, 1982; 73 pages £6.50
Environmental Carcinogens—Selected Methods of Analysis, Vol. 5: Mycotoxins	No. 44, 1983; 455 pages £20
Environmental Carcinogens—Selected Methods of Analysis, Vol. 6: N-Nitroso Compounds	No. 45, 1983; 508 pages £20
Directory of On-Going Research in Cancer Epidemiology 1982	No. 46, 1982; 722 pages £15
Cancer Incidence in Singapore	No. 47, 1982; 174 pages £10
Cancer Incidence in the USSR Second Revised Edition	No. 48, 1982; 75 pages £10
Laboratory Decontamination and Destruction of Carcinogens in Laboratory Wastes: Some Polycyclic Aromatic Hydrocarbons	No. 49, 1983; 81 pages £7.95
Directory of On-Going Research in Cancer Epidemiology 1983	No. 50, 1983; 740 pages £15
Modulators of Experimental Carcinogenesis	No. 51, 1983; 307 pages £25
Second Cancers Following Radiation Treatment for Cancer of the Uterine Cervix: The Results of a Cancer Registry Collaborative Study	No. 52, 1984; 207 pages £17.50
Nickel in the Human Environment	No. 53, 1984; 530 pages £30

Laboratory Decontamination and Destruction of Carcinogens in Laboratory Wastes: Some Hydrazines	No. 54, 1983; 87 pages £6.95
Laboratory Decontamination and Destruction of Carcinogens in Laboratory Wastes: Some N-Nitrosamides	No. 55, 1984; 65 pages £6.95
Models, Mechanisms and Etiology of Tumour Promotion	No. 56, 1985 (in press)

NON-SERIAL PUBLICATIONS

Available from WHO Sales Agents

Alcool et Cancer	1978; 42 pages Fr. fr. 35. —; Sw. fr. 14. —
Information Bulletin on the Survey of Chemicals Being Tested for Carcinogenicity No. 8	1979, 604 pages US$ 20.00; Sw. fr. 40. —
Cancer Morbidity and Causes of Death Among Danish Brewery Workers	1980, 145 pages US$ 25.00; Sw. fr. 45. —
Information Bulletin on the Survey of Chemicals Being Tested for Carcinogenicity No. 9	1981, 294 pages US$ 20.00; Sw. fr. 41. —
Information Bulletin on the Survey of Chemicals Being Tested for Carcinogenicity No. 10	1982, 326 pages US$ 20.00; Sw. fr. 42. —

IARC MONOGRAPHS ON THE EVALUATION OF THE CARCINOGENIC RISK OF CHEMICALS TO HUMANS

Available from WHO Sales Agents.

Some Inorganic Substances, Chlorinated, Hydrocarbons, Aromatic Amines, N-Nitroso Compounds, and Natural Products
Volume 1, 1972; 184 pages (out of print)

Some Inorganic and Organometallic Compounds
Volume 2, 1973; 181 pages US$ 3.60; sw. fr. 12.– (out of print)

Certain Polycyclic Aromatic Hydrocarbons and Heterocyclic Compounds
Volume 3, 1973; 271 pages (out of print)

Some Aromatic Amines, Hydrazine and Related Substances, N-Nitroso Compounds and Miscellaneous Alkylating Agents
Volume 4, 1974; 286 pages US$ 7.20; Sw. fr. 18. –

Some Organochlorine Pesticides
Volume 5, 1974; 241 pages US$ 7.20; Sw. fr. 18.– (out of print)

Sex Hormones
Volume 6, 1974; 243 pages US$ 7.20; Sw. fr. 18. –

Some Anti-thyroid and Related Substances, Nitrofurans and Industrial Chemicals
Volume 7, 1974; 326 pages US$ 12.80; Sw. fr. 32. –

Some Aromatic Azo Compounds
Volume 8, 1975; 357 pages US$ 14.40; Sw. fr. 36. –

Some Aziridines, N-, S- and O-Mustards and Selenium
Volume 9, 1975; 268 pages US$ 10.80; Sw. fr. 27. –

Some Naturally Occurring Substances
Volume 10, 1976; 353 pages US$ 15.00; Sw. fr. 38. –

Cadmium, Nickel, Some Epoxides, Miscellaneous Industrial Chemicals and General Considerations on Volatile Anaesthetics
Volume 11, 1976; 306 pages US$ 14.00; Sw. fr. 34. –

Some Carbamates, Thiocarbamates and Carbazides
Volume 12, 1976; 282 pages US$ 14.00; Sw. fr. 34. –

Some Miscellaneous Pharmaceutical Substances
Volume 13, 1977; 255 pages US$ 12.00; Sw. fr. 30. –

Asbestos
Volume 14, 1977; 106 pages US$ 6.00; Sw. fr. 14. –

Some Fumigants, the Herbicides 2,4-D and 2,4,5-T, Chlorinated Dibenzodioxins and Miscellaneous Industrial Chemicals
Volume 15, 1977; 354 pages US$ 20.00; Sw. fr. 50. –

Some Aromatic Amines and Related Nitro Compounds – Hair Dyes, Colouring Agents and Miscellaneous Industrial Chemicals
Volume 16, 1978; 400 pages US$ 20.00; Sw. fr. 50. –

Some N-Nitroso Compounds
Volume 17, 1978; 365 pages US$ 25.00; Sw. fr. 50. –

Polychlorinated Biphenyls and Polybrominated Biphenyls
Volume 18, 1978; 140 pages US$ 13.00; Sw. fr. 20. –

Some Monomers, Plastics and Synthetic Elastomers, and Acrolein
Volume 19, 1979; 513 pages US$ 35.00; Sw. fr. 60. –

Some Halogenated Hydrocarbons
Volume 20, 1979; 609 pages US$ 35.00; Sw. fr. 60. –

Sex Hormones (II)
Volume 21, 1979; 583 pages US$ 35.00; Sw. fr. 60. –

Some Non-nutritive Sweetening Agents
Volume 22, 1980; 208 pages US$ 15.00; Sw. fr. 25. –

Some Metals and Metallic Compounds
Volume 23, 1980; 438 pages US$ 30.00; Sw. fr. 50. –

Some Pharmaceutical Drugs
Volume 24, 1980; 337 pages US$ 25.00; Sw. fr. 40. –

Wood, Leather and Some Associated Industries
Volume 25, 1980; 412 pages US$ 30.00; Sw. fr. 60. –

Some Anticancer and Immunosuppressive Drugs
Volume 26, 1981; 411 pages US$ 30.00; Sw. fr. 62. –

Some Aromatic Amines, Anthraquinones and Nitroso Compounds and Inorganic Fluorides Used in Drinking-Water and Dental Preparations
Volume 27, 1982; 341 pages US$ 25.00; Sw. fr. 40. –

The Rubber Industry
Volume 28, 1982; 486 pages US$ 35.00; Sw. fr. 70. –

Some Industrial Chemicals and Dyestuffs
Volume 29, 1982; 416 pages US$ 30.00; Sw. fr. 60. –

Miscellaneous Pesticides
Volume 30, 1983; 424 pages US$ 30.00; Sw. fr. 60. –

Some Feed Additives, Food Additives and Naturally Occurring Substances
Volume 31, 1983; 314 pages US$ 30.00; Sw. fr. 60. –

Chemicals and Industrials Processes Associated with Cancer in Humans (IARC Monographs 1–20)
Supplement 1, 1979; 71 pages (out of print)

Long-term and Short-term Screening Assays for Carcinogens: A Critical Appraisal
Supplement 2, 1980; 426 pages US$ 25.00; Sw. fr. 40. –

Cross Index of Synonyms and Trade Names in Volumes 1 to 26
Supplement 3, 1982; 199 pages US$ 30.00; Sw. fr. 60. –

Chemicals, Industrial Processes and Industries Associated with Cancer in Humans (IARC Monographs Volumes 1 to 29)
Supplement 4, 1982; 292 pages US$ 30.00; Sw. fr. 60. –

Polynuclear Aromatic Compounds, Part 1, Chemical, Environmental and Experimental Data
Volume 32, 1983; 477 pages US$ 35.00; Sw. fr. 70. –

Polynuclear Aromatic Compounds, Part 2, Carbon Blacks, Mineral Oils and Some Nitroarenes
Volume 33, 1984; 245 pages US$ 25.00; Sw. fr. 50. –

Polynuclear Aromatic Compounds, Part 3, Industrial Exposures in Aluminium Production, Coal Gasification, Coke Production, and Iron and Steel Founding
Volume 34, 1984; 219 pages US$ 20.00; Sw. fr. 48.–

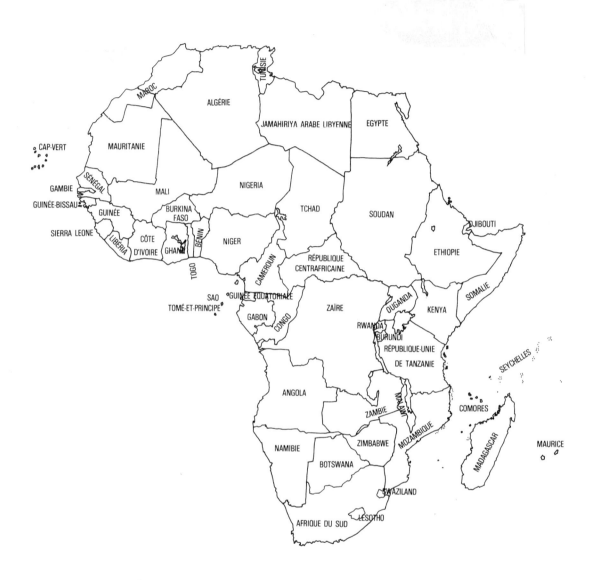

CAP-VERT

MAROC

ALGÉRIE

TUNISIE

JAMAHIRIYA ARABE LIBYENNE

EGYPTE

MAURITANIE

GAMBIE

SÉNÉGAL

GUINÉE-BISSAU

GUINÉE

SIERRA LEONE

LIBÉRIA

MALI

NIGERIA

TCHAD

SOUDAN

DJIBOUTI

BURKINA FASO

CÔTE D'IVOIRE

GHANA

BÉNIN

NIGER

TOGO

CAMEROUN

RÉPUBLIQUE CENTRAFRICAINE

ETHIOPIE

SOMALIE

SAO TOMÉ-ET-PRINCIPE

GUINÉE ÉQUATORIALE

GABON

CONGO

ZAÏRE

OUGANDA

KENYA

RWANDA

BURUNDI

RÉPUBLIQUE-UNIE DE TANZANIE

SEYCHELLES

ANGOLA

ZAMBIE

MALAWI

COMORES

MADAGASCAR

MAURICE

NAMIBIE

ZIMBABWE

MOZAMBIQUE

BOTSWANA

SWAZILAND

AFRIQUE DU SUD

LESOTHO